Jadhg P E
Mater M
Hospital

Reanimation of the paralyzed face
NEW APPROACHES

Reanimation of the paralyzed face

NEW APPROACHES

Edited by

Leonard R. Rubin, M.D., F.A.C.S.

Diplomate, American Board of Plastic Surgery;
Clinical Professor of Plastic Surgery,
State University of New York at Stony Brook,
Stony Brook; Director, Plastic and Maxillofacial
Surgery and the Burn Center, Nassau County
Medical Center, East Meadow; Attending Plastic
Surgeon, North Shore University Hospital, Manhasset;
Nassau Hospital, Mineola, New York

Contributions by international researchers and surgeons

WITH 352 ILLUSTRATIONS

The C. V. Mosby Company

Saint Louis   1977

Copyright © 1977 by The C. V. Mosby Company

All rights reserved. No part of this book may be reproduced in any manner without written permission of the publisher.

Printed in the United States of America

Distributed in Great Britain by Henry Kimpton, London

The C. V. Mosby Company
11830 Westline Industrial Drive, St. Louis, Missouri 63141

Library of Congress Cataloging in Publication Data

Main entry under title:

Reanimation of the paralyzed face.

    Bibliography: p.
    Includes index.
    1. Paralysis, Facial—Surgery. 2. Facial nerve—Surgery. 3. Nerve grafting. 4. Facial muscles—Surgery. 5. Muscles—Transplantation. I. Rubin, Leonard R. [DNLM: 1. Facial paralysis—Surgery. 2. Plastic surgery. WL330 R288]
RD595.R4   617'.52   77-13172
ISBN 0-8016-4210-8

GW/U/B 9 8 7 6 5 4 3 2 1

Contributors

H. ANDERL, M.D.
University Professor for Plastic and Reconstructive Surgery, Universitätsklinik für Plastische und Wiederherstellungschirurgie, Innsbruck, Austria

NAHUM BEN-HUR, M.D., F.A.C.S.
Professor of Plastic Surgery, Hebrew University, Hadassah Medical School; Director, Department of Plastic and Maxillofacial Surgery, Shaare Zedek Hospital, Jerusalem; Consultant, Israel Defense Force, Israel; Professor of Plastic Surgery, State University of New York at Stony Brook, Stony Brook, New York

LEWIS BERGER, M.D.
Staff Surgeon, Plastic and Maxillo-facial Surgery, Nassau County Medical Center, East Meadow, New York

BLOYCE HILL BRITTON, M.D.
Associate Clinical Professor of Otolaryngology, University of Southern California, Los Angeles, California

JOHN CONLEY, M.D., F.A.C.S.
Professor of Otolaryngology, Columbia University, College of Physicians and Surgeons; Attending Otolaryngologist, Chief, Head and Neck Service, Columbia Presbyterian Medical Center; Chief, Head and Neck Service, St. Vincent's Hospital and Medical Center of New York; Chief, Head and Neck Department, Pack Medical Foundation, New York, New York

VINCENT R. DiGREGORIO, M.D.
Plastic and Maxillo-facial Surgeon, Nassau County Medical Center, East Meadow, New York

LARS HAKELIUS, M.D.
Assistant Professor, Department of Plastic Surgery, University Hospital, Uppsala, Sweden

KIYONORI HARII, M.D.
Attending Plastic Surgeon, Chief of Microsurgery Unit, Tokyo Metropolitan Police Hospital, Tokyo, Japan

LEE A. HARKER, M.D.
Associate Professor of Otolaryngology and Maxillofacial Surgery, University of Iowa College of Medicine, University of Iowa Hospitals and Clinic, Iowa City, Iowa

SYDNEY LOUIS, M.D., M.R.C.P.E.
Professor of Neurology, State University of New York at Stony Brook, Stony Brook; Director of Neurology, Nassau County Medical Center, East Meadow, New York

LEONARD MALIS, M.D., F.A.C.S.
Professor and Chairman, Department of Neurosurgery, Mt. Sinai School of Medicine of the City University of New York; Director, Department of Neurosurgery; Neurosurgeon-in-Chief, The Mt. Sinai Hospital, New York

BRIAN F. McCABE, M.D., F.A.C.S.
Professor and Chairman, Department of Otolaryngology and Maxillofacial Surgery, University of Iowa College of Medicine, University of Iowa Hospitals and Clinic, Iowa City, Iowa

WILLIAM H. McCOY, III, M.D.
Staff Surgeon, Plastic and Maxillofacial Surgery Nassau County Medical Center, East Meadow, New York

Contributors

HANNO MILLESI, M.D.

Professor of Plastic Surgery, University Clinic in Surgery, Vienna, Austria

KITARO OHMORI, M.D.

Attending Plastic Surgeon, Tokyo Metropolitan Police Hospital, Tokyo, Japan

BERNARD S. POST, M.D.

Director, Department of Physical Medicine and Rehabilitation, St. John's Episcopal Hospital, Brooklyn, New York

CALVIN RASWEILER, M.D., F.A.C.S.

Associate Professor of Surgery, State University of New York at Stony Brook, Stony Brook; Attending Head and Neck Surgeon, Nassau County Medical Center, East Meadow; Attending Surgeon, Nassau Hospital, Mercy Hospital, New York

LEONARD R. RUBIN, M.D., F.A.C.S.

Diplomate, American Board of Plastic Surgery; Clinical Professor of Plastic Surgery, State University of New York at Stony Brook, Stony Brook; Director, Plastic and Maxillofacial Surgery and the Burn Center, Nassau County Medical Center, East Meadow; Attending Plastic Surgeon, North Shore University Hospital, Nassau Hospital, Mercy Hospital, Kings County Hospital Center, New York

JOANNA HOLLENBERG SHER, M.D.

Associate Professor of Pathology and Director, Neuropathology Laboratory; State University of New York Downstate Medical Center, Brooklyn, New York

To my wife, Annette, whose devotion, encouragement, and understanding have permitted me to divert most precious time from her and our family to write and edit these chapters.

We hope that the effort in compiling the information contained in these writings will stimulate others to seek the perfect cure for the patient afflicted with facial paralysis.

Preface

No animal in the evolutionary tree has attained the range of facial expression displayed by man. Man's face is a mirror of his inner emotions, conveying love and hate and a myriad of subtle, fleeting gradations from joy through indifference to deep despair. A catastrophe occurs when the human face can no longer move.

The seventh nerve innervates the facial muscles. Impulses starting in the higher centers of the brain pass on to the seventh nerve nuclei and from there outward to the muscular periphery. Any interruption in the pathway results in facial paralysis. The surgical restoration of complete facial function has been not only difficult but also, in most cases, totally inadequate. During the past decade, the majority of restorative surgeons have been content to use fascia lata or plastic slings to hold the drooping paralyzed face at an elevated level, disregarding dynamic function. Ophthalmological surgeons have placed springs and weights into the eyelids to aid closure. None of these procedures has restored function; in contrast, they have accentuated malfunction.

The past decade has seen tremendous interest in dynamic restoration of facial muscle function. Challenging innovations are opening up vistas for restorative surgeons. Research into the histopathology of nerve and muscle degeneration has helped to overcome previous failures of striated muscle grafting and has facilitated the surgical deciphering of the mysteries of free nerve grafting. The growing use of the microscope to visualize accurate nerve grafting has enabled the surgeon to use the most minute of sutures to limit fibrous scar formation. Emphasis is now being placed on the prevention of facial paresis, either by immediate or delayed (3 weeks) nerve grafting when the efferent seventh nerve axons are interrupted surgically in the cranium, temporal canal, parotid gland, or the periphery. When immediate bridge nerve grafting cannot be performed, the use of the microscope has stimulated cross-face nerve grafting from the normal side to help synchronize facial activity on the paralyzed side. If the facial muscles have degenerated, substitute muscle transpositions, free muscle grafting, and free muscle neurotization are being surgically performed to give dynamic activity to the paralyzed face. Even for the patient with congenital paralysis, who is usually immobile on both sides, the surgeon now has recourse to restoration of facial expression through muscle transposition.

Many treatises have been written on the facial nerve. Some have been romantic, some scientific, some wishful thinking, many very pedantic, a few pragmatic. The function of this volume is to present realistically how and why we can reanimate the face using more effective techniques, either immediately or at a later period. I have

Preface

invited contributions from a number of physicians who have been outstanding in pioneering these concepts. It is hoped that the surgeons reading this book will be inspired to strive for nothing less than total restoration of facial function in those who have suffered the agony of facial nerve disruption.

Leonard R. Rubin

Contents

PART I MECHANISM OF FACIAL EXPRESSION AND PATHOPHYSIOLOGY OF DEGENERATION

1. Anatomy of facial expression, 2
   LEONARD R. RUBIN

2. Surgical anatomy of the facial nerve, 21
   LEE A. HARKER and BRIAN F. McCABE

3. Pathophysiology of denervation in facial neuromuscular motor unit, 28
   JOANNA HOLLENBERG SHER

PART II ETIOLOGY OF DISRUPTION OF THE FACIAL NEUROMUSCULAR MOTOR UNIT

4. Congenital facial paresis (Möbius syndrome), 44
   LEONARD R. RUBIN

5. Medical causes of facial paresis including Bell's palsy, 53
   SYDNEY LOUIS

6. Surgical causes of facial paresis in the cranium, 57
   LEONARD MALIS

7. Surgical causes of facial paresis in the temporal canal, 71
   LEE A. HARKER and BRIAN F. McCABE

8. Surgical causes of facial paresis in the parotid gland, 79
   CALVIN RASWEILER

9. Diagnosing the site of nerve disruption by electronic methods, 81
   BERNARD S. POST

10. Diagnosing the site of nerve disruption by anatomical location, 98
    VINCENT R. DiGREGORIO

PART III CONTEMPORARY CONCEPTS IN FREE NERVE AND MUSCLE GRAFTING

11. Reinnervation and regeneration of striated muscle, 110
    JOANNA HOLLENBERG SHER

12. Technique of free nerve grafting in the face, 124
    HANNO MILLESI

Contents

13 Free whole muscle grafting: a survey, 136
LARS HAKELIUS

14 Free minced-muscle grafting, 156
LEWIS BERGER and LEONARD R. RUBIN

15 Nerve-end implantation into a denervated muscle, 166
WILLIAM H. McCOY, III, and LEONARD R. RUBIN

16 Fundamentals of microvascular suturing, 174
KIYONORI HARII and KITARO OHMORI

PART IV REANIMATION OF THE PARALYZED FACE

Section one Immediate or early treatment

17 Value of galvanic muscle stimulation immediately after paresis, 194
BERNARD S. POST

18 Medical treatment for Bell's palsy, 201
SYDNEY LOUIS

19 Present-day concepts of surgical treatment for Bell's palsy, 204
BLOYCE HILL BRITTON

20 Nerve grafting by microscope in the cranium, 211
LEONARD MALIS

21 Establishing facial nerve continuity in the temporal canal, 217
BRIAN F. McCABE and LEE A. HARKER

22 Management of facial nerve paresis in malignant tumors of the parotid gland, 224
JOHN CONLEY

23 Primary nerve suturing of severed motor nerves in facial trauma, 235
NAHUM BEN-HUR

Section two Intermediate surgical treatment for facial paresis—4 months to 1 year

24 Cross-face nerve grafting—up to 12 months of seventh nerve disruption, 241
H. ANDERL

Section three Late surgical treatment for facial paresis—after 12 months

25 Free muscle and nerve grafting in the face, 278
LARS HAKELIUS

26 Entire temporalis muscle transposition, 294
LEONARD R. RUBIN

27 Free muscle grafts by microneurovascular techniques, 316
KITARO OHMORI and KIYONORI HARII

28 Surgical treatment of bilateral facial paresis (Möbius syndrome), 328
LEONARD R. RUBIN

29 Partial facial paresis, 340
LEONARD R. RUBIN

Introduction

This book has been divided into four sections to facilitate the reader's comprehension of the problems associated with facial paralysis.

The first section is concerned with the mechanism of facial expression, the surgical anatomy of the facial nerve, and the pathophysiology of the degenerating facial neuromuscular motor unit, when the seventh nerve pathway is interrupted.

The second section describes the etiology of disruption of the nervous pathways to the face from the brain to the periphery.

The third section presents to the reader the contemporary concepts in free nerve and muscle grafting and some of the experimental work done with muscle that might be of importance in restoring atrophic facial muscle.

The fourth section describes in detail the therapy of facial paralysis, unilateral, bilateral, and partial. The time factor (the lag period from the moment of nerve interruption to the time of surgical intervention) is of great importance in picking the therapy of choice. Accordingly, this section has been subdivided into (1) immediate or early treatment after paralysis, (2) the intermediate treatment, which covers approximately 4 months to 1 year, and (3) the treatment after 16 months, when muscle degeneration probably thwarts efforts of nerve grafting to restore normal muscle function.

PART I

MECHANISM OF FACIAL EXPRESSION AND PATHOPHYSIOLOGY OF DEGENERATION

1 Anatomy of facial expression

LEONARD R. RUBIN

The muscles of the face serve a dual purpose: (1) to act as a cover for the mouth cavity and to produce protection for the eyeballs and (2) to open and close the oral cavity and the eyelids. The contractions and relaxations of these muscles throw the overlying skin into many folds, supplying a bonus of facial expressions, which can mirror the inner emotions. The patterns created make the variations in smiles. The subtle portrayal of emotions by delicate gradations of muscle contractures is made possible by the intimate relationship of the superficial fascia with the muscles and the overlying skin.

The human face, most highly developed of the primate line, has been gifted by evolution with an additional specialized function beyond that of providing a cover for the orifices of feeding, breathing, and seeing. The face of man is capable of portraying a vast range of emotions through its facial expressions.

The mechanisms for expression is provided by delicately balanced, coordinated muscles. Single muscles in various areas of the face have the capacity of contracting and relaxing in controlled, minimally graded degrees. The muscles of the face are concerned primarily with opening and closing the eyelids and compressing and relaxing the cheeks and lips. The relative strength, length, and line of directions these take from their origin to their insertion vary from individual to individual and determine differences in facial expression. The subtle nuances, however, exhibited by the human face could never take place were it not for the intricate relationship of the muscles with their investing superficial fascia, which is the means of transmitting contracting forces to the overlying skin.

The muscles of the face are intimately connected with the superficial fascia. *Gray's Anatomy* describes them as "cutaneous muscles lying within the layers of superficial fascia."[1] Muscles and fascia send attaching filaments to the overlying dermis. When the muscles contract, the skin is pulled into multiple folds, better known as Langer's lines.[2] These wrinkles make up the more subtle aspects of facial expression.

The deep fascia coming up from the neck splits into deep and superficial layers as it encounters the mandible. The superficial layer invests the platysma and then advances to the cheeks where the superficial facial muscles are enveloped. In the cheeks, the fascia, which adheres to the muscles, sends fibrous septa to the overlying dermis, thereby making the latter responsive to the slightest muscle contracture. Deep to this layer, pockets of fat make up the space between the buccinator and the rest of the facial muscles.

The importance of the superficial fascia cannot be overemphasized. It acts as a distributor of the facial muscles movements to the skin.[3] Since different muscles contract with varying strength, the number of facial movements becomes infinite and the extent is wide ranging, especially because the transmissions of these forces are blended by the network of overlying facial skin attachments. This allows for a smooth interplay of controlled motion that creates shades of expression (Fig. 1-1).

I have conducted an extensive study of the variations of Langer's lines in the human face.[4] Using a police fingerprinting service, I was able to determine facial patterns of individuals that differed considerably from textbook Langer's lines. Each individual has his own facial wrinkle design, which is determined by the skin's being thrown into folds at right angles to the resultant muscle pull, transmitted to the skin by the superficial fascia. Thus the forehead wrinkles would be at right angles to the line of frontalis muscle contracture and, of course, would run horizontally. Variations would occur by forceful contractures of other muscles about the forehead.

Examination of numerous facial patterns reveals, however, certain prevalent types. In regard to the cheeks, one finds individuals with upward-curving horizontal lines that create a "happy face." In contrast, a "sad face" is one where the wrinkles curve downward. In a similar fashion, two common variations are found in the upper lip and two in the lower lip (Fig. 1-2). From the surgical viewpoint, individual variations must be carefully determined before any incision is made in the face.

As the aging process continues, fat is lost from the subcutaneous tissue through which the fibrous filaments run from the muscles to the dermis. The thin skin appears to become attached more firmly to the deep muscles. Offering less resistance, it is thrown into deeper and more numerous folds or wrinkles.

No paper on facial expression would be complete without mention of the nasolabial folds. The variations of deep to thin folds and the infinite varieties of smiles cannot be explained by muscle attachment. At this line, where the lip joins the cheek, the fat is almost absent on the lip side and quite abundant on the cheek, whereas the superficial fascia is very thin in this area. The facial muscles do not attach to the fold but rather pass under it. This fold appears to be a cutaneous thickness that fades out over the nose and cheek superiorly and the mouth and cheeks inferiorly. It is deepened when the facial muscles about the mouth and lips contract, and it returns to normal when they relax. The facies of smiling is modified by the fold depths. The mystery of facial muscle control of the fold is heightened by the disappearance of the fold in facial palsy, however, in death, when all nerve stimulation is gone, the fold persists.

The muscles of expression are innervated by the seventh nerve. Any interruption in the pathway from the brain to the motor receptors in each individual muscle will paralyze the latter and alter the coordinated facial movements. Severance can occur in the cerebral cortex, the motor pathways in the brain, the facial nucleus, the facial nerve in the cranium, the temporal canal, and finally portions of the face.

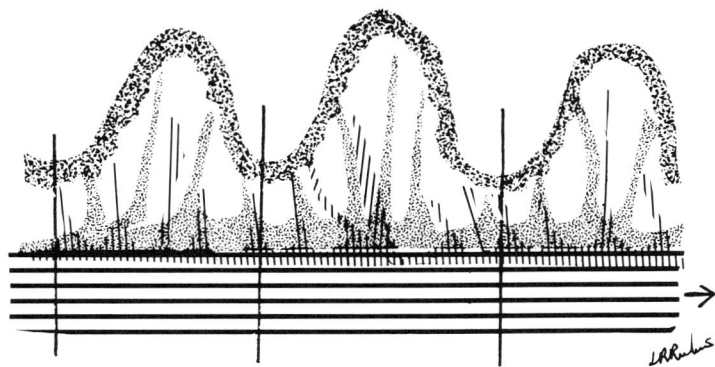

Fig. 1-1. Diagrammatic illustration of skin lines formed at right angles to the direction of resultant muscle contractions. The fascia and fine muscle fibrils pierce the subcutaneous tissue to insert into the dermis. Contracture of the muscles bunch the skin like an accordian into the lines of the face. The superficial fascia is the transmission and blender of many muscle contractions, allowing gradations of subtle facial movements.

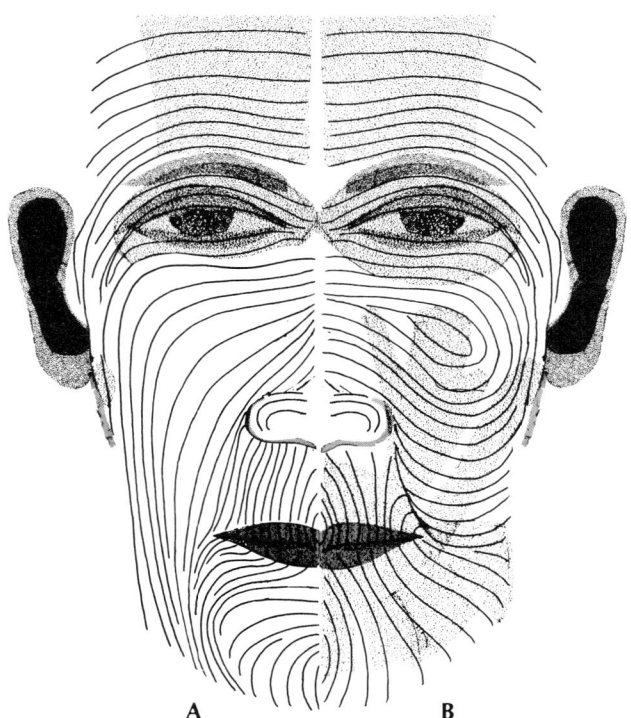

Fig. 1-2. Variations in the facial lines. Note **A,** the sad face, and **B,** the happy face. In the former, all lines curve downward. In **B,** the lines curve upward. The variation is an individual factor and is caused by contraction forces of different muscles blended by the superficial fascia.

Dissections of cadavers have demonstrated the most frequent directions taken by facial muscles and their lines of contraction. The most consistent departure from the standard textbook description can be found in the insertion of the major elevators of the upper lip.[5] The dominance of different lip muscles can alter lip movements and, secondarily, affect the smile.

Knowing these variations makes it possible for one to plan the surgical repair of chronic facial paralysis by properly placing new motor tendons into paralyzed sites so that the movements on the healthy side may be imitated.

The remainder of this chapter will deal with a description of the muscles of the face and how they affect the expression.

The foundations of facial muscle expression are found in the major circular muscles, the two around the orbit openings, and the one about the mouth. The orbicularis oculi (Fig. 1-3, *A*) coordinates the muscles about the eyelids, forehead, and zygomatic malar region, whereas the orbicularis oris (Fig. 1-3, *B*) correlates lip and cheek movements.

Region of the forehead and eyelids

There are tremendous variations in forehead and eyelid movements. These are determined by four separate muscles on each side. Despite the coordinated bilateral action usually seen, it is possible for one side to move independently. The four muscles involved are as follows:
1. Orbicularis oculi
2. Epicranius, which contains the frontalis muscles (left and right) and the occipital muscles with their connecting fasciae (Fig. 1-4)
3. Corrugator supercilii (Fig. 1-5, *A*)
4. Procerus muscle (Fig. 1-5, *B*)

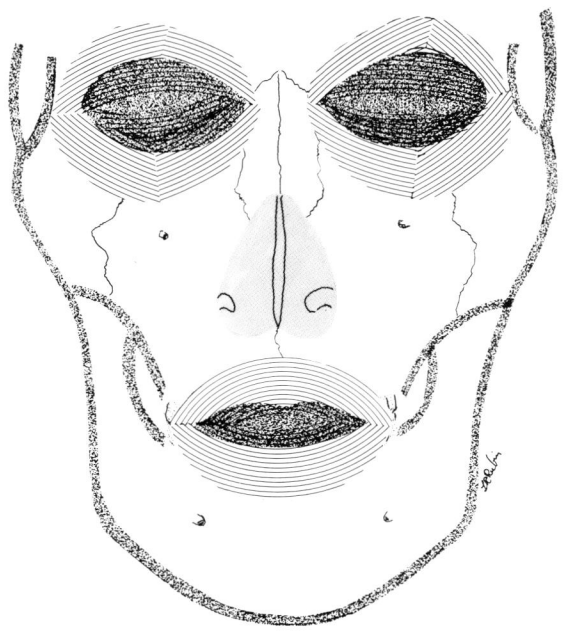

Fig. 1-3. The orbicularis oculi, *A*, makes up the bulk of the eyelids, surrounding the palpebral opening, and extends to the forehead, cheeks, and temporal region. It arises from the nasal part of the orbital bone, from the frontal process of the maxilla, and from the medial palpebral ligaments, which intersect its long attachment. The muscle fibers run through the eyelid laterally, blending with the frontalis and corrugator muscles, and some insert into the skin.

The fibers at the palpebral margin run from the medial canthal ligament and the surrounding frontal bone laterally to interlace and form the lateral canthal ligament or raphe. The portion very close to the palpebral lid margins is known as the ciliary bundle.

The anatomy books describe a lacrimal portion that lies behind the lacrimal sac. It is attached to the lacrimal bone and fascia medially and runs laterally to insert into the tarsus of the eyelids near the lacrimal carunculae, crossing laterally to help make up the lateral palpebral raphe.

Fig. 1-4. A, The epicranius consists of the frontalis, *A,* and the occipital, *B,* muscles with their connecting fasciae, which are intimately related to the overlying fasciae and skin. Posteriorly, the occipital arises by tendinous fibers from the lateral two thirds of the highest nuchal line of the occipital bone and the mastoid parts of the temporal bone. It runs anteriorly and becomes continuous with the galea aponeurotica.

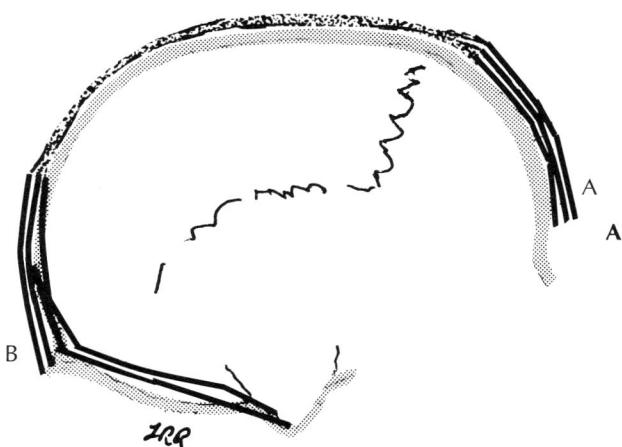

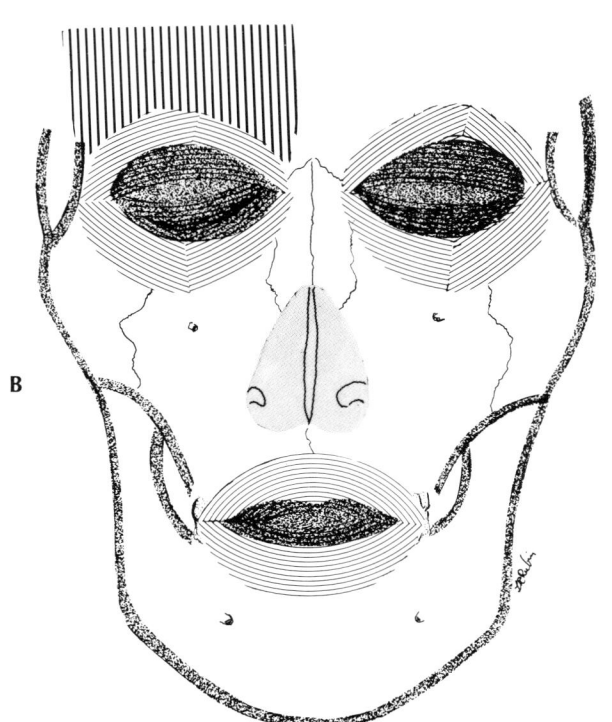

Fig. 1-4. B, In the forehead region, the frontalis muscles left and right continue anteriorly from the galea. The medial portions become continuous with the procerus, and the intermediate fibers become continuous with the corrugator supercilii and the orbicularis oculi. The lateral fibers of the frontalis, however, blend with the orbicularis laterally. Some of the frontalis fibers join each other medially above the nose.

NERVE SUPPLY

The frontalis muscle is supplied by the temporal branches of the facial nerve. The orbicularis, corrugator, and procerus are innervated by the temporal and zygomatic branches of the seventh nerve. The levator palpebrae superioris is supplied by the third cranial or oculomotor nerve. Some thin layers of the muscle are nonstriated and receive sympathetic innervation.

EFFECTS ON EXPRESSION

The occipital muscle draws the scalp backward and provides the resistance needed to allow the frontalis to contract. This results in raising the eyebrows and the superior part of the nose upward and backward, while also forming the transverse wrinkling of the forehead.

Constant contracture of the orbicularis throws the thin skin around the lateral canthal areas into radiating wrinkles known as "crow's-feet." When one smiles, the eyelids tend to close in varying degrees, creating a benign expression. When associated with a frown, the partial closing of the eyelids denotes a degree of anger.

The rapid opening and closing of the eyelids by the levator muscles can convey sexual "come hither" suggestions; whereas the lowering of the head and the fluttering of the eyelids associated with partial closing by the orbicularis can express to the opposite sex demure coyness. Wide opening of the eyelids by the levator on the other hand, when associated with contracture of the frontalis, can denote shock, fear, surprise, or despair.

The corrugator and the procerus combine to draw the eyebrows medially and downward, producing the vertical wrinkles in the midarea of the forehead, known as "frown lines."

The movements of the frontalis, corrugator, and procerus, acting in concert, can produce a tremendous range of emotional expressions. Raising the eyebrow can denote surprise, horror, or amusement. Raising one eyebrow can create the expression of surprise, playfulness, kindness, or tenderness.

A frown produced simultaneously with a wrinkling of the brows can express anger, sorrow, perplexity, or pain.

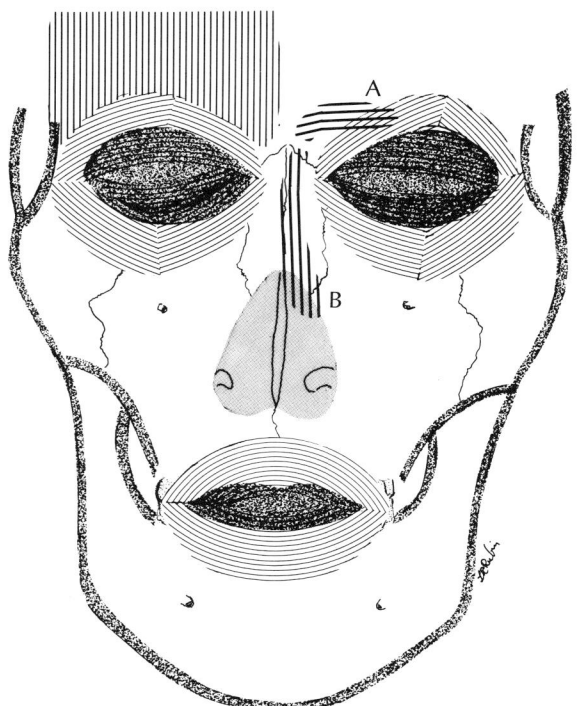

Fig. 1-5. *A,* The corrugator supercilii is a small muscle that arises from the medial end of the superciliary arch and passes its fibers laterally and upward to the deep surface of the skin above the middle of the supraorbital margins. *B,* The procerus muscle is a small pyramidal muscle that arises from the fascia covering the lower part of the nasal bone and the upper part of the lateral nasal cartilage. It is inserted into the skin over the lower part of the forehead and over the eyebrows.

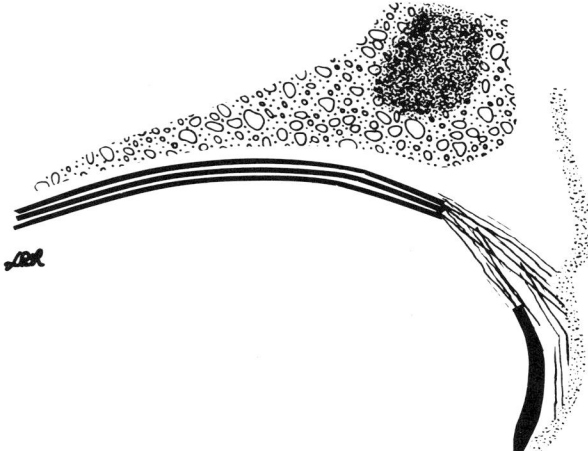

Fig. 1-6. The elevator of the eyelid, or the levator palebrae superioris, is not a muscle of expression in the strictest sense. When the muscle, however, is unable to function, as a result of either congenital or traumatic causes, the effect on expression is profound. That is why the elevator is included in this group of eyelid muscles.

The levator palpebrae superioris is a thin muscle arising from the inferior surface of the sphenoid bone. The muscle runs anteriorly, becoming a wide aponeurosis that splits into two lamellae, one of which is attached to the anterior surface of the superior tarsus while the other passes through the orbicularis to attach to the skin of the upper eyelid.

Region of the nose

The muscles of the nose are very distinctive in formulating facial expression. They are as follows:
1. Procerus
2. Nasalis
3. Depressor septi

The procerus has been described with the forehead muscles (Fig. 1-7).

NERVE SUPPLY

The nerve supply comes from the upper buccal branches of the facial nerve.

EFFECTS ON EXPRESSION

The functions of the nasalis and the depressor septi are to dilate and contract the nares, (nostrils), regulating the intake of air; however, combined with other facial muscles, they can express horror, anger, and rage by dilating the nostrils; physical pain and emotional agony are also conveyed by this dilation. Wrinkling and drawing the nose upward can demonstrate disgust or revulsion especially when associated with unpleasant odors and sights or intense dislike for an individual.

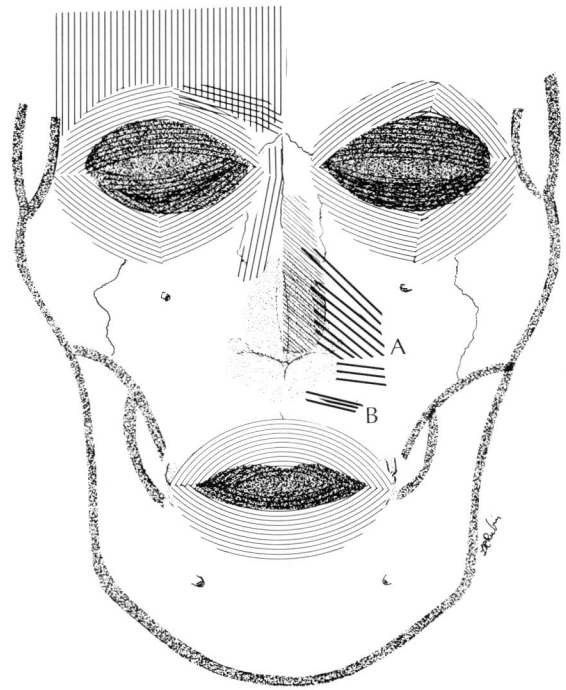

Fig 1-7. *A,* The nasalis consists of transverse and alar portions. The former, also known as the compressor naris, arises from the maxilla and blends anteromedially with its opposite and with the procerus over the bridge of the nose. The alar portion, known as the dilator naris, arises from the maxilla and runs medially to attach to the cartilaginous ala nasi.

B, The depressor septi arises from the maxilla and ascends under the mucous membrane of the upper lip to the membranous septum. It may be considered as part of the nasalis.

Region of the mouth and cheeks

The muscles in the mouth and cheeks serve as the container of the buccal cavity and guard its entrance by controlling the lips; their movements create the "smile," which is the keystone to facial expression.

The orbicularis oris makes up the bulk of the lips. The buccinator contributes fibers to the inner layers. These enter the muscles at the margins around the angle of the mouth. At a more superficial layer, the zygomaticus major and the depressor angularis add more muscle bulk. The elevators of the upper lip pass through the orbicularis and help swell its mass.

The muscle fibers of the orbicularis oris insert into the dermis of the lips. There are deeper muscles in the upper lip known as the incisivi labii superioris, which arise from the alveolar border of the maxilla opposite the lateral incisor tooth and run outward and downward toward the angle of the mouth. Similar muscles can be found in the lower lip, known as the incisivi labii inferioris. (See Fig. 1-8.)

NERVE SUPPLY

The lower buccal branches of the seventh nerve supply the muscles about the mouth.

EFFECTS ON EXPRESSION

The function of the orbicularis oris is to close the lips. Its deep fibers compress the lips against the teeth. The superficial fibers evert the lips into a pout or purse-string closure. The shades of emotion expressed by the lips are legion. The world's great writers and artists have described infinite variations of affection, lust, hatred, revulsion, anger—in short, the gamut of human emotions—all expressed by the lips. Lips are kissable, forbidding, inviting, sexually stimulating, and maddening. The full lips of a desirable woman are compared to a rosebud, whereas a miser has the lips drawn tight into a straight line. The lips have been used for every conceivable expressive purpose beyond guarding the entrance of the mouth.

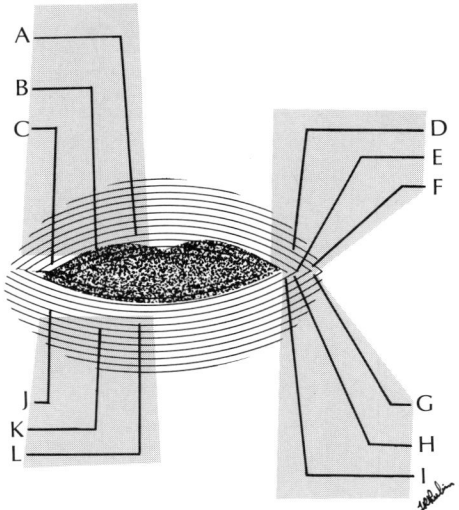

Fig. 1-8. The bulk and shape of the lips are made up of a complex of muscles consisting primarily of the sphincter orbicularis oris. The muscles of the cheeks contribute to its bulk and vary lip action. The muscles about the sphincter are grouped as follows:

ABC Elevators of the upper lip
DEF Elevators of the angle of the mouth
GHI Depressors of the angle of the mouth
JKL Depressors of the lower lip

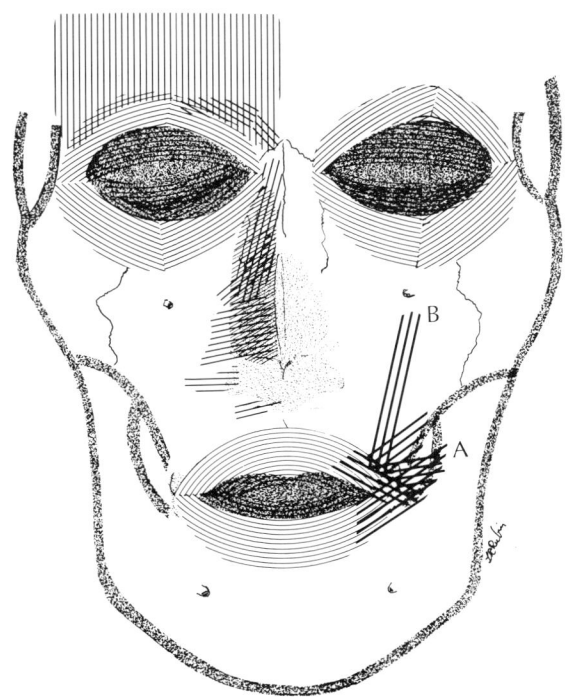

Fig. 1-9. *A*, The buccinator muscle arises from the outer surface of the alveolar process of the maxilla and mandible and the anterior border of the pterygomandibular raphe. A few fibers come from a tendinous band bridging the maxilla and the pterygoid hamulus.

The fibers of the buccinator converge on the corner of the mouth where the central fibers decussate to end in the orbicularis. The highest and lowest fibers continue medially into the upper and lower lips without decussating. Those from above decussate and pass through the orbicularis into the lower lip, while the lower fibers course through the angle to merge with the orbicularis fibers of the upper lip.

B, The caninus is a deep muscle that is associated with elevating the corners of the mouth. It arises from the maxilla in the canine fossa to travel downward and medially into the corner of the orbicularis where it adds to its bulk.

Elevators of the upper lip

The quadratus labii superioris is made up of the following three muscles, each taking part in elevating the upper lip and contributing to the bulk of the orbicularis oris (Fig. 1-10):
1. Caput angulare
2. Levator labii superioris
3. Zygomaticus minor

Elevators of the corner of the mouth

The elevators of the corner of the mouth are primarily made up of the following muscles. The last two have been described as deep muscles adding to the orbicularis oris.
1. Zygomaticus major (Fig. 1-11)
2. Upper part of the buccinator
3. Caninus

NERVE SUPPLY

The upper and lower buccal branches of the seventh nerve supply the elevators of the upper lip and angle of the mouth.

EFFECTS ON EXPRESSION

The elevators of the upper lip and the angle of the mouth contribute to the human smile. The exact direction the muscles take from their origin to their insertions into the orbicularis, the vermilion, and the mucocutaneous line determines the line of contracture. The line of contracture, point of insertion, and the varying strengths of each elevator muscle make up the different types of smiles. The effects of the muscle contractions are mediated by the investing superficial fascial attachments to the dermis. The types of smiles are described later in this chapter.

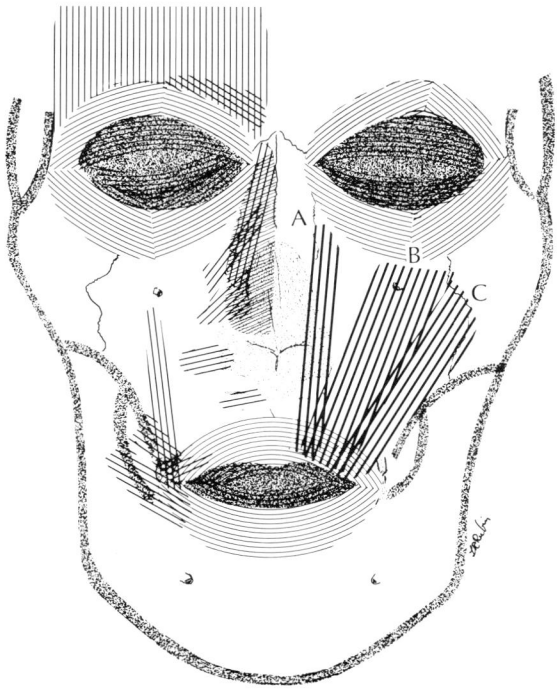

Fig. 1-10. *A,* The caput angulare crosses from the frontal process of the maxilla, traveling obliquely downward and laterally to insert some fibers into cartilage of the ala of the nose and a larger portion into the upper lip and finally passing through the orbicularis oris to insert into the skin, vermilion border, and mucocutaneous line of the upper lip.

B, The levator labii superioris is the major body of the quadratus labii superioris. It arises from the lower margin of the orbit above the infraorbital foramen, from the body of the maxilla, and from the prominence of the malar bone. The muscles converge into the upper lip, contributing to the bulk of the orbicularis, and pass through it to insert into the skin, mucocutaneous line, and the vermilion border. The mass of this muscle varies from individual to individual.

C, The zygomaticus minor arises from the lateral surface of the malar bone and passes downward and medially into the substance of the orbicularis mucocutaneous line, and vermilion.

Fig. 1-11. The zygomaticus major is the prime elevator at the angle. It arises in the zygomatic bone in front of the temporomalar suture and ranges forward to the angle of the mouth, where it blends and decussates with the orbicularis and the depressors of the angle of the mouth. It also sends fibers to the skin in that area.

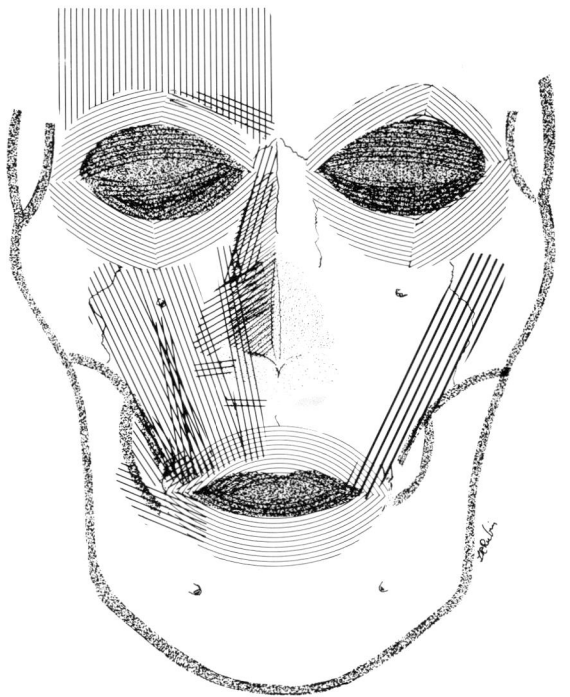

Depressors of the angle of the mouth

The depressors of the angle of the mouth are made up of the following:
1. Buccinator (lower fibers)
2. Depressor angularis (Fig. 1-12)
3. Risorius (Fig. 1-13)

Depressors of the lower lip

The depressors of the lower lip are made up of the following:
1. Mentalis
2. Depressor labii inferioris (Fig. 1-14)
3. Platysma

NERVE SUPPLY

The risorius and the lower buccal muscle fibers are supplied by the lower buccal branches of the facial nerve. The depressor angularis and the depressors of the lower lip are supplied by the marginal branch of the seventh nerve.

EFFECTS ON EXPRESSION

The pulling down of the angle of the mouth by the depressor angularis and the risorius is usually associated with anger, rage, sadness, depression, and sorrow. At its most extreme, the risorius pulls the angle of the mouth backward and downward to express the most intense emotions of rage and hate. In a less tight contraction, it can denote a sardonic smile.

The drooping of the lower lip by the quadratus labii inferioris and the mentalis can denote disappointment, sorrow, crying, and, in the extreme, rage and hate.

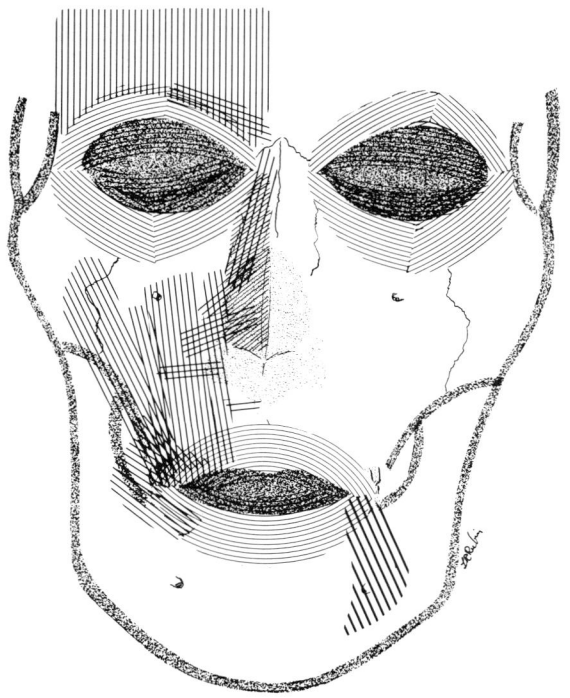

Fig. 1-12. The depressor angularis oris arises from the oblique line of the mandible and converges to enter the mass of the muscles of the angle of the mouth. It blends with fibers of the risorius and the platysma.

The lower portions of the buccinator decussate at the angle to help depress the latter.

Fig. 1-13. The risorius muscle, *R,* arises from the parotid fascia and inserts into the skin of the corner of the mouth.

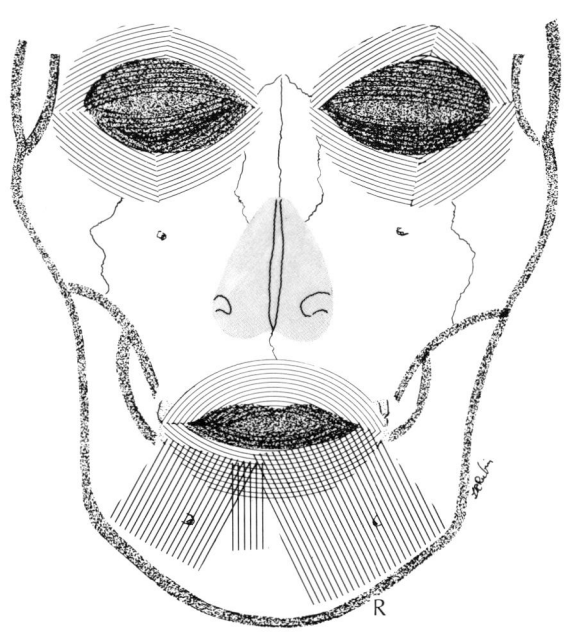

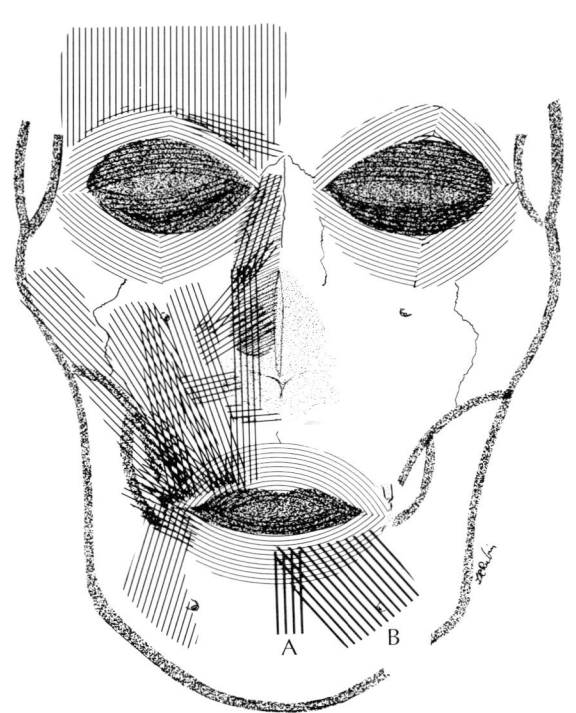

Fig. 1-14. *A,* The mentalis is a small muscle that arises from the incisor fossa of the mandible and passes upward through the orbicularis to insert into the lip skin and vermilion. *B,* The depressor labii inferioris, also known as the quadratus labii inferioris, arises from the lateral surface of the mandible deep and medial to the depressor of the mouth angle. It inserts into the orbicularis, the vermilion, and the skin of the lower lip. The medial fibers join with those of the opposite side and the angle depressor.

I have taken a narrow random sampling of 100 people, male and female, and classified their smiles.[5] Three basic forms are discernible (Figs. 1-15 to 1-17).

The factors influencing variations in a smile can be listed as follows:
1. Relative underdevelopment or overdevelopment of the elevators or depressors of the angles of the mouth and lower lip
2. Hereditary variation in width and length of the lips
3. Bony anatomical variations, such as protruding maxilla, underdevelopment or overdevelopment of the mandible, and high or low malar prominences
4. Variations in tooth structure, such as protruding or receding teeth or even absence of teeth
5. Hereditary factors making deep or shallow nasolabial folds
6. Pathological conditions
    a. Congenital absence or underdevelopment of muscles, as in the Möbius syndrome
    b. Muscular dystrophies
    c. Facial paresis, congenital or acquired
    d. Obesity
    e. Starvation
    f. Lipoid dystrophy
    g. Edema of soft tissues
    h. Bony tumors
    i. Tongue deformities
    j. Mouth tumors

Summary

The muscles of the face serve a double function, that is, to activate the orifices of the eyelids and mouth and to portray human emotion.

The facial nerve serves as the motor-stimulating nerve. Interruption of impulses along the pathway from the cortex to its destination can cause a paralysis of that muscle.

The muscles of the forehead and the orbicularis oculi serve as one unit. The muscles around the mouth focus about the orbicularis and not only contribute to its bulk, but also create expressions by their interplay of elevation and depression of the lips and the corners of the mouth.

The relative strength of individual groups of muscles about the mouth are responsible for variations of the smile, a uniquely human capability. In doing so, they create the expressions that differentiate the human from lower animals.

The subtle shades of human expression are possible because of the superficial faciae investing the facial muscles, acting as the transmission that blends the contractions of various facial muscles.

The human being is indeed the first and foremost of primates. He can express his deep inner emotions by an exquisitely controlled symphony of facial expressions.

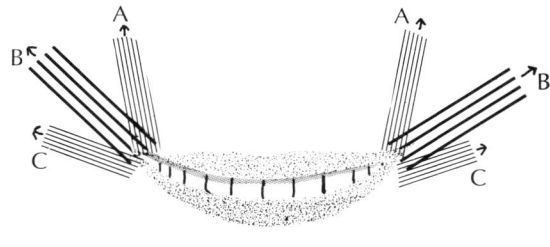 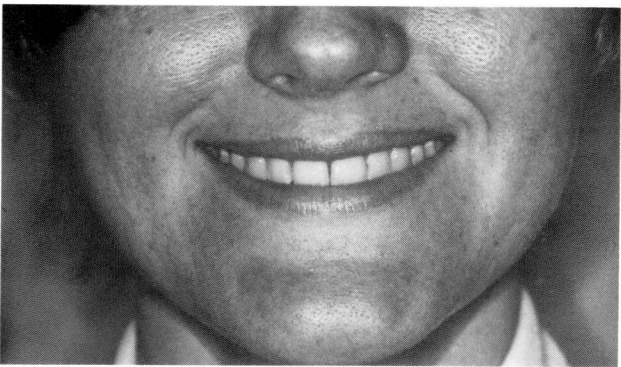

Fig. 1-15. The most common type (67%) (Mona Lisa smile). The corners of the mouth are elevated first, showing dominance of the muscles (zygomaticus major) lifting the angle of the mouth.

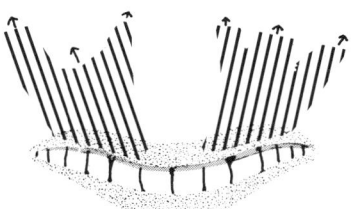 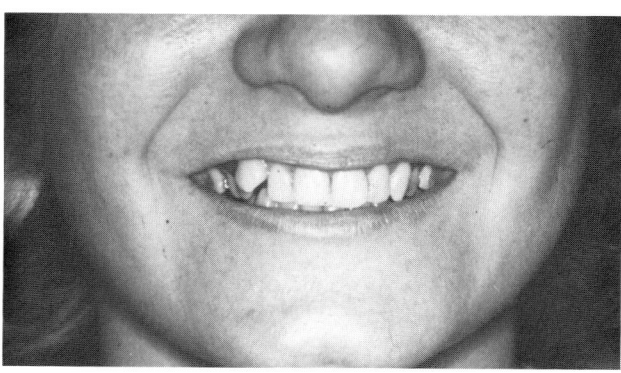

Fig. 1-16. The canine smile (31%) (Jimmy Carter smile). The dominance of the levator labii superioris was apparent. This muscle contracted first at the initiation of a smile, followed by the contracture of the elevators at the angle of the mouth.

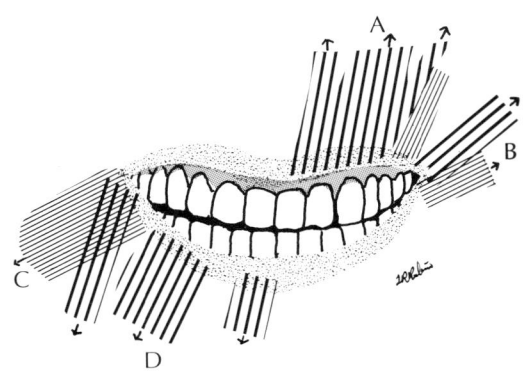 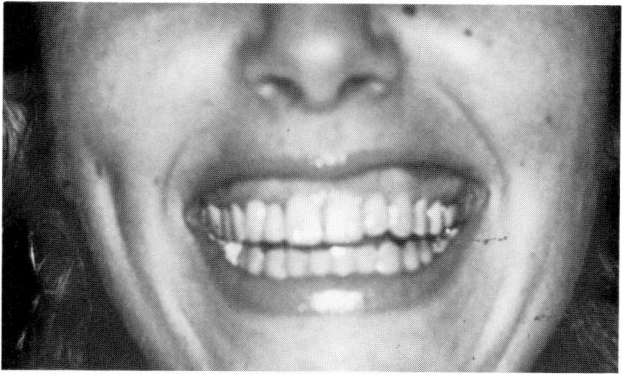

Fig. 1-17. The full-denture smile (2%) (Lena Horne smile). All the elevators and depressors of the lips and the angles contract at the same time, showing all the teeth.

19

REFERENCES

1. Converse, J. M.: Reconstructive plastic surgery, Philadelphia, 1964, W. B. Saunders Co., pp. 1154-1162.
2. Langer, K.: Cleavage of the cutis: anatomy and physiology of the skin, Royal Academy of Sciences Presentation, April 1861.
3. Mitz, V., and Peyronie, M.: The superficial musculo-aponeurotic system (SMAS) in the parotid and cheek area, Plast. Reconstr. Surg. **58:**20-88, 1976.
4. Rubin, L. R.: Langer's lines and facial scars, Plast. Reconstr. Surg. **3:**147-155, 1948.
5. Rubin, L. R.: The anatomy of a smile—its importance in the treatment of facial paralysis, Plast. Reconstr. Surg. **55**(4):384-387, 1974.
6. Sobotta, J.: Atlas of descriptive human anatomy, New York, 1954, Hafner Publishing Co., p. 242.
7. Warwick, R., and Williams, P. L., editors: Gray's anatomy, ed. 35, Philadelphia, 1973, W. B. Saunders Co., p. 490.

2 Surgical anatomy of the facial nerve

LEE A. HARKER
BRIAN F. McCABE

A concise surgical description of the anatomy of the facial nerve is outlined. Accurate knowledge of the surgical anatomy can pinpoint disruption along the nervous pathway from the brain to the peripheral muscles.

Otolaryngologic, neurologic, plastic, and general surgeons all deal with the facial nerve during surgical procedures; occasionally, through incomplete knowledge of its normal anatomy or common variations, unnecessary facial paralysis occurs. This chapter reviews the important features of the nerve's serpentine course, and its relationships from pontine emergence to muscular insertion. For purposes of convenient discussion, the nerve is divided into several arbitrary segments—cisternal, meatal, labyrinthine, tympanic, mastoid, parotid, and cervicofacial. Discussion topics include composition, course and relationships, and common variations.

Composition
FIBER TYPES AND DISPOSITION

The main root is composed of homogeneous 8 to 10 μm myelinated special visceral efferent fibers emanating from cell bodies in the facial nucleus of the pons. Except for a small branch to the stapedius muscle, these motor fibers course through the entire temporal bone to eventually innervate the superficial, skeletal, mimetic musculature of the face and scalp as well as the platysma, stylohyoid, and digastric (posterior belly) muscles.

The principle fiber components of the nervus intermedius and the functions they subserve are general visceral efferent (parasympathetic), special visceral afferent (taste), and general somatic afferent (general cutaneous sensation). The preganglionic parasympathetic fibers have cell bodies in the superior salivatory nucleus and innervate the lacrimal gland, submandibular and sublingual glands, and the glands of the mucous membrane of the nose and roof of the mouth. For the most part, fibers to the lacrimal and nasal glands leave the main trunk with the greater superficial petrosal nerve and synapse in the sphenopalatine ganglion. Those destined for the oral, submandibular, and sublingual glands course with the chorda tympani nerve and synapse in the submandibular ganglion. Taste fibers from the anterior two thirds of the tongue constitute the bulk of the chorda tympani nerve and join the facial nerve in its mastoid segment. Impulses are conducted to the cell bodies in the geniculate ganglion and conveyed by the central processes to the nucleus and tractus solitarius. The general sensory fibers, which are fewer in number, also have their cell bodies in the geniculate ganglion, and their central processes reach the nucleus and tractus solitarius. Their peripheral processes travel with the chorda tympani and then achieve their final destination as the auriculotemporal nerve.

NERVE COVERINGS

A peripheral nerve has three connective tissue investitures known as the epineurium, perineurium, and endoneurium. The epineurium is a fibrous sheath surrounding the nerve as a whole and serving as a conduit for its arterial supply and venous drainage. The perineurium is a similarly dense connective tissue sheath surrounding fascicles of fibers and also serves to transmit small blood vessels. The endoneurial sheath of Henle is a very delicate tubule that surrounds each individual myelinated fiber.[2] These three coverings can be easily identified in the parotid and cervicofacial portions of the nerve but not in all portions of the cisternal, meatal, and infratemporal segments. After the nerve roots leave the brainstem, a delicate layer of pia mater surrounds both the larger and smaller roots in the cisternal course, but there is no perineurium or epineurium. Near the porus of the meatus, these pial sheaths blend to encircle the two roots in a single covering. The dura of the posterior cranial fossa is densely adherent to the walls of the internal acoustic meatus and extends into that tunnel, becoming progressively thinner as it moves toward the fundus. This thin blend of periosteum and dura at the fundus is continuous with the coverings of the nerve in the fallopian canal. In this bony canal, the epineurium and the periosteum of the bony wall combine to form what is clinically referred to as the sheath of the facial nerve; these are sometimes distinguishable as separate layers and sometimes not. The diameter of the bony canal relative to that of the facial nerve, and the abundance of arteries and veins, are similarly variable. The nerve appears most cramped in the labyrinthine and tympanic segments, and the bony canal is most capacious in the mastoid segment as it funnels outward toward the stylomastoid foramen. There are local dilatations as perforating vessels join the nerve. The periosteal component of the sheath is thickest in the region of the stylomastoid foramen where it may approach the diameter of the nerve itself.

BLOOD SUPPLY

In its cisternal and meatal portions, the facial nerve is nourished by vessels arising from the vertebral artery usually reaching the nerve via the anteroinferior cerebellar artery. The complex vascular patterns in the internal auditory canal have recently been reviewed by Portman et al.[6] Once the nerve enters the fallopian canal, its arterial supply is derived from the external carotid system. There is an arterial arcade from the stylomastoid artery distally, and the petrosal branch of the middle meningeal artery proximally, which is the primary nourishment within the temporal bone. In the parotid and cervicofacial portions, there are numerous regional branches of the external carotid system to the nerve. Venous drainage, by and large, mirrors the arterial supply.

TOPOGRAPHIC LOCATION OF FIBERS

Several investigators have attempted to trace through the temporal bone the course of fibers to various muscle groups. With the microscope discrete fiber bundles can be dissected from their peripheral muscular terminations centrally to the geniculate ganglion, though proximal to the midmastoid segment dissection is difficult. There are communicating branches between the many ropelike fascicles.[9] No definitive topographic studies on humans have been performed, and recent topographic assignments are not in total agreement.[4,5] It is, however, a clinical observation that paralysis originating from inflammatory disease in the tympanum commonly affects the oral musculature initially, and it is also known that the nerve is devoid of a bony covering, most commonly just superior to the oval window in the mesotympanum. It is inferred that the superficial portion of the nerve just above the oval window often has a high density of fibers destined for the perioral musculature.

Course and relationships

At its pontine emergence the motor root is slightly rostral to the common trunk of the vestibulocochlear nerve in the recess between the olive and the inferior peduncle. The nervus intermedius lies between the ventral surfaces of the facial and vestibulocochlear nerves.

After entering the porus of the internal acoustic meatus, the main motor root courses to the anterior wall of the canal and occupies a shallow groove along its superior aspect. The inferior ledge of this groove is continuous at the fundus of the meatus, with a prominent transverse crest of bone separating the facial and superior vestibular nerves superiorly from the cochlear and inferior vestibular nerves inferiorly. A vertical wedge-shaped bony crest ("Bill's bar") serves as an important landmark separating the facial nerve anteriorly from the superior vestibular nerve posteriorly (unless the wedge is effaced by disease) (Fig. 2-1).

In the internal acoustic meatus, the nervus intermedius joins the main motor root. There is communication between fibers of the facial and superior vestibular nerves in the canal as they lie side by side; this makes gross distinction of their boundaries difficult at times. Also, in the internal acoustic meatus, the vestibulocochlear nerve divides into the cochlear nerve, the superior and inferior vestibular nerves, and the nerve to the singular foramen (Fig. 2-1).

As the facial nerve enters the fallopian canal, it is in close relationship anteroinferiorly with the basal turn of the cochlea; posteriorly, it is similarly close to the superior semicircular canal. As it approaches the tympanum, the nerve makes a U-shaped bend, coursing posteriorly and in a slight inferior direction within the bony confines of the middle ear. At the apex of this geniculum is the sensory ganglion (Figs. 2-2 and 2-3). The greater and lesser superficial petrosal nerves join the facial in this region. The tympanic segment almost always courses inferior to the lateral semicircular canal and superior to the oval window and stapes. The nerve then takes a more gentle turn inferiorly to descend through the mastoid portion proceeding inferiorly and slightly laterally giving off the branch to the stapedius muscle and receiving the fibers of the chorda

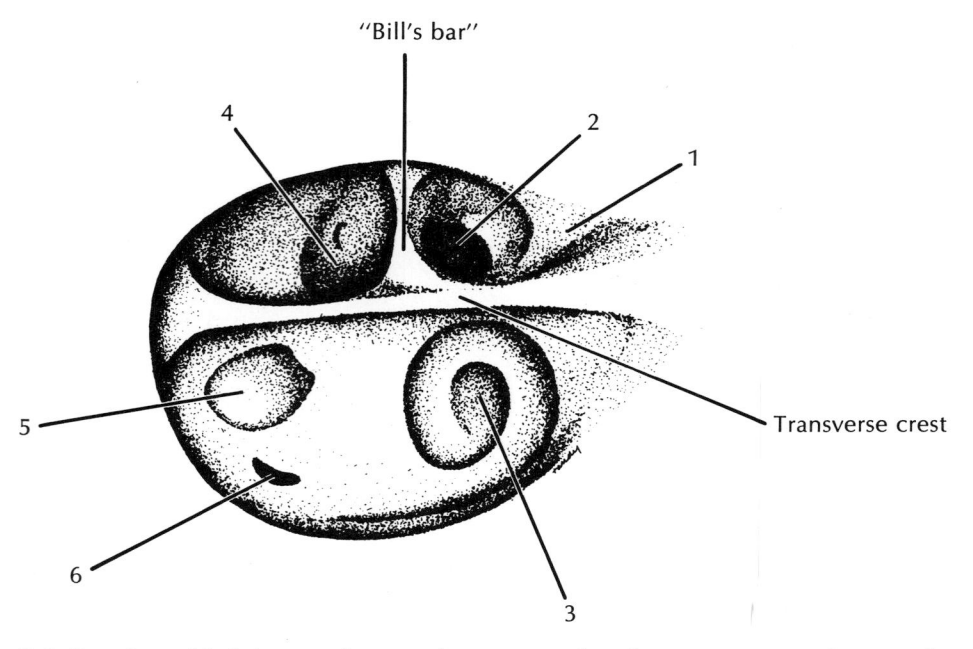

Mechanism of facial expression and pathophysiology of degeneration

Fig. 2-1. Fundus of left internal acoustic meatus showing anterosuperior canal wall groove for facial nerve, **1,** and foramina transmitting nerves: facial, **2;** cochlear, **3;** superior vestibular, **4;** inferior vestibular, **5;** and singular, **6.**

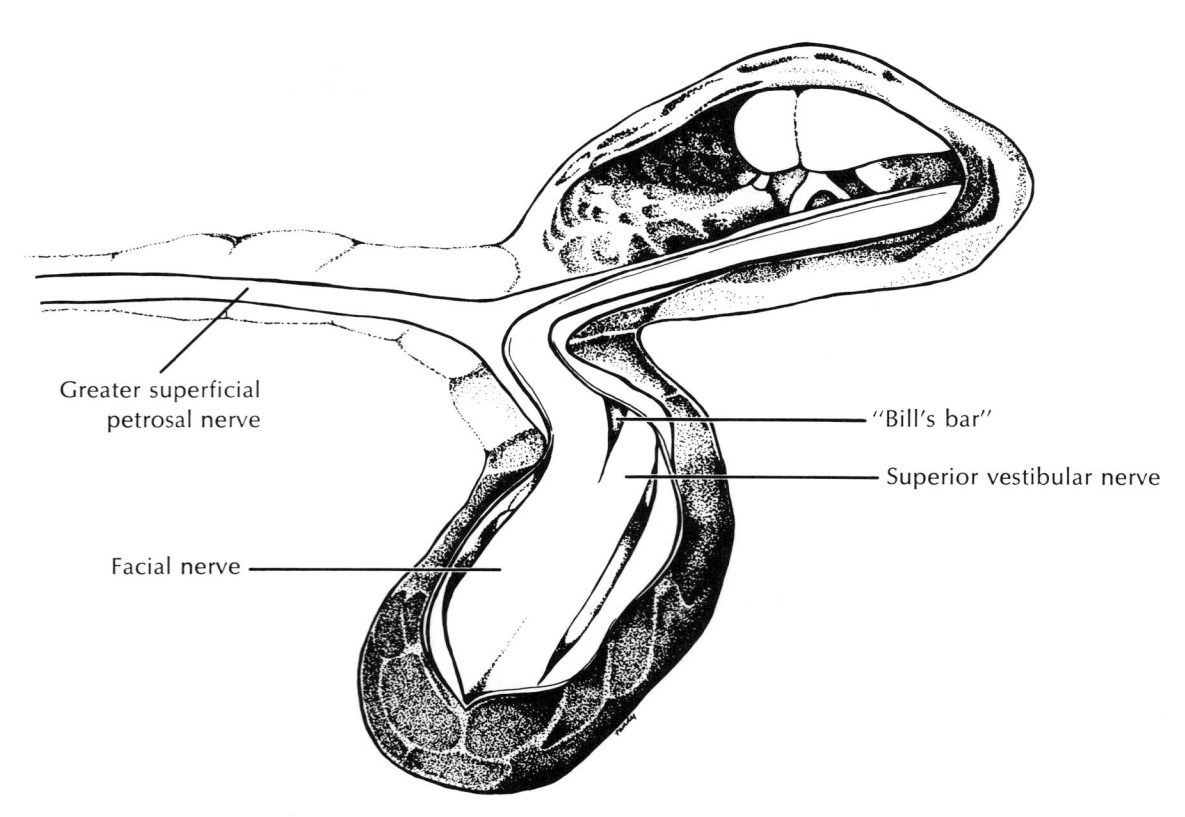

Fig. 2-2. Middle fossa exposure of right facial nerve showing meatal, labyrinthine, and tympanic segments.

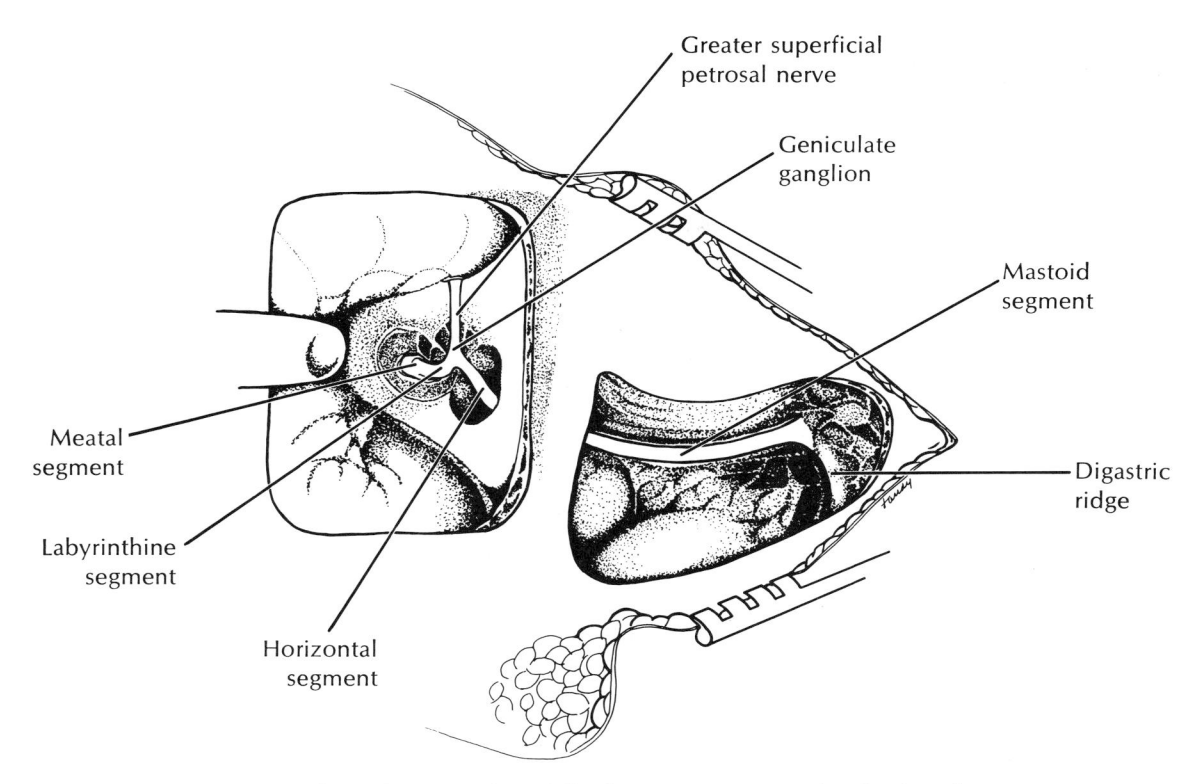

Fig. 2-3. Combined mastoid-middle fossa exposure of right facial nerve.

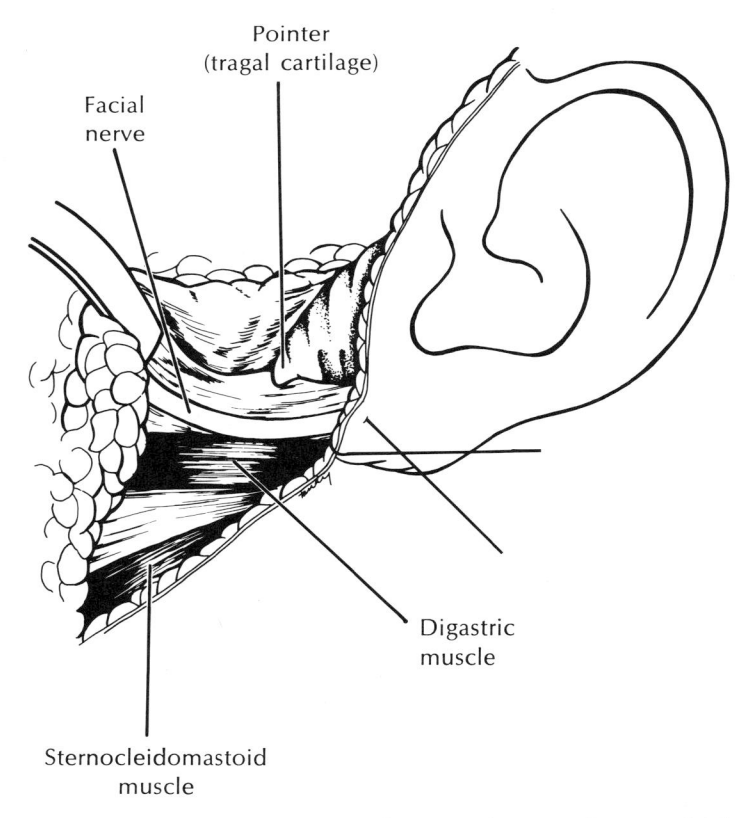

Fig. 2-4. Left facial nerve exposure after exit from stylomastoid foramen.

25

tympani. The posterior semicircular canal lies posterior to the facial nerve in its descending course, but the ampullate end of that canal dips medial to the nerve. The digastric ridge of the mastoid tip of pneumatized bones is a useful landmark to identify the nerve in its most inferior infratemporal portion (Fig. 2-3).

At the stylomastoid foramen, the nerve turns anteriorly and passes laterally through the substance of the parotid gland. At its stylomastoid emergence, it lies approximately 1 cm inferior and 1 cm medial to the tip of the pointer of the tragal cartilage. The nerve emerges just medial and superior to the posterior belly of the digastric muscle (Fig. 2-4). After 1 to 2 cm, it divides into an upper and lower division and, subsequently, ramifies into the well-known peripheral branching pattern.

As the branches course across the face toward their distal terminations, they become more superficial. This is a special surgical hazard in the region inferiolateral to the eye where the soft tissue is scanty and the branches lie just beneath the skin. A helpful relationship in the upper neck is that the ramus mandibularis branch consistently courses lateral to the posterior facial vein and facial artery and is found beneath the fascia medial to the platysma muscle.

VARIABILITY OF COURSE AND RELATIONSHIPS

The facial nerve exhibits a low incidence of significant anatomic variation in its exit from the brainstem and its course through the proximal portions of the temporal bone if there is normal development of the bony labyrinth. But if there exists dysplasia or aplasia of the osseus labyrinth, severe abnormalities of location and course usually occur. The extent of bony dysplasia generally portends the extent of the facial nerve abnormality. But with normal development of the cochlea and semicircular canals, the cisternal, meatal, and labyrinthine segments will usually have their normal relationships. Farther distally in the temporal bone, the nerve is more likely to stray from its normal course, especially if there is evidence of associated external ear or bony external auditory canal abnormality. In these situations, the nerve commonly makes an acute angle at the junction of the tympanic and mastoid portions, coursing anterolaterally, entering the temporomandibular joint and bypassing the mastoid tip.[3] Even when the external ear and canal are normal, more abnormalities appear in the tympanic and mastoid segments than elsewhere, but this does not necessarily reflect an excessively high incidence of these anomalies. The large number of surgical procedures that have visualized the nerve in these segments and the extreme importance of each variant to surgeons have resulted in many descriptions of variations of nerve position or course. The more commonly seen variants include bony dehiscences in the fallopian canal (sometimes with protrusion of a knuckle of nerve through the dehiscence), total absence of a bony covering for the nerve in the middle ear, duplication or even triplication of the main trunk in the middle ear or mastoid (with or without subsequent reunification), and a course across the promontory of the middle ear inferior to the oval window.[5,8]

The variability of the nerve's position at the inferior mastoid segment is greater than elsewhere in the temporal bone; variability of mastoid pneumatization is one factor affecting this. In the infant, the nerve exits on the lateral surface of the temporal bone before pneumatization of the developing mastoid tip displaces the stylomastoid foramen to a medial location protected by that cellular mastoid. It is at greatest risk in the first 2 years of life.[7]

Farther distally, the nerve almost always emerges from the stylomastoid foramen as a single trunk and divides into an upper and lower division after a centimeter or two. But the variability of the pes anserinus after this is well known to all surgeons operating on the face. Frontal, orbital, buccal, mandibular, and cervical branches are usually present, but their locations and interconnections are not predictable.

Another important relationship of the facial nerve is the fallopian canal itself. Dehiscences of this bone conduit occur in over 55% of temporal bones and, in one fifth of these, multiple areas are dehiscent.[1] By far, the most common site is the region of the tympanic segment just superior to the oval window, but in 10% to 15% of bones, the geniculate ganglion is separated from the middle cranial fossa only by dura.[1,8] Similar exposures occur in other parts of the tympanic and mastoid portions.

Appropriate surgical exposure and techniques, coupled with an understanding of the normal and aberrant course and relationships of the facial nerve, should result in an extremely low incidence of surgical injury.

REFERENCES

1. Baxter, A.: Dehiscence of the fallopian canal, J. Laryngol. Otol. **85**:587, 1971.
2. Carpenter, M. B.: Human neuroanatomy, ed. 7, Baltimore, 1976, The Williams & Wilkins Co.
3. Crabtree, J. A.: The facial nerve in congenital ear surgery, Otolaryngol. Clin. North Am. **7**(2):505, June 1974.
4. May, M.: Anatomy of the facial nerve; spatial orientation of fibers in the temporal bone, Laryngoscope **83**:1311, 1973.
5. Miehlke, A.: Surgery of the facial nerve, ed. 2, Philadelphia, 1973, W. B. Saunders Co.
6. Portman, M., Sterkers, J. M., Charachon, R., and Chouard, C. H.: The internal auditory meatus, Edinburgh, 1975, Churchill Livingstone.
7. Shambaugh, G. E.: Surgery of the ear, Philadelphia, 1967, W. B. Saunders Co.
8. Shuknecht, H. F.: Pathology of the ear, Cambridge, 1974, Harvard University Press.
9. White, A., and Verma, P. L.: Spatial arrangement of facial nerve fibers, J. Laryngol. Otol. **87**:957, 1973.

3 Pathophysiology of denervation in facial neuromuscular motor unit

JOANNA HOLLENBERG SHER

The interruption of nervous impulse to the facial muscles sets up a series of pathological reactions. A detailed description is given of how muscle fibers atrophy after loss of innervation. Of utmost importance is the fact that denervated atrophic muscle fibers may become reconstituted after reinnervation.

Pathophysiology of denervation in facial neuromuscular motor unit

The techniques for reanimation of paralyzed facial musculature described in Parts III and IV of this series depend on the regenerative capacity of peripheral nerve, motor end plates, and skeletal muscle, as well as upon the capacity of a denervated muscle fiber to become reinnervated and resume its normal contractile function. Recent electron microscopic and experimental studies have expanded knowledge of these processes, yet they leave some basic questions unanswered. The following review of normal muscle structure, and changes in denervation is offered to provide information on the basic cellular events occurring either as a result of disease, or as a consequence of surgical intervention. The basic research in these areas has not been done on facial muscle per se; however there is every reason to assume that the biological reactions of the striated muscles of the face do not differ from those of the other voluntary muscles.

Normal skeletal muscle structure and function

Striated muscle fibers are multinucleated cylindrical cells with tapered ends, measuring 30 to 100 μm in diameter in the large muscles of normal adults.[2a] They vary from a few millimeters to over 3 cm in length, and in long muscles the proximal and distal ends of fibers are joined by connective tissue. Facial and tongue muscle fibers may split at their insertions into membrane or skin. Within a given muscle, the fibers are arranged in groups or fasciculi of parallel fibers. These fasciculi are triangular or quadrangular in cross section.

MUSCLE CELL

Within the muscle fiber itself, bounded by the sarcolemmal membrane, the filaments of contractile proteins, arranged together in myofibrils, are surrounded by aqueous sarcoplasm, tubules of the sarcoplasmic reticulum, and mitochondria. The structures that make up the myofibril are alternating thick (myosin) and thin (actin) filaments. The thick filaments extend throughout the length of the A bands of the fibril.

I wish to thank Dr. S. A. Shafiq for advice and for the contribution of electron micrographs, Dr. Masazumi Adachi for permission to use some of the illustrations, Mr. R. Simowitz for photographic assistance, and Mr. Henry Veal for the histological and histochemical preparations.

Mechanism of facial expression and pathophysiology of degeneration

The thin filaments, containing actin, troponin, and tropomyosin, are attached to the dense Z lines, which are situated in the middle of the I bands. One A band is flanked by an I band on each side, and each I band ends at a Z line. One sarcomere is that part of the myofibril between two adjacent Z lines (Fig. 3-1). The thin filaments extend through the I band and into part of the A band. The central part of the A band containing only myosin is the H zone, which has a central faint M line because of focal thickening of the myosin strands. Thus a cross section of a myofibril at the level of the I band shows only thin filaments, whereas a cross section through the A band, except in the H zone, shows thick myosin filaments surrounded by thin filaments in a hexagonal arrangement. Myofibrils consist of many sarcomeres, and the cross striation of the muscle fiber is a result of the regular banded arrangement of these proteins. One muscle fiber has many such myofibrils within it.

Contraction of muscle is a result of sliding of the actin filaments between the myosin filaments; thus the I band and H zone are shortened.[25] Activated by the liberation of calcium ions from the sarcoplasmic reticulum, the positions of troponin and tropomyosin are altered. This allows the heads of the myosin molecules access to the actin; thus contraction of the myofibril is initiated.[11]

The aqueous sarcoplasm surrounds the myofibrils and contains glycogen granules, fat droplets, myoglobin, and enzymes such as phosphorylase. Mitochondria, oval

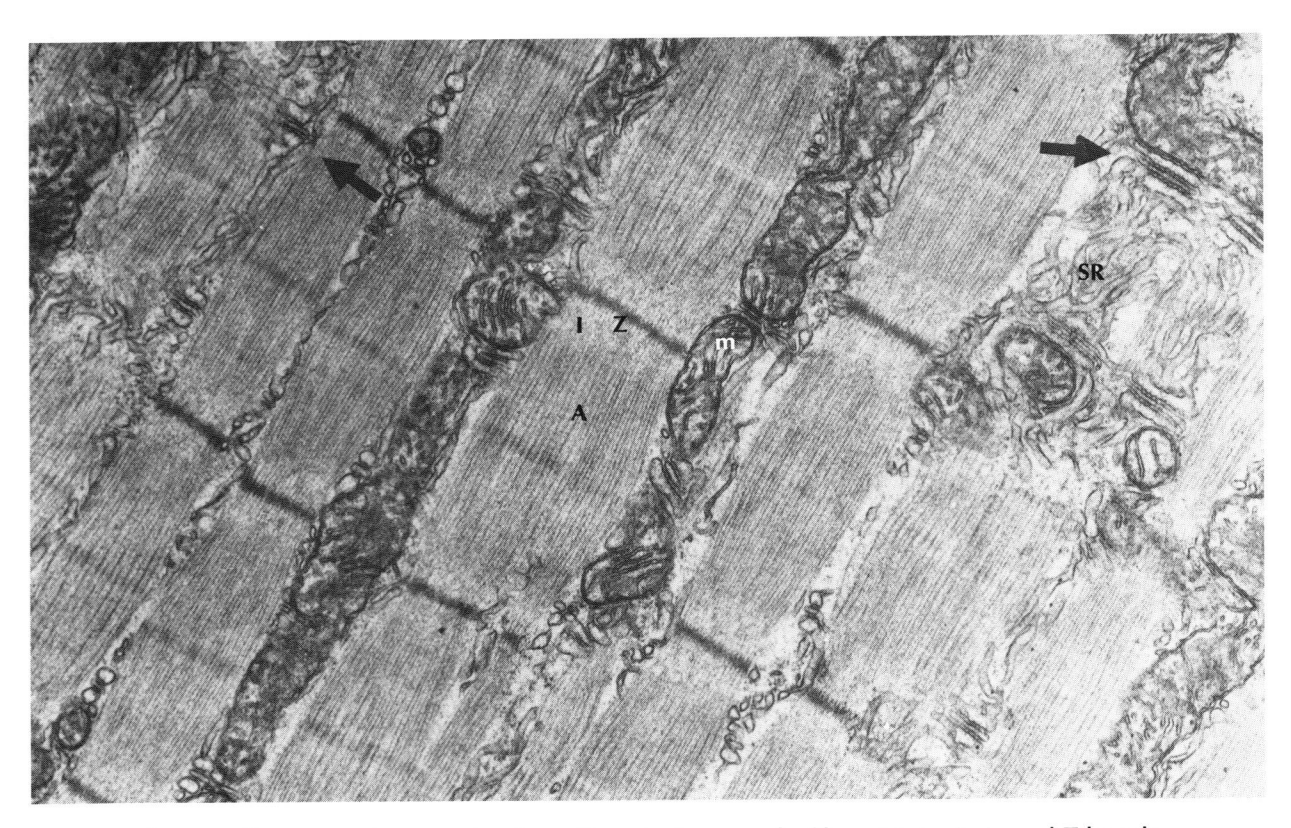

Fig. 3-1. Electron micrograph of small part of a muscle fiber. Note A, I, and Z bands of the myofibrils, mitochondria **(m)**, and sarcoplasmic reticulum **(SR)**. The arrows point to triads. (25,000×; courtesy Dr. S. A. Shafiq, New York.)

structures containing an inner membrane whose deep folds form characteristic cristae, are usually placed between myofibrils, on either side of the Z line. They contain the enzymes of the tricarboxylic acid cycle necessary for oxidative phosphorylation, and therefore provide energy for cellular metabolism. The tubules of the sarcoplasmic reticulum are arranged longitudinally, irregularly surrounding the myofibrils, whereas the transverse tubular system (T system) extends transversely across the fiber from its connection with the sarcolemma.[19,37] Projections of the vesicles of the T system weave between the outer filaments of the myofibrils. Tubules of the transverse system are usually seen at the A-I junction, where they are apposed to elements of the sarcoplasmic reticulum, forming "triads." The T system carries the depolarization impulse from the surface of the fiber to the interior; the sarcoplasmic reticulum releases calcium ions necessary for activation of the contraction mechanism and takes up calcium again to allow relaxation.[15] The relationships of myofibrils, mitochondria, and tubules within the muscle cell are illustrated in Fig. 3-1.

SARCOLEMMA

The sarcolemma, or the membrane surrounding each muscle fiber, consists of an inner trilaminate plasma membrane, dotted by invaginations (caveolae), and an outer basement membrane about 100 nm thick.[19] A network of collagen fibers (endomysium)

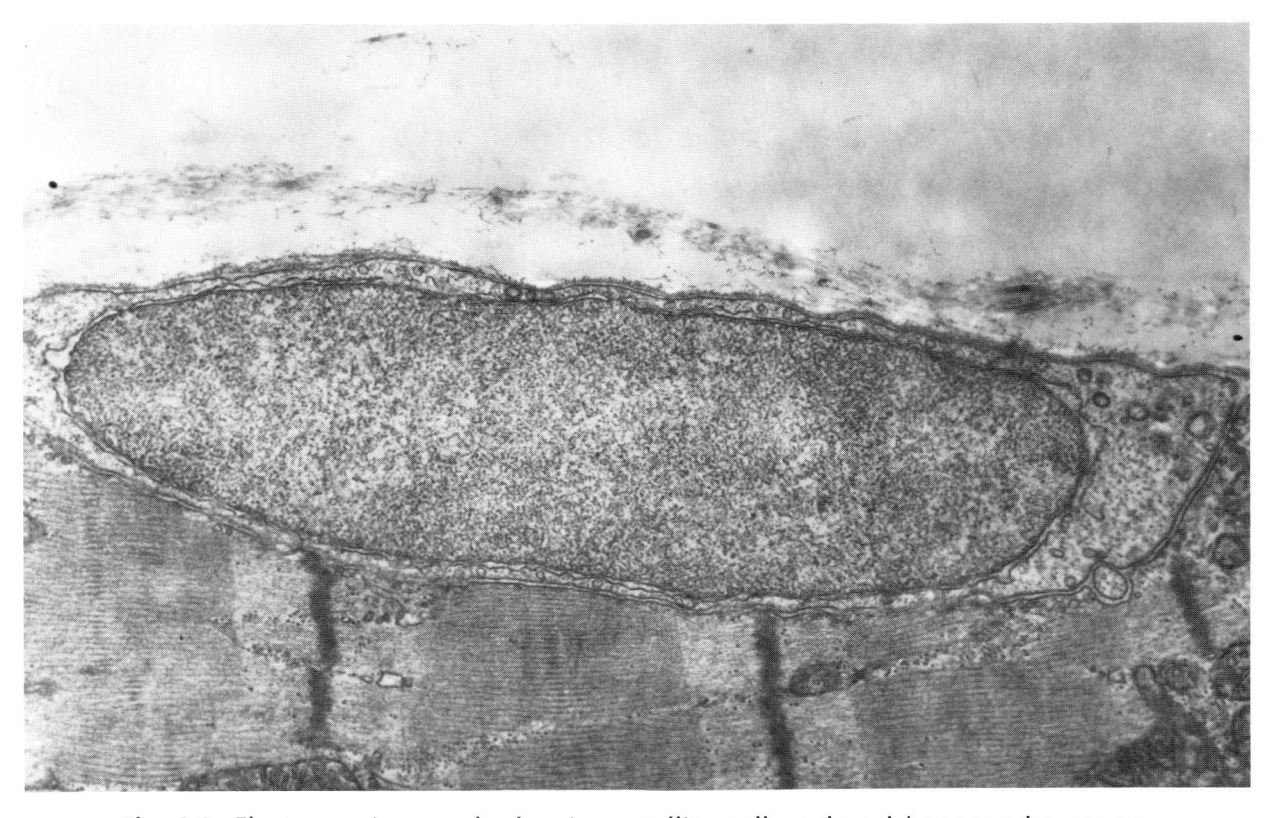

Fig. 3-2. Electron micrograph showing satellite cell enclosed between basement membrane and plasma membrane of muscle fiber. (25,000×; courtesy Dr. S. A. Shafiq, New York.)

Mechanism of facial expression and pathophysiology of degeneration

is present external to the basement membrane. Subsarcolemmal nuclei, or myonuclei, 5 to 10 μm long, are evenly spaced along the muscle fiber. Electron microscopic examination has revealed another nucleus associated with the muscle fiber, that of the satellite cell.[27,31] By definition, this cell is mononuclear, does not contain myofilaments, and lies enclosed between the basement membrane and plasma membrane of a muscle fiber (Fig. 3-2). It is fusiform, about 25 μm long and 4 μm wide, and its cytoplasm contains ribosomes, vesicles, and a few small mitochondria. Satellite cells, whose nuclei account for 4% to 10% of the nuclei of a muscle fiber, assume a possibly important and hotly debated role in muscle regeneration.

MOTOR END PLATE

At the neuromuscular junction, or motor end plate, there is an outpouching of sarcoplasm beneath the sarcolemma, containing several nuclei and many mitochondria. This sarcoplasm is indented in an synaptic trough to hold the nerve endings, and numerous secondary clefts are formed by sarcolemmal folds in this area (Fig. 3-3). This richly invaginated elevation of sarcoplasm, covered by a thickened plasma membrane, is known as the subneural apparatus. It contains cholinesterase, a feature used for the histochemical identification of neuromuscular junctions. The terminal unmyelinated

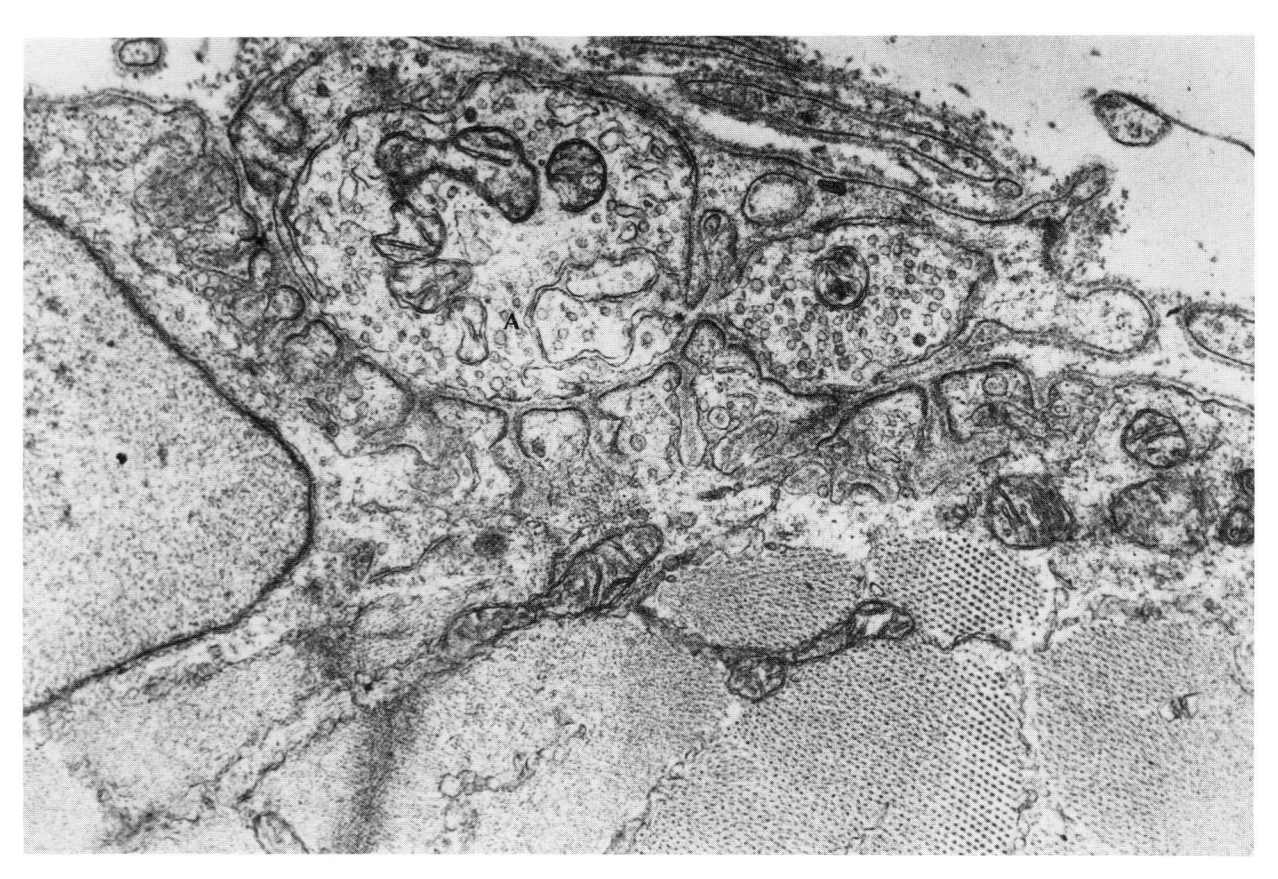

Fig. 3-3. Electron micrograph of motor end plate. The terminal axon, **A**, contains synaptic vesicles and is adjacent to the subneural apparatus with its radiating secondary synaptic clefts. (25,000×; courtesy Dr. S. A. Shafiq, New York.)

branches of the motor nerve occupy the synaptic troughs and are surrounded by a Schwann cell process that closes the top of the trough and by an external connective tissue sheath (of Henle). The narrow space between the axolemma and sarcolemma forms the synaptic cleft, which extends into the invaginated sarcolemmal folds as secondary clefts and which contains basement membrane material. The deepest parts of the synaptic clefts are connected to rows of vesicles. The nerve ending contains mitochondria, smooth reticulum, microtubules and filaments, and numerous synaptic vesicles adjacent to the axolemma.

CORRELATION OF STRUCTURE WITH FUNCTION

Each component of the muscle fiber serves its special function. The motor end plate receives the neural stimulus, generating an action potential, which is transmitted inward along the T system. Calcium ions are released from the sarcoplasmic reticulum, initiating the contractile process by changing the configuration of the proteins of the thin filaments, allowing the heads of the myosin molecules access to the actin, with activation of myosin adenosine triphosphatase (ATPase).[2b] Bonds between actin and myosin are formed, and in the process, the thin filaments are pulled toward each other, sliding between the thick filaments, thus shortening the myofibril. The sarcolemma, with its caveolae, is concerned with transport of ions, sugars, fats, and amino acids into the muscle fiber, and the transport of metabolites out of the fiber. The aqueous sarcoplasm contains the enzymes and glycogen necessary for energy production from anaerobic glycolysis, whereas the enzymes present in the mitochondria carry on the oxidative processes needed for recovery from oxygen debt and for cell metabolism.

MUSCLE SPINDLE

The muscle fibers are bound into fascicles by endomysial and perimysial connective tissue. Small arteries, veins, and nerves run between the fascicles. A rich capillary network ramifies between the fascicles, surrounding the muscle fibers. Muscle spindles are distributed throughout striated muscles, often between the fascicles, and consist of small groups of specialized fibers containing nuclear "bags" or "chains" within a connective tissue capsule. They are richly supplied with specialized sensory nerve endings, and their motor innervation is by the gamma efferent fibers that arise from small neurons in the anterior horns of the spinal cord. The spindles serve as stretch and position receptors. Encapsulated stretch and position receptors (Golgi tendon organs and Golgi-Mazzoni corpuscles) are also present at the musculotendinous junctions, and free nerve endings, which act as pain receptors, are found mainly associated with the blood vessels within muscle tissue.

FIBER TYPES

As a tissue, human striated muscle is not homogeneous but consists of a mixture of fiber types. Two main types have been distinguished histochemically: the type I fiber with high oxidative (dehydrogenase) and low glycolytic (phosphorylase) activity, and the type II fiber with relatively low oxidative and high glycolytic activity.[14] In animal studies, rough correlation between physiological and histochemical attributes has been made, although great variation among species and even among different muscles renders the enumeration and characterization of muscle fiber types extremely complex. In investigations of guinea-pig muscles, fast-twitch fibers are strongly reactive for ATPase

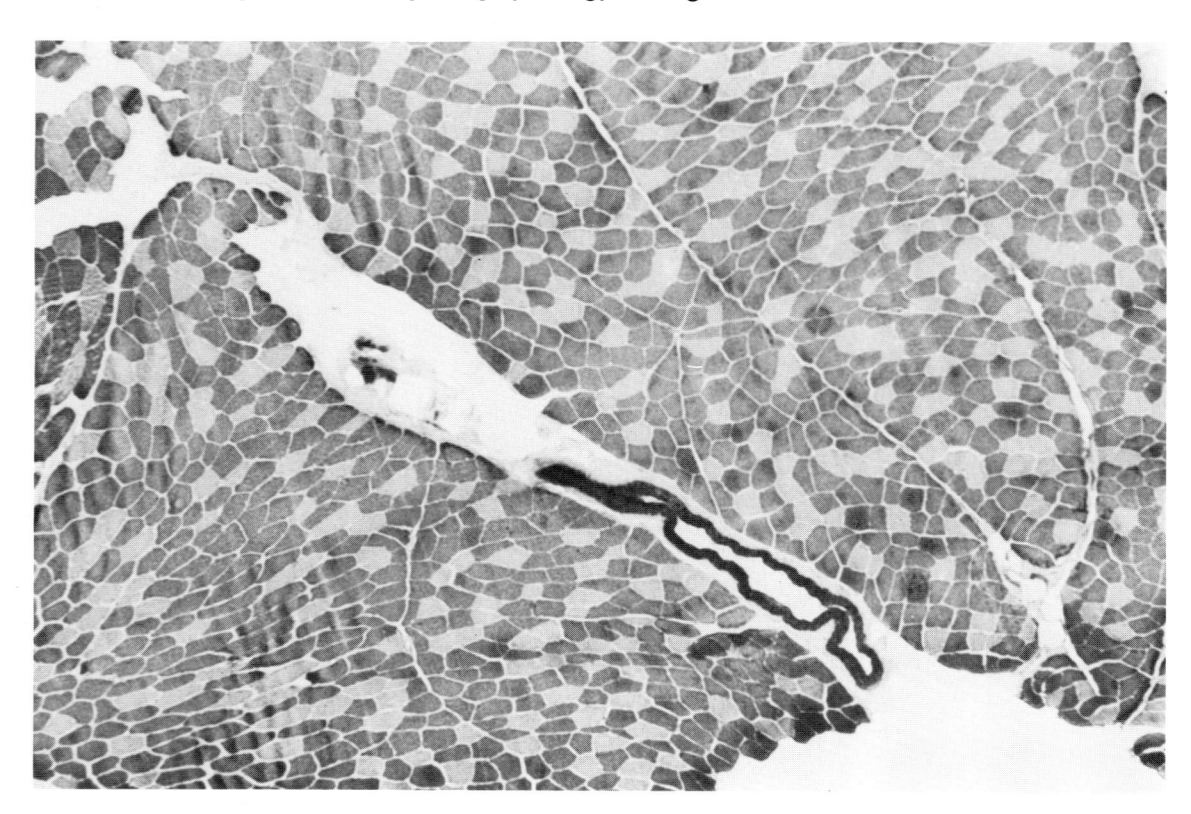

Mechanism of facial expression and pathophysiology of degeneration

Fig. 3-4. Cross section of normal human muscle stained for ATPase, showing "checkerboard" or mosaic pattern of dark (type II) and light (type I) fibers. (125×.)

and glycolytic activity but may have low or high oxidative enzyme content, whereas slow-twitch fibers react weakly for ATPase and have low or intermediate oxidative enzyme reactivity.[5,36] In human muscle, it appears likely that the type I fiber is comparable to the "slow oxidative fiber" of animal studies, and the type II fiber seems comparable to the "fast glycolytic" and "fast oxidative glycolytic" animal fibers. Human muscle stained for myosin ATPase and phosphorylase shows a checkerboard pattern of light (type I) and dark (type II) staining fibers (Fig. 3-4). Serial sections demonstrate that the type I fibers react strongly for mitochondrial oxidative enzymes (succinic dehydrogenase and reduced nicotinamide adenine dinucleotide–tetrazolium reductase) whereas the type II fibers stain lightly for these enzymes. Further studies of the ATPase-staining reactions in these fibers show that the ATPase in type I fibers stains lightly in the routine stain, done at pH 9.4, because it is alkali-labile. Preincubation at acid pH causes the ATPase of type I fibers to react strongly. Type II fibers can be divided into three subtypes on the basis of the acid lability of their myosin ATPase. Type IIA fibers are the most acid-labile, IIB are intermediate, and IIC the least susceptible to acid preincubation.[9,13]

MOTOR UNIT

A motor unit consists of the motor neuron in the anterior horn of the spinal cord, its axon, and the muscle fibers it innervates. The number of muscle fibers in a motor unit varies from as few as 10 in small muscles such as those of the eye, to several hundred, in most muscles, to as many as 1000, in deltoid and biceps.[2c] Ingenious experiments allowing mapping of motor unit fibers in histological sections (by glycogen depletion secondary to repetitive stimulation of single nerve fibers) have shown that fibers of one motor unit are of the same histochemical type and that they are not contiguous, but scattered over a limited area of the muscle section. This work confirmed inferences made from prior cross-innervation experiments regarding the homogeneity of the motor unit and provided a background for understanding of the changes occurring in denervated and reinnervated muscle.

Postdenervation changes in the muscle fiber and motor end plate

ATROPHY AND DEGENERATION

When a striated muscle fiber loses its motor innervation, whether it be caused by interruption of the axon in the peripheral nerve or nerve root, or caused by degeneration of the motor neuron in the anterior horn of the spinal cord or in the brainstem, profound changes result. There is a progressive decrease in fiber size, so that a denervated muscle may be reduced to half its original weight as early as 2 weeks after denervation.[34] Chronic denervation atrophy studies in the opossum[43] showed that after a loss of 50% of muscle weight by 60 days, the atrophy then was slower, reaching 80% by 120 days and not progressing much beyond that point. The question of whether chronically denervated muscle fibers eventually degenerate, become necrotic, and disappear, was investigated by Denny-Brown in a study of femoral nerve section in cats.[2d] By 8 months he observed not only severe atrophy of the remaining fibers, but also loss of many fibers in some areas of the denervated muscles. It was of interest that parts of the muscles (such as the lateral sartorius and the shorter head of the vastus lateralis) showed only moderately severe atrophy, without noticeable loss of fibers. In a review of this problem, Gutmann and Zelená[23] note that postdenervation degeneration occurs only to a minor degree in rat and rabbit muscle and was not observed in mouse and opossum. They conclude that postdenervation necrosis of muscle fibers does not occur in some species and that when it does occur, it is not progressive. It is of obvious importance to the surgeon attempting reinnervation procedures to know whether denervated human muscle loses significant numbers of fibers through degeneration. Bowden and Gutmann,[7] in a study of muscle changes after nerve trauma in humans, saw no degeneration of fibers until 3 years after nerve interruption. Hyalinization and fragmentation of some fibers was noted at this point. At late stages, 20 to 26 years after denervation, most fibers were fragmented, and only a very few thin fibers retaining their cross-striations were evident. It is apparent from this study and from observations on human muscle biopsies in various denervating diseases that atrophic denervated muscle fibers retain their architecture and cellular integrity for long periods. Eventual degeneration and loss of fibers takes place after several years. As atrophy occurs, fat and fibrous tissue infiltrate between muscle fascicles and later between muscle fibers. Recent observers have not confirmed an earlier impression that metaplasia of muscle fibers into fibroblasts might occur.[2e]

EARLY CELLULAR CHANGES

At a cellular level, the first noticeable change after loss of innervation occurs in the subsarcolemmal nuclei of the muscle fiber. By 2 days, these nuclei are rounded and enlarged, and in very early experimental work an increase in both number and size of these nuclei was noted.[44] This is correlated with a large increase in DNA, peaking at 14 days.[23] Electron microscopic study of this phenomenon shows chromatin changes as early as 4 hours after denervation, with rounding of the nuclei, peripheral aggregation of chromatin, and dispersal of the nucleolar substance by 24 hours.[26] By 1 to 2 weeks, the number of nuclei had increased, although mitoses were not seen, and by 3 weeks, deep infoldings of the nuclear membrane appeared. These changes reached a maximum by 3 months and then regressed. More recently it has been reported that satellite cells increase in number in denervated muscle by as early as 1 week after nerve section.[33] These were described as originating by "pinching off" of subsarcolemmal nuclei along with their adjacent sarcoplasm. By the third week, these cells showed many microtubules and polyribosomes, a little rough endoplasmic reticulum, and microfilaments. The same phenomenon has been observed in pigeon breast muscle, without observed mitosis. It has been suggested that the presence of this increased number of satellite cells in denervated muscle accounts for its enhanced ability to regenerate after transplantation and is the morphological reflection of the so-called plastic state of recently denervated muscle.

In the motor end plates, 1 week after axonal interruption, the terminal axons have fragmented and degenerated and the Schwann cell processes have retracted from the

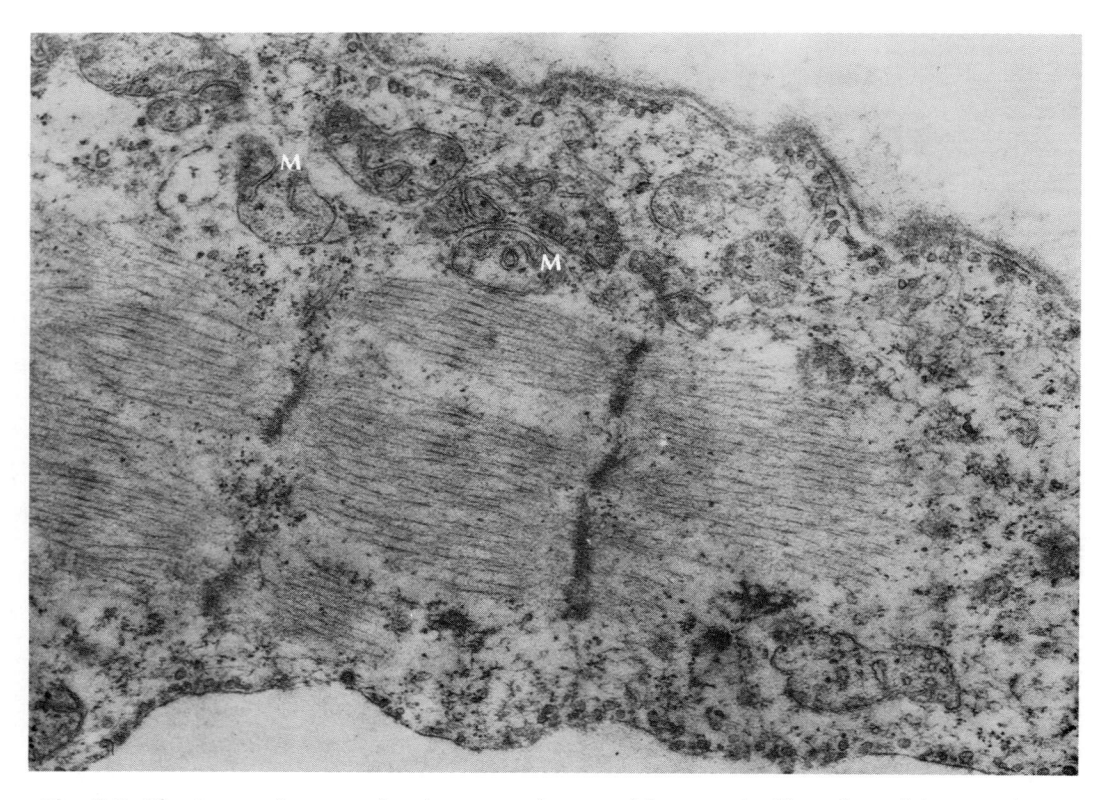

Fig. 3-5. Electron micrograph of extremely atrophic muscle fiber from biopsy of patient with motor neuron disease. (23,400×; from Adachi, M., Torii, J., Sher, J., Ratinoff, E., Aronson, S. M., and Lapovsky, A.: J. Neurol. Sci. **13**:13, 1971.)

Pathophysiology of denervation in facial neuromuscular motor unit

subneural apparatus. Flattening of the primary synaptic clefts and shortening and widening of the secondary synaptic clefts progresses over a 3-week period, and collagen appears in the shallow clefts if reinnervation does not occur.

Loss of myofilaments and eventually whole myofibrils is perhaps the most prominent feature of denervation atrophy (Fig. 3-5). In denervated rat leg muscle, a rapid autolytic process occurs at 7 to 14 days, correlated with loss of cell striations and a 50% loss of muscle weight.[34] The first change appears at the Z lines, followed by disruption of myofilaments, eventually leaving areas of the fiber with only sarcoplasm, vesicles, and mitochondria remaining. Lysosomes containing masses of lipoproteins are seen, and "waste" sarcoplasm is discarded into the intercellular space. In this study, after 2 weeks, a slower phase of atrophy began, during which myofilaments were observed to become detached from the periphery of fibrils and then to be broken down in the interfibrillary spaces. Similar extensive loss of peripheral myofilaments associated with Z line dissolution has been described in human muscle biopsies from patients suffering from diseases such as spinal muscular atrophy and amyotrophic lateral sclerosis.[4,39,41] Adachi et al.,[1] in a study of the Wohlfart-Kugelberg-Welander syndrome (a form of

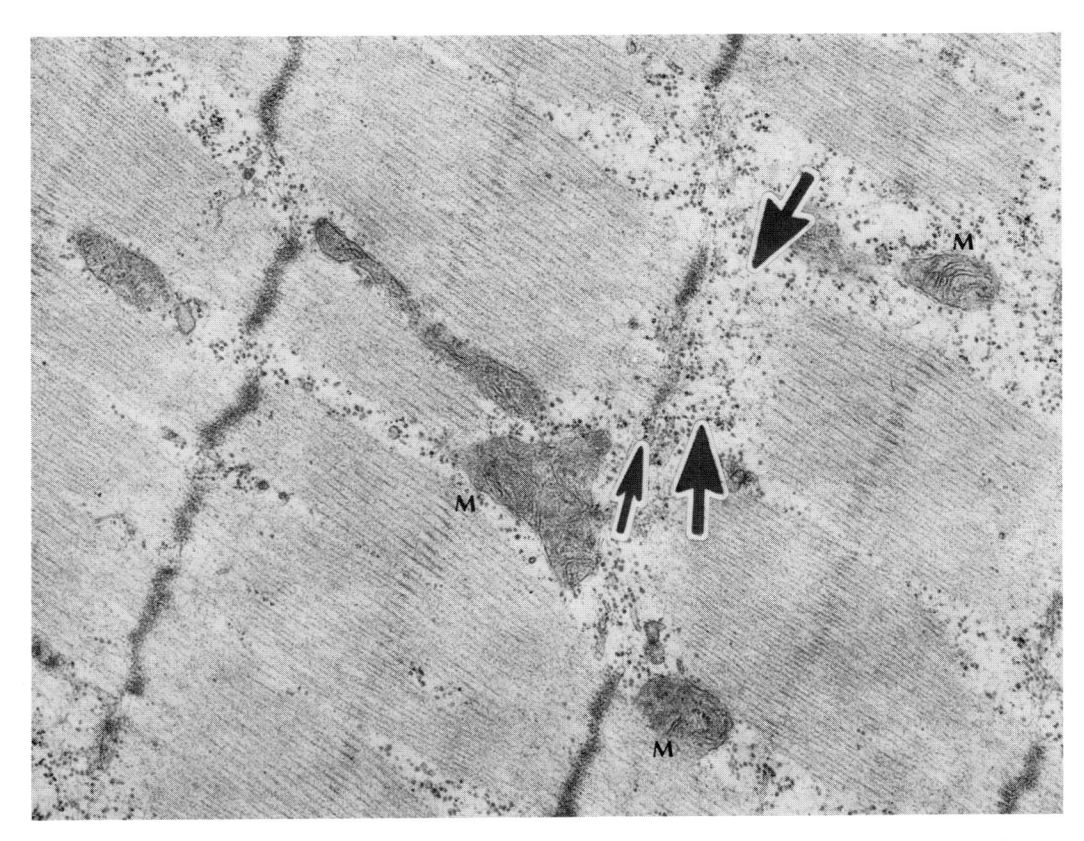

Fig. 3-6. Electron micrograph of early denervation changes in a muscle fiber, from biopsy of patient with motor neuron disease. *Arrows,* Focal dissolution of an I band and a Z line. The mitochondria, **M,** appear elongated. (30,300×; from Adachi, M., Torii, J., Sher, J., Ratinoff, E., Aronson, S. M., and Lapovsky, A.: J. Neurol. Sci. **13:** 13, 1971.)

Mechanism of facial expression and pathophysiology of degeneration

slowly progressive spinal muscular atrophy), demonstrated the earliest changes in the myofibril at the level of the I bands and postulated that this occurred prior to changes in the Z lines (Fig. 3-6).

The fate of the mitochondria of the muscle fiber after denervation has been the subject of some debate. Experimental work in the rat[34] and some observations in human muscle[39,44] showed a decrease of mitochondria in parallel with the disappearance of myofilaments, so that they appeared either decreased in number, or present in about normal concentrations. Other studies of human material[1,4] suggested that, at least in the early stages, mitochondria were actually increased in number and size. In the early stage of atrophy of frog muscle, which undergoes denervation atrophy at a slower rate than does mammalian muscle, there was a definite increase in numbers of mitochondria and in mitochondrial protein.[32] An elegant and detailed morphometric study of denervated rat leg muscle has shown definitively that there is an increase in mitochondrial volume during the first few days after denervation and then a decrease after the first week. Reorientation of the mitochondria so that their long axes became parallel with the myofibrils was also described.[16]

In both rat and frog muscle, the sarcoplasmic reticulum appeared hypertrophied after nerve section.[32,34] Morphometric analysis confirmed an increase in sarcotubular surface concentration, although the arrangement of these abundant sarcotubular components became more irregular after denervation.[16] This increase in sarcotubules has been correlated with a transient postdenervation increase in total calcium ion uptake by fragmented sarcoplasmic reticulum.[42] However, observations on human muscle have not shown this hypertrophy of sarcotubular elements in denervating diseases.[4,39,41] Abnormal aggregates of tubular structures in lamellar arrays or concentric cisternae have been described in both human and animal denervated muscle fibers and are believed by some to arise from the sarcoplasmic reticulum.[30,40,41]

Another membrane change associated with loss of innervation occurs in the sarcolemma. A dissociation of the plasma membrane from the basement membrane is observed, since the plasmalemma appears to shrink with the shrinking cell. As a result, the basement membrane is thrown into scallops or pleats around the fiber.[6,40,41]

A finding of great interest but uncertain significance in early denervation is the increase in muscle ribonucleic acid content, correlated morphologically with accumulation of ribosomes and rough endoplasmic reticulum in subsarcolemmal regions.[20] Engel and Stonnington[16] observed an increase in ribosomal particles in subsarcolemmal and perinuclear locations and between myofibrils, beginning after the first week and persisting for 6 weeks after denervation. Increased RNA content of denervated fibers has also been shown histochemically in human muscle biopsies.[35] It has been postulated that this observed increase in materials necessary for protein synthesis, happening at a time when breakdown of the contractile proteins is predominant, may be responsible for production of hydrolytic enzymes concerned in cell catabolism. An alternative interesting suggestion is that the ribosomes may be synthesizing a protein receptor substance for acetylcholine.[20] It is known that after denervation the phenomenon of sensitivity to acetylcholine spreads from its normal localization at the neuromuscular junction to involve the entire surface of the muscle fiber and that this spread of sensitivity can be prevented by blocking protein synthesis.[21,22,28] The fact that ribosomes tend to accumulate in the first few days, prior to the spread of the acetylcholine sensitivity, adds credence to this hypothesis, as does the demonstration that denervated muscle membrane binds neurotoxins that act by blocking acetylcholine receptors, outside the neuromuscular junctions.[29]

POSTDENERVATION HYPERTROPHY

Under peculiar specific circumstances, that is, in the rat hemidiaphragm and the chick anterior latissimus dorsi muscles, denervation results in transient hypertrophy of muscle fibers during the first week.[30] Under these conditions there is increased DNA and RNA content of the muscle fibers and increased myofibril synthesis.[8,30] In the case of the hemidiaphragm the denervation hypertrophy is associated with continued passive stretch of the muscle and indicates the large capability of the denervated fiber to synthesize protein. Rare instances of hypertrophy of human muscle occurring after nerve injury have been reported but never explained.[3,24]

HISTOCHEMICAL CHANGES

Postdenervation changes occur in the histochemical attributes of different muscle fiber types. In studies of phosphorylase and oxidative enzymes in both rat and pigeon

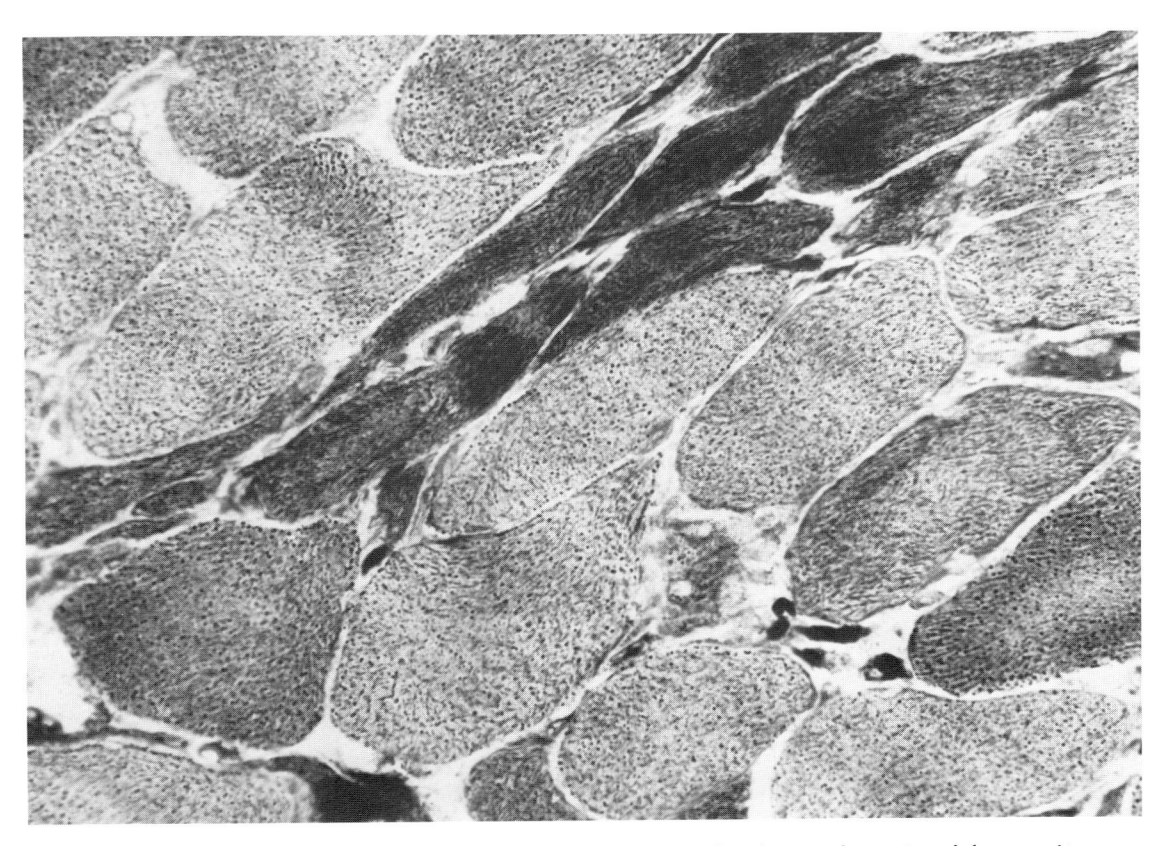

Fig. 3-7. Oblique section of partially denervated skeletal muscle stained for a mitochondrial oxidative enzyme, showing a group of angular atrophic fibers with increased staining. (400×; from Adachi, M., Torii, J., Sher, J., Ratinoff, E., Aronson, S. M., and Lapovsky, A.: J. Neurol. Sci. **13**:13, 1971.)

skeletal muscle, fibers tended to lose most quickly the enzyme activity highest in that particular fiber type, resulting in a decrease or disappearance of enzymatic differences between fiber types. Parallel biochemical studies confirmed a similar "metabolic dedifferentiation", showing, for example, greater loss of oxidative enzymes of the tricarboxylic acid cycle in type I than in type II fibers.[10,38] Loss of phosphorylase after denervation and the presence of very small fibers staining dark for all oxidative enzymes were reported in studies on totally denervated cat muscle.[17] Human muscle biopsies from patients with either motor neuron diseases or peripheral neuropathies show groups of small atrophic angular fibers that lack phosphorylase but stain intensely for mitochondrial oxidative enzymes[1,13b] (Fig. 3-7).

TARGET FIBERS

A peculiar "target fiber" change is associated with human denervation atrophy. These fibers, which are usually not atrophic, show loss of mitochondrial and ATPase staining in their centers, sometimes surrounded by a deeply stained intermediate zone. Electron microscopy shows that the center of these fibers contains clumped filaments with interspersed dense material, without mitochondria or sarcoplasmic reticulum.[44] The significance of this target fiber change is unknown; it may possibly represent a result of reinnervation rather than denervation.[12]

Conclusions

A few points gleaned from the foregoing may be useful to those attempting to apply laboratory knowledge for human benefit in the area of neuromuscular function. Muscle fibers are profoundly affected by denervation, and eventually atrophy severely, but they do not degenerate for years and are presumably capable of being reinnervated for some time. The early stages of denervation are characterized by an increase in protein-manufacturing machinery (ribosomes) and in mitochondria, sarcoplasmic reticulum, and satellite cells. These changes are associated with what has been termed a "plastic state," which allows muscle fibers at this stage to regenerate faster and to be transplanted more successfully than normally innervated muscle.

REFERENCES

1. Adachi, M., Torii, J., Sher, J., Ratinoff, E., Aronson, S. M., and Lapovsky, A.: Ultrastructural and histochemical features of skeletal muscle in the Wohlfart-Kugelberg-Welander syndrome, J. Neurol. Sci. **13:**13, 1971.
2. Adams, R. D.: Diseases of muscle, ed. 3, New York, 1975, Harper & Row, Publishers, Inc., a, pp. 9-15; b, p. 84-85; c, pp. 54; d, pp. 121-131; e, pp. 127-129.
3. Adams, R. D., Denny-Brown, D., and Pearson, C. M.: Diseases of muscle, ed. 2, New York, 1962, Harper & Brothers, p. 669.
4. Afifi, A. K., Aleu, F. P., Goodgold, J., and MacKay, B.: Ultrastructure of atrophic muscle in amyotrophic lateral sclerosis, Neurology **16:**475, 1966.
5. Barnard, J., Edgerton, V. R., Furukawa, T., and Peter, J. B.: Histochemical, biochemical, and contractile properties of red, white, and intermediate fibers, Am. J. Physiol. **220:**410, 1971.
6. Birks, R., Katz, B., and Miledi, R.: Dissociation of the surface membrane complex in atrophic muscle fibers, Nature (London) **184:**1507, 1959.
7. Bowden, R. E. M., and Gutmann, E.: Denervation and reinnervation of human voluntary muscle, Brain **67:**273, 1944.
8. Bowman, D. C., and Martin, A. W.: Nucleic acids and protein synthesis after denervation of the rat hemidiaphragm, Exp. Neurol. **33:**256, 1970.
9. Brooke, M. H., and Kaiser, K. K.: Muscle fiber types: how many and what kind? Arch. Neurol. **23:**369, 1970.

10. Cherian, K. M., Bokdawala, F. D., Vallyathan, N. V., and George, J. C.: Effect of denervation on the red and white fibers of the pectoralis muscle of the pigeon, J. Neurol. Neurosurg. Psychiatry 29:299, 1966.
11. Cohen, C.: The protein switch of muscle contraction, Sci. Am. 233:36, 1975.
12. Dubowitz, V.: Pathology of experimentally reinnervated skeletal muscle, J. Neurol. Neurosurg. Psychiatry 30:99, 1967.
13. Dubowitz, V., and Brooke, M. H.: Muscle biopsy, a modern approach, Philadelphia, 1973, W. B. Saunders Co., a, pp. 49-60; b, pp. 105-167.
14. Dubowitz, V., and Pearse, A. G. E.: A comparative histochemical study of oxidative enzyme and phosphorylase activity in skeletal muscle, Histochemie 2:105, 1960.
15. Ebashi, S., and Lipmann, F.: Adenosine triphosphate linked concentration of calcium ions in a particulate fraction of rabbit muscle, J. Cell Biol. 14:389, 1962.
16. Engel, A. G., and Stonnington, H. H.: Morphological effects of denervation of muscle. A quantitative ultrastructural study. In Drachman, D. B., editor: Trophic functions of the neuron, Ann. N.Y. Acad. Sci. 228:68-88, 1974.
17. Engel, W. K., Brooke, M. H., and Nelson, P. G.: Histochemical studies of denervated or tenotomized muscle, illustrating difficulties in relating experimental animal conditions to human neuromuscular diseases. In Bajusz, E., editor: Experimental primary myopathies and their relationship to human muscle diseases, Ann. N.Y. Acad. Sci. 138:160-185, 1966.
18. Fardeau, M.: Normal ultrastructural aspect of human motor end-plate and its pathologic modifications. In Pearson, C. M., and Mostofi, F. K., editors: The striated muscle, Baltimore, 1973, The Williams & Wilkins Co., pp. 342-363.
19. Franzini-Armstrong, C.: Membranous systems in muscle fibers. In Bourne, G. H., editor: The structure and function of muscle, ed. 2, Vol. II, New York, 1973, Academic Press, Inc., pp. 533-535.
20. Gauthier, G. F., and Dunn, R. A.: Ultrastructural and cytochemical features of mammalian skeletal muscle fibers following denervation, J. Cell. Sci. 12:525, 1973.
21. Grampp, W., Harris, J. B., and Thesleff, S.: Inhibition of denervation changes in skeletal muscle by blockers of protein synthesis, J. Physiol. 221:743, 1972.
22. Guth, L.: Trophic influences of nerve on muscle, Phys. Rev. 48(4):645, 1968.
23. Gutmann, E., and Zelená, J.: Morphological changes in denervated muscle. In Gutmann, E., editor: The denervated muscle, Prague, 1962, Publishing House of the Czechoslovak Academy of Sciences, pp. 57-102.
24. Krabbe, K. H.: The myotonia acquisita in relation to postneuritic muscular hypertrophies, Brain 57:184, 1934.
25. Huxley, H. E., and Hanson, J.: Changes in the cross-striations of muscle during contraction and stretch, and their structural interpretation, Nature (London) 173:973, 1954.
26. Lee, J. C., and Altschul, R.: Electron microscopy of the nuclei of denervated skeletal muscle, Z. Zellforsch. 61:168, 1963.
27. Mauro, A.: Satellite cell of skeletal muscle fibers, J. Biophys. Biochem. Cytol. 9:493, 1961.
28. Miledi, R.: The acetylcholine sensitivity of frog muscle fibers after complete or partial denervation, J. Physiol. 151:1, 1960.
29. Miledi, R., and Potter, L. T.: Acetylcholine receptors in muscle fibers, Nature 233:599, 1971.
30. Miledi, R., and Slater, C. R.: Electron microscopic structure of denervated skeletal muscle, Proc. Roy. Soc. Lond. (B) 174:253, 1969.
31. Muir, A. R.: The structure and distribution of satellite cells. In Mauro, A., Shafiq, S. A., and Milhorat, A. T., editors: Regeneration of striated muscle, and myogenesis, Amsterdam, 1970, Excerpta Medica Foundation (ICS 218, pp. 91-100).
32. Muscatello, U., Margreth, A., and Aloisi, M.: On the differential response of sarcoplasm and myoplasm to denervation in frog muscle, J. Cell. Biol. 27:1, 1965.
33. Ontell, M.: Effects of denervation on satellite cell population of rat striated muscle, Anat. Rec. 172:376, 1972.
34. Pellegrino, C., and Franzini, C.: An electron microscope study of denervation atrophy in red and white skeletal muscle fibers, J. Cell. Biol. 17:327, 1963.
35. Perl, D. P., Sher, J., and Aronson, S. M.: Acridine orange fluorochrome staining of RNA in atrophic and regenerating skeletal muscle, J. Neuropath. Exp. Neurol. 27:110, 1968.
36. Peter, J. B., Barnard, J., Edgerton, V. R., Gillespie, C. A., and Stempel, K. E.: Metabolic profiles of three fiber types of skeletal muscle in guinea pigs and rabbits, Biochemistry 11:2627, 1972.
37. Porter, K. R., and Palade, G. E.: Studies

of endoplasmic reticulum, J. Biophys. Biochem. Cytol. **3**(suppl.):269, 1957.
38. Romanul, F. C. A., and Hogan, E. L.: Enzymatic changes in denervated muscle. I. Histochemical studies, Arch. Neurol. **13**:263, 1965.
39. Roth, R. G., Graziani, L. J., Terry, R. D., and Scheinberg, L. C.: Muscle fine structure in the Kugelberg-Welander syndrome (chronic muscular atrophy), J. Neuropath. Exp. Neurol. **24**:444, 1965.
40. Schrodt, G. R., and Walker, S. M.: Ultrastructure of membranes in denervation atrophy, Am. J. Pathol. **49**:33, 1966.
41. Shafiq, S. A., Milhorat, A. T., and Gorycki, M. A.: Fine structure of human muscle in neurogenic atrophy, Neurology **17**:934, 1967.
42. Sreter, F. A.: Effect of denervation on fragmented sarcoplasmic reticulum of white and red muscle, J. Neuropath. Exp. Neurol. **29**:52, 1970.
43. Sunderland, S., and Ray, L. J.: Denervation changes in mammalian striated muscle, J. Neurol. Neurosurg. Psychiatry **13**:159, 1950.
44. Tower, S. S.: Atrophy and degeneration in skeletal muscle, Am. J. Anat. **56**:1, 1935.

PART II

ETIOLOGY OF DISRUPTION OF THE FACIAL NEUROMUSCULAR MOTOR UNIT

4 Congenital facial paresis (Möbius syndrome)

LEONARD R. RUBIN

There are several current etiological theories concerning the origin of congenital facial paresis. The consensus is that a hypoplasia of ectoderm as well as mesoderm exists in varying degrees. Most cases of bilateral facial paresis exhibit a loss of function of the zygomatic and buccal branches of the facial nerve. It appears that muscle and nerve deficiencies are involved. Microanatomical sections of Möbius specimens have shown that most often the seventh nerve is totally intact and that there is an extreme hypoplasia of facial muscles, which causes the expressionless face. Other specimens have demonstrated deficiency of nerve elements both in the brain and in the periphery. The term "Möbius syndrome" has been enlarged to encompass unilateral facial paresis as well as those cases where deformities of extremities are not involved but congenital facial paresis exists.

Congenital facial paresis (Möbius syndrome)

His good hand nervously crossed over his lap to clutch his fingerless left wrist. Wide-open eyes seemed to penetrate me. The deep stare was interrupted by his eyeballs rolling upwards for a quick movement, only to return. His upper lids were motionless, but the lower ones drooped to expose conjunctivae reddened from chronic inflammation. His face was blank with no movement except when, every now and then, the corners of his mouth were pulled downward and outward to expose his mandibular dentition. There were no nasolabial folds, no facial wrinkles, no facial movements—this was a vacant face. When he spoke, his words were difficult to understand. Listening intently, I recognized that he was speaking full sentences, that the words were slurred and poorly enunciated. He consistently sucked in and swallowed his ever-forming saliva.

Fourteen years old, he was a well-built, big adolescent. His mother and father, a handsome couple, looked on, making an obvious effort to avoid speaking for their child.

This young man is suffering from congenital bilateral facial diplegia, commonly known as the Möbius syndrome (Figs. 4-1 and 4-3). In this chapter the characteristics of this bizarre and tragic congenital deformity are fully described. The clinical and pathological findings are so complex that multiple conflicting theories have been put forth to explain the baffling etiology.

Present-day definition of the Möbius syndrome

It has been commonly accepted in the past that bilateral facial diplegia associated with cranial nerve palsies that have shown one or more deformities of the extremities could be classified as belonging to the Möbius syndrome. Now, however, the syndrome has been broadened to include unilateral congenital facial paresis (Fig. 4-2) and those cases that do not have extremity deformities associated with congenital facial paresis.

Historical background

Möbius[12] published his well-known series on congenital facial paralysis in the years 1888 and 1892, lending his name to this established syndrome. Von Graefe,

Etiology of disruption of the facial neuromuscular motor unit

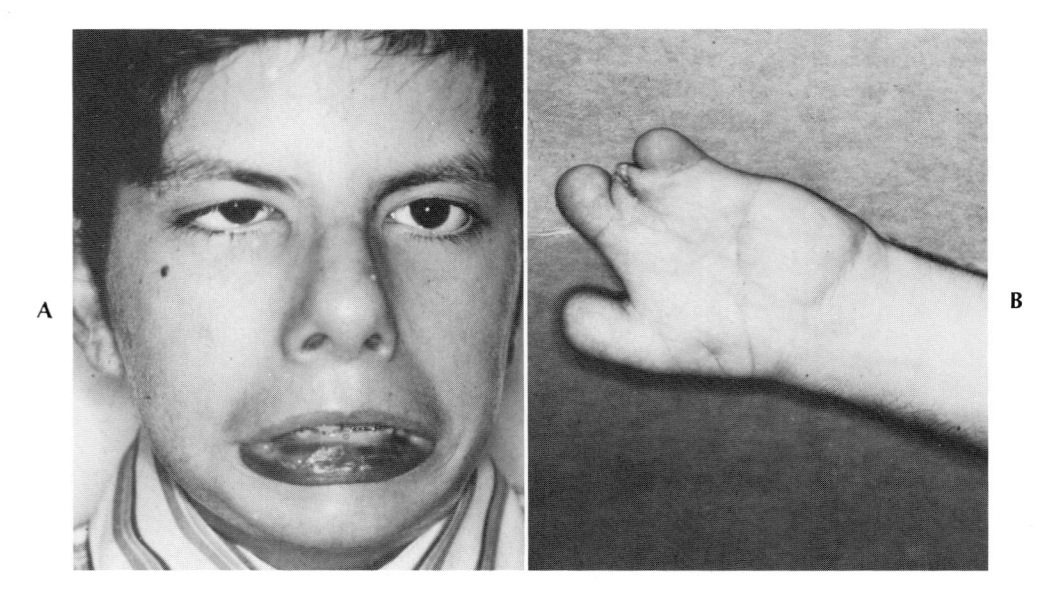

Fig. 4-1. Bilateral facial paralysis (Möbius syndrome) with malformed hand. Note the lower lip function showing the presence of good lip muscles and intact seventh nerve.

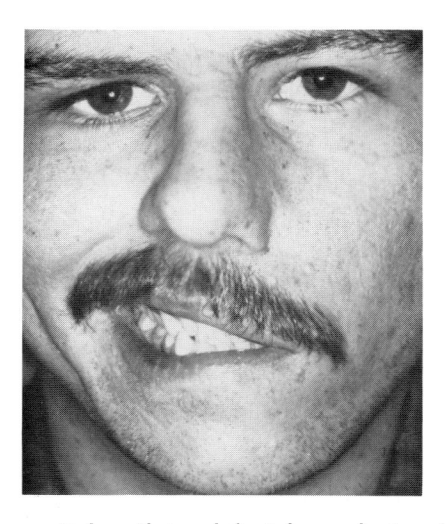

Fig. 4-2. Right-sided congenital unilateral facial paralysis with no other deformity. Weakness involved entire left side of face. Patient is shown trying to smile.

however, has been credited with reporting on congenital bilateral facial paresis in the year 1880. In 1881, Harlan[6] described a case who had a facial paralysis and difficulty with eye movements because of external rectus paresis. In 1882, Chisholm[3] reported a facial paralysis case. Möbius characterized his syndrome as one that includes congenital bilateral diplegia, limitation of eye movements, notably difficulty in the lateral gaze, cranial nerve defects, and deformities of the extremities. A number of authors have since reported small series of cases describing the condition and broadening the range of accepting deformities to be included under the name "Möbius syndrome." The extensive review of previously published cases by Henderson[7] in 1939 helped to

Congenital facial paresis (Möbius syndrome)

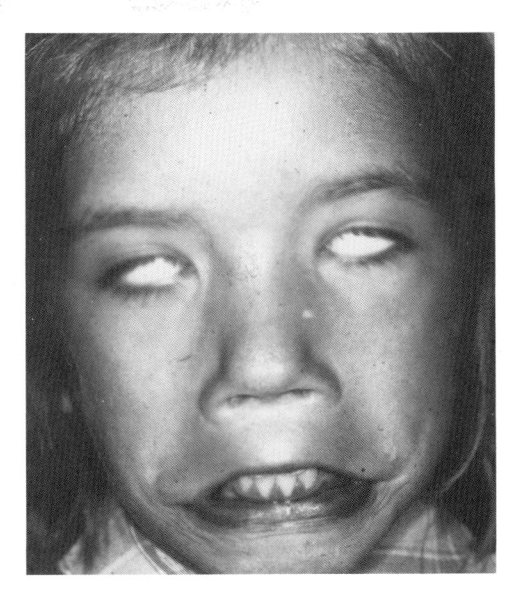

Fig. 4-3. Congenital bilateral facial paralysis with paresis of upper portion of face but normal lower lip function.

familiarize the public with the condition and brought to the foreground the controversy concerning the etiology of the disease. In 1967 I[17] reported a definitive surgical treatment for the relief of this bilateral facial paralysis.

Clinical characteristics

Approximately 150 cases of the Möbius syndrome have been described by various authors in the past 100 years. I am contributing nine additional cases. It is most likely that only several hundred victims of this rare disease exist at any one given time.

The facial paralysis can be accompanied by various associated disorders. The deformities are complex, multiple, and, at times, seemingly unrelated:

1. Facial paresis of the entire, or segments, of the face. Most often, the lower lips and the necks are normal.
2. Nerve palsies of the third, fourth, sixth, seventh, ninth, tenth, and twelfth nerves. On rare occasions, some weakness of the fifth nerve has been reported, although the reports may be considered inaccurate.
3. Deformities of the chest wall, including the pectoral girdle.
4. Deformities of the upper extremity, involving the arm, forearm, and hand.
5. Deformities of the lower extremity, involving the legs, ankles, and feet.

FACIAL NERVE AND MUSCLE INVOLVEMENT

The one constant factor in describing the "Möbius face" is the masklike expression that never varies except for lower lip movements, in some cases, when the patient attempts to speak. This created a grimace in most of our cases. None of our cases could close their lower eyelids. Many had constant epiphora. The exposed conjunctivae at the lower eyelids were reddened from irritation. Although none of our patients drooled, they constantly attempted to suck in the excess saliva that accumulated in the lower

Etiology of disruption of the facial neuromuscular motor unit

buccal sulcus. In contrast to our seven cases with actively contracting lower lips, observations made by Henderson in analyzing 61 cases of the Möbius syndrome reported by numerous authors before 1938 described 19 cases of total paralysis of the entire face including the lower lip. In 13 cases the lower lips were free of paralysis, and in nine one side or the other of the lower lips was involved. As in all of our patients, his 61 suffered paresis of the forehead, eyelids, and the maxillary regions. In the series of nine cases reported by Evans, four showed unilateral facial involvement whereas the other five had varying degrees of bilateral paresis. Richards reported three cases where the upper parts of the face showed paresis and the lower portions were normal or partially normal.

Total electrical stimulation was completed in only four of our nine cases. The four, tested extensively, showed various activities of the facial nerve at the trunk but no activity of the forehead, upper face, or upper lip. Stimulation elicited contraction of the lower lips and of the risorius muscles. Henderson related that of his 61 reported cases, 23 were tested. His report that he found no qualitative changes, only diminished reaction in the facial muscles, must be considered inaccurate. We recorded normal electromyography in the muscles of the lower lip. Those in the upper portions of the face showed no muscular galvanic reaction. Our one case of total paresis showed no reaction anywhere in the face.

OCULAR INVOLVEMENT

Eight of our nine cases showed no disturbances of the sixth nerve. Only one was free of any ocular disease. This was consistent with Henderson's finding that 31 cases out of 61 showed various signs of eye afflictions. None of our cases had ptosis. In six of Henderson's cases the third nerve was involved, causing not only ptosis but medial and inferior rectus disturbances.

LINGUAL NERVE INVOLVEMENT

Henderson reported 18 cases of tongue weakness in varying degrees. None of our cases had tongue involvement.

TRIGEMINAL NERVE INVOLVEMENT

None of our cases showed disturbances of the trigeminal nerve. Henderson reported four cases showing some weakness. We doubt the accuracy of this report because the description of the weakness seemed to be rather inconsistent with the rest of the problems.

SOFT-PALATE PARESIS

Four of our cases showed weakness of the soft palate and the fauces, resulting in poor speech. None had dysphagia. This contrasts to Henderson's four palate and six dysphagia cases. The palates showed poor elevation and failed to meet the posterior pharyngeal wall. Passavant's cushion formation was absent on the posterior pharyngeal wall of all our patients.

Congenital facial paresis (Möbius syndrome)

MANDIBLE DEFORMITIES

Many authors have described patients with mandibular deformities, most micrognathia. Only one of our cases showed any mandibular deformity. This patient's occlusion was pathological, with a projecting maxilla and a moderate crossbite.

MALFORMATION OF THE EXTREMITIES

The defects of the extremities have been varied and multiple. They include complete and partial absence of the limbs, which reveals defects of ectoderm and mesoderm.

1. Pectoral girdle
   a. Defects such as absence of scapula and its muscles
   b. Absence of mammae
2. Upper extremity
   a. Absence of deltoid
   b. Absence of radius
   c. Elbow joint deformities
   d. Ankylosis of finger and wrist joints
   e. Absence of fingers
   f. Syndactyly of fingers
   g. Microdactylia of fingers
3. Lower extremities
   a. Absence of limbs below the knees
   b. Hypoplasia of thigh muscles
   c. Ankylosis of ankle and interphalangeal joints
   d. Clubfoot deformities
   e. Equinovarus
   f. Absence of phalanges and toes
   g. Absence of portions of feet

Two of the eight cases had deformities of the extremities. One case had ankylosis of the wrist with absent fingers. The remaining hand was greatly underdeveloped. One boy had both legs and feet missing, distal to the upper third of the legs. In Henderson's series of 61 cases, 19 patients had clubfeet, with 16 being bilateral. Thirteen had hands affected in various degrees. Henderson reported eight cases with pectoral mammary hypoplasia.

ASSOCIATED DEFORMITIES

Cases have been reported with hypertelorism, ear deformities, and deafness.

MENTAL DEFECTS

Only one of our cases was a clear-cut mental defective. All the others were normal. At first glance, these children appeared to have diminished intelligence. The appearances, however, were indeed deceiving. With careful investigation, most demonstrated normal intelligence, with one or two having somewhat lower intelligence quotients. The multiple deformities plus poor speech and vacant facies of these patients required diligent testing for the proper evaluation of their intelligence.

Etiology of disruption of the facial neuromuscular motor unit
Discussions on etiological factors causing defects in Möbius syndrome

I have not received the opportunity to perform an autopsy on any Möbius case. The confusing picture of multiple congenital deformities has led to extensive speculation as to their cause. Two theories have evolved, each with its adherents:

1. A mesodermic defect, resulting in a primary aplasia of the muscles, with the muscle anlage being deficient and causing secondary nerve atrophy.
2. An ectodermal defect being primarily located in the brain, involving the nuclei, the brainstem, and the peripheral nerves with secondary muscle dysplasia.

Möbius believed that the disease was a degeneration of the brainstem with secondary degeneration of the muscles and other tissues. He believed that the cause was probably toxic in nature.

Heubner examined the brain and spinal cord of a patient with the Möbius syndrome. The nuclei of the sixth, seventh, and twelfth cranial nerves were abnormal, with lesser abnormalities being found in the third and eleventh cranial nerves. The ganglion cells were absent in each sixth nucleus. The rest of the nerves were lacking or degenerated. The entire lower part of the medulla was underdeveloped.

Rainy and Fowler[16] examined the entire neuromuscular unit of the seventh nerve. They found atrophy of the facial muscles. The seventh nerve trunk and the nuclei were also degenerated. They found a few fragments of muscle, which they believed to be normal, histologically. Entire muscle bundles, however, were missing.

Spatz and Ullrich[19] found histological changes in the nuclei of the third, fourth, sixth, and seventh nerves, with the sixth being most affected. These authors supported the view that nuclear hypoplasia accounted for the cranial nerve palsies in the Möbius syndrome with secondary mesodermic changes.

A better understanding of the pathological condition in the Möbius syndrome has been presented by Pitner et al.,[13] who were fortunate in being able to completely section a month-old child who had died from bronchial pneumonia. The patient had suffered from a primary syndrome of bilateral facial paralysis. By shedding light on the pathological microanalysis of the facial nerve, facial muscles, and brain, they have clarified some of the confusing findings. Their conclusions are summarized as follows:

1. The patient had aspiration bronchial pneumonia. Except for the brain, face, and palate, none of the patient's organs were abnormal.
2. A relative increase in the subcutaneous fat and almost total absence of the facial muscles were found. Some muscle fibers were in the orbicularis, buccinator, and zygomaticus. A hemiatrophy of the tongue was discovered. The myofibers of the facial muscles were greatly decreased in number and size. Adipose replacement of the muscle was severe, with moderate fibrosis. *Nerve fibers were present in the identifiable muscles.* The changes were believed to be a primary failure of formation of the involved muscles rather than changes secondary to neuronal dysplasia.
3. The left olivary prominence of the brainstem was missing, and there was a moderate hypoplasia of the right cerebellar hemisphere, the ansiform lobule, and the biventer. All cranial nerves on gross inspection appeared normal. The gross findings were congenital hypoplasia of the cerebellum and facial musculatures. Microscopic examination showed numerous neurons in multiple areas under-

going eosinophilic (anoxic) necrosis, particularly in the frontal gyri and the hippocampal gyri. The neurons of the right dentate nucleus were greatly reduced in number. The left inferior olivary nucleus was absent on the left side, with moderate decrease in the prominence of the restiform body on the right and pronounced hypoplasia of various portions in the pontine and mesencephalic sections. All cranial nerve nuclei appeared to be well preserved. *The facial nuclei were of equal size, and the neurons were normal.*

The final microscopic neuropathological diagnosis was congenital cerebellar hypoplasia with associated changes in the midline cerebellar nuclei, pons, and olives.

All previous discussions of the etiology have evolved from two theories:
1. Was the disorder primarily degenerative?
2. Was it aplastic?

Concerning the latter, the question has been asked whether a primary defect of the brainstem existed with secondary mesodermal changes, *or* did we have a primary muscular defect with secondary changes, causing neurological deficiencies.

The clinical courses after birth show no continuous degeneration taking place. Despite their writings, Möbius, Rainy, and Fowler have presented no evidence to further their hypothesis that degeneration is a primary cause. It is difficult to prove the accuracy of their theory that the brainstem is involved first, causing secondary muscular changes, or that the reverse is true. Many authors, like Lennon, have used the fact that muscular skeletal defects are absent as evidence of the mesodermal primary dysplasia; others have advocated that the syndrome is attributable to primary developmental defects in the brainstem as evidence. Pitner et al. have held that their evidence in the one case that they dissected points definitely to the Möbius syndrome as being caused by a primary dysplasia of the facial muscles. They believe, however, that there is sufficient proof in other cases to show that brain defects are the primary culprit. They conclude that more than one cause may be present in this syndrome. With the incomplete state of knowledge of how nervous structures and their peripheral fields are related during the development of the embryo, no conclusions at present can be made on a primary etiology.

Summary

The Möbius syndrome can be defined as a bilateral facial dysplasia with associated cranial nerve palsies accompanied by one or more deformities of the extremities. Variations can include unilateral congenital facial paresis and can occur in those who do not have extremity deformities.

The etiology has been most complex to understand. The present consensus is that there are two basic defects responsible. One is an ectodermal dysplasia of the midbrain with secondary mesodermal defects, whereas a second is primary mesodermal dysplasia, which accounts for the neurological findings. It appears that both explanations are correct and the defects probably exist side by side. The basic cause is still unknown and may depend on environmental influences during the development of the fetus. The culprits may be infections, bacteria or viruses, effects of drugs, alcohol, cigarette smoking, or poor placental placement. There also is a possibility that built-in hormonotrophic influences may have gone astray in triggering ectodermal and mesodermal maldevelopment.

Etiology of disruption of the facial neuromuscular motor unit

REFERENCES

1. Andersen, J. G.: Surgical treatment of lagophthalmos in leprosy by the Gillies temporalis transfer, Br. J. Plastic Surg. **14:**339-345, 1961.
2. Bedrossian, E. H.: The Möbius syndrome, Arch. Ophthalmol. **54:**137, 1955.
3. Chisolm, J. J.: Congenital paralysis of the sixth and seventh cranial nerves in an adult, Arch. Ophthalmol. **11:**332, 1882.
4. Evans, P. R.: Nuclear agenesis: Möbius' syndrome; congenital facial diplegia syndrome, Arch. Dis. Child. **30:**237-242, 1955.
5. Gillies, H. D.: Experiences with fascia lata grafts in operative treatment of facial paralysis, Proc. Roy. Soc. Med. **27:**1372-1378, 1934.
6. Harlan, G. C.: Congenital paralysis of both abducens and facial nerves, Trans. Am. Ophthalmol. Soc. **3:**216-218, 1881.
7. Henderson, J. L.: Congenital facial diplegia—clinical features, pathology and etiology, Brain **62:**381-403, 1939.
8. Heubner, O.: Ueber angeborenen Kernmangel (infantiler Kernschwund Moebius), Charité Am., **25:**211-243, 1900.
9. Kirby, D. B.: Congenital oculo-facial paralysis, Arch. Ophthalmol. **52:**452-459, 1923.
10. Lennon, M. B.: Congenital defects of the muscles of the face and eyes. Report of 3 cases of Möbius, Calif. State J. Med. **8:**115-117, 1910.
11. McLaughlin, C. R.: Surgical support in permanent facial paralysis, J. Plastic Reconstr. Surg. **11:**203-214, 1953.
12. Möbius, P. J.: Ueber angeborene doppelseitige Abducens facialis Lahmung, Munch. Med. Wochenschr. **39:**17-21, 41-43, 55-58, 1892.
13. Pitner, S. E., Edwards, J. E., and McCormick, W. F.: Observations on the pathology of the Moebius syndrome, J. Neurol. Neurosurg. Psychiatry **28:**362-374, 1965.
14. Richards, R. N.: The Möbius syndrome, J. Bone Joint Surg. **35-A:**437-444, 1953.
15. Richter, R. B.: Unilateral congenital hypoplasia of facial nucleus, J. Neuropathol. Exp. Neurol. **19:**33-41, 1960.
16. Rainy, H., and Fowler, J. S.: Congenital facial diplegia due to nuclear lesion, Rev. Neurol. Psychiatry **1:**149-155, 1903.
17. Rubin, L. R.: Congenital bilateral facial paralysis; surgical animation of the face, Transactions of the Fourth International Congress on Plastic and Reconstructive Surgery, Amsterdam, 1969, Excerpta Medical Foundation, pp. 740-746.
18. Rubin, L. R.: The anatomy of a smile: its importance in the treatment of facial paralysis, Plastic Reconstr. Surg. **53**(4):384-387, 1974.
19. Spatz, H., and Ullrich, O.: Klinischer und anatomischer Beitrag zu den angeborenen Beweglichkeits-defeckten im Hinnervenbereich, Z. Kinderheilkd. **51:**579-597, 1931.
20. Sprofkin, B. E., and Hillman, J. W.: Moebius's syndrome—congenital oculofacial paralysis, Neurology **6:**50-54, 1956.
21. Ullrich, O.: Turner's syndrome and status Bonnevie-Ullrich, Am. J. Hum. Genet. **1:**179-202, 1949.
22. Yasuna, J. M., and Schlezinger, N. S.: Congenital bilateral abducens facial paralysis (Möbius syndrome), Arch. Ophthalmol. **54:**137-139, 1955.

5 Medical causes of facial paresis including Bell's palsy

SYDNEY LOUIS

There are numerous medical causes for facial palsy, including Bell's palsy. Bell's palsy still remains an enigma. To this day, no etiological factors have been identified consistently. However, the overwhelming impression is that the susceptible patient has a swollen nerve associated with compression in the epineurium or in a congenitally small or narrow facial bony canal, leading to a loss of nerve conduction when afflicted with a virus.

Paralysis, or palsy, of one side of the face can be divided into two major categories. The first occurs with damage above the lower motor neuron, and the second involves the lower motor neuron and its distal termination upon the facial musculature. Supranuclear palsy is easily recognized, as the frontalis muscle of the forehead is spared from paralysis by virtue of its nucleus having bilateral innervation from both cerebral hemispheres. Such palsies are quite often inconsistent and may affect either voluntary or mimetic movements, or sometimes both. The causes of supranuclear facial palsy are protean. In most such syndromes the facial involvement is the least part of the patient's problem when associated with the accompanying corticospinal deficits of hemiplegia or dysphasia, or both.

Palsies caused by damage of the lower motor neuron are easily recognized in that they usually involve the entire face to all types of movement, voluntary or mimetic. Nuclear lesions are usually recognized by the concurrent involvement of adjacent brainstem structures, particularly the abducent and trigeminal nerves, as well as long tracts, motor, sensory, or sympathetic. The part of the nerve most commonly damaged appears to lie within the facial canal and at each end of the canal.

The etiology of facial palsy is complex and in many senses uncertain. Perhaps the largest etiological category is Bell's palsy, also called "idiopathic facial palsy" in the European literature. This entity cannot, however, be defined etiologically or even diagnosed by exclusion of other etiologies. It is, however, easily recognized by its clinical presentation, that is, the relatively rapid onset of an isolated facial palsy unilaterally, involving the lower motor neuron and affecting the forehead, orbicularis oculi, the muscles about the mouth, and the platysma. Paralysis of the ipsilateral digastric muscle, defect of taste sense on the ipsilateral anterior two thirds of the tongue, and hyperacusis as a result of damage to the nerve to the stapedius muscles, may or may not occur. The remaining neurological examination is normal. Modest pain in or about the ear or side of the face may or may not be present for a few days before and during early stages of onset of palsy. The key features are therefore an isolated paresis or paralysis of one complete side of the face of relatively rapid onset.

The etiology of Bell's palsy is still almost as obscure as when Bell described it in 1821[1] and attributed it to a "rheumatic" cause. To this point no etiologic factors have been identified consistently. Pathological material is quite rare and only 10 autopsied cases are available, with death in each having occurred from an incidental cause some weeks or months after Bell's palsy. No consistent changes have been seen in this pathological material. Inflammation seen in a few patients may have been attributable to unrecognized herpes zoster. In two patients with hemorrhages in the canal, or in the nerve, hypertension was present. In one case degenerative changes were seen. In studies at the time of surgical decompression, the overwhelming impression is of swollen nerve, associated with compression in epineurium or in a congenitally small or narrow facial bony canal, usually close to the stylomastoid foramen. Inflammatory changes have been rare and poorly documented. When the variability of the time of surgery after onset and the general lack of experience of normal facial nerve appearance are considered, it becomes clear that great care has to be exercised in interpreting these results.

At a strictly clinical level the only factor raised with any consistency is exposure to cold, to draughts, or to sudden temperature changes. It is hard to interpret these observations; they are uncontrolled and statistically unreliable; animal experiments to test the role of cold have been inconclusive.

Mononeuritis involving almost any of the cranial nerves may occur in patients with diabetes. Certainly facial palsy does happen in diabetic patients, but the precise statistical correlation has been quite varied in a groups of sufferers from Bell's palsy because of the variable diagnostic categories used in the proof of a diagnosis of diabetes, prediabetes, chemical diabetes, etc.[5]

Hypertension has been found associated with Bell's palsy in 8% to 36% of patients, in large part related to the age of the sample. Of most interest, however, is the report of Lloyd, Jewitt, and Still,[6] who found that 20% of children with severe hypertension in a children's hospital had a facial palsy. It has been suggested that its occurrence is related to the severity of the hypertension and that the palsy results from hemorrhage into the facial canal or nerve.

The etiology of lower motor neuron facial palsy other than Bell's palsy includes the five following groups.

1. Infections
    a. *Geniculate herpes zoster (cephalic herpes, or Ramsay Hunt syndrome)*. The distribution of weakness and the degree of the facial paralysis in geniculate herpes zoster are indistinguishable from that of Bell's palsy.[8] Distinctive, however, may be the severity and duration of pain in the side of the neck or ear areas preceding the onset of paralysis. Pain may be present for periods of 2 to 10 days before weakness or vesicles appear. Vesicles often appear in the

external auditory canal or on the earlobe itself, in the so-called sensory field of the seventh nerve. Antibodies to herpes zoster are found in blood in the majority of such patients. The prognosis of geniculate herpes zoster is not different from that of Bell's palsy.
   b. *Other viral disorders.* Facial paralysis of one side of the face of lower motor neuron type can occur in anterior poliomyelitis though this cause is quite rare today. There have been some suggestions that facial palsy may occur in association with infectious mononucleosis though the frequency of this cause in groups of patients with facial palsy is low. Facial palsy, albeit bilateral, is found fairly commonly in patients with Guillain-Barré syndrome. This is usually associated with many other features of the disorder and therefore rarely constitutes a problem in diagnosis. The possible role of herpes simplex and other viruses in the etiology of facial paralysis have not been satisfactorily defined.
   c. *Chronic granulomatous infections.* Facial paralysis occurs commonly with sarcoidosis of the nervous system. It is commonly bilateral but may occur on one side prior to the other.
   d. *Association with ear infections.* In the preantibiotic era this association was found more commonly than it is presently. The facial nerve runs superomedially in proximity to the middle ear and may be involved transiently in acute otitis media. It is more frequently involved with chronic otitis media. Miehlke[7] has suggested that facial palsy in association with chronic middle ear infection strongly suggests the presence of cholesteatoma.
   e. *Dural inflammation.* Facial palsy alone or with dysfunction of other cranial nerves is often seen in patients after contracting infectious meningitis and is believed to be caused by dural inflammation.
2. *Traumatic facial palsy.* Lower motor neuron facial paralysis has resulted from head injury, especially injuries in which the petrous or temporal bones are fractured. The facial paralysis in such closed head injuries may be immediate or delayed. Figures as high as 38.5% to 46% have been recorded in patients with closed head injuries who have fractured the petrous or temporal bones. The percentage of such patients showing recovery is not essentially different from that of Bell's palsy. Surgery, either operations on the middle ear or more rarely operations on the parotid gland, has produced facial paralysis, fortunately infrequently.
3. *Congenital facial paralysis.* Facial paralysis appearing at birth is usually said to result from compression of the facial nerve by forceps. Other explanations for this phenomenon have related to compression of the facial nerve by the birth canal, according to the fetal head presentation.
4. *Möbius syndrome.* Möbius syndrome is a rare entity in which facial paralysis is present bilaterally, from birth, often associated with paralysis of the external rectus muscles on the two sides. More rarely associated congenital anomalies, including mental defect, may occur. The entity has been found in some instances to be attributable to agenesis of the cranial nerve nuclei. Other instances have been found in which the muscles of the face have been absent because of either a primary agenesis of muscle or because of a progressive early facial myopathy.

5. *Melkersson-Rosenthal syndrome.* This rare and poorly understood syndrome is characterized by recurrent lower motor neuron facial paralysis, in no way different from Bell's palsy. This is associated with two other features—lingua plicata and swelling of the face, particularly of the upper lip. The swelling of the face is initially transient and recurrent but may ultimately become permanent. The etiology is obscure; it has been suggested to be congenital and perhaps inherited though inflammatory and allergic theses have also been advanced. Disorders of the autonomic nervous system have been suggested as another cause, possibly because of its frequent association with migraine. Reports that steroids are effective in both the paralytic phase and against the edema may strengthen the notion of an immune basis.

REFERENCES

1. Bell, C.: On the nerves of the face, Trans. Roy. Soc. London (Philosophical) **3:**398, 1821.
2. Fisch, U., and Esslen, E.: Total intratemporal exposure of the facial nerve: pathological findings in Bell's palsy, Arch. Otolaryngol. **95:** 400, 1972.
3. Hamstein, O. P.: Melkersson-Rosenthal syndrome. In Vinken, P. J., and Bruyn, G. W., editors: Handbook of clinical neurology, Amsterdam, 1970, North Holland Publishing Co., vol. 8, pp. 205-240.
4. Karnes, W. E.: Diseases of the seventh cranial nerve. In Dyck, P. J., Thomas, P. K., and Lambert, E. H., editors: Peripheral neuropathy, Philadelphia, 1975, W. B. Saunders Co., vol. 1, pp. 570-603.
5. Korczyn, A. D.: Bell's palsy and diabetes mellitus, Lancet **1:**108, 1971.
6. Lloyd, A. V. C., Jewitt, D. E., and Still, J. D. L.: Facial paralysis in children with hypertension, Arch. Dis. Child. **42:**292, 1966.
7. Miehlke, A.: Die Chirurgie des Nervus facialis Munich, 1960, Urban & Schwarzenberg, Verlag.
8. Tomita, H., Hayakawa, W., and Honda, R.: Varicella-zoster virus in idiopathic facial palsy, Arch Otolaryngol. **95:**364-368 1972.
9. Zülch, K. J.: "Idiopathic" facial paresis. In Vinken, P. J., and Bruyn, G. W., editors: Handbook of clinical neurology, Amsterdam, 1970, North Holland Publishing Co., vol. 8, pp. 241-302.

6 Surgical causes of facial paresis in the cranium

LEONARD MALIS

Described here are the common causes of facial nerve disruption in the cranium. The acoustic nerve tumor so closely associated anatomically with the seventh nerve is the most common cause of unilateral facial paresis.

The neurosurgeon has been in the unfortunate situation that the surgical treatment of neoplasms of the cerebellopontine angle has been one of the major causes of facial palsy. The most common tumor of the area is the acoustic neuroma, with angle meningioma, jugular foramen neuroma (originating from the ninth, tenth, or eleventh nerves), fifth nerve neuromas, and epidermoid tumors, occurring in decreasing order of incidence. An occasional pontine glioma may extend into the angle and cause facial nerve problems.

The cerebellopontine angle normally contains the somewhat kite-shaped pontocerebellar cistern and is bounded in an oblique anterosuperior lateral plane by the tentorium, in an anteroinferior lateral plane by the petrous pyramid and medially by the cerebellum, pons, and medula, which fill its concavity. The ninth, tenth, and eleventh nerves cross laterally from the medulla to exit in the jugular foramen. The seventh and eighth nerves traverse the cistern anterior to the flocculus from the junction of the medulla and pons to exit through the internal auditory meatus. The critically important anteroinferior cerebellar artery originates from the basilar artery, crosses inferior to the sixth nerve, and appears in the pontocerebellar cistern anteriorly to the ninth nerve and then frequently has a loop around the seventh and eighth nerves before it returns to give the vital supply to the brainstem. More anteriorly, the fifth nerve traverses the apex of the cistern from its pontine origin in relation to the superior cerebellar artery and exits through the entrance to Meckel's cave.

Acoustic neuromas, if seen at a time early enough so that their origin can be determined, nearly always arise from the superior vestibular nerve in the internal auditory canal (Fig. 6-1, *A*). They usually enlarge slowly, though their rate of growth is extremely variable despite essentially the same pathologic appearance for both slowly growing and rapidly growing tumors. Hearing deficit (most often characteristically

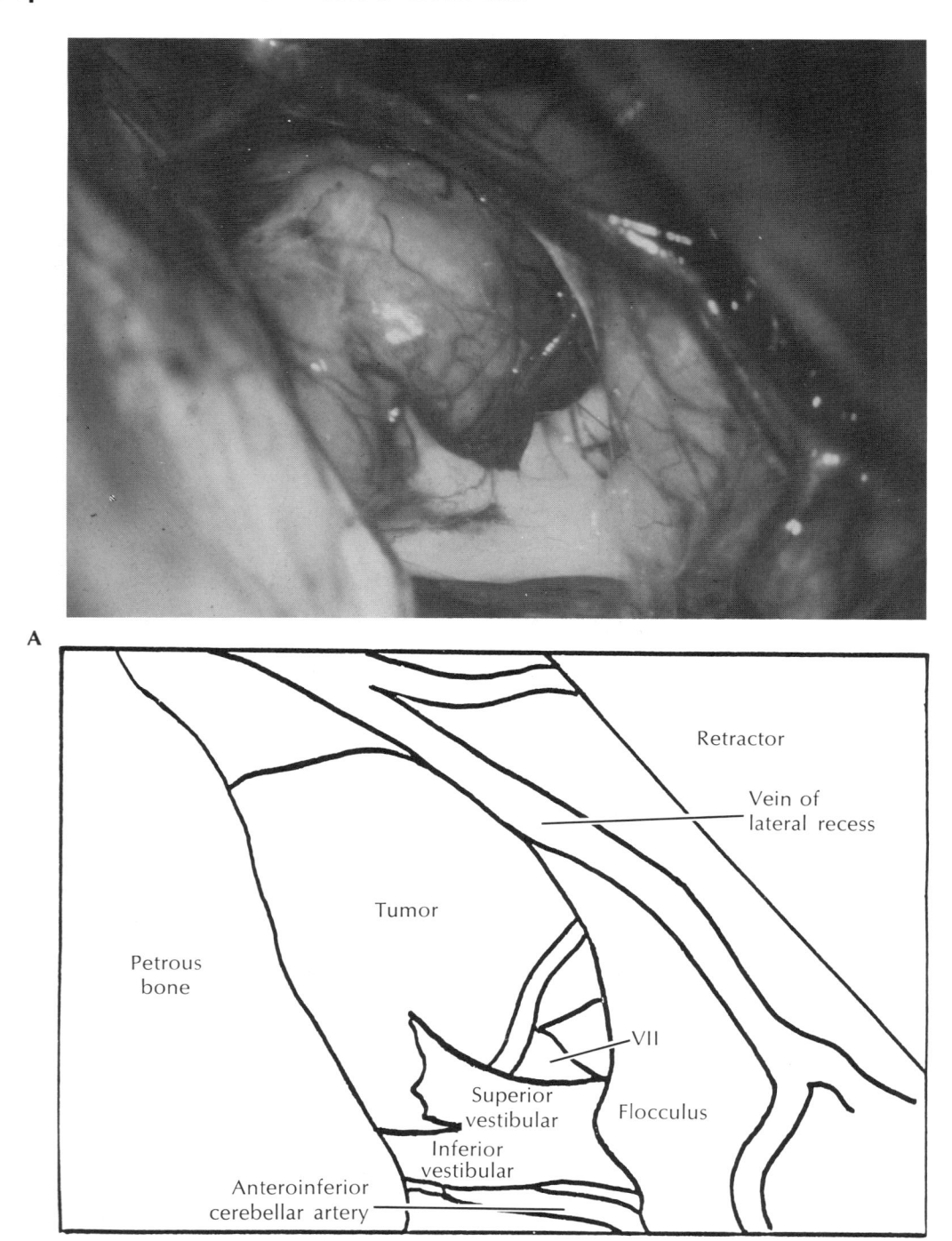

Etiology of disruption of the facial neuromuscular motor unit

Fig. 6-1. A, Left retrolabyrinthine suboccipital craniectomy. A 2 cm acoustic neuroma can be seen arising from the superior vestibular nerve, extending toward the brainstem from the internal auditory meatus. Inferior vestibular nerve is pushed downward and auditory and facial nerves are anteroinferior to the tumor. **B,** Same patient as in **A.** Posterior wall of internal auditory canal has been removed with a diamond drill. Tumor has been removed with sparing of facial and auditory nerves as well as arterial supply to labyrinth. Patient has normal facial movement and functional hearing.

Surgical causes of facial paresis in the cranium

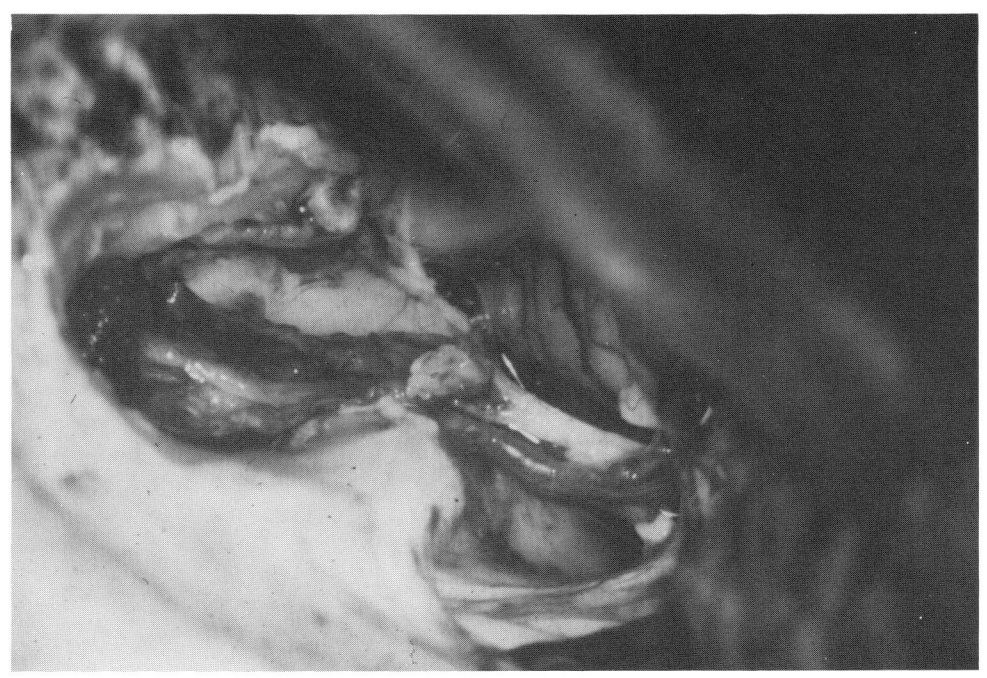

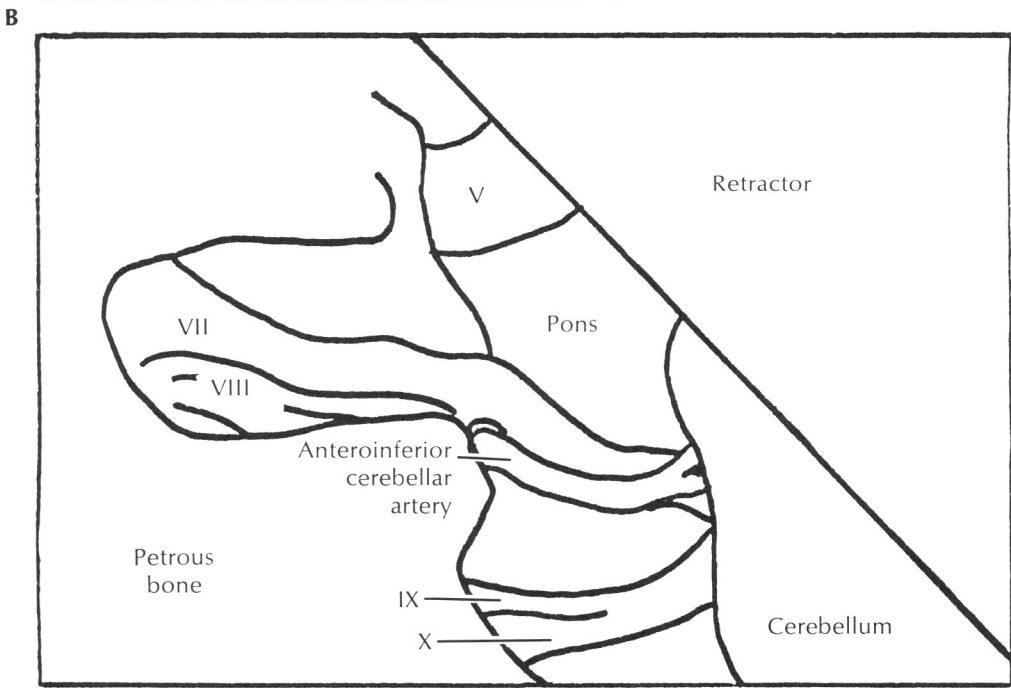

B

Diagram labels: V, Pons, Retractor, VII, VIII, Anteroinferior cerebellar artery, Petrous bone, IX, X, Cerebellum

Fig. 6-1, cont'd. For legend see opposite page.

sensorineural in type) appears first, since the vestibular dysfunction is rarely recognized unless episodes of vertigo occasionally occur. Despite bony erosion and widening of the canal by the tumor, facial nerve dysfunction is virtually never present at this stage. As the tumor grows up through the enlarging internal auditory canal to now become a posterior fossa mass, it pushes the cerebellar flocculus backward and the cerebellar hemisphere medially and upward and grows across the jugular foramen and ninth, tenth, and eleventh nerves posteriorly, while anteriorly it begins to distort the fifth nerve into a forward curve. It then progressively cups into the pons and medulla and may also elevate portions of the pons and medulla, growing across the basilar artery and compressing the sixth nerve between the basilar artery and the tumor. In the meantime, the facial nerve has been stretched out in a long course, most usually passing medially on the tumor capsule along the deep cup in the brainstem and then around either the superior or anteroinferior apex of the tumor to finally turn backward. It then runs beneath the petrosal vein and just beneath or along the fifth nerve to pass the fifth nerve and then turn abruptly laterally as it enters the anterior part of the internal auditory meatus. By the time the tumor has reached a diameter of 5 cm, the patient generally is totally deaf as well as having severe ataxia, dysarthria, and papilledema, and the distortion of the facial nerve is extreme. The rate of loss of hearing is somewhat variable, but most patients have no significant hearing left by the time the tumor is 2.5 cm in diameter. Nevertheless, facial nerve dysfunction even in the very large tumors is usually minimal and not particularly disturbing to the patient because the retained function is adequate. Decreased corneal reflex, present by the time there is significant distortion of the fifth nerve is generally accompanied by a mild decrease in sensation in the fifth nerve distribution and is related to fifth nerve dysfunction rather than to facial nerve damage. It appears probable that the relative resistance of the facial nerve (like the motor fifth) is related to the fact that these motor nerves are composed of postganglionic regenerable fibers, whereas the sensory fifth and the auditory nerves are preganglionic and therefore part of the central nervous system.

Historically, these tumors, though benign, have not provided statistically happy results. In the era between World War I and World War II, Cushing's[1] dictum that total removal of these tumors would not be possible and that only intracapsular partial removal was feasible, began to be abandoned mainly as a result of Dandy's demonstration that total removal could be successfully carried out.[2] It had become apparent that two thirds of patients with partial removal had recurrence within the next 5 years, leading either to the death of the patient or the need for a second operation or both. On the other hand, the preservation of the facial nerve, frequently accomplished with partial removal, was rarely possible with total removal. Most neurosurgeons prior to the advent of the microneurosurgical approach accepted the idea of routine total facial paralysis after a successful total removal. There were some exceptions; Olivecrona[6] had been able to save the facial nerve function in 20% of his 415 patients. Eighty-four percent of his patients had total removals with an overall mortality of about 20%. One should note that results as good as these in terms of the facial nerve and the total mortality were being achieved by very few surgeons and that a significant number of patients were also disabled because of brainstem and cerebellar damage.

It was routine to explain preoperatively to the patients that if they recovered sufficiently from the tumor removal and if the total removal had been achieved, spinofacial anastomosis or hypoglossal anastomosis would be carried out.

Although neurosurgery had been rather slow to enter the microsurgical era, the otologists, with a much wider and earlier experience at microsurgery, particularly in the middle ear,[3] pioneered the approach to the acoustic neuromas through the microscope. House[4] demonstrated that in the small acoustic neuromas, one could achieve facial nerve preservation in the majority of patients by use of a transtemporal approach for the intracanalicular tumors and a translabyrinthine approach for those that bulged slightly into the posterior fossa. The further refinement of the posterior fossa unilateral microsurgical approach[7,8] with its retrolabyrinthine extension[5] reaffirmed the neurosurgical treatment of these tumors by being able to bring the mortality of even the large tumors down below 3% or 4%, with regular achievement of total removal and approximately 80% of the patients having satisfactory preservation of facial nerve function.[5,8] An additional advantage of the retrolabyrinthine posterior fossa approach, besides its ability to maintain low mortality in the large tumors with good functional result, has been the ability to preserve useful hearing in an appreciable percentage of those patients who still had useful preoperative hearing at the time of surgery. This, of course, cannot be accomplished with the translabyrinthine approach.

I have routinely carried out the operation with the patient in semisitting position and the head fixed with a steel-pin headrest. The patient's body is encased in a Gardner pressure suit, and a Doppler ultrasonic monitor is in use over the right atrium. All our patients are curarized and given mechanical respiration with controlled P_{O_2} and P_{CO_2} levels, with visual control preferred to prevent brainstem damage rather than observation of changes in spontaneous respiration. The operative approach has been through a vertical linear incision just medial to the mastoid process. A lateral suboccipital craniectomy has been carried out, with removal of the mastoid process crossing the sigmoid sinus. The exposure stops short of the jugular foramen and the stylomastoid foramen as well as the external auditory canal. After the dura is opened, the sigmoid sinus is drawn out over the cut surface of the mastoid by traction sutures, so that a direct approach along the plane of the petrous bone is permitted without going around the corner of the remaining mastoid and sinus. This more lateral approach has permitted less retraction and a more direct and better visualization of the tumor.[5]

Although there is no question that preservation of life is the important criterion in the removal of an acoustic tumor so that preservation of the arterial supply and care in dissection of the brainstem are the most crucial parts of the operation, nevertheless preservation of facial nerve function can be achieved without loss of the other requisites in the majority of patients. In addition, the approach to the seventh nerve is in a way the basis for a number of different techniques in handling acoustic neuromas. Two major directions of approach have been generally promulgated; one is to first open the internal auditory meatus and see the facial nerve in the canal and then to remove the tumor, beginning at the most lateral portion of the facial nerve and progressing in the medial direction along the facial nerve as the facial nerve is dissected from the capsule.[7] Almost the opposite approach has been suggested; i.e., one begins medially on the brainstem viewing the facial nerve just anterior and above the flocculus after viewing the choroid plexus at the lateral recess, then follows the facial nerve forward as it is pressed against the brainstem, and separates it from the capsule from this all the way out to the lateral margin.[8]

I have preferred still a different approach. Separation of the capsule superiorly as internal removal of the tumor content is carried out is usually reasonably safe, since the dissection is against the tentorium or a cap of cerebellum. One must separate the capsule inferiorly to free the vascular structures. I continue these two directions of separation around the superior margin and the inferior margin of the capsule, collapsing the capsule down between, until I see the facial nerve (usually anteroinferiorly), and bisect the capsule, leaving both a medial and a lateral portion of the tumor in place so that the tumor has been cut in half in the sagittal plane. Removal of the medial half of the tumor is then carried out usually with a little more freedom of movement because of the fact that it is detached from the lateral part in the meatus. Since these tumors begin to grow from the superior vestibular nerve out in the meatus, as they grow into the posterior fossa they carry with them an invaginating layer of arachnoid membrane. Although these layers may become adherent and even partially fused, it is often possible to stay between the two layers in the dissection, and this provides an internal layer of arachnoid to protect the rest of the posterior fossa structures. The facial nerve generally is both splayed out and weakest at its apex of the distorted curve, which is the area where it has first been visualized in this bisection technique. Dissection, therefore, carried from the point of origin on the brainstem toward this weak point does not stress the point of maximum thinning so badly. After the removal of the medial half of the tumor, attention is now turned to the lateral part, and this is approached by the opening of the internal auditory meatus. Using the high-speed diamond burr, one drills away the posterior wall of the meatus. In the small tumors where hearing may be present and an attempt is being made to preserve this hearing, it is important not to perforate the labyrinth in the course of the bony removal. As the bone is cut away laterally, most of the tumors will be seen to reach the crista that divides the canal usually at a depth of about 1.25 cm. Since a few of the tumors do not go quite this far, it may be easier to open the dura of the canal at each step of the drilling in order to recognize the lateral end of the tumor as soon as possible. The superior vestibular nerve is then cut, the facial nerve and perhaps the auditory nerve are visualized, and the tumor is separated from these structures (Fig. 6-1, *B*). There is a significant risk to the facial nerve at this part of the procedure, since the tumor has totally filled the canal, destroyed the crista, and become more adherent to the nerves, vessels, and dura. At the lateral end of the canal, the arrangement of the nerves is such that the facial nerve is anterosuperior, the auditory nerve is anteroinferior, and the two vestibular nerves, superior and inferior, are posterior. The vestibular nerves remain in this position as they are followed to the medial aspect of the internal auditory meatus. Usually the facial and auditory nerves rotate in their relationship to each other, with the facial nerve eventually crossing the medial lip of the canal at its anteroinferior margin and the auditory nerve lying just below and slightly posterior to the facial nerve. The facial nerve takes many courses; sometimes it deviates higher up along the fifth nerve or it may be down to actually contact the basilar artery as part of a much-displaced medial anteroinferior course. The alterations in the appearance of the facial nerve are also great, with some bundles looking quite like a nerve and others splayed out in multiple fibers almost like the posterior root of the fifth nerve, and still other facial nerves may look almost membranous (Fig. 6-2).

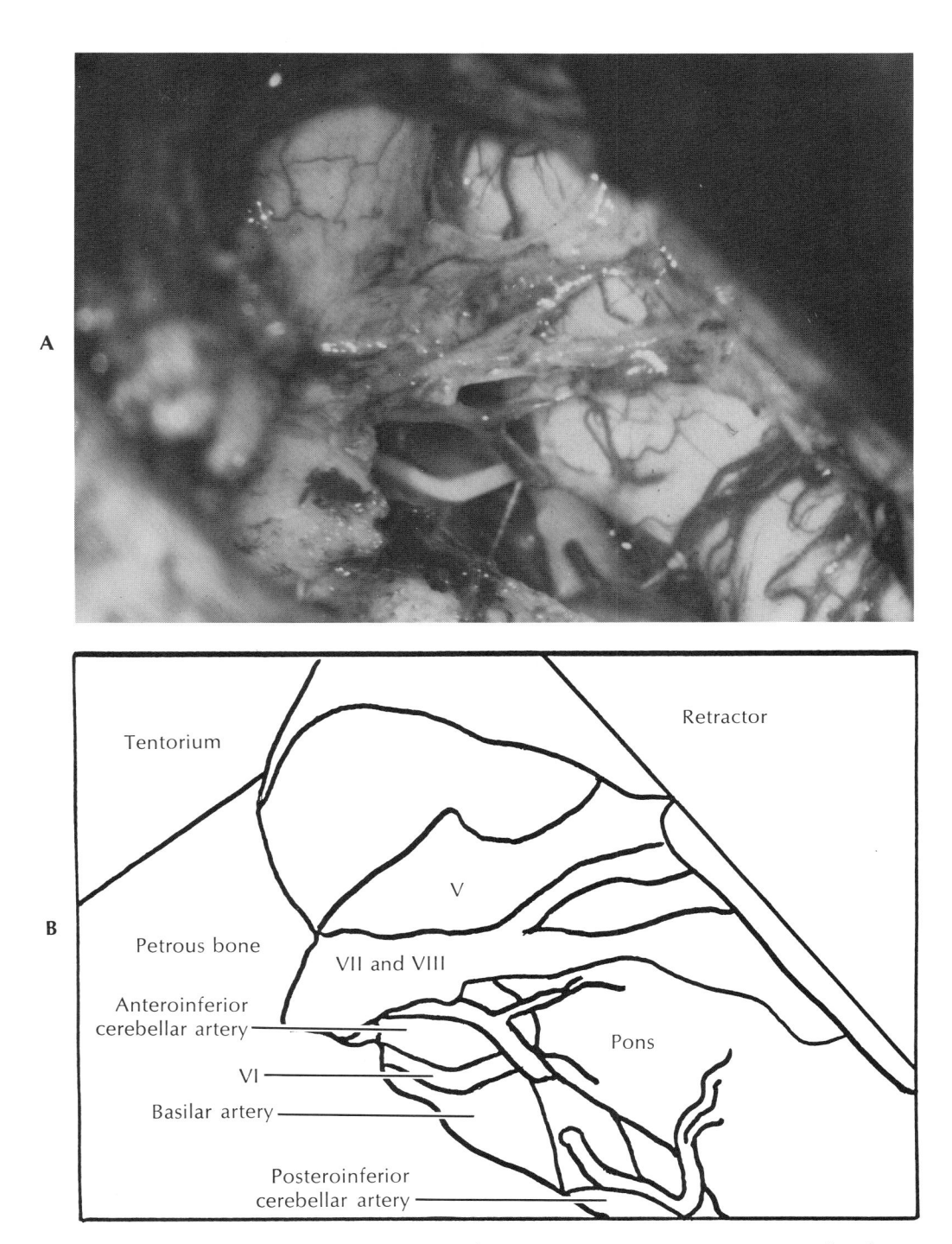

Surgical causes of facial paresis in the cranium

Fig. 6-2. Left retrolabyrinthine suboccipital craniectomy. A 5.5 cm neuroma has been removed. Despite ragged and tremendously distorted appearance of auditory and facial nerves, this patient has excellent hearing and normal facial movement. Patient works full time and has no disability.

Etiology of disruption of the facial neuromuscular motor unit

As indicated in the previous paragraphs, in a certain percentage of patients, it has been impossible to save the facial nerve regardless of precautions. In one large tumor, the extension forward in the auditory meatus had gone through the anterior wall of the petrous pyramid, with the dome of the tumor in the middle fossa incorporating the facial nerve at the geniculate ganglion, and the facial nerve was surgically lost at this point. In some of the tumors, the facial nerve will be lost on the capsule and yet the proximal and distal portions may be sufficiently well preserved to permit anastomosis. The most likely area of such damage to the facial nerve occurs just at the medial margin of the meatus where the sharp angle is formed, as the facial nerve may turn anteriorly. The segment from the lip of the canal to the thinned-out portion at the apex of the tumor is indeed the last portion removed, with maximum visualization and the clearest tracing of the direction of displacement of the facial nerve fibers.

Angle meningiomas arising generally from the petrous pyramid dura or from the tentorial surface have in general been easier to separate from the involved nerves, since they do not ordinarily invade the auditory meatus. However, I have had a case of one totally intracanalicular meningioma that had enlarged the canal to more than 1.5 cm in diameter without entering the posterior fossa. This is the only tumor where I was unable to spare the facial nerve and yet was able to preserve excellent hearing. The tumor had eroded the crista and invaded slightly upward for several millimeters into the facial canal and had actually incorporated the neural sheath in the tumor capsule. Other angle meningiomas may be unremovable because they have surrounded all the neural elements from the eleventh nerve to the fifth nerve or have completely incorporated the anteroinferior cerebellar artery within their bulk. Nevertheless, in the meningiomas the prognosis for maintenance of facial nerve function has been better than 80%.

Neurofibromas growing from the ninth, tenth, or eleventh nerves (Fig. 6-3) or from the fifth nerve (Fig. 6-4) have been encountered approximately 10% as often as acoustic neuromas in our series. Again, because these tumors do not enter the internal auditory meatus, their separation from the seventh nerve is easier and preservation of both seventh nerve function and hearing has been essentially routine.

Ependymomas arising from the fourth ventricle have been found in the angle on a number of occasions. They have either reached the angle by dilating the lateral recess of the fourth ventricle and growing directly out, or by growing out of the fourth ventricle posteriorly and filling the cisterna magna and then extending out often into both angles. Separation of these tumors from the seventh and eighth nerves has been the least difficult part of the removal.

Epidermoid tumors of the angle deserve a special mention. These tumors growing as they do often to a very large size consist of a thin neoplastic membrane filled with an avascular cholesterin cheeselike material (Fig. 6-5, *A*). Since they grow around most structures and insinuate glovelike through the cisterna, they often cause minimal symptoms until they have reached a size when there is no further room in the cisterns. Although they do indeed cause neural deficits, these are often minimal compared to the anatomic stretching and involvement of the nerves that are present within them (Fig. 6-5, *B* and *C*). Precise microdissection allowing progressive removal of the contents of these tumors and then meticulous separation of the thin capsular layer has prevented loss of function and avoided recurrence of these lesions. Epidermoid tumors tend to be irritative and in the angle most often present with a painful syndrome that may not be

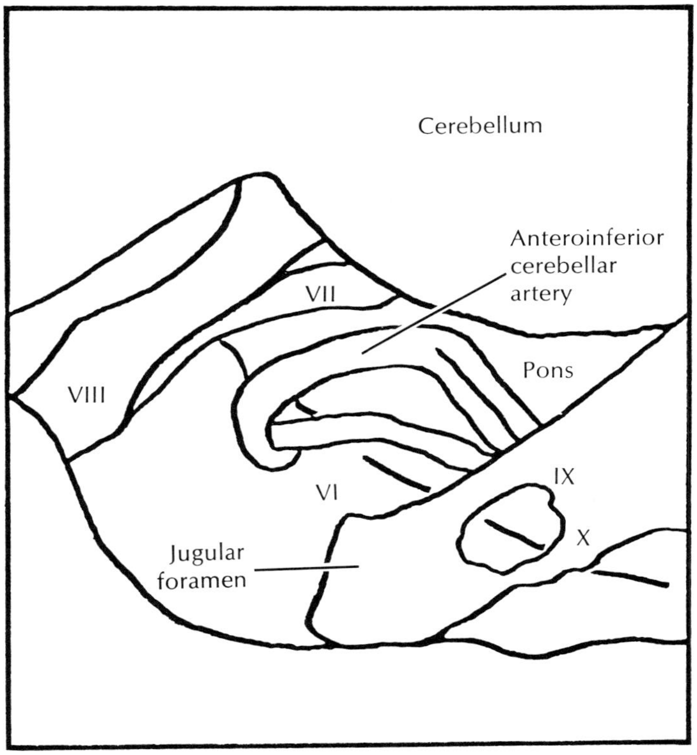

Fig. 6-3. Left retrolabyrinthine suboccipital craniectomy. A 4.5 cm neuroma of eleventh nerve has been removed. Although this tumor had filled cerebellopontine angle, it has not entered auditory meatus nor grown out through jugular foramen. Displacement and preservation of seventh and eighth nerves can be seen. Patient has no neurological deficit.

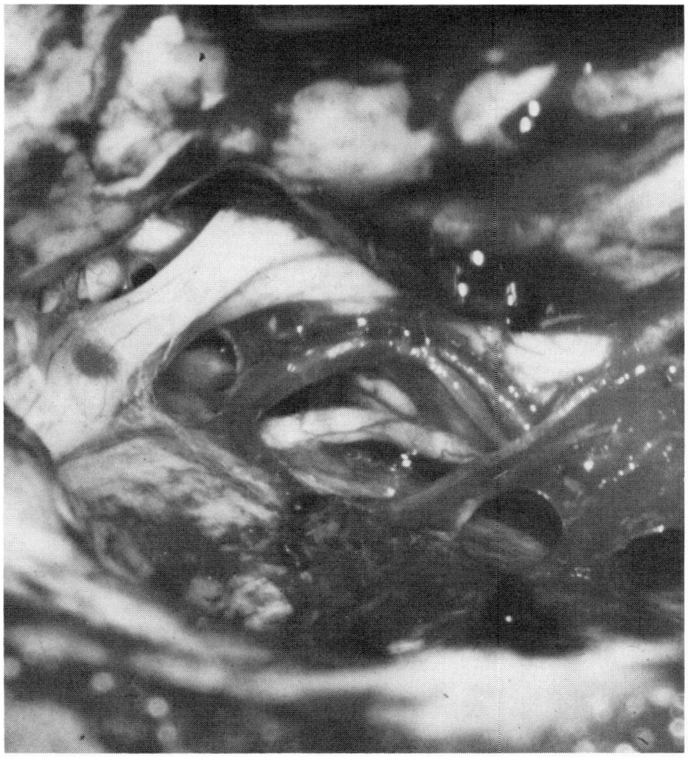

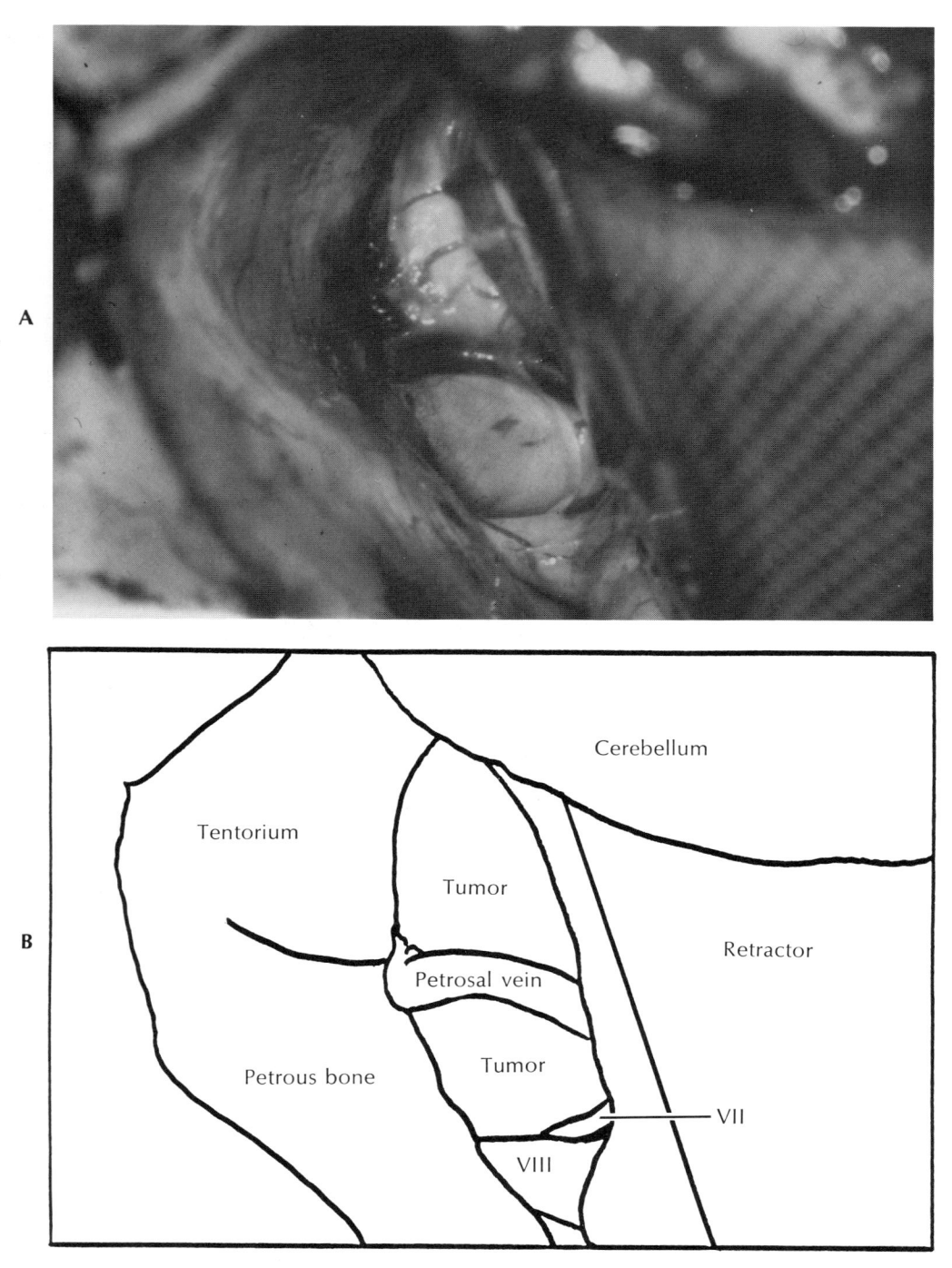

Etiology of disruption of the facial neuromuscular motor unit

Fig. 6-4. Left retrolabyrinthine suboccipital craniectomy. Large five nerve neurofibroma is present, stretching petrosal vein and seventh and eighth nerves posteriorly. Total resection of this tumor high in the cerebellopontine angle was carried out with preservation of full function except for sensory fifth, which had been destroyed by tumor.

Surgical causes of facial paresis in the cranium

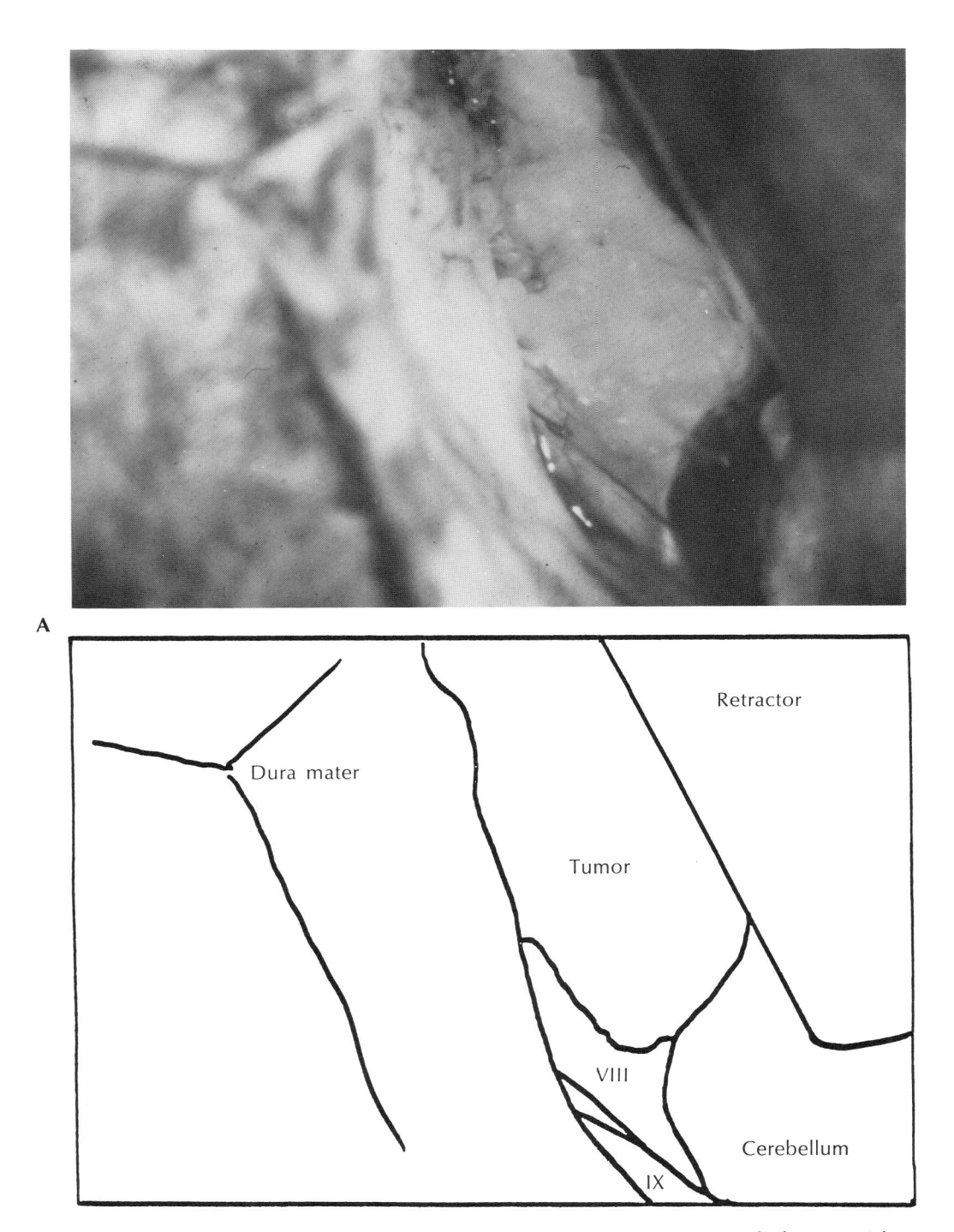

Fig. 6-5. A, Left retrolabyrinthine suboccipital craniectomy. Extremely large epidermoid tumor of cerebellopontine angle is seen. Seventh and eighth nerves are exposed partly within tumor and displaced downward and backward, actually crossing jugular foramen and contracting ninth and tenth nerves. Tumor extended posteriorly to level of foramen magnum.

Continued.

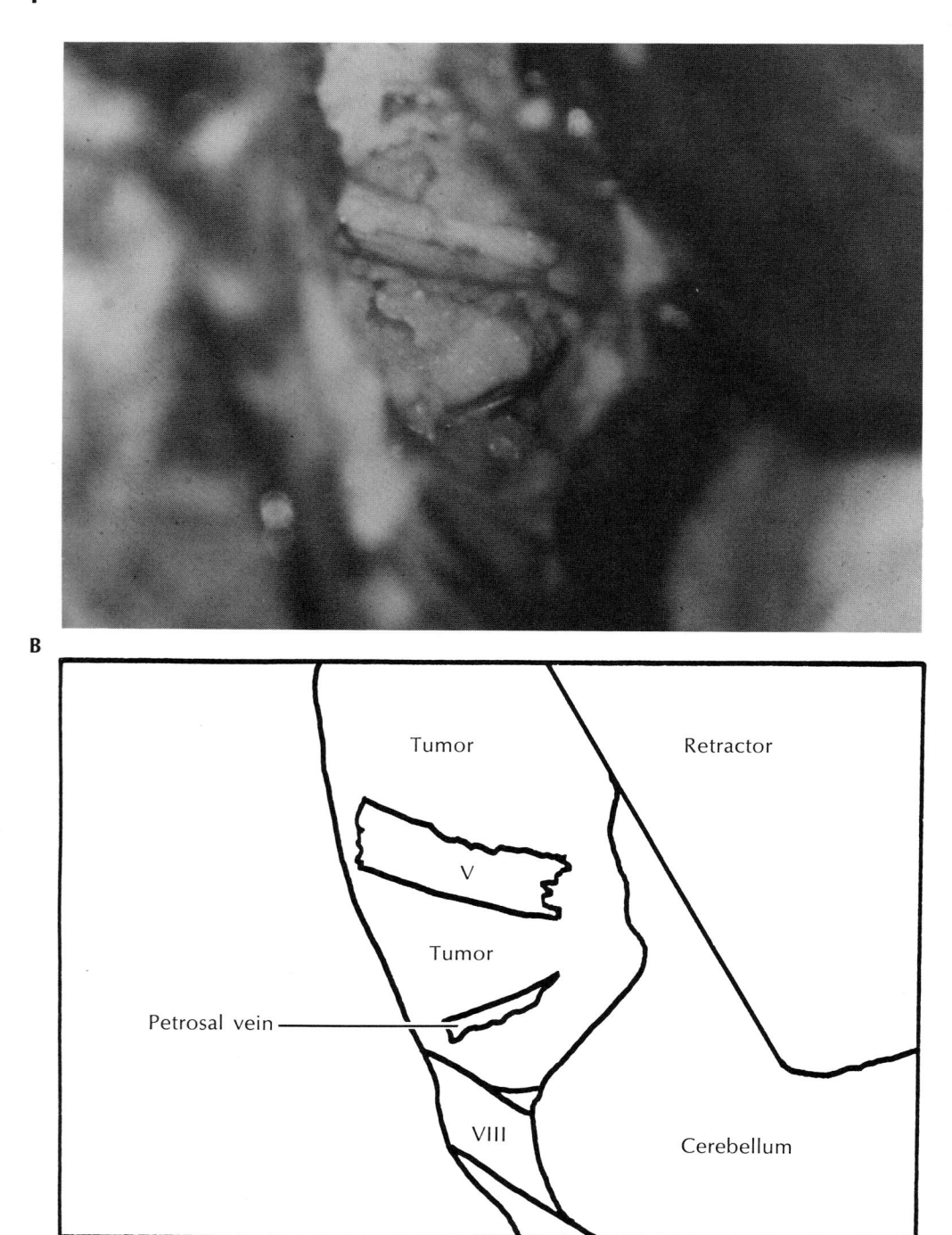

Etiology of disruption of the facial neuromuscular motor unit

Fig. 6-5, cont'd. B, Same patient as in **A.** Left retrolabyrinthine posterior fossa craniectomy. Further excavation within large epidermoid tumor shows fifth nerve entirely within tumor. This tumor, which extended forward through tentorium to reach carotid artery, was completely removed in 16-hour microsurgical procedure.

Surgical causes of facial paresis in the cranium

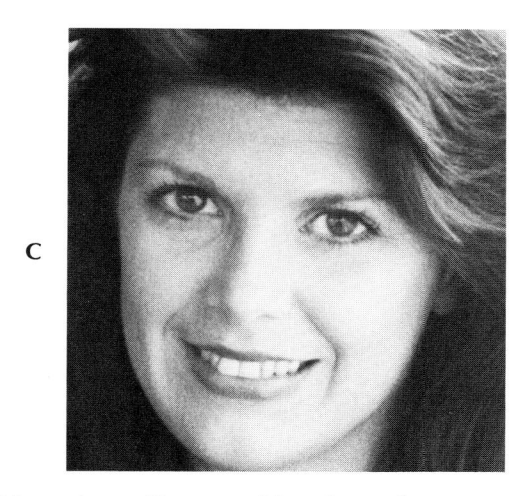

Fig. 6-5, cont'd. C, This patient, 19 years old at time of surgery, now 7 years later, is a successful television actress. There is no deficit of ocular or facial movement or expression even to the close-up camera lens.

distinguishable from trigeminal neuralgia. The contents may also cause a chemical meningitis if part of the tumor is left in place after opening the capsule, and it is therefore important that the removal be complete in one operative stage.

Finally, metastatic tumors of the angle arising from petrous bone metastases may present with a syndrome quite like an acoustic neuroma. In general, these are best subjected to radiation therapy, particularly if they arise from the breast or other significantly radiosensitive areas and are not dealt with surgically.

Pontine gliomas tend to involve cranial nerve nuclei and usually remain relatively symmetrical within the pons during a long period of their growth. However, I have had several that presented as angle tumors with growth of the pontine tumor often with a cystic component out into the angle so that the presentation was that of an acoustic tumor, even with dilatation of the internal auditory meatus and the auditory canal. This rarity is not surgically curable, but one can easily resect the extrinsic bulk and cyst, thereby achieving a better opportunity for radiotherapeutic control.

In conclusion, it is rather remarkable that despite the great strides in diagnostic techniques and the increased ability to deal with these tumors, the average size of the angle tumors that we face is not appreciably smaller than the average size of tumors that I saw at the beginning of the microsurgical era some 10 years ago. Certainly, the most important and gratifying treatment of facial palsy from one of these tumors is its prevention. The rather minimal mortality and morbidity of the operation in the smaller tumors as well as the opportunity to save hearing in these lesions should hopefully lead to an earlier diagnosis, permitting another major step forward in achieving still better results.

REFERENCES

1. Cushing, H.: Tumors of the nervus acusticus, Philadelphia, 1917, W. B. Saunders Co.
2. Dandy, W. E.: An operation for the total removal of cerebellopontine (acoustic) tumors, Surg. Gynecol. Obstet. **41**:139-148, 1925.

3. Holmgren, G.: Some experiences in the surgery of otosclerosis, Acta Otolaryngol. **5:** 460-466, 1923.
4. House, W. F.: Monograph II: acoustic neuroma, Arch. Otolaryngol. **88:**576-715, 1968.
5. Malis, L. I.: Microsurgical treatment of acoustic neurinomas. In Handa, H., editor: Microneurosurgery, Baltimore, 1975, University Park Press, pp. 105-120.
6. Olivecrona, H.: The removal of acoustic neurinomas, J. Neurosurg. **26:**100-103, 1967.
7. Rand, R. W., and Kurze, T.: Facial nerve preservation by posterior fossa transmeatal microdissection in total removal of acoustic tumors, J. Neurol. Neurosurg. Psychiatry **28:**311-316, 1965.
8. Yaşargil, M. G.: Microsurgery applied to neurosurgery, Stuttgart, 1969, Georg Thieme Verlag, pp. 154-164.

7 Surgical causes of facial paresis in the temporal canal

LEE A. HARKER
BRIAN F. McCABE

Without otological, neurological, and often roentgenological examination, many patients with facial paralysis secondary to disease processes within the temporal bone are diagnosed as having Bell's palsy. Paresis may occur from infectious disease states, benign and malignant tumors, and traumas such as fracture of the temporal bone and sharp and blunt trauma to the nerve.

Without otologic, neurologic, and often roentgenographic examination, many of the patients with facial paralysis secondary to disease processes within the temporal bone are diagnosed as having Bell's palsy until the true nature of their diseased state becomes obvious. This chapter reviews infectious disease states, tumors, and traumatic etiologies that can result in intratemporal facial nerve paralysis. Bell's palsy, more appropriately termed "idiopathic facial nerve paralysis," is treated in a separate chapter.

Infectious processes
HERPES ZOSTER OTICUS

The varicella-zoster DNA virus is the agent responsible for the Ramsay Hunt syndrome. A deep-seated, aural pain is followed in a few days by a vesicular eruption, usually of the external ear canal and concha, sensorineural hearing loss, vertigo, and a complete or partial facial paralysis (Fig. 7-1). Pathologic studies have failed to substantiate Hunt's hypothesis that a herpetic geniculate ganglionitis was etiologic. Current opinion, based on the few available postmortem studies, is that the disease represents an encephalomeningomyelitis that occurs after the virus gains entry to the cerebrospinal fluid and spreads from the meninges to the motor and sensory nerve roots and end organs.[12] The facial nerve fares poorly with this disease. Over half of all patients affected have some permanent motor disturbance and some remain permanently paralyzed. A complete paralysis is more likely to have severe residua.[2] Steroids or nerve decompression are recommended by some, but controlled studies are lacking.

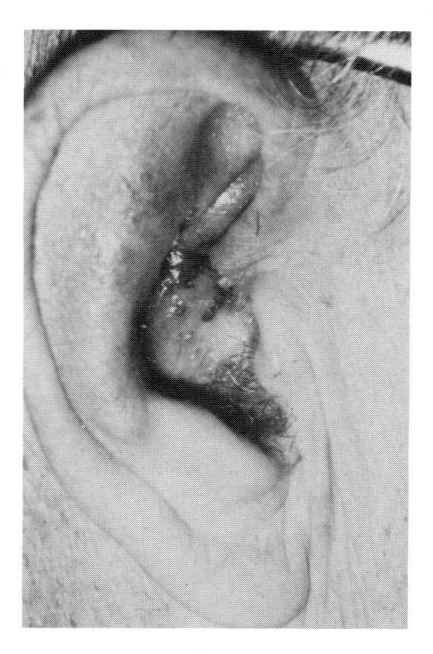

Etiology of disruption of the facial neuromuscular motor unit

Fig. 7-1. Vesicular eruption 1 week after onset in herpes zoster oticus.

ACUTE SUPPURATIVE OTITIS MEDIA

Facial paralysis secondary to acute suppurative otitis media is usually seen in children with ear pain and an inflamed bulging tympanic membrane. It seems likely that a combination of a dehiscent fallopian canal, a middle ear suppuration with a particularly virulent organism or organisms, and a susceptible host are necessary. In addition to appropriate antibiotic treatment, myringotomy (either daily or with insertion of a ventilating tube) is indicated to quickly decrease the number of microorganisms in contact with the nerve.

CHRONIC SUPPURATIVE OTITIS MEDIA

Chronic suppurative otitis media may affect the facial nerve anywhere within the temporal bone and may or may not have associated keratoma (cholesteatoma). To reach the nerve, the organisms need fallopian canal dehiscence, bone resorption, or bone infection adjacent to the nerve. The facial paralysis is commonly indolent and of gradual onset over hours to days. Frequently, the perioral musculature is initially affected, and the pathologic processes are involving the nerve in its tympanic segment. The flora is usually multiple and contains both aerobic and anaerobic organisms.[5] Treatment dictates surgical removal of keratoma or infected granulation tissue, or both, from the nerve, with distal and proximal surgical exposure of normal-appearing nerve, as well as appropriate cultures and antibiotics.

MALIGNANT EXTERNAL OTITIS

Special mention need be made of facial nerve involvement with this unusual variant of temporal bone infection. This process usually occurs in elderly diabetic patients and begins in the floor of the external canal where bone meets cartilage, extends to the

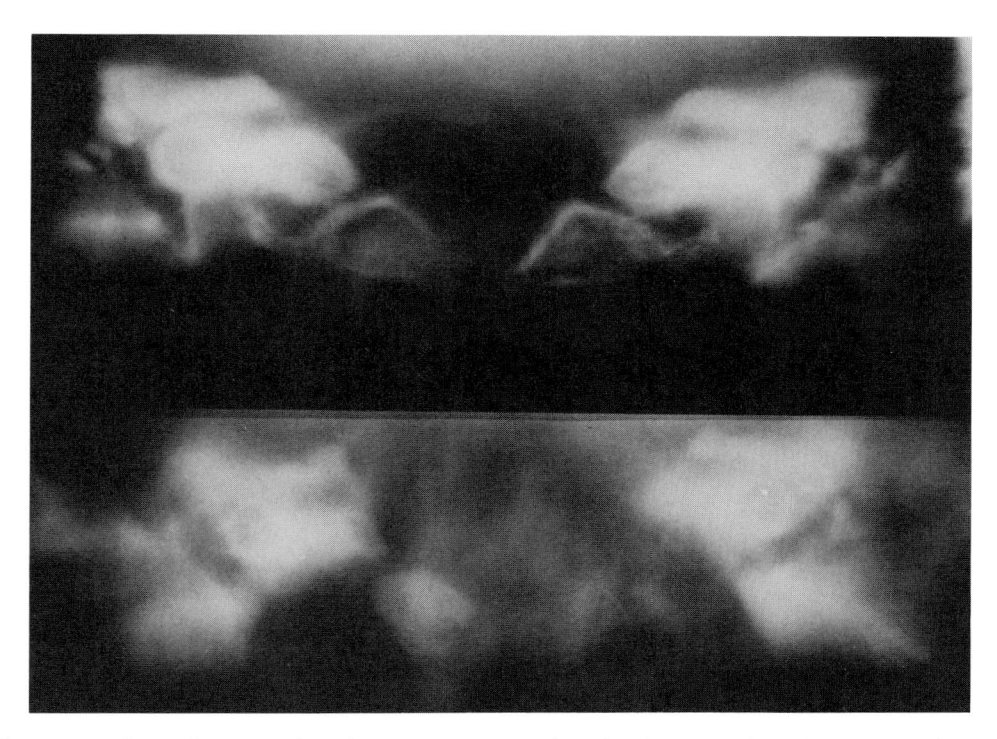

Fig. 7-2. Bilateral coronal polytomograms at level of internal auditory canals and occipital condyles in a normal patient (above), and one with malignant external otitis. Extensive destructive changes evident, even in occipital condyle. Patient had paralysis of seventh to twelfth cranial nerves on that side and sixth nerve on opposite side.

subjacent bony external auditory canal and soft tissue, and thereafter throughout the temporal bone and adjacent bone and soft tissue. *Pseudomonas aeruginosa* is the prevalent organism. Facial nerve paralysis is the most common complication of the disease and occurs in nearly 40% of patients. The nerve may be involved anywhere from the parotid gland to the petrous apex (most commonly at the stylomastoid foramen) and frequently is involved with a suppurative neuritis. Once involved, the prognosis for facial nerve recovery is guarded. The other cranial nerves at the base of the skull have also been involved with advancing disease. With cranial nerve involvement, the prognosis for life drops to less than 50%.[1] Terminal problems include meningitis, sepsis, renal failure (secondary to aminoglycoside antibiotics), and medical complications commonly seen in this age group. Treatment is aggressive, being surgical excision of diseased bone coupled with intensive antibiotic therapy. All necrotic bone cartilage and soft tissue need be excised,[1] but this is not always feasible (Fig. 7-2).

Tumors
FACIAL NERVE TUMORS

Schwannomas and less commonly neurofibromas can involve the facial nerve, usually in patients in the second, third, and fourth decades. Some believe the two tumors represent different ends of a continuum. Facial nerve symptoms may be en-

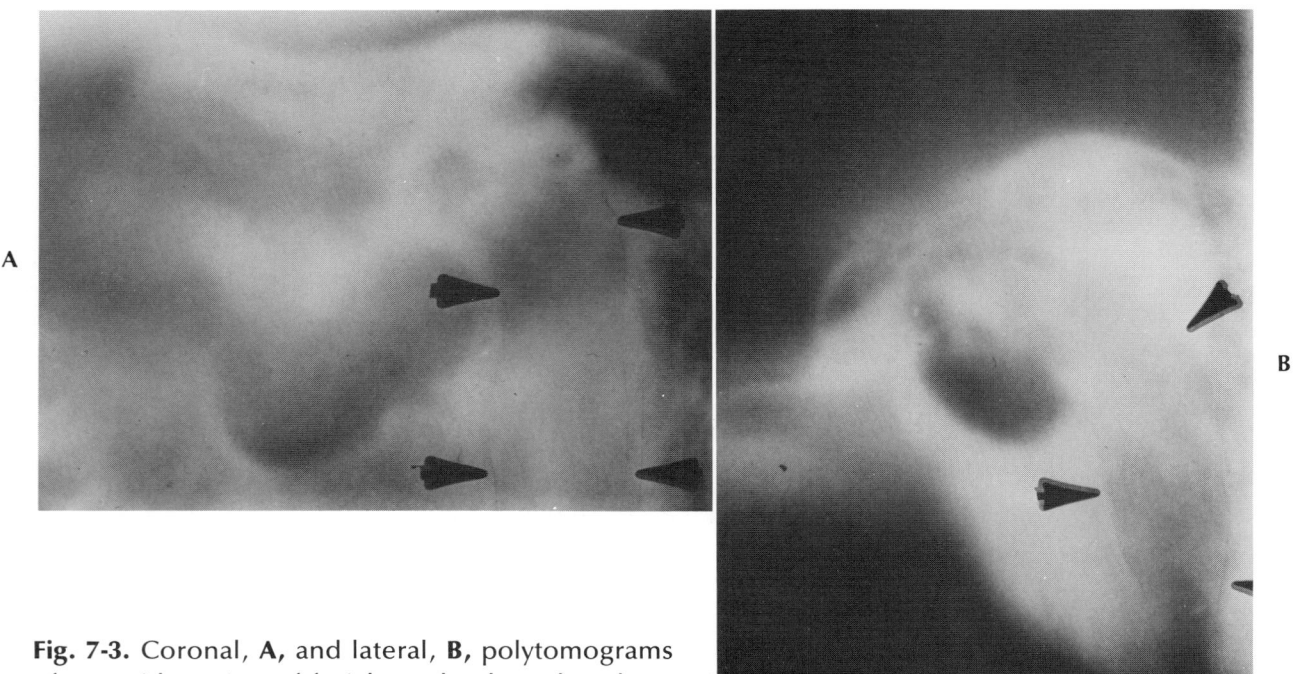

Etiology of disruption of the facial neuromuscular motor unit

Fig. 7-3. Coronal, **A,** and lateral, **B,** polytomograms of mastoid portion of facial canal enlarged to three times normal diameter by facial neuroma.

tirely absent, but usually there is a painless, partial, or complete paralysis that comes on gradually over a period of months. In a significant proportion of cases, there is a facial tic initially. Associated symptoms depend on the location of the tumor. Those arising in the mastoid segment are silent until quite large, when they present as a deep mass palpable in the region of the stylomastoid foramen, or they may erode the overlying mastoid cortex, or the bony external auditory canal. Those originating in the tympanic segment cause an early conductive hearing loss and are usually visible behind an intact tympanic membrane. In the internal auditory canal additional symptoms are those seen with vestibular schwannomas in that location. Cerebellopontine angle or brainstem symptoms may be added. Growth of these tumors is slow and occurs along the course of the nerve, enlarging the fallopian canal in the process. That enlargement provides the most helpful radiographic sign (Fig. 7-3). Simultaneous or sequential involvement of other cranial or spinal nerves suggest the autosomal dominant neurofibromas of von Recklinghausen, as does the presence of café-au-lait spots.

EXTRINSIC TUMORS

Benign tumors

Glomus tumor. Whether they arise from the glomus bodies in the dome of the jugular bulb or those along the nerves on the middle ear promontory, these tumors may paralyze the facial nerve. It is, however, late in the course of the disease and occurs in only 11% of cases.[4] By the time the facial nerve is involved, these tumors can almost always be visualized as a red (frequently pulsatile) mass behind an intact tympanic membrane or, even later, as an infected mesotympanic mass visible through a

Surgical causes of facial paresis in the temporal canal

perforation. As the tumor grows, it invades the temporal bone air cell system usually proceeding medial to the facial nerve into the mastoid air cell system, and infracochlearly toward the petrous apex cells, rather than eroding bone in a smooth advancing interface as schwannomas or apical keratomas do. This sometimes makes the assessment of preoperative tumor size difficult. The appearance and location are typical, and biopsy is not advocated until the definitive surgical procedure, which follows an extensive radiographic evaluation. Through the efforts of House, Glasscock, and others,[3,7] surgical treatment has greatly improved in the past 15 years. Even with extensive tumors arising from and occluding the jugular bulb, complete tumor removal with low risk of mortality and morbidity is now possible. The areas of surgical failure are the carotid artery and medial base of the skull. Radiotherapy offers good palliation and tumor shrinkage but is reserved for those patients in whom surgical removal is not desirable or possible.

Acoustic neuroma. The acoustic neuroma (more appropriately vestibular schwannoma) and neurofibromas of the eighth cranial nerve rarely cause facial paralysis. In 1938, long before current diagnostic techniques for detecting small tumors, the incidence was believed to be only 4%.[8] The nerve is involved in the cisternal and meatal segments and, despite its rare paresis, is often thinned and splayed by the adjacent, enlarging tumor. The presence of facial paralysis with a lesion in the internal acoustic meatus or the cerebellopontine angle immediately arouses suspicion that a less common lesion than the schwannoma is present. Treatment of acoustic tumors is excision except in the elderly where serial evaluation for tumor growth rate may be appropriate. Prognosis for preservation of facial nerve function is good to excellent.

Meningioma. The arachnoid villi, from which meningiomas are believed to arise, are most common in the major dural venous sinuses but are also present in smaller venous sinuses, tributary veins, and dural prolongations of the cranial nerves. Although less than 10% of all meningiomas occur in the temporal bone, they occur sporadically in the internal auditory canal and cerebellopontine angle, and rarely near the jugular bulb, the geniculate ganglion, and the sulci of the greater or lesser superficial petrosal nerves.[9] In the internal canal and cerebellopontine angle, they more commonly occur as the ovoid, firm, lobulated, *en globe* type than the flat, spreading, investing, *en plaque* type. Radiographic studies demonstrate tumor location and size. Intratumor calcification, surrounding osteoblastic reaction, and a higher incidence of facial nerve involvement help differentiate these tumors from schwannomas. Although the treatment is surgical, the tendency to encircle blood vessels rather than displace them renders surgical removal more hazardous as does the propensity to adhere to the adjacent central nervous system.

Congenital keratoma. Embryologic epidermal rests grow and expand into soft, pearly cysts that become clinically significant in the basilar cysterns, petrous apex, and cerebellopontine angle. There exists a curious predilection for these lesions to cause total dysfunction of the cranial nerves with which they come into contact. The clinical variety most commonly affecting the facial nerve arises at the petrous apex and gradually causes facial paralysis (sometimes preceded by a tic), cochlear and vestibular nerve deficits, and an abducens paralysis as the tumor expands to occupy the entire petrous apex. It is not uncommon for facial nerve function to return after removal of the tumor.[10] Radiographically there is the appearance of a smooth, concave bite from

Etiology of disruption of the facial neuromuscular motor unit

the medial portion of the temporal bone. Surgical excision is curative, but the tumor frequently is adherent to the brainstem, and so complete removal is made difficult. Occasionally, large tumor size makes adequate exposure difficult as well.

Chordoma. Cranial axis notochord remnant tumors commonly become syptomatic between ages 20 and 40 years. Characteristic clinical features include cranial nerve paralysis and headache. Often the cranial nerve involvement is unilateral, and the nerves most commonly affected are the second to the eighth. When the facial nerve is involved, the involvement of more rostral cranial nerves helps to distinguish this disease process from other tumors, as does the presence of severe headache. Radiographically the hallmark is bony destruction with or without evidence of a soft-tissue mass. The amount of bony destruction is variable and reflects the origin and spread of the tumor (as does the clinical picture). Although combinations of surgery and radiotherapy are the best current therapy, tumor recurrence (more appropriately recrudescence of residual tumor) and ultimate death from the disease are almost universal.

Malignant tumors

Squamous cell carcinoma. Over half of all malignant tumors of the external auditory canal and temporal bone are epidermoid carcinomas, which usually arise in the external auditory canal. Approximately one fourth of these patients will develop facial paralysis, but pain and otorrhea are the customary presenting symptoms. An infected polyp resembling granulation tissue is often present in the external canal. The scope of surgical resection depends on the extent of location of the primary and regional tumor; adjunctive radiotherapy is advocated by some. The overall prognosis however is poor, with over two thirds of these patients ultimately dying of their disease.[4]

Other primary tumors. Adenoid cystic carcinoma, basal cell epithelioma, adenocarcinoma, embryonal rhabdomyosarcoma, and other tumors also occur in the temporal bone and can occasionally paralyze the face. Treatment usually involves surgery but is individualized according to type and extent of tumor.

Metastatic tumors. Although distinctly uncommon, special features warrant separate mention of secondary temporal bone tumors. These characteristically are described as representing hematogenous extensions to the marrow-containing spaces at the petrous apex or retrofacial areas medial to the mastoid tip, but other metastatic sites include the external auditory canal and middle ear.[4] Pain is quite common. Adenocarcinoma of the breast is the most common primary tumor, but metastases from kidney, lung, bladder, and stomach are also seen.

Trauma
TEMPORAL BONE FRACTURE

Fractures of the temporal bone are commonly classified as transverse, longitudinal, or tympanic. Transverse fractures account for only 10% of temporal bone fractures and derive their name from the fact that the line of fracture is perpendicular to the long axis of the petrous portion of the temporal bone. They are usually the result of a severe blow to the occiput or occipitomastoid region. Facial nerve paralysis occurs in nearly 50% of these fractures, and the paralysis is likely to be complete and of immediate onset. As a rule, the prognosis for complete recovery spontaneously is considerably poorer than with longitudinal fractures.[6]

Up to 90% of all temporal bone fractures are longitudinal in type and result from forces applied to the temporoparietal region. The fracture then passes along the longitudinal aspect of the temporal bone to the apex. These fractures always involve the middle ear and usually the external canal as well. Facial nerve paralysis is seen in 10% to 20%.

Extensive comminution often occurs with both longitudinal and transverse fractures, and frequently the site of comminution and injury to the facial nerve is in the region of the geniculate ganglion. Damage can occur, however, at any point from the porus of the internal auditory canal to the stylomastoid foramen.

Tympanic bone fractures are the least common and do not often result in facial nerve paralysis. The facial nerve can occasionally be damaged in the region of the stylomastoid foramen.

There are a variety of mechanisms whereby the nerve can be injured. Particularly with transverse fractures, complete disruption of the nerve occurs. Although there may be little or no evidence of a fracture visible radiographically, at the time of the injury the two fragments may shear some distance apart and tear the facial (and cochlear and vestibular) nerve. Contusion of the nerve with intraneural hematoma and edema (with or without penetration by bony fragments) is a common mechanism of injury. A third type of injury is by extrinsic compression. This is seen most commonly with longitudinal temporal bone fractures, as the edema and hematoma in the surrounding tissues compress the nerve and interrupt transmission across the compressed segment. Finally, a suppurative neuritis may involve the nerve after a temporal bone fracture.

The most important aspect of assessment of the facial nerve in temporal bone fractures is serial assessment of the functional state of the nerve. It is essential to determine whether the preponderance of fibers are in a state of functional block, or are degenerating; multiple assessments over time are necessary to ensure that the physiological state of the fibers is not deteriorating with time. The clinical assessment of the patient alone is not sufficient to give this information and electrical testing (see Chapter 9) is necessary. The therapeutic goal is to allow those nerves that exhibit predominantly a functional block to recover without surgery, and to utilize surgery both to prevent impending degeneration from occurring and to restore anatomic continuity of a disrupted nerve.

Operative techniques are available to reestablish the continuity of the nerve within the temporal bone (with or without grafting or rerouting), to explore the areas of contusion and remove bone fragment, and to unroof compressed segments before degeneration ensues.

Special mention should be made of the patients who clinically seem to initially recover from traumatic facial paralysis but then exhibit a plateau in recovery rate, with incomplete recovery and failure of additional improvement over 3 to 4 weeks. Surgical exploration is advised in these patients. Findings have often included the partial penetration of the nerve by fragments of bone. Reduction in the surrounding edema has allowed partial recovery, which cannot further progress until removal of fragments.

FACIAL TRAUMA

Blunt and sharp injuries to the facial nerve after it leaves the stylomastoid foramen are easier to diagnose than those in the temporal bone. Although the same basic types of injuries to the nerve occur, traumatic disruption of the nerve is the most common.

Etiology of disruption of the facial neuromuscular motor unit

With disruption, integrity of the nerve or the involved branches must be reestablished for maximum opportunity for return of function.

With blunt injuries, paralysis can result from compression of a nerve branch on the underlying bony skeleton, or stretching of the nerve or its branches can occur when underlying fracture occurs. If the entire facial nerve is paralyzed after a nonpenetrating injury and the nerve degenerates, facial nerve exploration should be undertaken because of the possibility of avulsion at the stylomastoid foramen.

REFERENCES

1. Chandler, J. R.: Malignant external otitis and facial paralysis, Otolaryngol. Clin. North Am. **7**(2):375, June 1974.
2. Devriese, P. P.: Facial paralysis in cephalic herpes zoster, Ann. Otol. Rhinol. Laryngol. **77**:1101, 1968.
3. Glasscock, M. E., and Miller, G. W.: Glomus tumors, diagnosis and treatment, Instructional course at the American Academy of Ophthalmology and Otolaryngology, October 1976.
4. Greer, J. A., Cody, D. T. R., and Weiland, L. H.: Neoplasms of the temporal bone, J. Otolaryngol. **5**(5):391, 1976.
5. Harker, L. A., and Koontz, F. P.: The bacteriology of cholesteatoma. In: McCabe, B. F., Abramson, M., and Sadé, J., editors: First international conference on cholesteatoma, Birmingham, Ala., 1977, Aesculapius Publishing Co.
6. Harker, L. A., and McCabe, B. F.: Temporal bone fractures and facial nerve injury, Otolaryngol. Clin. North Am. **7**(2):425, June 1974.
7. House, W. F., and Glasscock, M. E.: Glomus tympanicum tumors, Arch. Otolaryngol. **87**:124, May 1968.
8. Jefferson, G., and Smalley, A. A.: Progressive facial palsy produced by intratemporal epidermoids, J. Laryngol. **53**:417, 1938.
9. Nager, G. T.: Meningiomas involving the temporal bone, Springfield, Ill., 1964, Charles C Thomas, Publisher.
10. Neely, J. G.: Neoplastic involvement of the facial nerve, Otolaryngol. Clin. North Am. **7**(2):June 1974.
11. Pulec, J.: Facial nerve neuroma, Laryngoscope **82**:1160, 1972.
12. Shuknecht, H. F.: Pathology of the ear, Cambridge, Mass., 1974, Harvard University Press.

8 Surgical causes of facial paresis in the parotid gland

CALVIN RASWEILER

The parotid gland envelops the peripheral facial nerve. It serves as a protection against injury. However, penetrating wounds and surgical procedures to the parotid account for the majority of nerve injuries in that region.

The anatomy of the parotid gland and the facial nerve has been discussed in a previous chapter. To fully understand disruption of the facial nerve within the parotid gland, one must fully consider and appreciate the anatomical nature of this area. Surgery upon the parotid gland would be a relatively easy process if it were not for the existing relationship between the gland and the facial nerve. Consequently, here is one area where surgical intervention is truly a challenge to the surgeon's skill.

Anatomists have tried to help the operating surgeon by dividing the gland into superficial and deep lobes. At times this seems to be more arbitrary than real. Embryologically the facial nerve is formed prior to the gland, which then grows around the nerve and envelops it. The first reaction from the operating surgeon is to abuse the originator of this design. However, we must be cognizant of the fact that this relationship was not established with the surgeon in mind, but rather as a way of protecting a motor nerve.

The parotid gland, in its position behind and overlying the mandible, is massaged during mastication, producing a flow of saliva into the oral cavity. Within the gland the facial nerve is protected from injury. See Fig. 8-1.

There are various forms of trauma associated with disruption of the nerve within the gland.
1. Sharp injuries to the face can be caused by knives and glass, which can penetrate the skin and the gland and traumatize the facial nerve.
2. Penetrating wounds caused by a bullet or shot can result in nerve disruption.
3. Blunt trauma to the face may result in an avulsion type of injury to the nerve.
4. Third-degree thermal, chemical, and electrical burns to this facial area, which result in deep tissue destruction, may have adverse affects on the nerve.
5. Surgical intervention of the parotid gland may also result in disruption of the

Etiology of disruption of the facial neuromuscular motor unit

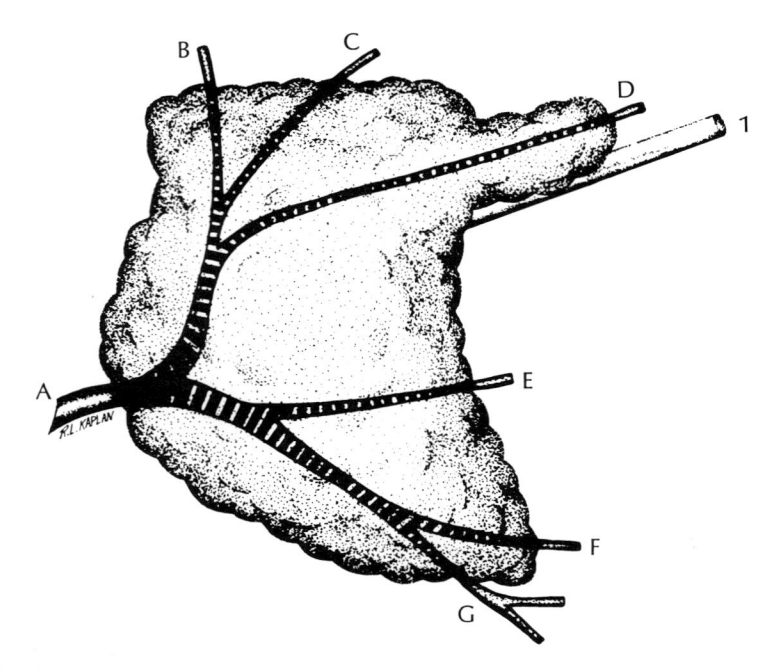

Fig. 8-1. Diagram shows portions of facial nerve that are enveloped by parotid gland. Main trunk, **A,** enters the gland and divides into two divisions: temporofacial and cervicofacial. Terminal branches shown: temporal, **B**; zygomatic, **C**; infraorbital, **D**; buccal, **E**; inframandibular, **F**; and cervical, **G.** Salivary duct also shown, **1.** (Illustrated by Ronnie L. Kaplan, Plainview, N.Y.)

neuromuscular unit of the facial nerve. This can occur during the drainage of a parotid abscess, with removal of a calculus, or with the surgical removal of lesions of the gland parenchyma.

The physical examination of these patients must include a careful evaluation of the function of the facial nerve, particularly before an anesthetic is administered.

The recommended surgical approach in this area is to identify the main trunk of the nerve first and then its divisions and branches as a surgical dissection.

During this surgical procedure the nerve can be injured inadvertently. It may become necessary to sacrifice the facial nerve or sections of it because of the involvement by a recurrent mixed tumor or because of the presence of a malignancy.

After dissection of the facial nerve and its branches, weakness or paralysis of the facial muscles can occur. This may be caused by nerve fatigue or edema. In either case, the operating surgeon, knowing that disruption has not occurred, need not be concerned about a secondary procedure for nerve repair.

In conclusion, disruption of the facial neuromuscular motor unit within the parotid gland may occur after traumatic injuries or during surgery. Although the anatomical relationship of the nerve and the gland provide protection against traumatic injury, it makes surgery upon the parotid gland difficult.

REFERENCES

1. Conley, J. J.: Salivary glands and the facial nerve, New York, 1975, Grune & Stratton.
2. McCabe, B. F.: Injuries to the facial nerve, Laryngoscope **82:**1891, 1972.
3. Ward, C. M.: Injury to the facial nerve during surgery of the parotid gland, Br. J. Surg. **62:** 401, 1975.

9 Diagnosing the site of nerve disruption by electronic methods

BERNARD S. POST

Elaborate methods, including the use of computors, are now used to pinpoint the site of disruption to the nervous pathway of the facial nerve. Not only is the site of disruption identified but, by the plotting of curves of electronic data, the examiner also can prognosticate recovery or degeneration of the seventh nerve.

Many studies by various researchers seem to establish that the questions posed by facial paralysis cannot be answered on the basis of clinical examinations alone.[3,10,11,16,19] Additional information is needed and is generally acquired by various forms of electrical exploration. Since natural healing is so common in many of the facial paralyses and since plastic procedures are undertaken mainly to correct the severe asymmetry of the face produced by permanent paralysis, it is most important to determine whether the disorder is in a reversible stage, or whether the nerve is completely or partially degenerated. Electrodiagnostic testing is the means by which these functions of the neuromuscular structure are disclosed. To coin a phrase, they may be considered the "microscopic" method of studying abnormalities in the neuromuscular structure. In many instances, these studies are quantitative and therefore very useful for prognostication.

The causes of various facial palsies have been discussed in the previous chapters and therefore will not be reiterated in this discussion. I will also assume that the reader has digested the expositions on the structure and physiology of the motor unit, which is the basic element in electrodiagnosis. An excellent history of the development of electrodiagnosis throughout the centuries is available in Licht's *Electrodiagnosis and electromyography*.[15] Most of the data obtained from the various forms of electrodiagnosis consist of wave trains, made up of either algebraically summated single motor unit potentials or exceedingly complex evoked potentials. The invention of the amplifier and the cathode ray oscilloscope made accurate recording possible. The rapid advances in space technology were accompanied by the solid state and then the integrated circuit, both of which form the foundation for the modern minicomputer. The natural development of the modern digital and analog computer systems created techniques for complete and automatic mathematical analysis of the on-line data taken from the patient.[5,6]

Etiology of disruption of the facial pathophysiology of degeneration

Various computer softwear techniques of programming made available numerous new avenues of investigation, such as automatic pattern identification and autocorrelation and cross-correlation studies. Additional examples of diagnostic techniques derived from computer technology are the following:

1. Use Fourier analysis by both fast and slow theorems for the determination of harmonic content in muscle potential output.
2. Supply capability for studying mathematical models of the physiologic activity.
3. Operate devices that can transduce temperature and physical motion of muscle into electrical patterns, thereby making muscle-excitability studies easier and more accurate.
4. Give capability of doing on-line, continuous signal averaging with histograms.

Suffice it to say that the more primitive equipment used in earlier years is being rapidly replaced with computer technology capable of performing all the complicated analysis mentioned above. Some of the newest programs can do pattern identification of wave forms and histographic outputs to develop power spectrums and integrations automatically.

Procedures for investigation of the facial nerve fall into two categories:

1. Those methods using stimulation with currents to produce evoked potentials that are analyzed and studied.
2. Those methods in which electromyographic recordings of various configurations of electrical activity are made from the muscles, analyzed, and then studied.

Testing by stimulation

The capability of tissues to respond to stimuli is referred to as their excitability. Nerve-excitability studies are measurements of change in threshold level. Stimuli are applied to motor nerves, and the readout of excitation is visible muscle movement. We will confine our definition of stimulus to electrical pulses. The threshold response, or rheobase, is the minimal intensity of current with a duration necessary to excite the tissue. This rheobase is measured in volts or milliamperes. The state of excitability of nerve or muscle tissue can be investigated in a number of different ways.

CHRONAXY

Measurement of chronaxy is one way of comparing the state of excitability from time to time or from one subject to another. This method has value but has fallen out of favor because it is time consuming. However it is a test that can be accurately carried out by a technician, using a chronaximeter. Lapicque[14] arbitrarily defined chronaxy as the duration of a shock of twice rheobase strength that will just produce a threshold response. The value is stated in milliseconds. Chronaxies, therefore, depend on the relationship between stimulus duration and intensity. Denervation is characterized by a rise in chronaxy. Reinnervation is associated with a fall in chronaxy value.

The chronaximeter is a stimulator dedicated to the special purpose of producing square or rectangular pulses of various amplitudes and duration over a wide range, starting with those of short duration and of high amplitude (voltage or milliamperage) and extending down to long pulses of low amplitude. These machines are electronically configured to produce either constant voltage or constant current pulses for the purpose of uniformity throughout the examination. Constant current pulses are better tolerated by patients and produce smoother response. The constant voltage type is more painful and produces a jolt in the subject, causing movement that can affect the recording. Its use also requires much more skin preparation.

With the chronaximeter one first determines the rheobase of a specific muscle, after which one turns a dial, doubles the current (or voltage), and determines the chronaxy determined by finding the smallest pulse duration that maintains the contraction. The muscles presumed to be normal are tested first, followed by those that are suspect. In innervated muscle, the response to the stimulus depends on the integrity of the motor nerve supplying it. Muscle fibers without nerve supply are far less excitable than is nerve tissue. Consequently the chronaxy of denervated muscle is nearly 100 times larger than that of the innervated fibers.[9] The great increase in chronaxy found in denervated muscle is not caused by any alterations in the time constants of muscle fibers, but is really attributed to the fact that the nerve is no longer there to conduct and stimulate the muscle membrane depolarization through the neuromuscular junction apparatus.[21] The information assimilated from this type of electrical testing is in terms of degree of denervation or regeneration and, therefore, helps in prognostication. The rheobase value in denervated muscle usually falls below the normal in from 10 to 20 days after the insult and tends to remain low. If reinnervation does not occur within a reasonable time, the muscle atrophies and is gradually replaced by fibrous tissue. This is sometimes accompanied by a temporary gradual rise in rheobase, and then, later, the tissue loses excitability. Chronaxy value of completely denervated muscle, not atrophied, is between 50 and 200 times that of normal muscle. As fibrous tissue replacement of muscle takes place, chronaxy comes down to 100 times normal and usually remains at this level until the muscle becomes totally inexcitable. The presence of a chronaxy of over 50 times normal means denervation or complete muscle death.

In partially denervated muscle, the accuracy of values of chronaxy and rheobase obtained will depend on the relative depth of position of the affected fibers in relation to the stimulating electrodes. In the case of muscles supplied by the facial nerve, they are accessible and there is not nearly so much separation of affected and unaffected muscle fibers as there can be in a larger and deeper muscle.

During reinnervation of muscle, chronaxy begins to fall from the denervated value of about 100 times normal toward the normal level. This fall is sometimes preceded by a sharp rise to 200 or more times the normal. The fall in chronaxy does not usually happen until reinnervation is well advanced. It may fall gradually or abruptly. However, a considerable number of nerve fibers must have regenerated before chronaxy falls toward normal. In some cases, therefore, clinical signs of improvement can precede the drop in chronaxy. Some investigators[17] claim that a sudden rise in rheobase to two to three times the normal value precedes clinical recovery. These claims have been vehemently controverted, but Harris[9] believes that a rising rheobase in denervated muscle in good condition (without atrophy) often indicates impending recovery. After reinnervation, the rheobase falls slowly to normal levels.

Technique is very important in this type of objective study. Different examiners might disagree on the point of response, one seeing movement and the other not. This is the area of importance for the newer kind of equipment which may use transducers in the form of accelerometers or force gauges to read movement of muscle that is in-

Etiology of disruption of the facial pathophysiology of degeneration

visible to the naked eye. The light source during the testing can be critical too, when the eye alone is being trusted to observe.

STRENGTH-DURATION CURVE PLOTS

By far a more complete method of measuring excitability is the plotting of strength-duration (S-D) curves, which is no more difficult technically but is far more time consuming than chronaximetry. This curve relates the parameters of current amplitude and duration of pulse. Since the complete curve gives the rheobase and the chronaxy as well as a lot of other information, it is more useful. This makes chronaximetry, by itself, impractical, and so most electrodiagnosticians have taken to plotting the S-D curves for each of the facial muscles studied. Where there is any doubt, pure chronaximetry can be used to support the S-D curve accuracy. A normal nerve produces a characteristic curve with slight variations depending on whether the stimulator is constant current or constant voltage. If the impulse propagation in a nerve is impaired, the general level of the curve rises and its slope steepens. Each reduction in shock duration calls for a sharp increase in intensity needed for threshold response. For the very short duration pulses, the threshold becomes so high that response to the very shortest pulse is not obtained. If the impulse conduction is lost, as in degenerated nerve fibers, no response is obtained at tolerable intensities.

The S-D study is made by determination of the current required to produce minimal contraction at each of a wide range of pulse durations. One usually starts with the long-duration pulses of low amplitude in order to obtain the rheobase. The duration of the impulse is progressively shortened while the intensity is increased just enough to produce a contraction. The S-D curve is plotted with these pairs of values. The intensity of current is plotted as the ordinate, and the duration is laid out on the abscissa. This curve usually takes the form of a parabola (Fig. 9-1). In normal muscle, the nerves remain the most excitable component and the curve reflects the excitability characteristics of nerve. In denervated muscle, the curve reflects the excitability of muscle fibers rather than of the nerve components. One can read chronaxy directly from the curve by finding the rheobase and then referring to the duration (ordinate), which is at the point in the curve that is twice the rheobase. This is also useful.

Since alterations in the threshold values of excitation are most easily demonstrated with stimuli of short duration, one can confine the examination to these points only. This point of view was first propounded by Bauwens and constituted the basis of the nerve-excitability testing, which is a simple and sensitive study providing data that are reproducible and comparable.

S-D curves have the same applicability in facial nerve problems as they do in peripheral nerve injuries. They are particularly useful in Bell's palsy (Fig. 9-2) for indicating whether recovery is likely to be rapid or slow. This can prepare the patient for a long wait until regeneration and recovery take place. Changes involving facial nerve occur more rapidly than those in the limbs, and therefore the electrical tests can offer usable and valuable information earlier. If nerve conduction is still strong on the fifth day after the onset of paralysis and if the S-D curve shows no more than slight abnormality, a rapid recovery is to be expected since the lesion is mainly a neurapraxia. This was substantiated by C. B. Wynn Parry,[22] who studied a series of 54 patients with Bell's palsy by means of detailed electrodiagnostic examinations. The average duration

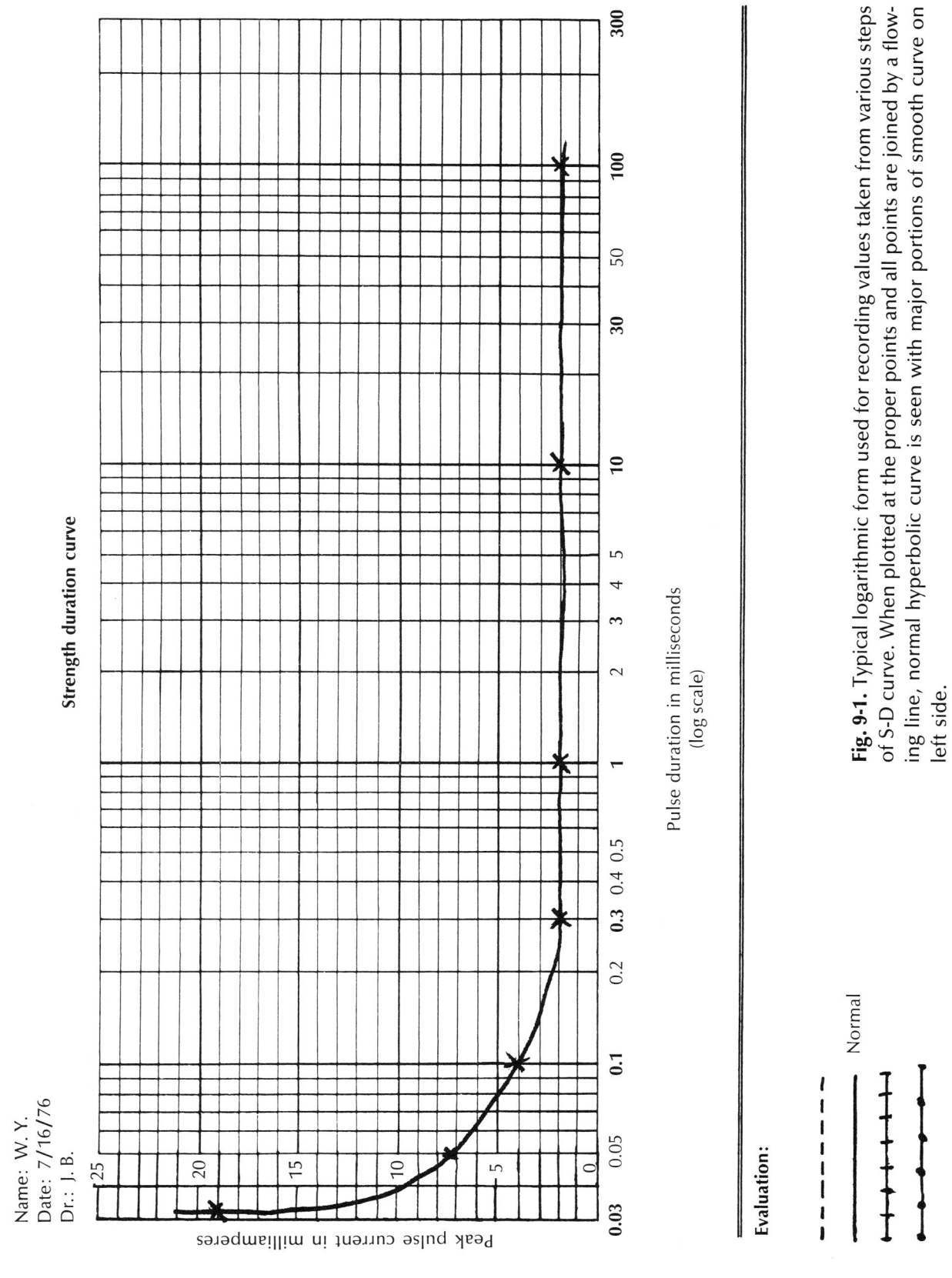

Diagnosing the site of nerve disruption by electronic methods

Fig. 9-1. Typical logarithmic form used for recording values taken from various steps of S-D curve. When plotted at the proper points and all points are joined by a flowing line, normal hyperbolic curve is seen with major portions of smooth curve on left side.

Etiology of disruption of the facial pathophysiology of degeneration

Strength duration curve

Name: P. E.
Date: 6/28/75
Dr.: T. P.

Peak pulse current in milliamperes

Pulse duration in milliseconds (log scale)

Evaluation: ------ Abnormal (Bell's palsy)

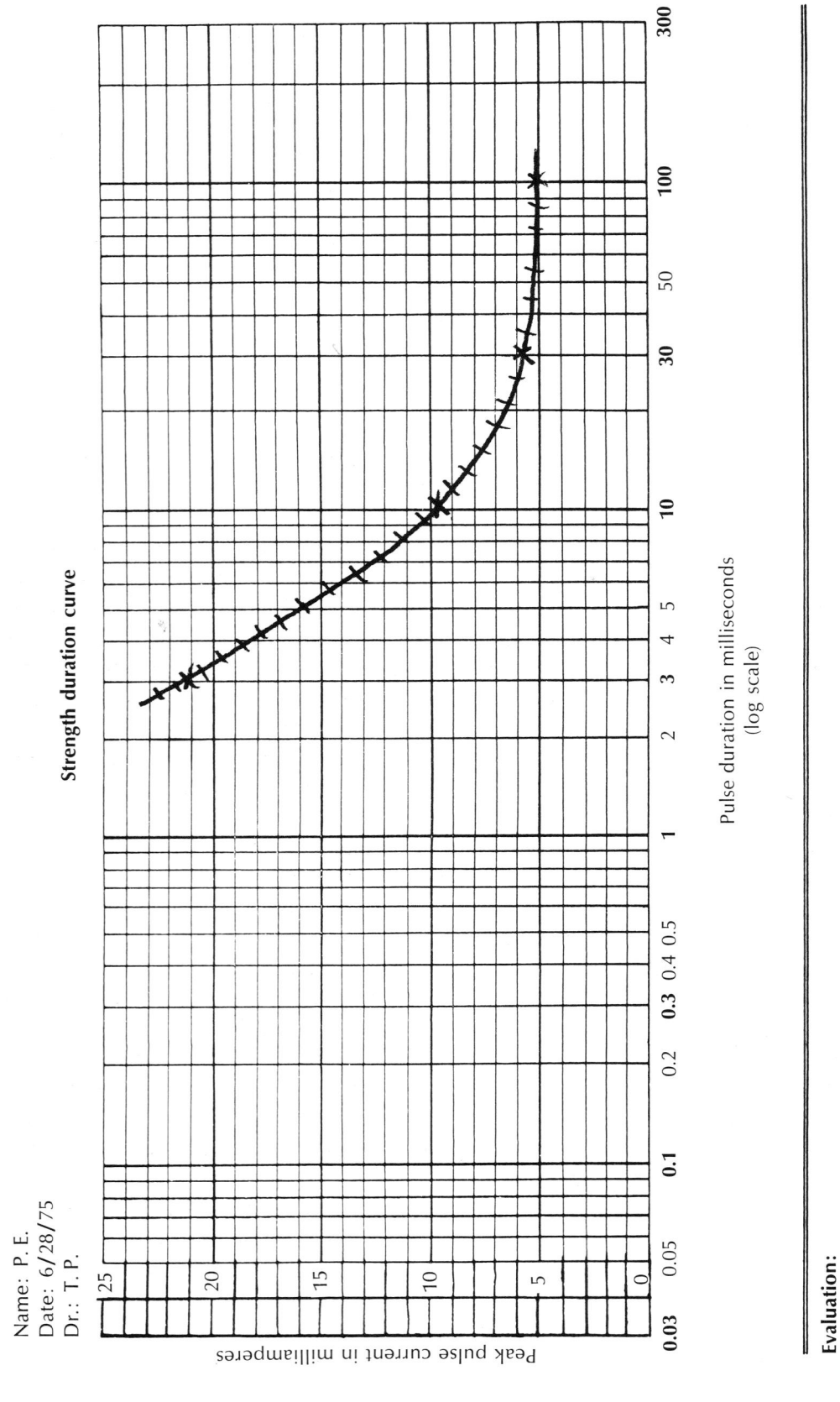

Fig. 9-2. Typically abnormal S-D curve plot made on same type of form as that in Fig. 9-1. In this instance, note higher threshold, pronounced shift of curve to right side, since there is no response to the very short duration pulses. Shortest pulse that produced a response was 2.6 milliseconds as compared to fractional durations noted in Fig. 9-1.

of illness from start to full recovery was 6.3 weeks. Voluntary movement appeared on an average in 16 days after onset. Twenty-five of these subjects showed normal S-D curves throughout the illness, 19 showed a higher slope of the left-hand part of the curve than normal, and 10 showed kinks and raises in threshold. To recapitulate, 29 of these patients showed some evidence of denervation despite rapid clinical recovery.

Fibrillations (to be discussed later) were found in one third of these patients. Serial curves demonstrate that degeneration is not progressive. Patients with complete degeneration show the usual changes in S-D curve during the regeneration period. The average time between first signs of reinnervation on the curve and the first signs of clinical recovery is 21 days. The rheobase of facial muscles is normally low, and because of this, denervated curves tend to be shifted more to the left than such curves in limb muscles.

CONDUCTION-LATENCY MEASUREMENTS

If injury to the nerve causes degeneration of the fibers, stimulation of the nerve distal to the lesion fails to elicit evoked potentials in the subservient muscles. Degenerative nerve lesions result in cessation of conduction in the peripheral part within 3 to 4 days.[7,18]

If injury causes neurapraxia, only transient, reversible paralysis is produced. Stimulation of the nerve trunk below the level of the lesion results in brisk contraction of the muscle throughout the period of paralysis. Collier[4] believes that when this happens, any lesion proximal to the stylomastoid foramen is nondegenerative or causes only minimal degree of denervation. Richardson and Wynn Parry[18] believe that if normal nerve conduction remains beyond 3 days of paralysis, it carries a good prognosis. If it extends beyond a week of paralysis, the outlook is excellent. This point of view is more valid in cases of trauma. In Bell's palsy, the onset is slower and a few weeks should go by before a bad prognosis is declared. Serial measurements should be made before one gets too optimistic.

To measure the latency, proceed as follows, starting on the normal side first. Place two monopolar or a single concentric needle electrode into the orbicularis oris or frontalis muscle, according to individual preference. Then stimulate the facial nerve percutaneously with a bipolar electrode placed over the pretragal or stylomastoid area. Use a supramaximal stimulus only. The purpose of this is to get all the functioning axons to conduct. The current is turned up slowly so as not to overtax the tolerance of the subject. If there is no further increase in the amplitude of the evoked potential with further increase in current applied, then that point starts the level of being supramaximal. Then you may advance the intensity of the stimulating current another bit to be sure that it is supramaximal. Readout on a storage oscilloscope or moving chart provides the record. A time base is inserted for measurements in milliseconds. Then repeat the same procedure on the affected side.

Conduction measurements provide relatively early evidence of denervation, since it has been shown that all conduction ceases in the distal segment of the nerve by the seventh day after nerve section.[7] Failure to obtain an evoked potential during the second week after the development of facial paralysis is strong evidence that denervation is complete. Of course, this conclusion is predicated on elimination of the possibility of equipment failure, which is, indeed, a rare occurrence. The presence of an evoked potential in a patient with facial palsy implies neurapraxia, even after a normal latency. Where the conduction latency is prolonged, careful examination during the following number of weeks usually demonstrates the presence of fibrillation potentials of denervation. In general, an increased latency means partial denervation, but the prognosis is ordinarily good in this type of case. This impression has been supported by reports from Langworth and Taverner[13] and Taverner.[20] In the early evaluation of Bell's palsy, the presence of an evoked potential with either normal or prolonged latency during the second week indicates a good prognosis, with partial or complete recovery. If there is no evoked potential, complete denervation is probably present and the prognosis is poor.

Taverner[20] reported a study in which a population of 167 patients were examined. They all had in common the fact that they had suffered with spontaneous facial nerve palsy. Also included were 16 cases of herpes zoster with facial nerve palsy. The following procedures were carried out on each:

1. Conduction-time (latency) measurements
2. Size of evoked potential
3. Threshold to stimulation
4. Presence of fibrillation potentials searched for

The first group of patients were examined at weekly intervals, but the later patients were seen daily from the day of onset of the paralysis. Later in the course of study, they were examined at weekly intervals and then monthly until the condition became static. Taverner divided this group into three subdivisions:

1. Those with no denervation
2. Those with complete denervation
3. Those with partial denervation

The first results established from these studies demonstrated that in a total of 254 observations, the mean value of latency for the right side was 2.7 milliseconds with a standard deviation (SD) of ±0.37. For the left side 2.7 msec (SD, ±0.35), and for the total observation 2.7 msec (SD, ±0.36). The mean plus three times the standard deviation is 3.8 msec. A round number of 4 msec. was then chosen as the upper limit of normal for the conduction times.

In the first group, in which there was no denervation, there were 47 patients. In each of them, the conduction time was less than 4 msec. every time it was measured. No fibrillations were found in any of the electromyographic samplings. Clinical recovery was complete after 6 months, and there was no "blink burst" (associated movements) activity noted or reported. In this group, movement began to reappear in from 1 to 11 days after the onset of paralysis. Mean time for this group to reach 25% recovery was 10 days, for 50% recovery it was 15 days, and for 75% recovery it was 18 days.

In the second group, in which denervation was complete, there were 57 patients, 22 of whom were seen during the first 2 weeks of the illness. The others were examined at intervals up to 14 months from the onset. In this group, excitability was completely lost after 4 days. The level of excitability remained near normal for the first 4 days, and then during the 24 to 48 hours of the fifth and sixth days the amplitude of the response dropped away rapidly and was followed by total loss of conduction. In none of the cases in this group was an evoked potential seen in response to stimulation on the seventh day or later. An important point to note was that the amplitude of the evoked

Diagnosing the site of nerve disruption by electronic methods

potential falls first, followed by the loss of conduction. Only after several months of recovery time was any response noted again. Twenty-six patients were seen more than 7 days from the onset. They all had complete paralysis and an inexcitable facial nerve. Another nine patients were first seen after they began recovering from paralysis, presumably after complete denervation had occurred. In them, the nerve was still inexcitable or delayed conduction was evident. In this group with complete denervation, the earliest return of a normal conduction time was at 11 months after the onset of the paralysis. In one patient the latencies were 6 msec at 6 months, 5 msec at 8 months and 3.5 msec at 11 months. Conduction time (Fig. 9-3) always returns to normal if the patients are followed up long enough (in Bell's palsy). The latency may become normal while the evoked potential is very low in amplitude, very widely dispersed in time, and quite abnormal. Clinical recovery of the orbicularis oris muscles varied from almost nothing to 40%. Many had strong contracture and associated movements ("blink burst" activity). Despite this, 16 of the 22 (73%) followed up for more than 1 year were very satisfied with the results.

For best results in early detection in the group developing total denervation, the first electrical examination should take place within 3 days from the onset of the palsy and thereafter daily, in order to observe that there is a rapid loss of response to electrical stimulation.

In the third group, sustaining partial denervation, there were 63 patients. The presence of denervation was established by the detection of fibrillation potentials or was inferred when associated movements appeared later on. In these people, a response to

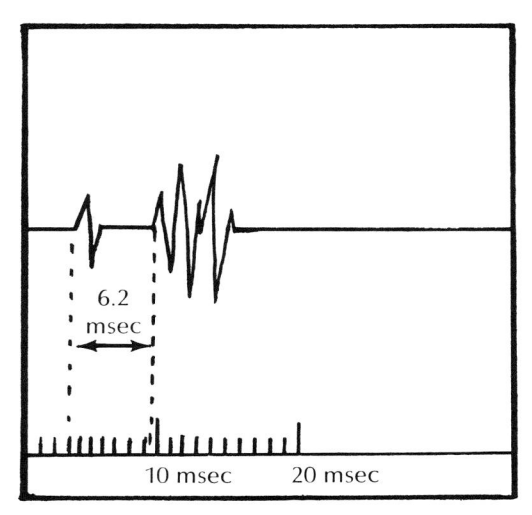

Facial nerve latency measurements
Latency = 6.2 milliseconds (abnormal)

Fig. 9-3. Schematic drawing of face of storage oscilloscope (Tektronix 564 series) recording during latency measurements. Upper line shows recording of an electrical stimulating pulse on left side and evoked muscle potential to right of it. Lower line is a display of calibrating signal in milliseconds. Every tenth one is taller. By projecting calibration signals upward to beginning of each potential, one can measure the delay in milliseconds. This one is 6.2 msec (abnormal) (up to 4 msec is normal).

Etiology of disruption of the facial pathophysiology of degeneration

electrical stimulation was always present and the conduction time remained unchanged or slowed considerably. The amplitude of the evoked potential was unaffected or decreased greatly for days or weeks. There was a tendency for the lengthening of conduction time from the second to the fourth weeks of the illness in the partial denervation group to be more striking and prolonged than in those patients with no denervation. When the conduction time is prolonged, it usually returns to normal within 4 weeks after the onset of the paralysis.

GROSS NERVE EXCITABILITY

In laboratories where there is minimal equipment, some form of gross nerve-excitability testing can be done. The facial nerve is percutaneously stimulated in the region of the stylomastoid foramen with square pulses of short duration, gradually made to increase in intensity. The amount of current required to obtain the minimum visible muscle contraction is recorded. The test is first carried out on the normal side. The threshold values of the affected side are compared to those of the normal side. Adequate equipment is necessary. It is also possible to use electrical transducers to sense the contraction in muscle and thereby to obtain a more accurate response. Any stimulator that can deliver short-duration square pulses may be used, provided that the intensity of the current may be measured. Automatic repetitive pulsing may be of some further help. A stimulator with high impedance, capable of producing at least 20 milliamperes (ma), and preferably of the constant current type is most desirable. Various observers use different pulse durations in their testing. Gilliatt and Taylor use 0.1 msec, Campbell and Cawthorne stimulate with pulses of 1 msec duration, and Richardson and Wynn Parry prefer 0.3 msec. However, it is agreed that differences in the threshold value of excitation become more observable at shorter durations. Stimulating electrodes may be monopolar with a distant inactive electrode, or they may be bipolar with an optimum separation of 2.5 to 3.5 cm. The commonplace differences of skin resistance and temperature as well as the variations in thickness of soft tissues between the electrodes and the nerve being studied, plus the few anomalies in anatomic course of the facial nerve, which occur in different patients, make it very difficult to set a standard for threshold intensity. In fact, it is virtually impossible. It not only is different from patient to patient, but also varies in the same patient from examination to examination. The best way to reach an acceptable technique is to compare the abnormal to the normal side at each examination. Laumans reported the average threshold intensity for the normal facial nerve in 459 patients as being 6.5 msec. Campbell reported his normals to vary between 3 and 8 msec in the normal facial nerve.

The absence of motor nerve excitability indicates an unfavorable prognosis, whereas normal excitability suggests the possibility of a good recovery. Since the excitability of a nerve is not lost abruptly and completely, one cannot merely assume that either one end of the gamut or the other is the true situation. Even the most severe lesions show only a decrease in excitability in the beginning and as the condition progresses, stronger and stronger stimuli are needed to elicit a response until a time may be reached where none is forthcoming even at 20 ma levels (the strongest that can usually be tolerated). In transection of a nerve, the process is very rapid, and excitability may disappear completely in 2 to 4 days. In the case of less serious lesions such as Bell's palsy, the progression is much slower or even may begin at a later time. Laumans reports observing complete loss of excitability in a case of Bell's palsy 11 days after the onset of the paralysis.

THRESHOLD TO ANODAL SIMULATION OF THE TONGUE

The sensation of taste is initiated in the taste buds on the tongue and palate. The afferent nerve fibers from these travel along several pathways to the brain. The majority of nerve fibers arising from the taste buds on the anterior two thirds of the tongue are found in the chorda tympani nerve and they pass with the facial nerve into the proximal part of the eustachian canal. Changes in taste associated with lesions of the facial nerve give additional information about the severity of the lesions. Krarup[10,15] described an apparatus that he developed and used that implements anodal unipolar stimulation of the lateral borders of the anterior two thirds of the tongue. The anode is applied to the lateral border of the tongue while the cathode is held in the hand. The apparatus can deliver varying currents up to 300 microamperes at a fixed potential gradient of 100 volts, direct current. The standard sensation in a normal subject is a sour, metallic taste at a current of 20 microamperes.

It has been demonstrated that in patients who suffer section of the chorda tympani at operation, 85% are unable to feel the stimulus on the affected side. Where a facial nerve has been severed during a parotid gland operation, the threshold to anodal stimulation is unaffected. In those who have Bell's palsy with neurapraxia and partial denervation, transient changes in the taste threshold may occur, but these are usually slight and the threshold rarely rises above 50 microamperes. In the series of patients described by Taverner, all patients in this group did not show loss of taste on the affected side. In his group of patients showing complete denervation, six of the eight people seen during the first 7 days after the onset of paralysis showed total loss of taste on the affected side, from the first observation. In these patients, complete loss of taste always preceded the failure of the facial nerve to respond to electrical stimulation. After 9 weeks, the taste threshold had returned to normal in most of the subjects in this group. There was some variation in two or three of the patients.

In those who suffered facial palsy after severe head injury, total loss of response to anodal stimulation may occur and is a guide to the severity of the lesion. If the threshold remains normal, satisfactory recovery of facial nerve function can be expected.

Electromyographic recording

The recording and analysis of electrical activity of contracting muscle provides information concerning the structure and functioning of the motor units. This permits one to possibly localize the site of the lesion affecting either the muscle or its innervation. Evidence is also frequently provided concerning the nature of the pathological process.

Muscle is used as the readout device for nerve in this type of testing. The nerve fibers that supply muscle are each the extension of a neuron within the gray matter of brain or cord, the terminal branches of which supply a large number of muscle fibers. The nerve cell and the muscle fibers it supplies are known as the motor unit, which also includes the neuromuscular junction. Upon contraction, the surface membrane of a muscle fiber undergoes depolarization, resulting in an electrical action potential, which can be recorded. The fibers of a motor unit contract fairly synchronously, but not quite because of the varying lengths of the terminal filament arborizations. This, therefore,

Etiology of disruption of the facial pathophysiology of degeneration

produces an algebraic summation of all the individual fiber diphasic waves. The end result can be fairly complex, nonsinusoid wave forms, which must be interpreted, and are known as motor-unit action potentials.

When the structure and function of the motor unit is affected by trauma or disease, the action potentials may have an abnormal configuration and the pattern of motor-unit activity during voluntary contraction may vary from the normal. In the healthy state, muscle fibers contract in response to activation by neurons and produce motor-unit action potentials. In neuromuscular disease, single muscle fibers may fire spontaneously, in which case, the potential recorded is closer to the diphasic wave form produced by cell membrane depolarization. The function of electromyography is to record and display the action potentials of contracting muscle fibers or motor units. The analysis of these potentials can be performed by the examiner on an "eyeball" basis plus the interpretation of sounds, or it can be done by employing sophisticated apparatus designed for the purpose (Fig. 9-4). It is, by chance, that all the electrical impulses recorded from muscle are within the audible frequency range of the human ear. Since the ear is a reasonably good frequency analyzer, it is possible to listen to the audio output

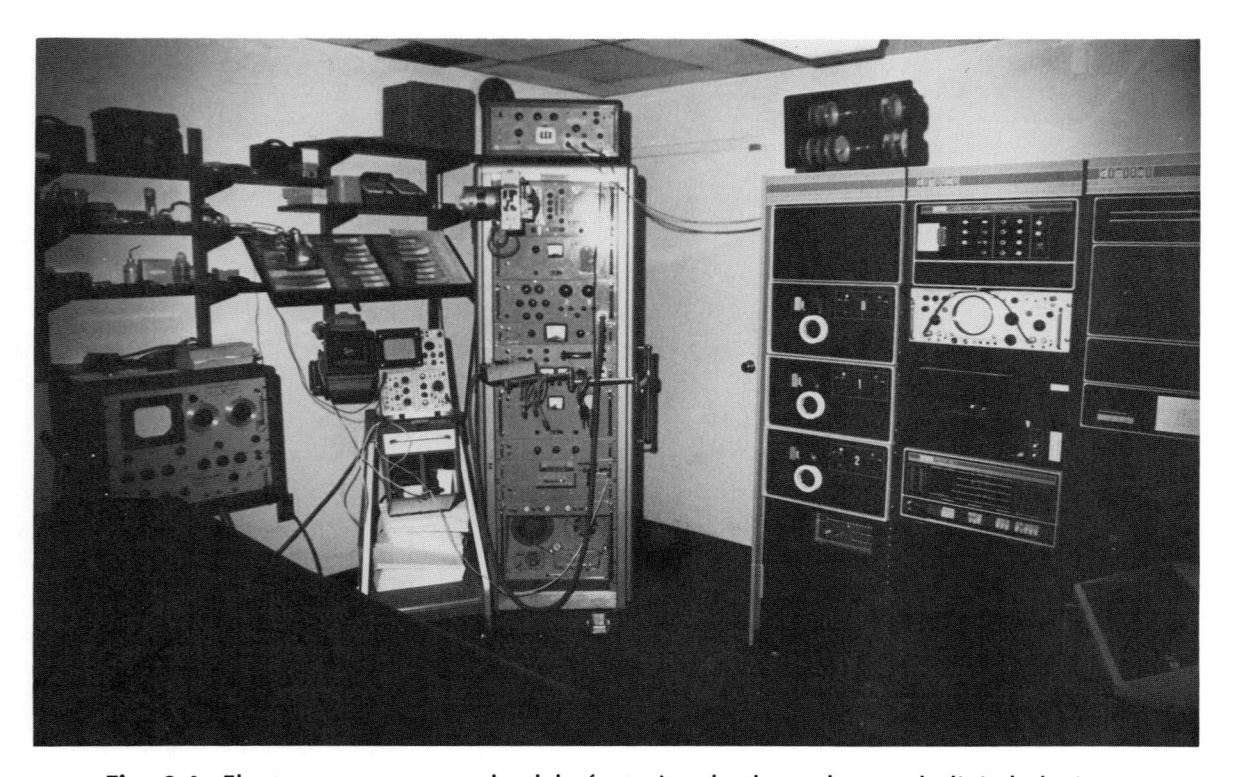

Fig. 9-4. Electroneuromyography lab featuring both analog and digital devices. PDP8I computer on right side of room does all mathematical analysis, pattern identification, autocorrelation and cross-correlation studies, Fourier series, integrations, averaging, and so forth. To the left of this instrument is analog device, which accepts data in analog form from patient and prepares it for digital conversion. Other instruments include a synthesizer for producing mathematical models, spectrum analyzer, amplitude discriminator, and calibrating instruments to maintain accuracy.

from the electromyographic equipment and to empirically differentiate different action potentials by identifying the sound while at the same time looking at the wave shapes on an oscilloscope that monitors that output.

Single muscle fiber output can be recorded with proper microelectrodes by fairly advanced techniques. In clinical practice, muscle action potentials can be more readily recorded through extracellular electrodes that are placed very close to the muscle cells. Potentials obtained in this manner are much lower in amplitude than those taken intracellularly. Therefore, amplification is necessary before the potentials can be displayed on an oscilloscopic screen. Skin electrodes may be used to record electrical activity from muscle, but one must remember that, in this case, one is summating the output of many motor units that are in the neighborhood. Surface electrodes are useful in spectral studies of large muscle areas, where no details of individual units are necessary. Individual units are best studied with extracellular electrodes during minimal contraction, which calls for the activity of only one or a few motor units.

The basic equipment required is available commercially and consists of one or more channels of differential amplification supported by a proper preamplifier up front, an audio amplifier with loudspeaker, a built-in constant-current stimulator, some sort of recording device such as a camera, tape recorder, or light writing paper plotter. Permanent tracings or photographs can only depict wave trains of very limited length, for study. Photography is mainly useful where a storage oscilloscope is part of the system. Moving picture cameras may be used to photograph longer wave trains if the transport speed of the film can be controlled. In recent years, computers have been implemented more frequently because of their tremendous capability to do rapid, complicated, mathematical analysis of the various wave forms and trains of potentials that occur in the functioning neuromuscular apparatus. Some of the newer laboratories have become quite advanced, as noted in Fig. 9-4, which is a picture of my personal installation. Note the complete computer with discs, tape transports, high-speed reader and punch, Decwriter, analog to digital converter, and laboratory peripherals. With proper softwear (programming), these machines are capable of fast on-line analyses such as pattern identification, amplitude measurements, autocorrelation and cross-correlation studies of individual potentials or trains, statistical mathematics as well as that of trend and resolution. Mathematical models can be worked out; evoked potentials can be quantified and averaged; phase and integration studies can be performed. The problem of using synchronization as a factor in determining the presence or absence of control losses is much facilitated by computer softwear application. There is no doubt that the future increase in accuracy and ease of application of complex investigations will be mediated through such apparatus, which can make a very competent examiner of a physician not versed in engineering and mathematics.

There are two types of activity recorded during electromyographic sampling. The first is spontaneous and the other is the result of voluntary activity.

Spontaneous activity. In the relaxed normal muscle, fibers are not in a state of contraction and there should be no electrical activity. If a few motor units are recorded, one must concede that there is incomplete relaxation. On occasion, there can be some small action potentials if the electrodes are near the end-plate zone. See Fig. 9-5.

1. A needle electrode inserted into a muscle evokes a discharge of action potentials that lasts for only a very brief period of time, no longer than a few seconds.

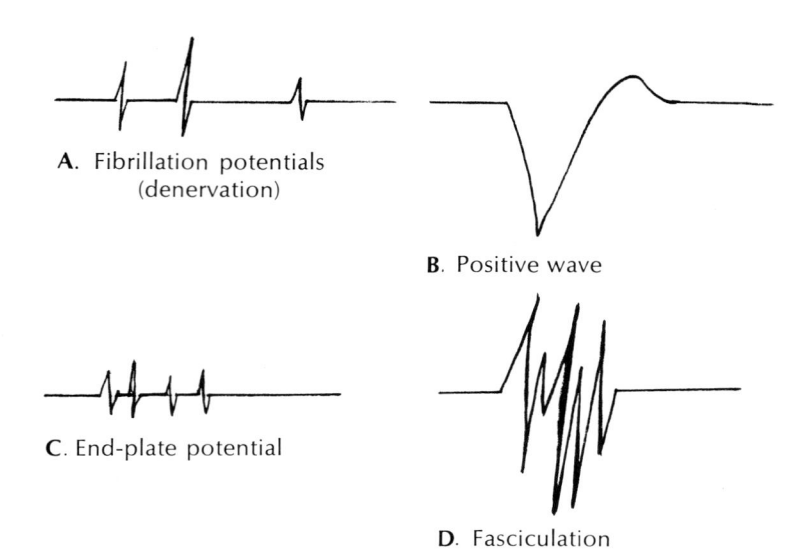

Etiology of disruption of the facial pathophysiology of degeneration

Fig. 9-5. Drawings of most important spontaneous potentials. **A,** Denervation potentials (fibrillations), low in amplitude and short in duration. **B,** Positive sharp waves. These have same significance as fibrillation potentials and indicate denervation. **C,** End-plate potentials occur around the neuromuscular junctions. They are normal and are result of physiochemical processes at this junction. **D,** Fasciculations are spontaneous polyphasic contractions usually associated with anterior horn cell disease, such as amyotrophic lateral sclerosis.

These are of low amplitude and short duration and are probably attributable to mechanical excitation of the muscle fibers as the electrode passes through. They are generally noted in normal muscle but are more pronounced in denervated muscle and last much longer. Certain of the myopathies demonstrate prolonged insertional activity.

2. The end-plate zone of muscle corresponds roughly to the point at which the nerve enters. When extracellular electrodes are placed in this area, two types of potentials may be recorded. The first is a short, rapidly recurring potential of up to 2 msec duration and 100 microvolts amplitude in the form of a monophasic negative discharge. These represent miniature end-plate potentials. They occur independently of the nerve impulse in a random manner. The other type of potential recorded from this area may be in the form of diphasic waves of longer duration and larger amplitudes. These may represent groups of nearly synchronous miniature end-plate potentials (Buchtal and Rosenfalk[1]).

3. Certain forms of spontaneous activity are of important clinical value. Perhaps the commonest is known as fibrillation. These forms are considered to be the electrical potential resulting from the spontaneous contraction of single muscle fibers and are particularly characteristic of denervated muscle. This potential is also reputed to be occasionally recorded from normal muscle or from myopathic fibers. However, because of their form, amplitude, and duration, they can be very easily misinterpreted in the clinical setting. The determination of whether or not a subject is completely relaxed makes it very difficult to establish what is spontaneous and what is volitional because of tenseness and fear. The fibril-

lation potential is small and has a duration of 0.5 to 1 msec and an amplitude of about 30 to 150 micro-volts. The waveform is diphasic and usually starts with an initial positive phase.[18] To appear, fibrillations usually require approximately 3 weeks after the onset of pathology. However, in the facial muscles, the time may be 7 to 8 days shorter.

4. Positive sharp waves are potentials that occur spontaneously and are of longer duration than the fibrillation but do have about the same amplitude. They consist of an initial positive phase followed by a prolonged negative phase. Total duration may be in the region of 10 msec. In general, they have the appearance of the standard sawtooth wave. Their origin is still a matter of debate.

5. Fasciculations are spontaneous contractions of groups of muscle fibers or of motor units large enough to produce visible contraction of muscle. They are associated mainly with degeneration of the anterior horn cells in conditions such as amyotrophic lateral sclerosis. However, there are some instances in which they are found in the healthy state, such as in myokymia. Fasciculations are frequently found in facial muscles, where they may be a sign of severe fatigue.

6. A spontaneous discharge of action potentials can occur in the condition called "myotonia," which is a form of myopathy. These are characterized by a waxing and waning of the sounds so as to create the sound of a dive bomber. They can occur at needle-electrode insertion, or when one plucks at the needle while it is in the muscle. It is also not uncommon to record these characteristics potentials during relaxation after a voluntary contraction. Rapidly changing pulse repetition rate is the outstanding feature of the electrical activity in myotonia. The individual potentials that make up the myotonic discharge vary considerably in parameters. Some are of short duration and low amplitude, whereas others are hard to differentiate from motor-unit action potentials recorded during volition. Some of these potentials can resemble the positive waves that are seen frequently in denervation. One source of difficulty encountered while facial muscles are examined is that occasional spasms can resemble myotonic activity.

The identification of spontaneous potentials is extremely important in electrodiagnostic work, especially about the facial muscles. The low-amplitude, short-duration muscle action potentials in the facial muscles strongly resemble the spontaneous fibrillation potential and must be carefully evaluated before a decision as to which they are is made. The computer analysis of these potentials makes it far easier and more dependable. End-plate noise may also be mistaken for fibrillation activity if the electrodes are near the motor point.

Voluntary activity. Motor-unit action potentials are the main product of volitional contraction while electrodes are in place in the muscle. They are the result of the slightly asynchronous firing of all the muscle fibers (cells) in a single motor unit. All these potentials algebraically summate with the potentials formed by other motor units, and these together form a large mass of wave forms that completely obliterates the isoelectric line in the sweep of the beam across the oscilloscopic screen. The result of this process is the interference pattern, which indicates that contraction is good and strong or weak, with all shades and degrees in between. The parameters of the patterns recorded are directly affected by electrode geometry capacitance and structure as well as by the wave-shaping circuitry within the amplifiers. The innervation ratio of the motor unit also predetermines the wave shape. This ratio is determined by the number of muscle cells that are supplied by a single axon. Large muscles whose function is mainly antigravitational have a large innervation ratio; as many as 1500 to 2500 cells per axon. Muscle that have critical function, such as the external ocular muscles, have small innervation ratios; as few as 4 to 6 cells per axon. This latter arrangement better synchronizes all the individual cellular potentials and is the probable reason for the fine control prevalent in these structures.

It might be well to repeat that healthy muscle is electrically silent immediately after the insertion potentials cease. In disease states, the action potentials are altered in a fashion so as to demonstrate the particular pathological condition, for example, the case of various myopathies, specifically muscular dystrophy. The pathological condition causes the degeneration and loss of some of the muscle fibers of the motor units, thereby lowering the innervation ratio that is effective. As a result, fewer fiber potentials combine to form the motor-unit action potential and it becomes smaller in amplitude. Duration of this action potential also diminishes because fewer potentials are being summated from the cells. Another effect from the pathological disorder is a loss of pulling strength in each of the motor units. Therefore, to perform a given action, more units must be recruited and as many more action potentials are recorded from relatively weak movements. If 10 motor units were required to perform a given motion during the normal state, now three times the number of motor units must be used to produce the same strength. This is manifested in the recording of full interference patterns during minimal contractions. The patterns demonstrate low amplitudes. This is referred to as dystrophic activity. In the normal muscle, the pattern increases only as the volitional contraction increases. The rise in amplitude and the increase in complexity of the interference patterns are not linearly related, but there is some correlation. Quantitative methods for such comparisons are available but are not useful for work in the facial muscles. Only in the case of studying a muscle for possible transposition, such as the temporalis, does one use quantitation in the face.

When a peripheral or cranial nerve supplies peripheral muscle and becomes affected for whatever the reason, it becomes no longer possible for the maximum number of motor units to fire during volitional contraction. Thus the interference pattern is altered in a degree referable to the depth of involvement of the nerve. In a mild peripheral neuropathy, only some of the fibers are affected. In a neurapraxia, most of the cells may be unable to contract. Where many of the axons of a nerve are involved in the pathological condition, the electrical output varies in many ways. If the disease is on the rise, less and less motor unit activity will be forthcoming, resulting in poor interference patterns, combined with a neuropathic type of activity that is of high amplitude and short duration. If regeneration is taking place in the nerve and new axons are being formed, their conduction velocity will be slow, and therefore the duration of the resulting potentials will be increased and the number of phases greater. The latter are referred to as polyphasic forms. Many varying shades of interpretation can be made by the expert electromyographer and valuable information concerning the state of the condition propounded. The finer details of the interpretation of the electrical parameters is available in some of the texts previously referred to.[15]

A common finding in a recovering facial paralysis in which regeneration is occurring is crossed innervation, which is also referred to as "blink burst." This phenomenon occurs when regenerating axons fail to achieve the same pathway to the muscle innervated before the episode and, instead, grow to another muscle supplied by the same trunk. When a particular facial muscle needs to contract, the somal cell that supplies the axon, fires, but if the axon goes to a different muscle, then associated movements result. For instance, blinking an eyelid may also cause quivering of the lip or movement of the platysma or frontalis muscle. These uncalled for movements can be monitored by placing electrodes in all three muscles at the same time and asking the patient to contract one of the muscles chosen. By recording from all muscles at the same time, one can identify the associated movements.

Summary

One may use electrodiagnostic testing to great advantage in the evaluation of the patient with a paralyzed face. The applications are as many as the imagination of the examiner and his knowledge of neurophysiology. There are some pitfalls in a number of the techniques used if the greatest care and the most conservative approach is not used in interpretation.[1]

REFERENCES

1. Buchtal, F., and Rosenfalk, P.: Spontaneous electrical activity of human muscle, Electroencephalogr. Clin. Neurophysiol. **20**:321-336, 1966.
2. Campbell, E. D. R., et al.: Value of nerve excitability measurements in prognosis of facial palsy, Br. Med. J. **2**:7, July 1962.
3. Cawthorne, T., and Haynes, D. R.: Facial palsy, Br. Med. J. **2**:1197, 1956.
4. Collier, J.: Symposium on facial paralysis: rationale for operative treatment, Proc. Roy. Soc. Med. **52**:1075, Dec. 1959.
5. Cromwell, L., Weibell, F. J., Pfeiffer, E. A., and Usselman, L. B.: Biomedical instrumentation and measurements, Englewood Cliffs, N.J., 1973, Prentice-Hall, Inc.
6. Geddes, L. A., and Baker, L. E.: Principles of applied biomedical instrumentation, New York, 1968, John Wiley & Sons, Inc.
7. Gilliatt, R. W., and Taylor, J. C.: Electrical changes following section of facial nerve, Proc. Roy. Soc. Med. **52**:1080, 1959.
8. Greiner, G. F., Klotz, G., and Gaillard, J.: Le traitement de la paralysie faciale après fracture du rocher, Ann. Otolaryngol. **78**:89, Jan.-Feb. 1961.
9. Harris, R.: A study of electrical excitability of muscle. Doctoral thesis. Leeds, 1950.
10. Jonkees, L. B. W.: The causes and surgical treatment of intratemporal facial paralysis, Germ. Med. Monthly **3**:77, 1958.
11. Kettel, K.: Peripheral facial palsy, Copenhagen, 1959, Munksgaard.
12. Krarup, B.: Electrogustometry: method for clinical taste examinations, Acta Otolaryngol. **49**:294-305, 1958.
13. Langworth, E. P., and Taverner, D.: The prognosis in facial palsy, Brain **86**:465-480, 1963.
14. Lapicque, L.: La chronaxie et ses applications physiologiques. In Physiologie générale du système nerveux, Paris, 1938, vol 5, p. 23.
15. Licht, S.: Electrodiagnosis and electromyography, ed. 3, New Haven, Conn., 1971, Elizabeth Licht.
16. Laumans, E. P. J.: Nerve excitability tests in facial paralysis, Arch. Otolaryngol. **81**(5): 478-485, May 1965.
17. Pollock, L. J., Golseth, J. G., and Arieff, A. J.: Changes in chronaxie during degeneration and regeneration of experimentally produced lesions, Surg. Gynecol. Obstet. **81**: 451, 1945.
18. Richardson, A. T., and Wynn Parry, C. B.: Theory and practice of electrodiagnosis, Ann. Phys. Med. **4**:41, Feb.-May, 1957.
19. Taverner, D.: Prognosis and treatment of spontaneous facial palsy, Proc. Roy. Soc. Med. **52**:1077, 1959.
20. Taverner, D.: Electrodiagnosis in facial palsy, Arch. Otolaryngol. **81**:470-477, May 1965.
21. Watts, C. F.: Effect of curare and denervation upon electrical excitability of striated muscle, J. Physiol. **59**:143, 1924.
22. Wynn Parry, C. B.: Strength-duration curves. In Licht, S.: Electrodiagnosis and electromyography, ed. 3, New Haven, Conn., 1971, Elizabeth Licht.

10 Diagnosing the site of nerve disruption by anatomical location

VINCENT R. DiGREGORIO

A careful analysis of the seventh nerve innervation to muscles and organs can lead to pinpointing of the site of nerve disruption. A chart accompanying this chapter facilitates the localization of the signs and symptoms of facial palsy and the site of nerve obstruction.

Diagnosing the site of nerve disruption by anatomical location

The accurate diagnosis of a site of disruption in the facial nerve requires thorough knowledge of the anatomy and function of the seventh nerve. A precise anatomical localization of the site of the lesion can be made by a careful history and a thorough clinical examination. The clinical correlation between the physical findings and the findings at operation or pathological examination is accurate. In the following pages the anatomy, motor, sensory, secretory, and reflex functions of the seventh nerve are correlated with the clinical findings of lesions at various levels of the facial nerve pathways.

Anatomical description

The facial nerve, as it exits from the brainstem at the caudal border of the pons, has two roots—the motor division or facial nerve proper, and the sensory division or nervus intermedius. These two divisions have little in common from a physiological viewpoint. The motor division supplies the muscles of the face, scalp, and auricle; the buccinator, platysma, stapedius, and stylohyoid; and the posterior belly of the digastric muscle. The sensory division transmits fibers of taste from the ipsilateral anterior two thirds of the tongue by the chorda tympani, transmits fibers of taste from the soft palate by the palatine and greater petrosal nerves, and transmits preganglionic parasympathetic fibers to the submandibular and sublingual salivary glands, the lacrimal gland, and the glands of the nasal and palatine mucosa.

The facial nerve, together with the nervus intermedius and the eighth cranial nerve (vestibulocochlear nerve), then passes through the internal auditory meatus to gain access to the temporal bone. It passes through the bony facial canal or fallopian aqueduct, has a characteristic bend (genu) at the mastoid where the geniculate ganglion appears, and exits through the stylomastoid foramen. Within the facial canal, the nerve to the stapedius muscle and the chorda tympani are given off. As the facial nerve emerges from the stylomastoid foramen, it passes through the parotid gland dividing into terminal branches that supply the muscles of facial expression, platysma, and stylohyoid and the posterior belly of the digastric muscle. The levator palpebrae superioris muscle is the only superficial muscle of the face not supplied by the seventh nerve.

Etiology of disruption of the facial pathophysiology of degeneration

At the geniculate ganglion, the greater superficial petrosal nerve is given off to carry two groups of fibers—taste fibers, which are distributed to the mucous membranes of the palate, and preganglionic parasympathetic fibers, which proceed to the pterygopalatine ganglion and which stimulate lacrimation. The nervus intermedius continues along with the facial nerve and gives off the chorda tympani just prior to the emergence of the facial nerve at the stylomastoid foramen. The chorda tympani proceeds medial to the incus through the middle ear and finally joins the lingual branch of the trigeminal nerve to reach the tongue. In addition to supplying taste to the anterior two thirds of the tongue, it also carries secretory motor fibers originating in the superior salivary nucleus for the submandibular and sublingual glands.

Appraisal of facial nerve function

In examination of the seventh nerve function, with particular reference toward ultimate facial reanimation, we are primarily concerned with motor function. However, an evaluation of the sensory, secretory, and reflex function may also contribute to localization of the precipitating lesion and perhaps modify the surgical approach and objectives.

EXAMINATION OF MOTOR FUNCTION

Examination of motor function essentially consists of an appraisal of the action of the muscles of facial expression. The face is first examined in repose for asymmetry or abnormality of muscle mass. The height and width of the palpebral fissure is estimated as is height of the corners of the mouth. Furrows of the brow are inspected for equality of depth and length. The nasolabial fold is examined from both anterior and lateral orientation for suggestion of flatness.

A dynamic examination of facial musculature is made in which the patient is asked to activate various muscles individually and then in unison. The patient is asked to frown, to wrinkle his forehead, and to raise his eyebrows. Next he is asked to close his eyes individually and then bilaterally, tightly, and then against resistance. He is asked to smile as hard as he can, show his teeth, grimace, blow out his cheeks, purse his lips, whistle, and then retract his chin. Some patients may be able to voluntarily wiggle their ears and scalp. The contractions of the platsyma may be tested by having the patient open his mouth against resistance. In all of these maneuvers, the tone of the muscle is evaluated by palpation and any atrophy or fasciculations are noted. Clinical evaluation of the function of the stylohyoid muscle and the posterior belly of the digastric muscle is difficult, but weakness or paralysis of these muscles may be suggested by a history of regurgitation of food.

EXAMINATION OF SENSORY FUNCTION

Clinical examination of sensory function of the seventh nerve is difficult and is limited to evaluation of taste and an appreciation of low tones. There are four basic pure tastes—sweet, salty, sour, and bitter—and all are closely associated with sense of smell.[2] When the need to test taste arises, this can simply be performed by assessment of an appreciation for salt. A few grains of salt are placed on the protruded tongue and gently massaged into the tongue. The patient cannot be allowed to talk or to swallow, as in each of these maneuvers the tongue is retracted into the mouth, a movement that

Diagnosing the site of nerve disruption by anatomical location

allows saliva to bathe the tongue, carrying salt to the opposite side of the tongue or to its posterior third. The patient then indicates when he has perceived a taste by holding up a finger and nodding yes or no to each of several tastes suggested.

Stapedius muscle dysfunction may also be inferred if the patient claims increased sensitivity to sounds, especially low tones (hyperacusis). However, this is a very subjective observation and may not be perceived even with complete central seventh nerve paralysis.

EXAMINATION OF SECRETORY FUNCTION

Disorders of secretory function can usually be evaluated by history and by observation. Increased lacrimation is usually apparent, and decreased lacrimation usually elicits bitter complaints from the patient. Relative amounts of lacrimation may be tested clinically by insertion of strips of filter paper in each lower lid and observation of the amount of moisture elicited (Schirmer's test).

Reflex secretion of tears may be elicited by stimulation of the cornea or by mechanical or chemical stimulation of the nasal mucosa (the nasolacrimal reflexes).

Decreased salivary secretions by the submandibular or submaxillary glands is usually elicited by history. There are also methods of clinically stimulating submaxillary or submandibular secretion by placement of flavored substances on the tongue and observation of secretions beneath the tongue. However, these are awkward examinations that require subjective interpretation of taste by the patient and relative unilateral estimations of the quantity of saliva by the examiner.

EXAMINATION OF REFLEX FUNCTION

Numerous reflex activity in which the facial nerve participates has been described.[17] The activity may be tested in a thorough examination of the facial nerve.

The *orbicularis oculi reflex* may be elicited by percussion of the glabella, outer aspect of the supraorbital ridge, or the margin of the orbit. A reflex bilateral contraction of the orbicularis oculi follows. The afferent portion of the reflex is mediated by the trigeminal nerve or by the facial nerve as proprioceptive impulses, and the efferent portion is by the facial nerve. A sudden loud noise may elicit reflex bilateral closure of the eyes. This is known as the *auditory-palpebral reflex* and may be more noticeable in the lid closest to the noise. The afferent loop of the reflex is mediated by the vestibulocochlear nerve and the efferent loop by the facial nerve. A reflex closing of the eyes in response to a strong light or a menacing gesture is known as the *blink reflex,* with the afferent loop dependent on an intact optic nerve and visual cortex. A painful stimulus to the face also produces reflex closing of the eyes, known as the *trigeminal reflex,* and is mediated through the afferent trigeminal nerve.

Percussion of the upper lip or the side of the nose stimulates a reflex contraction of the ipsilateral quadratus labii superioris and caninus muscle. This is known as the *orbicularis oris reflex.*

Diagnosis of impaired seventh nerve function

Armed with a thorough knowledge of the anatomy and the motor, sensory, secretory, and reflex functions of the intact seventh nerve, one can make an accurate diagnosis of the site of the lesion in impaired seventh nerve function. I shall discuss abnor-

Etiology of disruption of the facial pathophysiology of degeneration

mal facial nerve function from a central to a peripheral orientation. Clinical findings are summarized in Table 1.

Central or supranuclear lesions

In central or supranuclear facial paralysis, there is paresis of the lower portion of the face with relative sparing of the upper portion. The paresis is rarely complete and the site of the lesion is always in the contralateral cerebral cortex to the clinically involved musculature. The sparing of the upper facial musculature is explained by the bilaterality of the cortical representation of forehead and eyelid musculature in the cerebral cortex (Fig. 10-1).[6,11] In most instances the orbicularis oculi always contracts simultaneously. In fact, unilateral winking must be learned and may be impossible for some in-

Table 1. Signs and symptoms denoting site of facial nerve interruption

Signs and symptoms	Location of lesion
I Contralateral signs in face Limited to one side of face Upper face not affected Volitional and emotional types of paralysis	1. Supranuclear lesions
II Complete ipsilateral peripheral paralysis Decreased lacrimation Hyperacusis Loss of taste, anterior two thirds of tongue Decreased salivary secretion Clinical complex modified by adjacent structures involved in midbrain	2. Nuclear or intrapontine lesions (Fig. 10-2, A)
III Complete ipsilateral peripheral paralysis findings similar to II Usually associated with middle-ear signs	3. Cerebropontine angle lesions (Fig. 10-2, B)
IV Complete ipsilateral peripheral paralysis findings similar to II	4. Lesions between internal auditory meatus and geniculate ganglion (Fig. 10-2, C)
V Complete ipsilateral peripheral paralysis Normal lacrimation Usually associated with pain at tympanic membrane	5. Lesions at the geniculate ganglion (Fig. 10-2, D)
VI Complete ipsilateral peripheral paralysis findings similar to II Normal lacrimation	6. Lesions between geniculate ganglion and nerve to stapedius (Fig. 10-2, E)
VII Complete ipsilateral peripheral paralysis Normal lacrimation Normal hearing	7. Lesions between nerve to stapedius and chorda tympani (Fig. 10-2, F)
VIII Complete ipsilateral peripheral paralysis Normal lacrimation Normal hearing Normal taste Normal salivary secretion	8. Lesions distal to origin of chorda tympani (Fig. 10-2, G to I)

Diagnosing the site of nerve disruption by anatomical location

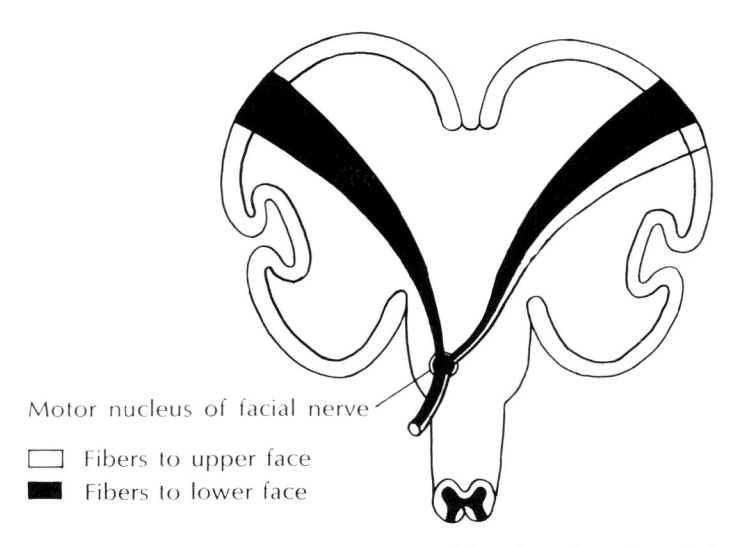

Fig. 10-1. Bilaterality of cortical representation of forehead and eyelid musculature, the pathway of different neurons from cerebrum to seventh nerve nucleus. In supranuclear facial paralysis there is paresis of lower portion of face with relative sparing of upper portions. Site of lesion is always in contralateral cerebral cortex to clinically involved musculature.

dividuals. The musculature of the lower face, however, is represented in the contralateral cortex only; thus the tremendous variety of activity and expression elicited by these lower muscles, which are often used asymmetrically, is accounted for.

As a result, a cortical or subcortical lesion in one cerebral hemisphere will result in paralysis of the lower face on the contralateral side with relative sparing of the upper portion. There is, however, a great deal of variation in facial innervation and central types of lesions may affect from one third to one half the lower facial musculature in any individual. The frontalis is almost always spared. The lower portion of the orbicularis oculi, however, may be weakened, and a widened palpebral fissure may be produced on the affected side. Lagophthalmos and epiphoria may be the only sign of dysfunction in the upper face. The lower portion of the face is smoother than normal, and the nasolabial fold is flattened out.

There are two distinct types of central facial paresis, a volitional and an emotional type. The volitional type is most pronounced in attempts at volitional contraction and becomes most apparent on attempts to bare the teeth or to smile. However, there is preservation of motion associated with involuntary spontaneous activity such as smiling or crying. The lesion producing this variety of central paresis is located in the cerebral cortex or in the subcortical pathways. In the emotional type of central paresis, the deficit is apparent only upon spontaneous emotional activity such as smiling and crying. The patient has no difficulty with voluntary motion of the lower face. The etiology of this type of lesion remains obscure but is probably a deep-seated lesion located in the basal ganglia, thalamus, or hypothalamus, adjacent to the centers controlling emotional activity.[13] There is a wide variety of lesions responsible for both central type of paralysis such as neoplasms, vascular lesions, degenerative changes, and inflammatory lesions of the motor cortex, internal capsule, and basal ganglia.

Etiology of disruption of the facial pathophysiology of degeneration

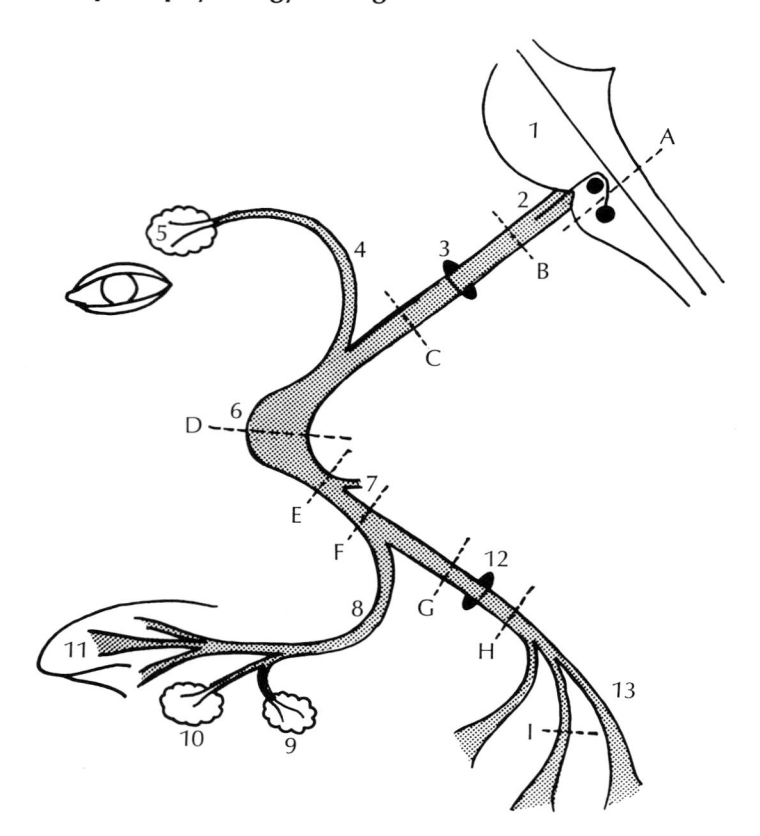

Fig. 10-2. **1**, Pons. **2**, Facial nerve. **3**, Internal auditory meatus. **4**, Greater superficial petrosal nerve. **5**, Lacrimal gland. **6**, Geniculate ganglion. **7**, Nerve to the stapedius muscle. **8**, Chorda tympani. **9**, Submaxillary salivary gland. **10**, Submandibular salivary gland. **11**, Tongue. **12**, Stylomastoid foramen. **13**, Peripheral motor distribution of the facial nerve.

A, Nuclear or intrapontine lesion. **B**, Lesion between pons and internal auditory meatus (cerebropontine angle lesion). **C**, Lesion between internal auditory meatus and geniculate ganglion. **D**, Lesion at geniculate ganglion. **E**, Lesion distal to the geniculate ganglion. **F**, Lesion distal to nerve to stapedius muscle. **G**, Lesion distal to chorda tympani. **H**, Complete peripheral nerve lesion. **I**, Peripheral intrafacial lesion.

NUCLEAR OR INTRAPONTINE LESIONS (Fig. 10-2, A)

Lesions with the substance of the pons may affect the facial nucleus, its intrapontine tract, or its contiguous structures. They produce complete, peripheral types of paralysis. The clinical picture is modified by the contiguous structures affected. For example, the abducens nucleus is in proximity to the facial nucleus in the pons, and its tract loops around the facial nucleus. Intrapontine lesions affecting both these structures result in a complete peripheral type of seventh nerve paralysis with an ipsilateral paralysis of lateral gaze. In pure seventh nerve lesions, sensory and secretory functions are intact. Nuclear lesions may be caused by a number of etiological factors.[4] Facial paralysis is seen in multiple sclerosis and is perhaps the only lower motor neuron manifestation of the disease. Poliomyelitis, the classical lower motor neuron inflammatory disease, may also involve facial palsy as the only manifestation of the disease.[12] Congenital aplasia or hypoplasia of the intracranial nuclei and neurons is seen in the peripheral type of palsy as in the Möbius syndrome.[9] Neoplasms, vascular lesions, and syringobulbia complete the etiological picture.

LESIONS BETWEEN THE PONS AND INTERNAL AUDITORY MEATUS (CEREBROPONTINE ANGLE LESIONS) (Fig. 10-2, B)

Between the pons and internal auditory meatus, the facial nerve lies within the meninges and in close association with the acoustic nerve. Lesions in this area produce a complete peripheral type of paralysis together with tinnitus, deafness, and vertigo. The nervus intermedius is frequently involved, producing loss of secretion of the submandibular and submaxillary gland with associated loss of taste in the anterior two thirds of the tongue.

Unilateral facial palsy originating in this area is most frequently caused by an acoustic neuroma. Other cerebropontine neoplasms such as meningioma may also be implicated. Bilateral facial palsy of this type is most commonly caused by basal meningitis such as meningeal carcinomatosis and tuberculous meningitis.

INTRACANALICULAR LESIONS

Clinical signs of facial nerve involvement within the facial canal are dependent on the level of interruption.

Lesions occurring between the internal auditory meatus and geniculate ganglion (Fig. 10-2, C). This distance is very small and lesions occurring at this exact junction are rare. A peripheral type of paralysis can be expected together with involvement of the nervus intermedius. There is, therefore, loss of ipsilateral taste to the anterior two thirds of the tongue and a loss of lacrimation and submandibular and submaxillary gland salivary secretion. There may also be hyperacusis, since the lesion is proximal to the branching off of the nerve to the stapedius muscle.

Lesions at the geniculate ganglion (Fig. 10-2, D). The Ramsay Hunt syndrome[10] is illustrative of a lesion at this location. This syndrome, also known as geniculate neuralgia, is a herpetic eruption (herpes zoster) of the geniculate ganglion. All the above symptoms are present in addition to pain in the region of the eardrum. Because the lesion is distal to the branching off of the greater superficial petrosal nerve, there is no disturbance in lacrimation. There may be vesicles present in the eardrum or external auditory meatus in the acute stages of Ramsay Hunt syndrome.

Lesions distal to the geniculate ganglion (Fig. 10-2, E). Lesions at this location are also manifested by peripheral facial palsy, loss of taste, and decreased salivation, but lacrimation is spared because the lesion is distal to the origin of the greater superficial petrosal nerve.

Lesions distal to the stapedius muscle (Fig. 10-2, F). In this situation there is again a peripheral type of facial palsy with loss of taste to the anterior two thirds of the tongue and decreased salivary secretion. However, hyperacusis and decreased lacrimation are not found.

Lesions distal to the corda tympani (Fig. 10-2, G). In this situation, there is only a peripheral type of facial palsy with no accompanying disability.

Lesions of the facial nerve between the internal auditory meatus and the stylomas-

Etiology of disruption of the facial pathophysiology of degeneration

toid foramen (intracanalicular lesions) are caused by a number of etiological factors.

Infectious processes from adjacent structures are common in this area. Facial palsies secondary to otitis media, chronic mastoiditis, or cholesteatoma are frequent.[13] The nerve is not rarely injured in mastoid or middle-ear surgery. Facial palsy secondary to hemorrhage into the facial nerve or facial canal in hypertensive adults and children has been described.[3]

Landry-Guillain-Barré syndrome, sarcoidosis, mumps, porphyria, leprosy, and osteitis fibrosa within the facial canal have all been described as causing facial palsy in this area.[7]

PERIPHERAL NERVE LESIONS (Fig. 10-2, H)

Lesions affecting the facial nerve after emerging from the stylomastoid foramen produce purely motor manifestations and are represented by total ipsilateral facial muscle paralysis. Lacrimation, hearing, and salivary secretion are intact. When complete, there is paralysis of the forehead and brow, drooping eyebrows, inability to close the eyes (lagophthalmos), escape of tears, epiphoria, Bell's phenomenon (in attempting to close the eye on the affected side, the eyeball is seen to turn upward and slightly outward), the nose is flattened or deviated to the opposite side, ironing out of the nasolabial fold, and sagging of the corner of the mouth. The patient is unable to raise his eyebrow, wrinkle his forehead, frown, close his eye, laugh, smile, show his teeth, whistle, pucker, blow out his cheek, or retract his chin on the affected side. The patient has difficulty retaining liquids in his mouth, and food tends to accumulate in the flaccid cheek while the patient is eating. Saliva may drip from the depressed angle of the mouth. All these deficiencies become much more pronounced upon animation of the face when any asymmetry would become more obvious.

Causes of seventh nerve paralysis distal to the stylomastoid foramen are trauma of various kinds, including surgical trauma, involvement with tumors (especially parotid tumors), and neuritis.

Idiopathic unilateral facial paralysis is classically known as Bell's palsy. Exposure to a cold draft such as riding in an open car or sleeping next to an open window has been implicated as an etiological factor, as has herpetic involvement. In Bell's palsy, the injury to the facial nerve occurs with edema and subsequent compression of the nerve at the stylomastoid foramen or within the facial canal.[14,15] Involvement of the chorda tympani and thus loss of taste may occur, although this is not usual (10% of cases in Miller's study).[12] Complete recovery is the rule, although partial or complete facial paralysis may occur. In Taverner's[16] series about half of the patients made a complete recovery.

PERIPHERAL INTRAFACIAL LESIONS (Fig. 10-2, I)

Peripheral intrafacial lesions of the facial nerve rarely result in appreciable permanent paralysis because of the numerous interconnections between branches and because the facial muscles receive innervation from the facial nerve at their posterior aspect. It is said that injuries to the facial nerve distal to a perpendicular dropped from the lateral canthus of the eye rarely produce permanent disability. Exceptions to this rule are the temporal branch to the frontalis muscle, which is vulnerable because of its great independent length, and the mandibular branch, which has few interconnections with other divisions of the facial nerve. Occasionally, an individual who has received and apparently recovered from a rather insignificant facial laceration develops a rather distressing syndrome of posttraumatic tics. These are involuntary contractions of the facial muscles not mediated by emotion. They are most commonly seen in involuntary contractions of the upper lip and cheek after trauma to the buccal branches and involuntary contractions of the upper and lower lids after trauma to the temporofacial branches. This phenomenon usually becomes manifest 2 to 3 months after injury when the initial laceration appears to be well healed without undue scar formation.

This is a difficult problem to treat, and complete relief may only be obtained by sectioning the involved branches and substituting complete or partial paralysis of the musculature involved. Nonsurgical therapy may include the use of an antispasmodic drug or tranquilizers in an effort to deal with what some consider a major emotional component of this syndrome. The use of local anesthesia or alcohol injection of the muscle units involved is frequently followed by a gradual recurrence of the symptoms.

An interesting allied clinical entity is the appearance of the *syndrome of crocodile tears*[8] after minor or major facial nerve trauma. In this syndrome, food or other gustatory stimulation results in paroxysmal lacrimation called "crocodile tears." The myth of crocodile tears refers to the remorseful shedding of tears by a crocodile when devouring its victim. The mechanism involved parallels posttraumatic tics, in that traumatized fibers that normally reached the submaxillary gland through the chorda tympani nerve are misdirected, during regeneration, to the lacrimal gland through the greater petrosal nerve. The misdirected fibers then mediate a misdirected clinical response to an appropriate stimulus.

Another clinical syndrome associated with previous injury to the facial nerve is the gustatory hyperhidrosis syndromes. In this disorder, reddening and profuse sweating occurs on half the face while the patient is eating. This has been called the auriculotemporal syndrome. When the same symptoms are widespread, involving half the face and, in addition, the neck, upper back, and chest associated with a sensation of warmth in the affected areas, the symptom complex is known as the chorda tympani syndrome. The auriculotemporal syndrome is common after supportive parotiditis or accidental or surgical trauma of the parotid gland.[5] The etiological mechanism of misdirected regeneration of fibers is postulated to be the same as in the syndrome of crocodile tears.

REFERENCES

1. Boyer, F. C., and Gardner, W. J.: Paroxysmal lacrimation and its surgical treatment, Arch. Neurol. Psychiatry **61:**56, 1949.
2. Clarke, E. C., and Dodge, H. W., Jr.: Extraolfactory components of flavor, J.A.M.A. **159:**1721, 1955.
3. Clarke, E., and Murphy, E. A.: Neurological manifestations of malignant hypertension, Br. Med. J. **2:**1319-1326, 1956.
4. Carter, S., Sciarra, D., and Merritt, H. H.: The course of multiple sclerosis as determined by autopsy—proven cases, Res. Publ. Assoc. Res. Nerv. Ment. Dis. Proc. **28:**471-511, 1950.
5. Converse, J. M.: Surgical treatment of facial injuries, ed. 3, Baltimore, Md., 1974, The Williams & Wilkins Co.
6. Daley, R. F.: New observations regarding the auriculotemporal syndrome, Neurology **17:**1159-1168, 1967.
7. Dandy, W. E.: Physiological studies following extirpation of the right cerebral hemisphere in man, Bull. Johns Hopkins Hosp. **53:**31-51, 1933.
8. De Wardener, H. E., and Lennox, B.: Cerebral beriberi (Wernicke's encephalopathy): review of fifty-two cases in a Singapore prisoner of war hospital, Lancet **1:**11-17, 1947.
9. Ford, R. F.: Paroxysmal lacrimation during

eating as a sequel of facial paralysis, Arch. Neurol. Psychiatry 29:1279-1288, 1933.
10. Henderson, J. L.: The congenital facial diplegia syndrome: clinical features, pathology and etiology. Brain 2:381-403, 1939.
11. Hunt, J. R.: On herpetic inflammation of the geniculate ganglion, J. Nerv. Ment. Dis. 34:73-96, 1907.
12. Lauer, E. W.: Ipsilateral facial representation in the motor cortex of macaque, J. Neurophysiol. 15:1-4, 1952.
13. Kettal, K.: Surgery of the facial nerve, Arch. Otolaryngol. 84:99-109, 1966.
14. Miller, H.: Facial paralysis, Br. Med. Bull. 3:815-819, 1967.
15. Monrad-Krohn, G. H.: On the dissociation of voluntary and emotional innervation in facial paresis of central origin, Brain 47:22, 1924.
16. Morris, W. M.: Surgical treatment of Bell's palsy, Lancet 1:429, 1938.
17. Morris, W. M.: Surgical treatment of facial paralysis, Lancet 2:558, 1939.
18. Taverner, D.: Bell's palsy: a clinical and electromyographic study, Brain 78:209, 1955.
19. Weingrow, S. M.: Facial reflexes, Arch. Pediatr. 50:234, 1939.

ADDITIONAL READINGS

Brain, Lord W. R., and Walton, J. N.: Brain's Diseases of the nervous system, ed. 7, New York, 1969, Oxford University Press.

Dejong, R. N.: The neurological examination, ed. 3, New York, 1970, Paul B. Hoeber Medical Division, Harper & Row Publishers, Inc.

Forster, F.: Clinical neurology, ed. 3, St. Louis, 1973, The C. V. Mosby Co.

Haymaker, W.: Bing's local diagnosis in neurological diseases, St. Louis, 1969, The C. V. Mosby Co.

Jacklin, H. N.: The gusto-lacrimal reflex (syndrome of crocodile tears), Am. J. Ophthalmol. 61:1521, 1966.

Luhan, J. A.: Neurology—a concise clinical textbook, Baltimore, 1968, The Williams & Wilkins Co.

PART III

CONTEMPORARY CONCEPTS IN FREE NERVE AND MUSCLE GRAFTING

11 Reinnervation and regeneration of striated muscle

JOANNA HOLLENBERG SHER

Described in detail is the reconstitution of striated muscle when the nerve impulse is restored. Regeneration of muscle fibers after degeneration is initiated by myoblasts, probably derived from the satellite cells normally present in muscle. These cells fuse to form tubules and eventually normal striated muscle fibers. Investigative evidence shows that muscles have great regenerative powers.

Reinnervation and nerve implantation

Reinnervation is the essential process whereby denervated muscle may be reanimated. The following review summarizes considerable evidence that experimentally denervated muscle will accept innervation by collateral sprouting from remaining intact axons or by an implanted nerve, and that reinnervation occurs commonly in human degenerative diseases of the motor neuron or peripheral nerve. Just as denervation severely affects the structure and function of the muscle fiber, reinnervation by a foreign nerve profoundly influences the physiological reactions of the fiber as well as the biochemical characteristics of the contractile protein itself.

EXPERIMENTAL REINNERVATION

The idea that muscle fibers might become reinnervated after losing their innervation was first proposed in 1885 by Exner,[16] who suggested that if a muscle is innervated by two nerves and one is sectioned, the denervated fibers become reinnervated somehow by the remaining intact nerve. Experiments in which muscles were partly denervated by sectioning of nerve roots at one level supported this thesis by showing recovery of function of some of the denervated fibers.[27,60] This recovery was not complete, but the muscles usually regained most of their lost weight and the majority of their contractile capacity. The early work of van Harreveld demonstrated an increase in the size of motor units in partially denervated muscle, substantiating the idea that the fibers were reinnervated by functioning nerve fibers from adjacent units.[56] That this occurred by collateral nerve sprouting was shown in a morphological study of partly denervated rat muscle.[12] The sprouting nerve fibers were seen to enter empty nerve sheaths and follow them down to their end plates. Hoffman suggested at this time that a chemical substance, possibly an unsaturated fatty acid arising from degenerating myelin, promoted axon sprouting.[28] The hypothesis that sprouting factors are manufactured by the denervated target tissue and are neutralized by substances brought to the nerve endings by axoplasmic transport, is supported by the fact that nerve sprouting

---

I wish to express gratitude to Dr. S. A. Shafiq for advice, to Mr. R. Simowitz for photographic assistance, and to Mr. Henry Veal for the histological and histochemical preparations.

ceases when the original number of nerve endings is restored. In work on reinnervation of salamander skin, interruption of axoplasmic flow by colchicine in one nerve allowed sprouting of fibers from adjacent nerves, demonstrating the presence of "antisprouting" factors, which are carried down the axon.[10] Correlation of collateral nerve branching with the development of large motor units, with absolute terminal innervation ratios increased to four or five, was reported by Hatsuyama.[25] Reinnervation of human muscle fibers undoubtedly occurs as a continuing process in denervating diseases. Spontaneous recovery of function of facial muscles after seventh nerve section has been observed in a few cases and was attributed to reinnervation by regenerating nerve fibers from injured masticator nerves.[55]

In 1953, Edds[13] concluded from the experiments done up to that time, that a few days after partial denervation of a muscle, subterminal branches sprout from the remaining intact intramuscular axons. These branches appeared to penetrate empty Schwann cell sheaths left by the degenerated nerve fibers and to grow down within them to the denervated end plates, resulting in neurotization of the muscle fiber.

DELAYED REINNERVATION

Gutmann and Young[23] investigated the effect of delayed reinnervation on the completeness of the process. They were able to show that enforced delay in reinnervation allowed increased fibrosis to occur in the muscle, diverting the sprouting axons and often preventing them from reaching the motor end plates. It was suggested that in this situation, new end plates might be formed. Reinnervation was less complete when delayed than when allowed to progress immediately and rapidly.

NERVE IMPLANTATION AND FORMATION OF NEW END PLATES

Some early work by Elsberg and Steindler[30,92] indicated that a nerve implanted into denervated muscle will form connections so that stimulation of the nerve causes muscle contraction. Further histological studies[1,22,36] showed that under these circumstances new end plates are formed. Although several end plates may be seen on one muscle fiber after reinnervation, only one contains cholinesterase and therefore presumably only one is functional. The cholinesterase is apparently induced by the arrival of a healthy terminal axon at the neuromuscular junction.

Usually, implantation of a nerve into an innervated muscle will not result in the formation of any new motor end plates. However, local injury of muscle fibers may induce them to accept additional innervation.[65] One may experimentally induce hyperneurotization, or the establishment of dual innervation of muscle, by injuring the original nerve to a muscle and simultaneously implanting a foreign nerve, or it may occur by collateral sprouting in a partly denervated muscle at a time when the original nerve is regenerating.[19] In a study of reinnervation in the tibialis anterior of the rat, Gwynn and Aitken[24] demonstrated both the formation of new end plates and the reinnervation of original ones. The time required for the formation of new motor end plates after experimental nerve implantation was as long as 120 days. However, in a study that may have considerable practical implication, Fox and Thesleff[17] found that if a nerve is implanted into a muscle several weeks before the muscle's own nerve is transected, new neuromuscular junctions may be formed as early as 2 days after denervation.

ELECTRON MICROSCOPY OF REINNERVATED MOTOR END PLATES

Electron microscopical observations on denervation and reinnervation of motor end plates in mouse foot muscle have shown that under the best conditions for reinnervation, new motor end plates are not formed.[44] In the first 3 weeks after nerve section the axon terminals disappeared from the synaptic clefts, which became flattened, and the Schwann cell processes retracted from the subneural apparatus. The secondary synaptic clefts became shortened and widened. After 3 weeks, axon sprouts surrounded by Schwann cell processes appeared in the neuromuscular junctions. Gradual reorganization of the regenerating end plates occurred over the next 12 weeks. Recovery of function was noted at 8 to 10 weeks, a time when the primary synaptic clefts still appeared shallow and the terminal axons remained morphologically immature. The formation of new end plates (in contrast to the reinnervation of old ones) has not been studied ultrastructurally. It has been postulated that they may follow the stages of embryonal development of neuromuscular junctions, with thickening of the muscle surface membrane in the future primary synaptic cleft, shallow new secondary clefts, and small terminal axons.[53]

EFFECT OF REINNERVATION AND CROSS-INNERVATION ON MUSCLE FIBER TYPES

An important aspect of reinnervation in striated muscle is the effect of the reinnervating nerve fibers on the physiological function and histochemical appearance of the reinnervated muscle fibers. Buller, Eccles, and Eccles[4] showed that reinnervation of a slow muscle (soleus) by the nerve to a fast muscle (flexor hallucis longus) and vice versa, in the cat, reversed the contractile properties of the reinnervated muscles. Thus, stimulation of the nerve of the flexor hallucis longus made to supply the soleus produced a fast contraction, and stimulation of the soleus nerve made to supply the flexor hallucis longus resulted in slow contraction of that previously fast muscle. Repetition of this experiment, with added histochemical characterization of the fibers, showed that the soleus muscle fibers were transformed from having strong staining for oxidative enzymes and relatively weak staining for glycolytic enzymes (type I) to having the staining characteristics of type II fibers, with "low oxidative and high glycolytic pattern."[43] Reverse changes occurred in the originally mainly type II flexor hallucis and flexor digitorum longus muscles. Control muscles in this study were simply reinnervated by their original nerves and showed no change in contraction speed or in proportions of fiber types. However, in both reinnervated and cross-innervated muscle, larger than normal groups of fibers of one type were observed (type grouping). Another study of guinea pig soleus reinnervated by nerves to fast muscles confirmed the speeding of isometric contractile properties of the muscle. Histochemically this was accompanied by the appearance of a variable number of type II fibers (as determined by ATPase staining) in the previously all–type I muscle. Stains for oxidative enzymes showed staining intermediate between type I and II intensities in many fibers.[42]

TYPE GROUPING

Human muscles are a mixture of type I and II fibers, which form a checkerboard or mosaic pattern in cross section (Fig. 11-1). "Type grouping," or the presence of larger than normal groups of fibers of the same histochemical type, is commonly seen in bi-

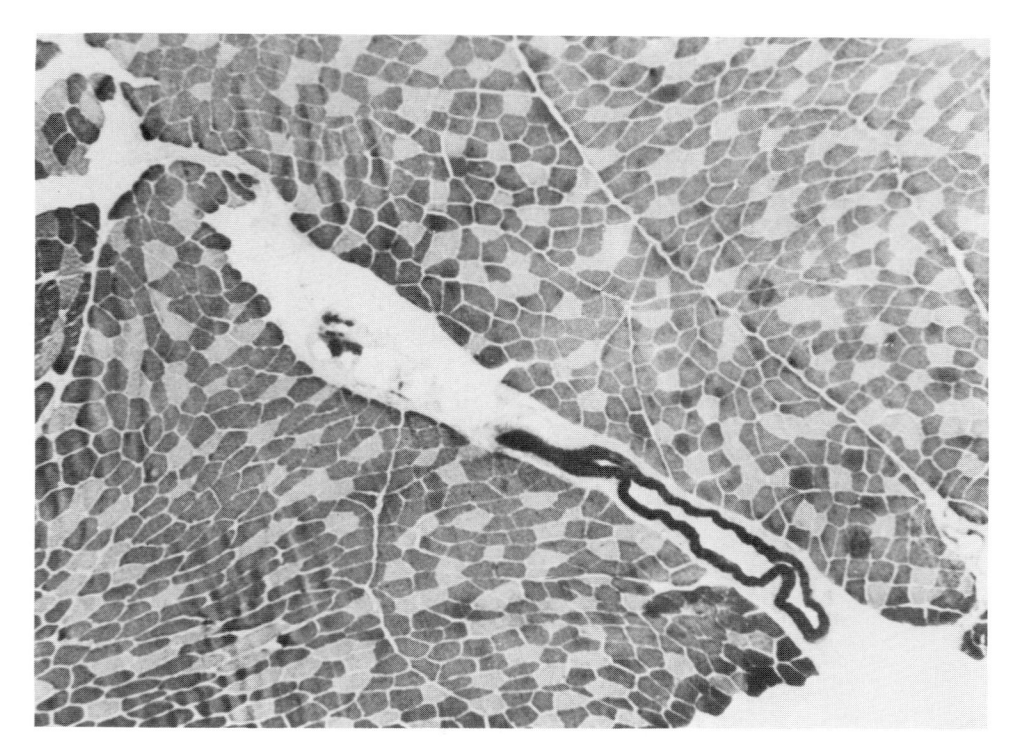

Fig. 11-1. Cross section of normal human muscle stained for ATPase showing checkerboard or mosaic pattern of dark (type II) and light (type I) fibers. (125×.)

opsies of human muscle in denervating diseases (Fig. 11-2). As we know from cross-innervation experiments that the axon determines the histochemical and physiological characteristics of the muscle fiber, and other experiments have confirmed that motor units are histochemically homogeneous,[14] it appears likely that type grouping is a result of collateral sprouting of healthy axons to reinnervate adjacent denervated fibers. This process would result in the formation of larger and larger groups of histochemically similar fibers as the motor units enlarged, because of the loss of axons with collateral sprouting of the few remaining ones to reinnervate the muscle fibers close by. The same mechanism explains the "size grouping," or presence of large groups of both atrophic and hypertrophic fibers, in muscle from patients with progressive denervating diseases (Fig. 11-3). As motor units enlarge by the addition of contiguous fibers, depending on whether they are finally denervated or remain reinnervated, they form large groups of small or large fibers respectively. Experimental support for this explanation of type grouping was provided by a study of reinnervation of guinea pig muscle, in which muscle reinnervated after nerve section and suture showed pronounced type grouping associated with extensive branching of subterminal axons.[31] Similar results were reported in experiments on rat leg muscle, after transection and resuturing of sciatic nerve.[61] Warszawski et al. followed regrowth of axons into leg muscle of rats after sciatic nerve crush and observed new axons reaching the muscle fibers by day 14, with complete reinnervation by day 33.[59] The normal checkerboard pattern did not disappear until day 28, and clear type grouping was not observed to be reestablished until 42 days after nerve crush. These experiments clearly demonstrated the lag period between reinnervation and the histochemical transformation of the muscle fibers.

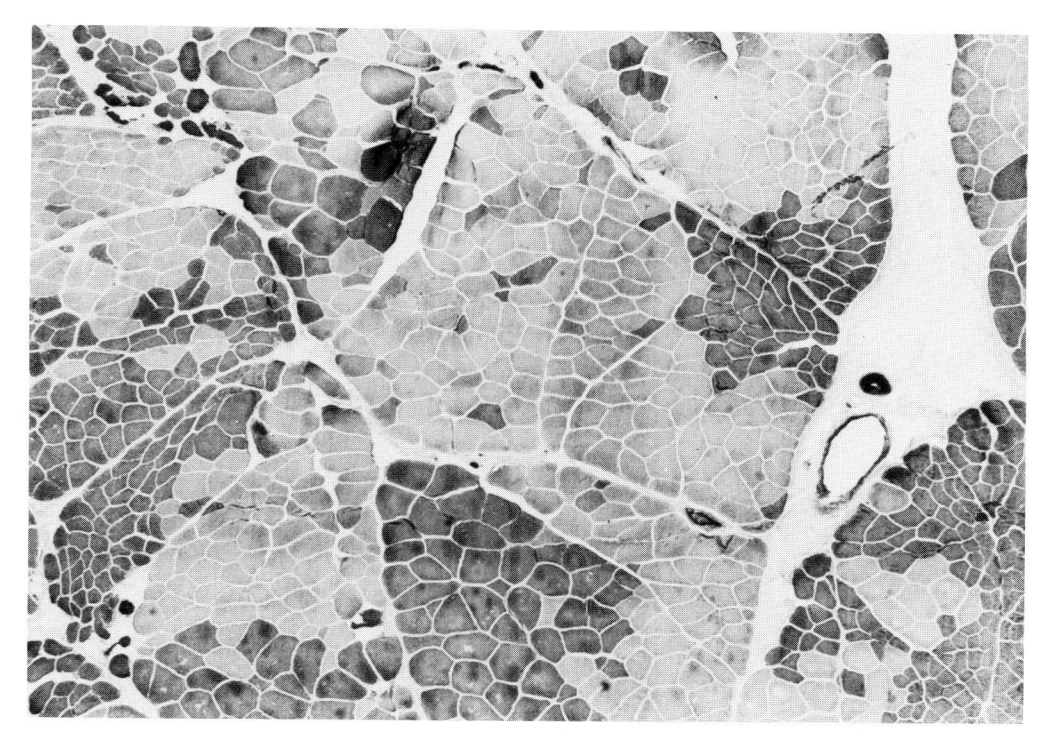

Fig. 11-2. Cross section of biopsy specimen of skeletal muscle stained for myosin ATPase from patient with peripheral nerve disease. Note absence of checkerboard pattern and presence of "type grouping," that is, large groups of both type I and type II fibers. (125×.)

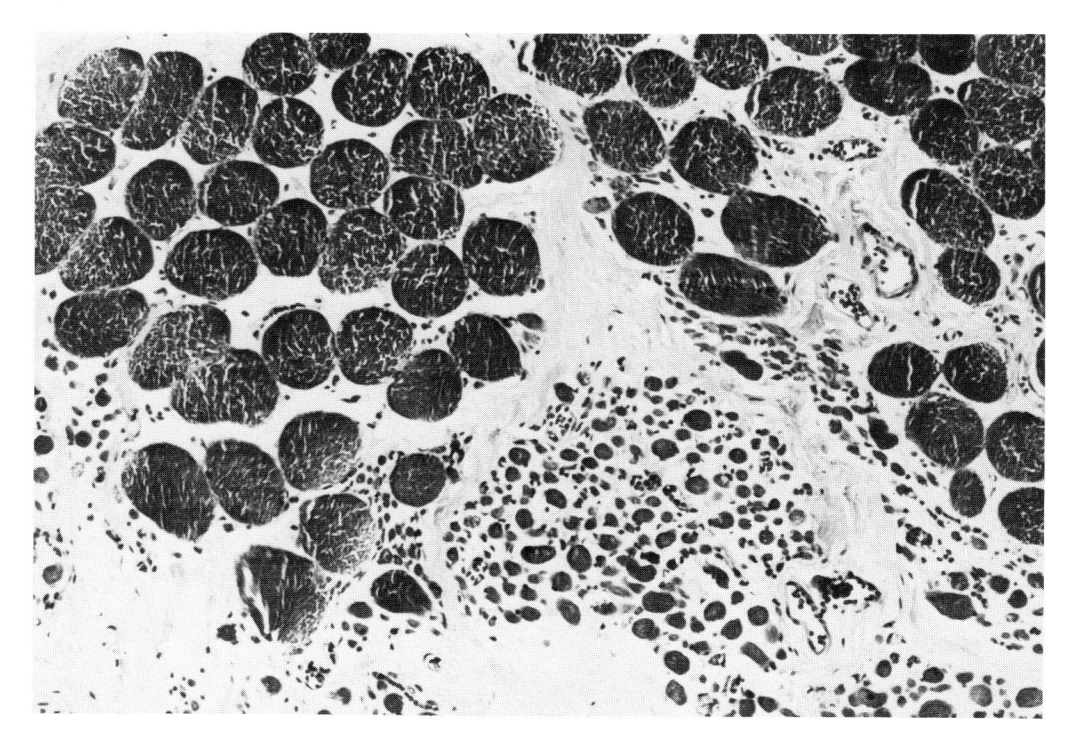

Fig. 11-3. Cross section of biopsy specimen of muscle showing groups of both large and atrophic fibers, from patient with motor neuron disease. (Trichrome stain, 500×.)

Kugelberg et al.[32] mapped motor units in denervated and reinnervated rat muscle. Their results, which are of great significance in understanding muscle biopsy changes in human denervating diseases, showed the expected correlation of type grouping with reinnervation. In muscle reinnervated and then redenervated (a circumstance probably happening frequently on a small scale in human neuromuscular disease), there was type grouping of both atrophic and normal-sized fibers. Without redenervation the atrophic fibers were histochemically heterogeneous.

A detailed study of human muscle biopsies, from patients with neuromuscular disease, confirmed the correlation of the presence of type grouping with an increase in the terminal innervation ratio, a measurement reflecting the size of the motor unit.[38] Thus in both human and animal studies, it has been established that the formation of larger than normal groups of muscle fibers of one histochemical fiber type is a result of collateral axon sprouting with reinnervation, and a corollary of enlargement of the motor unit in human neuromuscular disease.

EFFECTS OF CROSS-INNERVATION ON MYOSIN

The changes occurring in muscle after denervation and cross-reinnervation involve the biochemical structure of myosin itself. Guth et al.[20,21] showed that the myosin ATPase of fast muscle fibers in the rat is acid-labile and alkali-stable, whereas that of slow fibers was alkali-labile and acid-stable. After reinnervation of the slow fibers of the soleus by a nerve to a fast muscle, and vice versa, the pH lability of myosin ATPase changed in the reinnervated muscle. Further, electrophoretic analysis of myosin from fast and slow muscles shows distinct patterns, indicating that they are different proteins, each with its own characteristic subunits. Myosin from cross-reinnervated slow fibers becomes electrophoretically like fast muscle myosin, and, conversely, myosin from fast muscle reinnervated by the nerve to the slow soleus, changes to the slow type of myosin.[46] Thus myosin protein synthesis is altered by changing muscle innervation, demonstrating a neural effect on gene expression in the muscle cell. Jean, Guth, and Albers[30] showed that the observed change from slow to fast myosin is associated with the appearance of an additional peptide band (88,000 daltons) in cross-innervated soleus myosin (after tryptic digestion). This peptide is not normally seen in electrophoresis of soleus myosin but is characteristically released from fast myosin after tryptic digestion. These authors state that it is likely that there is a difference in the primary structure of the two types of myosin and that they are transformed from one to the other by a process of neural regulation of myosin synthesis.

REINNERVATION OF MUSCLE SPINDLES

Muscle spindles, which degenerate very slowly after denervation, will regenerate experimentally in newborn rats and become reinnervated in 14-day-old rats. If the denervation and reinnervation is done in mature animals whose muscle is fully differentiated, new spindles will not form, but those still present may be reinnervated.[64]

Regeneration of striated muscle
CONTINUOUS AND DISCONTINUOUS REGENERATION

That skeletal muscle may regenerate substantially after injury has been recognized since the early work of Volkmann[57] who emphasized the importance of integrity of the sarcolemma in promoting complete regeneration and suggested that regeneration might occur either by budding from surviving fiber segments (continuous type) or by proliferation and then fusion of myoblasts (discontinuous type). LeGros Clark[9] described regeneration by outgrowths from stumps of injured fibers and assumed that the observed increase in nuclei was the result of division of myonuclei by amitosis. Since that time many studies of regenerating muscle in humans and animals have shown the predominance of the discontinuous type of regeneration, in which myoblastic cells proliferate by mitosis prior to fusion.[3,18,34]

CELLULAR EVENTS IN MUSCLE REGENERATION

The cellular events leading to regeneration of muscle fibers may be summarized as follows[6]:

1. After injury, the sarcoplasm degenerates and is invaded by phagocytes. Depending on the type of injury, the sarcolemma may be focally destroyed or left intact.
2. Nuclei with a thin rim of basophilic cytoplasm, surrounded by a discrete plasma membrane, appear between the basement membrane and the degenerating sarcoplasm. These are the myoblastic cells, which undergo mitosis. They reach a peak 48 to 72 hours after trauma.
3. Myoblasts fuse into multinucleated myotubes 2 to 4 days after injury. Mitosis ceases and the formation of myofilaments proceeds.
4. Myofilaments are organized into myofibrils; the sarcoplasmic reticulum takes shape; the central nuclei migrate peripherally. At this point a young muscle fiber has been formed.

The myoblast contains many free ribosomes, some aggregated into polyribosome spirals, which are described as closely associated with newly formed myosin filaments in regenerating muscle.[33] Whether mononuclear cells can form myofilaments or whether myofilamentogenesis occurs only after the myotube is formed is debated. Okazaki and Holzer,[39] in a study of chick embryo myoblasts in tissue culture, saw incorporation of tritiated thymidine (indicating DNA synthesis) only in mononuclear cells and detected myofilament synthesis (by fluorescein-labeled antimyosin and antiactin antibodies) only after the mononuclear cells had fused into myotubes. Other observers have seen myofilaments developing in mononuclear myoblasts at the electron microscopic level.[47] It is clear that only the mononuclear cells undergo mitosis, which ceases once fusion has occurred.[18,34]

ORIGIN OF MYOBLASTIC CELL

The origin of the mononuclear myoblast is controversial. The experiments of Walker,[58] in which connective tissue nuclei were labeled radioactively prior to muscle injury, showed that myoblast nuclei are not of connective-tissue origin. It has been suggested by some that circulating cells might be the source of myoblasts. The observed inhibition of muscle regeneration by local irradiation prior to injury[41] disallows this possibility, as only cells previously present in muscle would be damaged by the radiation. However, some observers have noted that this inhibition by irradiation is incomplete and that the data presently available do not entirely rule out the possibility of a circulating cell participating in myogenesis.[49] Nevertheless, it is generally believed that the myoblastic cell originates in the muscle, and the debated question is whether it arises from the satellite cell or from myonuclei. Shafiq[47,48] showed a transition between satellite cells and myoblasts in regenerating human and mouse muscles, indicating the transformation of satellite cells to myoblasts after injury. In a study of crush lesions of web muscles of fruit bats, Church[8] showed increased numbers of satellite cells in the areas of injury. Certainly satellite cells appear to increase in number after injury of the muscle, and these new cells, which contain increased ribosomes, rough endoplasmic reticulum, mitochondria, and prominent nucleoli have been called activated satellite cells, or presumptive myoblasts. Others are of the opinion that the satellite cells are not numerous enough to perform this function and that the observed facts are consistent with origin of myoblasts from myonuclei. Reznik[40] has observed nuclei in injured muscle being separated off, along with a thin rim of sarcoplasm by fusion of multiple vesicles.

REGENERATION OF WHOLE MUSCLES FROM MINCED FRAGMENTS

The regeneration of entire muscles from minced fragments was first studied extensively by Studitsky[51] and is described in detail by Carlson.[5,6] The technique consists of complete removal of a muscle, mincing of it into tiny fragments, and replacement of the fragments in the muscle bed. After a week the fragments are molded into a homogeneous mass and connections to the original tendons develop. Eventually a small muscle that has normal gross relationships with its tendons, nerves, and blood vessels is formed. Histologically the muscle fragments undergo sarcoplasmic degeneration and invasion by macrophages, peripherally at first, as the tissue becomes vascularized. Myoblasts appear under the basement membranes of the old muscle fibers by 3 days (in the rat). The regenerating zone begins at the outside edges of the transplant and extends inward along with the vascularization. The capacity of the fragments in the center of the transplant to survive for a few days without a direct blood supply indicates that metabolic adaptations that allow traumatized muscle to remain viable under adverse conditions must occur. Fusion of myoblasts and maturation of myotubes then progresses. The fully regenerated rat gastrocnemius muscle at 30 days is much smaller than normal and often contains a considerable amount of connective tissue. Studitsky et al.[52] have observed reinnervation of these regenerated muscles. Physiological studies[45] have demonstrated normal contractile characteristics but decreased twitch tension in regenerated minced muscle. External pressure and tension along their long axes are important in the molding and orientation of these grafts.

FREE MUSCLE GRAFTS

Regeneration in free or whole muscle grafts of small leg muscles in rats (from one leg to the other) was investigated by Carlson and Gutmann.[7] In nondenervated grafted muscles there was a central degenerating zone that disappeared after a week. The peripheral zone showed a gradient of regeneration, most advanced on the outside. Grafts that had been denervated 14 days previously showed much more rapid disappearance of the central degenerating fibers (by 2 to 3 days) and fast development of regenerating fibers, so that cross-striations were visible at 5 days. Larger numbers of fibers survived at the periphery of the denervated grafts. Later stages of differentiation were the same in both types of graft. The demonstrated acceleration of early regeneration in muscle denervated prior to grafting may be a consequence of the observed

Reinnervation and regeneration of striated muscle

increase in satellite cells occurring after denervation.[3,26] Possibly these cells are potential myoblasts, ready to be activated upon transplantation of the muscle. These small free grafts of muscle develop more complete regeneration than is seen in other situations, even maturing histochemically and retaining their spindles. Unfortunately, larger muscles such as the gastrocnemius have not been successfully grafted.

Thompson[54] successfully grafted denervated pronator teres muscles of dogs' forelegs to sites in the face and hindleg, with 20 to 90% of the muscle fibers surviving. Reinnervation occurred. Similarly, small denervated foot or forearm muscle grafts were used as facial muscle transplants, around the mouth, in eight human cases with facial paralysis. The patients had voluntary muscular activity in the grafts by 3 months. The grafts had been denervated 2 to 3 weeks prior to transplantation. Apparently, the principles of free muscle grafts learned in laboratory experiments can be successfully applied to surgical procedures for remobilization of the face.

REGENERATION IN HUMAN MUSCLE DISEASE

In human muscle diseases, such as polymyositis and muscular dystrophy, regeneration occurs in a discontinuous fashion. Mononuclear myoblasts, possibly derived from satellite cells, line up under the sarcolemma around the degenerating sarcoplasm (Fig. 11-4). Mitoses are seen in these cells. Then they fuse to form syncytial masses, and then myotubes develop and mature into new fibers. The cellular events are similar to those described in animal models.[18,35,48]

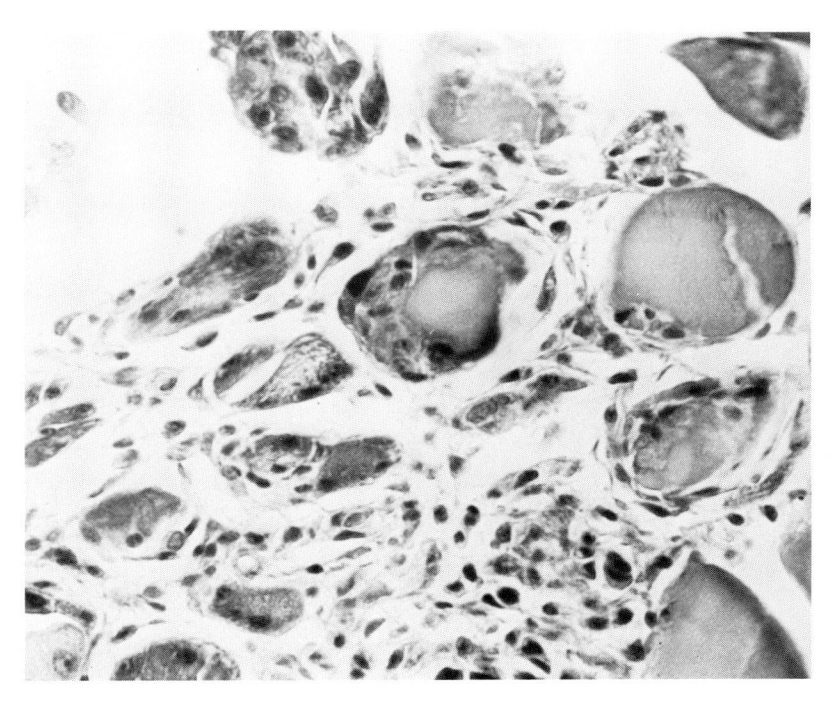

Fig. 11-4. Cross section of focus of regeneration in biopsy specimen of muscle from patient with rhabdomyolysis. Note large fibers with central sarcoplasmic degeneration, surrounded by mononuclear (myoblastic) cells. Other fibers are completely replaced by mononuclear cells. (Hematoxylin and eosin, 1250×.)

FACTORS NECESSARY FOR SUCCESSFUL MUSCLE REGENERATION

What has been learned in the laboratory that can be applied to techniques for promotion of muscle regeneration in humans?

1. Successful muscle regeneration in any system requires a good blood supply and lack of infection or the presence of irritants.[29]
2. Although an intact sarcolemma is not necessary for muscle regeneration, the presence of endomysial tubes results in better replacement of the fibers. The early stages of muscle regeneration occur within the residual basement membranes of the original fibers, which provide a scaffold upon which myoblasts can proliferate and fuse.[6]
3. Concerning the effect of denervation on muscle regeneration, certainly the development of myoblasts and their fusion happens without innervation. Prior denervation accelerates and promotes these early events in transplanted muscle. After the myotube stage, denervated muscle may mature more slowly[2] and eventually degenerate. In tissue culture experiments also, myotubes did not differentiate further until innervated (by explants of mouse fetal spinal cord), and histochemical differentiation of fiber types failed to occur without innervation.[11]
4. A source of myoblastic cells is necessary for regeneration of muscle fibers and can be provided by minced or small transplants.
5. Tension (stretch) helps regenerating muscle organize its architecture and may even promote the formation of new fibers.[6]

Conclusions

It is clear from the many experimental studies cited that reinnervation of muscle occurs either by growth of sprouting axons into existing motor end plates, or by the actual formation of new neuromuscular junctions. Nerve sprouting in denervated muscle is exuberant, apparently stimulated by the absence of factors that inhibit sprouting, which are normally carried down the axon by axoplasmic flow. In human disease, reinnervation of muscle fibers results in significant changes in the histochemical anatomy of the muscle, with the formation of large groups of one fiber type replacing the normal mosaic mixture of type I and II fibers. This "type grouping" reflects the increase in motor unit size, which occurs because of replacement of lost innervation by collateral sprouting of the remaining axons.

Regeneration of skeletal muscle occurs, with similar cellular events taking place in both human and animal muscle. The regenerated fibers once formed are morphologically and functionally normal. Small muscle transplants, if denervated 2 to 3 weeks previously, will regenerate well. A good blood supply, intact endomysial tubes, a source of myoblastic cells, and a degree of maintained tension or stretch are factors known to promote successful regeneration in voluntary muscle.

REFERENCES

1. Aitken, J. T.: Growth of nerve implants in voluntary muscle, J. Anat. **84:**38, 1950.
2. Allbrook, D. B., and Aitken, J. T.: Reinnervation of striated muscle after acute ischaemia, J. Anat. **85:**376, 1951.
3. Aloisi, M.: Patterns of muscle regeneration. In Mauro, A., Shafiq, S. A., and Milhorat, A. T., editors: Regeneration of striated muscle, and myogenesis, Amsterdam, 1970, Excerpta Medica Foundation (ICS 218, p. 180).
4. Buller, A. J., Eccles, J. C., and Eccles, R. M.: Interactions between motor neurons and muscles in respect of the characteristic speed

of their responses, J. Physiol. **150:**417, 1960.
5. Carlson, B. M.: 1. The regeneration of entire muscles from minced fragments. 2. Histological observations on the regeneration of striated muscle. In Mauro, A., Shafiq, S. A., and Milhorat, A. T., editors: Regeneration of striated muscle, and myogenesis, Amsterdam, 1970, Excerpta Medica Foundation (ICS 218), pp. 25-72.
6. Carlson, B. M.: The regeneration of skeletal muscle: a review, Am. J. Anat. **137:**119, 1973.
7. Carlson, B. M., and Gutmann, E.: Regeneration in free grafts of normal and denervated muscles in the rat: morphology and histochemistry, Anat. Rec. **183:**47, 1975.
8. Church, J. C. T.: Cell quantitation in regenerating bat web muscle. In Mauro, A., Shafiq, S. A., and Milhorat, A. T., editors: Regeneration of striated muscle, and myogenesis, Amsterdam, 1970, Excerpta Medica Foundation (ICS 218), pp. 101-121.
9. Clark, W. E. L.: An experimental study of the regeneration of mammalian striped muscle. J. Anat. **80:**24, 1946.
10. Diamond, J. Cooper, E., Turner, C., and MacIntyre, L.: Trophic regulation of nerve sprouting, Science **193:**371, 1976.
11. Dubowitz, V., Gallup, B., and Witkowski, J.: Normal and diseased muscle in tissue culture, J. Physiol. **231:**61P, 1973.
12. Edds, M. V., Jr.: Collateral regeneration of partially denervated muscles, J. Exp. Zool. **113:**517, 1950.
13. Edds, M. V., Jr.: Collateral nerve regeneration, Q. Rev. Biol. **28:**260, 1953.
14. Edstrom, L., and Kugelberg, E.: Histochemical composition, distribution of fibers, and fatiguability of single motor units in the anterior tibial muscle of the rat, J. Neurol. Neurosurg. Psychiatry **31:**424, 1968.
15. Elsberg, C. A.: Experiments on motor nerve regeneration and direct neurotization of paralyzed muscles by their own and foreign nerves, Science **45:**318, 1917.
16. Exner, S. (1885): Cited by Edds, M. V., Jr.: Collateral nerve regeneration, Q. Rev. Biol. **28:**260, 1953.
17. Fox, S., and Thesleff, S.: The time required for innervation of denervated muscle by nerve implants, Life Sci. **6:**635, 1967.
18. Gilbert, R. K., and Hazard, J. B.: Regeneration in human skeletal muscle, J. Pathol. Bacteriol. **89:**503, 1965.
19. Guth, L.: Neuromuscular function after regeneration of interrupted nerve fibers into partially denervated muscle, Exp. Neurol. **6:**129, 1962.
20. Guth, L., and Samaha, F. J.: Phenotypic differences between the actomyosin ATPase of the three fiber types of mammalian skeletal muscle, Exp. Neurol. **26:**120, 1970.
21. Guth, L., Samaha, F. J., and Albers, R. W.: The neural regulation of some phenotypic differences between the fiber types of mammalian skeletal muscle, Exp. Neurol. **26:**123, 1970.
22. Guth, L., and Zalewski, A. A.: Disposition of cholinesterase following implantation of nerve into innervated and denervated muscle, Exp. Neurol. **7:**316, 1963.
23. Gutmann, E., and Young, J. Z.: The reinnervation of muscle after various periods of atrophy, J. Anat. **78:**15, 1944.
24. Gwynn, D. G., and Aitken, J. T.: The formation of new motor end plates in mammalian skeletal muscle, J. Anat. **100:**111, 1966.
25. Hatsuyama, Y.: Histological studies on reinnervation of denervated muscle, with special reference to collateral branching, Electromyography **6:**71, 1966.
26. Hess, A., and Rosner, S.: The satellite cell bud and myoblast in denervated mammalian muscle fibers, Am. J. Anat. **129:**21, 1970.
27. Hines, H. M., Wehrmacher, W. E., and Thomson, J. D.: Functional changes in nerve and muscle after partial denervation, Am. J. Physiol. **145:**48, 1945.
28. Hoffman, H., and Springell, P. H.: An attempt at the chemical identification of "neurocletin" (the substance evoking axon sprouting), Aust. J. Exp. Biol. Med. Sci. **29:**417, 1951.
29. Hudgson, P., and Field, E. J.: Regeneration of muscle. In Bourne, G. H., editor: Structure and function of muscle, ed. 2, New York, 1973, Academic Press, Inc., pp. 312-363.
30. Jean, D. H., Guth, L., and Albers, R. W.: Neural regulation of the structure of myosin, Exp. Neurol. **38:**458, 1973.
31. Karpati, G., and Engel, W. K.: Type grouping in skeletal muscles after experimental reinnervation, Neurology **18:**447, 1968.
32. Kugelberg, E., Edström, L., and Abbruzzese, M.: Mapping of motor units in experimentally reinnervated rat muscle, J. Neurol. Neurosurg. Psychiatry **33:**319, 1970.
33. Larson, P. F., Hudgson, P., and Walton, J. N.: Morphological relationship of polyribosomes and myosin filaments in developing and regenerating skeletal muscle, Nature **222:**1168, 1969.
34. Lash, J. W., Holtzer, H., and Swift, H.: Regeneration of mature skeletal muscle, Anat. Rec. **128:**679, 1957.
35. Mastaglia, F. L., and Kakulas, B. A.: A his-

tological and histochemical study of skeletal muscle regeneration in polymyositis, J. Neurol. Sci. **10:**471, 1970.
36. Miledi, R.: Induced innervation of end-plate free muscle segments, Nature **193:**281, 1962.
37. Miledi, R.: Formation of extra nerve-muscle junctions in innervated muscle, Nature **199:**1191, 1963.
38. Morris, C. J.: Human skeletal muscle fiber type grouping and collateral reinnervation, J. Neurol. Neurosurg. Psychiatry **32:**440, 1969.
39. Okazaki, K., and Holzer, H.: Myogenesis: fusion, myosin synthesis, and the mitotic cycle, Proc. Natl. Acad. Sci. U.S.A. **56:**1484, 1966.
40. Reznik, M.: Satellite cells, myoblasts, and skeletal muscle regeneration. In Mauro, A., Shafiq, S. A., and Milhorat, A. T., editors: Regeneration of striated muscle, and myogenesis, Amsterdam, 1970, Excerpta Medica Foundation (ICS 218), pp. 133-156.
41. Reznik, M., and Betz, E. H.: Influence de l'irradiation locale préalable sur les capacités régénératrices du muscle strié squelettique, Pathol. Europ. (Brux.) **2:**69, 1967.
42. Robbins, N., Karpati, G., and Engel, W. K.: Histochemical and contractile properties in the cross-innervated guinea pig soleus muscle, Arch. Neurol. **20:**318, 1969.
43. Romanul, F. C. A., and Van der Meulen, J. P.: Slow and fast muscles after cross-innervation, Arch. Neurol. **17:**387, 1967.
44. Saito, A., and Zacks, S. I.: Fine structure observations of denervation and reinnervation of neuromuscular junctions in mouse foot muscle, J. Bone Joint Surg. **51:**1163, 1969.
45. Salafsky, B.: Studies on the physiology of skeletal muscle regenerates, J. Physiol. **231:**58P, 1973.
46. Samaha, F. J., Guth, L., and Albers, R. W.: The neural regulation of gene expression in the muscle cell, Exp. Neurol. **27:**276, 1970.
47. Shafiq, S. A.: Satellite cells and fiber nuclei in muscle regeneration. In Mauro, A., Shafiq, S. A., and Milhorat, A. T., editors: Regeneration of striated muscle, and myogenesis, Amsterdam, 1970, Excerpta Medica Foundation (ICS 218), pp. 122-132.
48. Shafiq, S. A., Gorycki, M. A., and Milhorat, A. T.: An electron microscopic study of regeneration and satellite cells in human muscle, Neurology **17:**567, 1967.
49. Sloper, J. C., Bateson, R. B., Hindle, D., and Warren, J.: Muscle regeneration in man and mouse: evidence derived from tissue culture and from the evolution of experimental and surgical injuries in the irradiated and non-irradiated subject. In Mauro, A., Shafiq, S. A., and Milhorat, A. T., editors: Regeneration of striated muscle, and myogenesis, Amsterdam, 1970, Excerpta Medica Foundation (ICS 218), pp. 157-164.
50. Steindler, A.: Direct neurotization of paralyzed muscles. Further study of the question of direct nerve implantation, Am. J. Orthoped. Surg. **14:**707, 1916.
51. Studitsky, A. N.: Cited by Carlson, B. M.: The regeneration of entire muscles from minced fragments. In Mauro, A., Shafiq, S. A., and Milhorat, A. T., editors: Regeneration of striated muscle, and myogenesis, Amsterdam, 1970, Excerpta Medica Foundation (ICS 218), p. 25.
51a. Studitsky, A. N.: Free auto- and homografts of muscle tissue in experiments on animals, Ann. N.Y. Acad. Sci. **120:**789, 1964.
52. Studitsky, A. N., Zhenevskaya, R. P., and Rumyantseva, O. N.: The role of neurotropic influences on the restitution of structure and function of regenerating muscles. In Gutmann, E., and Hnik, P., editors: The effect of use and disuse on neuromuscular functions, Prague, 1963, Publishing House of the Czechoslovak Academy of Sciences, pp. 71-81.
53. Teräväinen, H.: Development of myoneural junctions in the rat, Z. Zellforsch. **87:**249, 1968.
54. Thompson, N.: Autogenous free grafts of skeletal muscle. A preliminary experimental and clinical study, Plast. Reconstr. Surg. **48:**11, 1971.
55. Trojaborg, W., and Siemssen, S. O.: Reinnervation after resection of the facial nerve, Arch. Neurol. **26:**17, 1972.
56. van Harreveld, A.: Reinnervation of denervated muscle fibers by adjacent functioning motor units, Am. J. Physiol. **144:**477, 1945.
57. Volkmann, R.: Cited by Hudgson, P., and Field, E. J.: Regeneration of muscle. In Bourne, G. H., editor: The structure and function of muscle, ed. 2, New York, 1973, Academic Press, Inc., vol. II, pp. 312-313.
58. Walker, B. E.: The origin of myoblasts and the problem of dedifferentiation, Exp. Cell Res. **30:**80, 1963.
59. Warszawski, M., Tellerman-Toppet, N., Durdu, J., Graff, G. L. A., and Coers, C.: The early stages of neuromuscular regeneration after crushing the sciatic nerve in the rat. Electrophysiological and histological study, J. Neurol. Sci. **24:**21, 1975.
60. Weiss, P., and Edds, M. V.: Spontaneous re-

covery of muscle following partial denervation, Am. J. Physiol. **145**:587, 1946.
61. Yellin, H.: Neural regulation of enzymes in muscle fibers of red and white muscle, Exp. Neurol. **19**:92, 1967.
62. Zak, R.: Proteins in the denervated muscle, changes in their quantity, properties, and metabolism. In Gutmann, E., editor: The denervated muscle, Prague, 1962, Publishing House of the Czechoslovak Academy of Sciences, pp. 332-335.
63. Zak, R., Grove, D., and Rabinowitz, M.: DNA synthesis in the rat diaphragm as an early response to denervation, Am. J. Physiol. **216**:647, 1969.
64. Zelená, J.: Development, degeneration and regeneration of receptor organs. In Singer, M., and Schadé, J. P., editors: Mechanisms of neural regeneration, Prog. Brain Res. **13**:175-213, 1964.

12 Technique of free nerve grafting in the face

HANNO MILLESI

The technique of nerve grafting is described for teaching the optimal method that can allow regenerating axons to cross the scar barrier formed when nerve ends are sutured. A free nerve graft should be used whenever a severed nerve must be sutured with tension. Careful cutting away of all traumatized nerve and scar back to clean axons, and suturing of the nerve ends, will minimize interposing scars, which act as a barrier to new axon growth. The use of the microscope allows individual fascicular grafting with 10-0 nylon sutures instead of gross nerve end-to-end epineural anastomosis.

Technique of free nerve grafting in the face

The logical treatment of a transected nerve is restoration of continuity by an end-to-end nerve repair. If there is a defect of nerve tissue, we have in theory three possibilities:
1. Stretching the two nerve stumps to achieve union under tension
2. Use of a nerve graft
3. Achievement of neurotization of the distal stump by transfer of another nerve

The use of a nerve graft implies an important theoretical disadvantage. The regenerating axon sprouts have to cross two lines of union at the proximal and at the distal extremity of the graft, as compared with only one crossing in the case of an end-to-end neurorrhaphy. In consequence, nerve grafting did not become popular in peripheral nerve surgery, despite the fact that they have been in use for 100 years. Results of nerve grafting have been regarded as inferior to an end-to-end repair, and all attempts were made to perform a neurorrhaphy even if a defect was present. Only after all other possibilities of narrowing the extensive defect were exhausted would the distance between the two stumps be managed by a nerve graft. A nerve transfer is indicated when a proximal stump of injured nerve is not present. If a suitable stump is available, restoration of continuity is the better solution. The anatomical course of the facial nerve does not offer many possibilities to manage a defect by transposition with the exception of the area of the geniculum. Therefore, in facial nerve surgery, nerve grafts have been applied earlier than with other nerves.

Satisfactory nerve grafting results have been reported by Balance and Duel[1] (1932), Duel[5] (1934), Bunnel[2] (1927), and others at a period of time when nerve grafting of peripheral nerve defects was regarded with skepticism. The facial nerve showed a better tendency to recover than did other nerves. Facial nerve surgery could be successful by techniques that would fail with other peripheral nerves. This fact may have contributed to the more optimistic view on facial nerve grafts, compared with other nerves. However, the nerve graft is still regarded inferior to neurorrhaphy, despite the latter being performed under tension by stretching of the nerve stumps.

Contemporary concepts in free nerve and muscle grafting

Effects of local tension on nerve regeneration

Tension at the suture site has detrimental effects on nerve regeneration. This must be considered if a choice is to be made between end-to-end neurorrhaphy and nerve grafting in an actual clinical case. If there is no defect and no retraction, neurorrhaphy will be the technique of choice. But, if tension has to be applied to coapt the two stumps, one has to weigh the advantages and the disadvantages of each procedure. With increasing tension there is a moment when the consequences outweigh the disadvantages of the two suture sites of the nerve graft. We have good reasons to believe that only a very small amount of tension is tolerable to get an optimal result. If tension is avoided completely, one can exploit all the advantages of microsurgery and reduce the operative trauma to a minimum. A nerve graft is therefore indicated when coaptation of the nerve stumps without tension cannot be obtained.

After transection of a nerve, the two stumps spread apart because of the elasticity of the nerve tissue. To overcome the elasticity, a certain force is needed. In 1972, this force was measured in the sciatic nerve of the rabbit by Millesi, Berger, and Meissl[16] and was found to be between 6 and 10 grams. When a defect was present, the force necessary to achieve coaptation rose rapidly not only because of elasticity, which had to be overcome, but also because the nerve had to be stretched. With a defect of 5 mm, the force rose to a range of 40 to 60 grams. It is evident that under such tension, many sutures were needed to obtain a good union of the two stumps. This created surgical trauma and the use of more foreign material with increased foreign-body reaction. Despite the placement of an exact epineural suture, an internal gap might form by separation of the fascicles within the cross section. Such a gap is filled by proliferating connective tissue, forming a wide scar between the fascicular tissue. If a wound heals under tension, much more connective tissue proliferation occurs, resulting in a hypertrophic scar. Under continuous tension the scar is stretched, forming a wide gap between the nerve stumps filled with scar tissue. Histologic studies of suture lines after clinical or experimental nerve repairs under tension show such gaps filled with scar

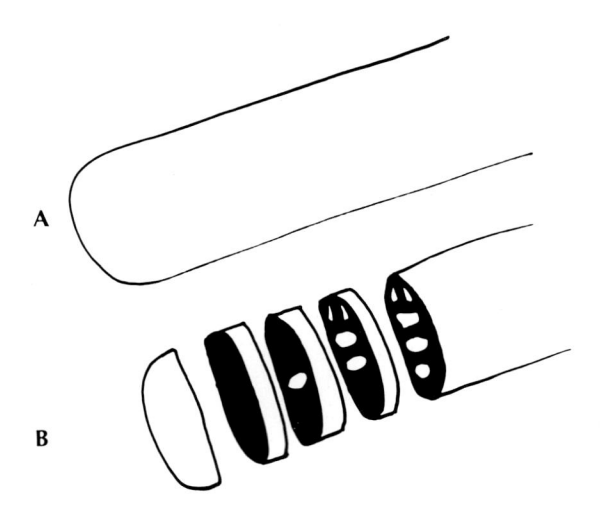

Fig. 12-1. Resecting the neuroma stump. **A,** Neuroma of proximal stump. **B,** Resection until normal tissue is met.

tissue without proper fascicular alignment. These gaps are obstacles for the axon sprouts. *They can be prevented if tension is avoided.* Tensionless coaptation results in an excellent fascicular alignment with virtually no scar tissue. In case of nerves sutured under tension, the continuous reaction of scar tissue causes hypertrophy, shrinking, or stretching, even at a later date. These reactions can damage axons that had already crossed the suture line. Studies of human nerve repairs, performed under tension, demonstrated axonolysis of the few axons that had reached the distal stump, even several months after the unsuccessful repair.

The handling of the nerve tissue is more difficult if coaptation has to be performed under tension. Proper resection of the damaged tissue at the proximal and distal nerve stump is essential for a satisfactory regeneration (Fig. 12-1). However, the necessary resection increases the size of the defect. Often something like a bulb suture without proper resection is performed to achieve an end-to-end coaptation. Proper resection and nerve grafting would be the better solution.

Basic considerations in autologous nerve grafting

After free grafting, the nerve graft is without any blood supply for a certain period of time. Vessels at the recipient site grow into the graft to make contact with the vessels of the graft. Circulation is reestablished. The interval between grafting and restoration of the blood supply is decisive for the survival. Within the graft wallerian degeneration takes place, but the original fascicular pattern is preserved and all cells, including the Schwann cells, can survive. The latter proliferate and form the so-called Hanke-Büngner bands. If the ischemic period is too long, the central tissue of the graft suffers and becomes fibrotic; the fascicular pattern is partially lost and the neurotization of the graft will be incomplete. Revascularization is the decisive factor. It depends on the vascularity of the recipient bed and of the relation between surface and tissue mass of the graft. Thinner grafts have better chances. If several grafts are used, they should not be packed together to form a cable, because part of the surface of each individual graft will then be in contact with another graft and not with the recipient bed.

To summarize, in a recipient site with normal vascularization, a thin nerve graft has a good chance for full cellular survival with preservation of its fascicular pattern. After wallerian degeneration, a free autologous nerve graft behaves like a distal nerve stump. In contrast to the autologous nerve grafts, preserved allografts consist of a collagen framework without cells. This framework has to be invaded by connective tissue cells. Neurotization occurs by the slow growth of axons along this framework. The results after the use of preserved allografts are inferior, compared with autografts, regardless of the technique of preservation. Lyophilization, irradiation, and storage in Cialite solution have been recommended. The results have been disappointing. Early optimistic reports have not been reproduced. Fresh allografts cause immunologic reactions, which have to be suppressed by immunologic suppressive therapy. Such treatment is not without danger and is not justified so long as other possibilities are available.

Autologous nerve grafts show wallerian degeneration. It was suggested to use predegenerated nerve grafts to facilitate neurotization. According to my experience, neurotization is not impeded by the process of wallerian degeneration and the use of predegenerated nerve grafts does not offer significant advantages.

Contemporary concepts in free nerve and muscle grafting

The length of the graft is, within certain limits, not a decisive factor for regeneration. It is preferable to use a longer graft and perform proper resection of the nerve stumps than do an inadequate resection and use a shorter graft. If the recipient site is scarred, it is better to use a longer graft and bypass the unfavorable area.

Technique of the nerve grafting

Several technical steps are necessary to perform a nerve graft. The two nerve stumps have to be prepared. The grafts must be provided and prepared. Coaptation between the proximal and the distal stumps of the nerve and the graft must be achieved. The union must be secured, and some surgeons believe that additional protection is necessary. The techniques currently in use allow one to try different approaches to manage the individual steps.

PREPARATION OF STUMPS

The classical technique to prepare the stumps is to cut slices of tissue until the cross section contains only normal nerve tissue. This may be sufficient in monofascicular nerves with a few very thin fascicles (Fig. 12-1). If the nerve contains several or many fascicles, it is much better to start the dissection between the fascicles (Fig. 12-2). Using the microscope and the microsurgical equipment, one can perform this with minimal surgical trauma. If there are few large fascicles, they are isolated individually. If the cross section consists of many fascicles, groups are isolated, each one consisting of several individual fascicles. These fascicle groups are separated from others by spaces filled with interfascicular epineural connective tissue and intraneural vessels. Following the course of the fascicles, the interfascicular dissection can be performed quite easily (Fig. 12-2, *C*).

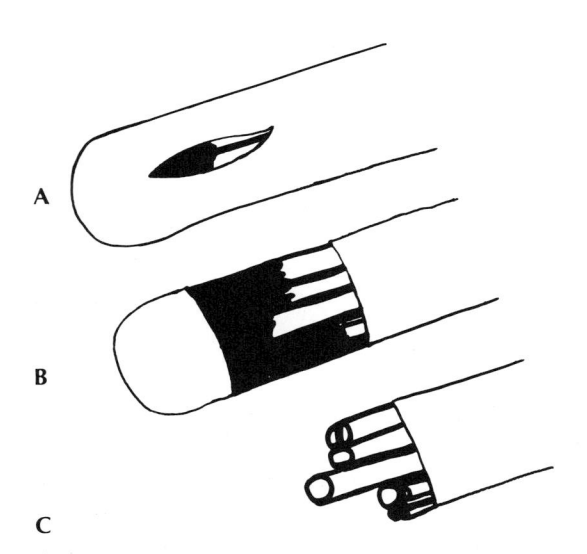

Fig. 12-2. **A,** Neuroma of proximal stump. Incision of epineurium, with epineurectomy starting from normal tissue. **B,** After resection of epineurium, fascicles are exposed. Interfascicular dissection to isolate fascicle groups and resection of neuromatous tissue. **C,** Three individual fascicle groups are isolated in this particular case: an upper one (three fascicles), a medium one (one fascicle), and an inferior one (five fascicles).

COAPTATION

The classical techniques achieve and maintain coaptation by *epineural sutures*. Several stitches are placed into the epineurium of the nerve stumps and the graft at various points of the circumference. The advantage of this technique is that it is simple, no additional dissection of the stumps is necessary and it may tolerate some tension. But the disadvantages outweigh the advantages: Graft and nerve stumps should be of similar size. The epineurium is very reactive. It is the main source of the connective tissue proliferation. The proliferation starts proximal and then distal to the suture line. The sutures, being an inorganic material, are passed on the outer aspect. After the epineural suture is performed, the behavior of the fascicles cannot be controlled. The fascicular alignment is not secured in the multifascicular nerves. The fascicles may buckle if the sutures are too tight, or separate if under tension. The facial nerve and its branches are rather thin nerves, and therefore the drawback of the epineural suture is more severe than in peripheral nerves. Conley[3,4] uses one stitch right across the nerve tissue, combined with *tubulization* of the suture site with silicone cylinders. Since it is impossible to control the fascicular alignment after the tube is placed, a *window* is cut into the tube at the suture site. After an exact coaptation through the window with fine silver probes is done, a drop of autologous serum is applied to the suture line. Miehlke[13] used the glue technique with *2-cyanobutylacrylate*. The danger of glue entering between the nerve ends was minimized by application of the glue at the end of the tube, far from the suture line. He made use of collagen tubes. Tubulization of the suture site is done to prevent aberration of axon sprouts and to avoid invasion of the suture line by connective tissue from the surroundings. Conley, Miehlke, and others achieved good results with this technique in facial nerve surgery. However, the technique failed with other nerves. The tube caused a reaction. The proliferation of epineural tissue inside the tube produced a thick layer of connective tissue between tube and nerve tissue.

Since 1964 the interfascicular technique of nerve grafting has been used by Millesi and others.[16-18] With this technique the two stumps are prepared by interfascicular dissection. A strip of epineurium is resected and with it the main source of connective tissue at the suture site is removed. The nerve graft epineurium is shifted away from the cross section. Each end of the nerve graft is brought into contact with one fascicle group of a multifascicular nerve by one 10-0 nylon stitch. The stitch is introduced into the perineurium of one of the fascicles or into the interfascicular connective tissue. The grafts have to be long enough to avoid any tension. If there is no tension and if the one stitch is well placed, broad contact over the whole surface within the cross section occurs. The coaptation is secured by natural fibrin clotting. The tensile strength of this fibrin clotting, which occurs in any wound, is very low but sufficient if tension is zero. Experimental measurements with the sciatic nerve of the rabbit demonstrated that after 24 hours the tensile strength ranges between 19 and 30 grams and reaches the values of 100 grams after 1 week. By this technique a maximum of exactness is achieved with a minimum of surgical trauma. Microsurgical equipment is essential. The size of the graft is selected according to the diameter of the fascicle groups (see below). If the nerve consists of only several major fascicles, each fascicle is united with one graft (fascicular coaptation). If the nerve consists of only one thick fascicle, several grafts are brought into contact with this single fascicle (fascicular coaptation

Contemporary concepts in free nerve and muscle grafting

1:2 or 1:3, etc.). Exact coaptation without tension makes aberration of axon sprouts and invasion of connective tissue from the surroundings unlikely and no further protection is necessary. The interfascicular grafting technique also proves its value with partial severed grafts. By interfascicular microsurgical dissection the whole fascicles can be saved and only the damaged ones repaired.

Intraneural topography of the extratemporal facial nerve

In the description of techniques, differentiation was made between multifascicular nerve and nerves with only a few or only one fascicle. I must discuss, at this time, the problem of intraneural orientation of the nerve fibers with the same function as in the extratemporal facial nerve, according to the following points:

1. Near the stylomastoid foramen the facial nerve consists of one big fascicle with a few small satellites. Interfascicular dissection is not possible. Fascicular coaptation usually with three nerve grafts (1:3) is performed. See Figs. 12-4 and 12-5, *A*.
2. Near its division, the facial nerve consists of up to 20 fascicles of different size (Fig. 12-5, *B*). Fascicular dissection of each individual fascicle would create too much trauma without functional advantage. Therefore, interfascicular dissection into three or even four fascicle groups should be performed and each group united individually with one graft (interfascicular coaptation) (Fig. 12-3, *B*).
3. Between these points, according to the changing fascicular pattern, different structures may be encountered.

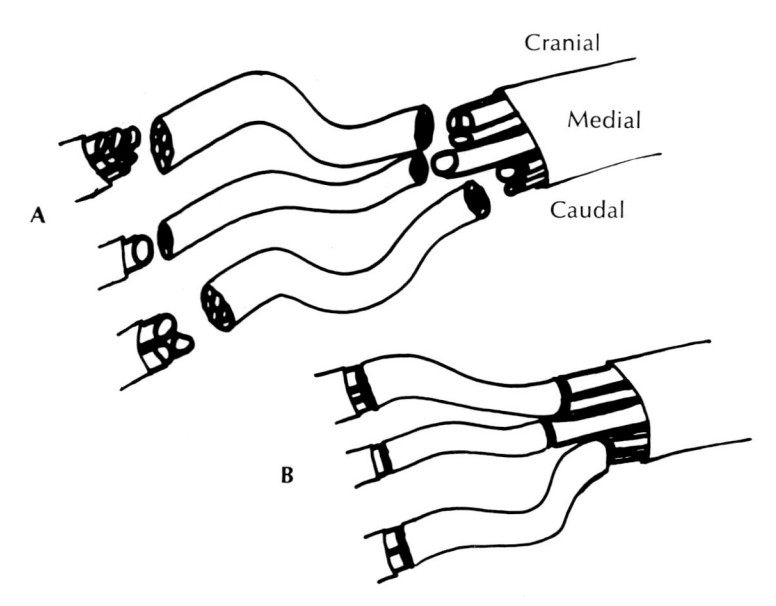

Fig. 12-3. Facial nerve near the stylomastoid foramen. **A,** At distal side three main branches of facial nerve are already well defined. Three grafts are used to reestablish continuity. **B,** Grafts are long enough and loosely connect the cranial fascicle group with upper branch, and the fascicle in the middle and the lower fascicle group with lower branch.

Technique of free nerve grafting in the face

Intraneural nerve fiber orientation

The facial nerve supplies muscles of different functions. The mimic expressions depend on the independent action of these muscles. The restoration of this independent function is our main goal. In fact, even after excellent motor recovery, the patient can perform mass movement only. This may partially be attributable to changes at the level of the ganglion cells.[8] But the main reason for this phenomenon is the irregular outgrowth of the axon sprouts. The axons that originally supply a certain muscle may branch into different muscles after regeneration. Thus each muscle is innervated by axons originally designated to supply another muscle. Mass movement results. It is evident that the quality of regeneration would be better if we would succeed in bringing at least a major part of the nerve fibers into the correct distal pathway. To achieve this, we must know how the fibers are distributed within the cross section. This problem has been discussed intensively during the last few years. Miehlke[14] gave a pattern of intraneural orientation of nerve fibers within the temporal bone. May[10] published patterns of intraneural fiber arrangements at different levels. He could differentiate topographical areas, where nerve fibers of the same function are more frequently located. Meissl studied this problem with serial sections. Before the division of the facial nerve, the nerve fibers to certain muscle groups are well separated within the fascicle groups. If one follows them in a central direction, one realizes that, in fact, much intermingling and cross-over occurs. However, there is still an area where the

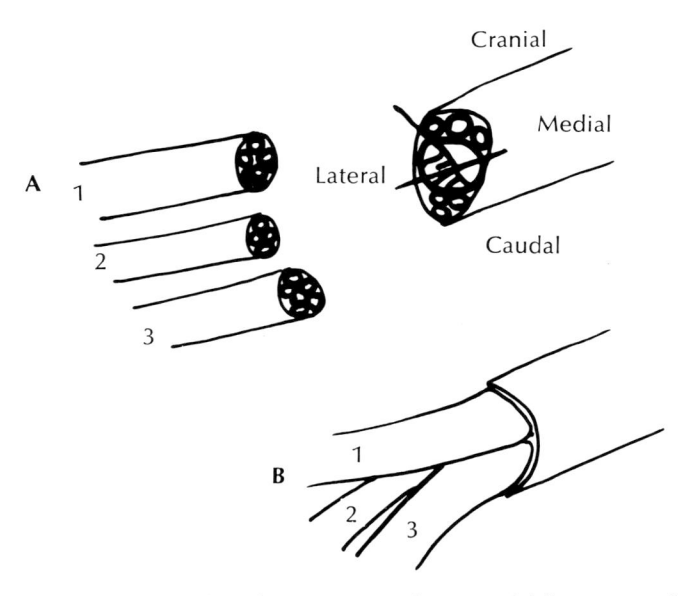

Fig. 12-4. Detail of grafting of facial nerve at stylomastoid foramen. **A,** At a proximal level the facial nerve consists of one big and several very small fascicles. The whole nerve is considered as one big fascicle group; three grafts are needed to satisfy the cross section. Note lines showing three sectors. **B,** First graft is used to cover cranial part of proximal stump. It will be connected with the cranial fascicle group of the distal stump. Second graft covers lateral portion. It will be connected with the medial fascicle group of the distal stump. Third graft covers inferior medial portion of proximal stump. It will be connected with the inferior fascicle group distally.

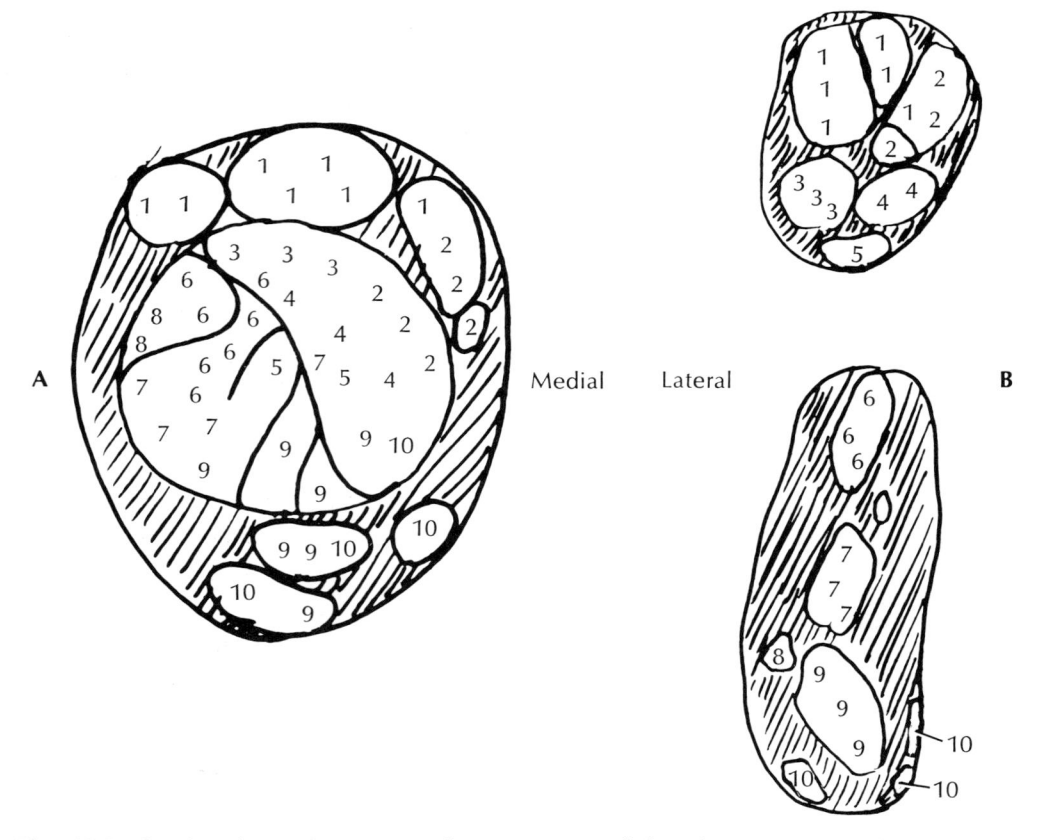

Contemporary concepts in free nerve and muscle grafting

Fig. 12-5. Study of serial section of extratemporal facial nerves in cadaver. **A,** Distribution of corresponding fibers near foramen stylomastoideum in the almost monofascicular nerve. **B,** Distribution of corresponding fibers near division of nerve. Here fibers are already arranged according to the division.

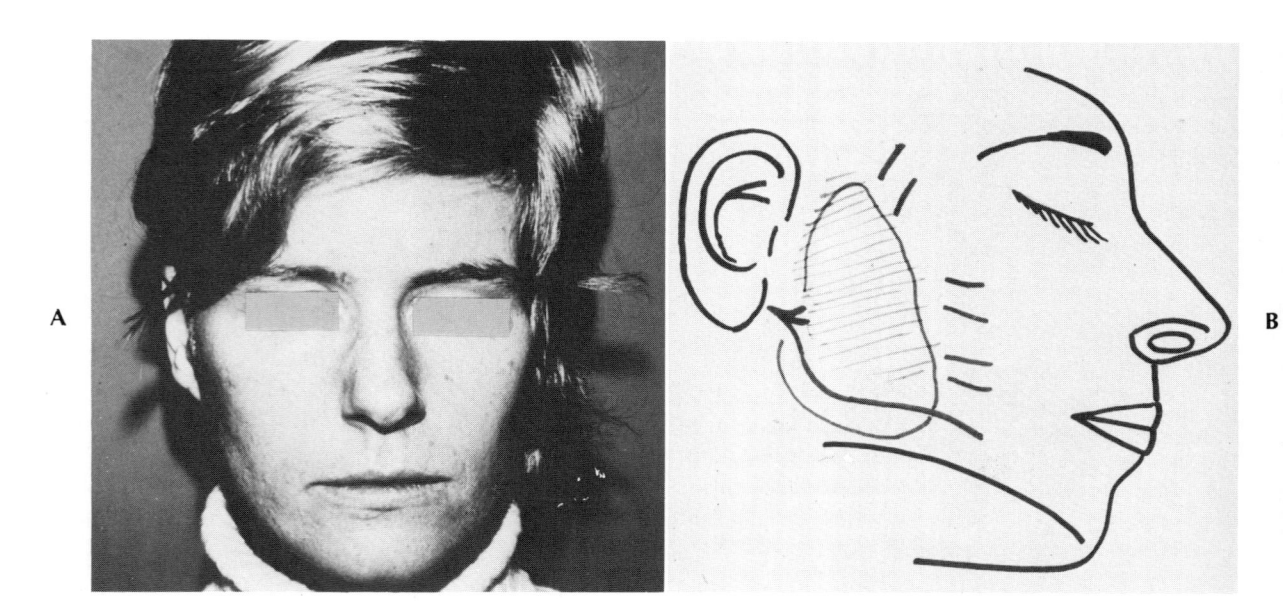

Fig. 12-6. For legend see opposite page.

Technique of free nerve grafting in the face

nerve fibers, for instance, for the frontal muscles and the eyelids, are predominant, especially near the stylomastoid foramen, where the cross section contains one big fascicle.

Therefore one should attempt to unite the corresponding parts of the cross section. In nerve grafting in the extratemporal segment, there usually is the proximal stump on one side and the individual branches on the other. The individual grafts are united at the distal end with the branches and at the proximal end with the fascicle group,

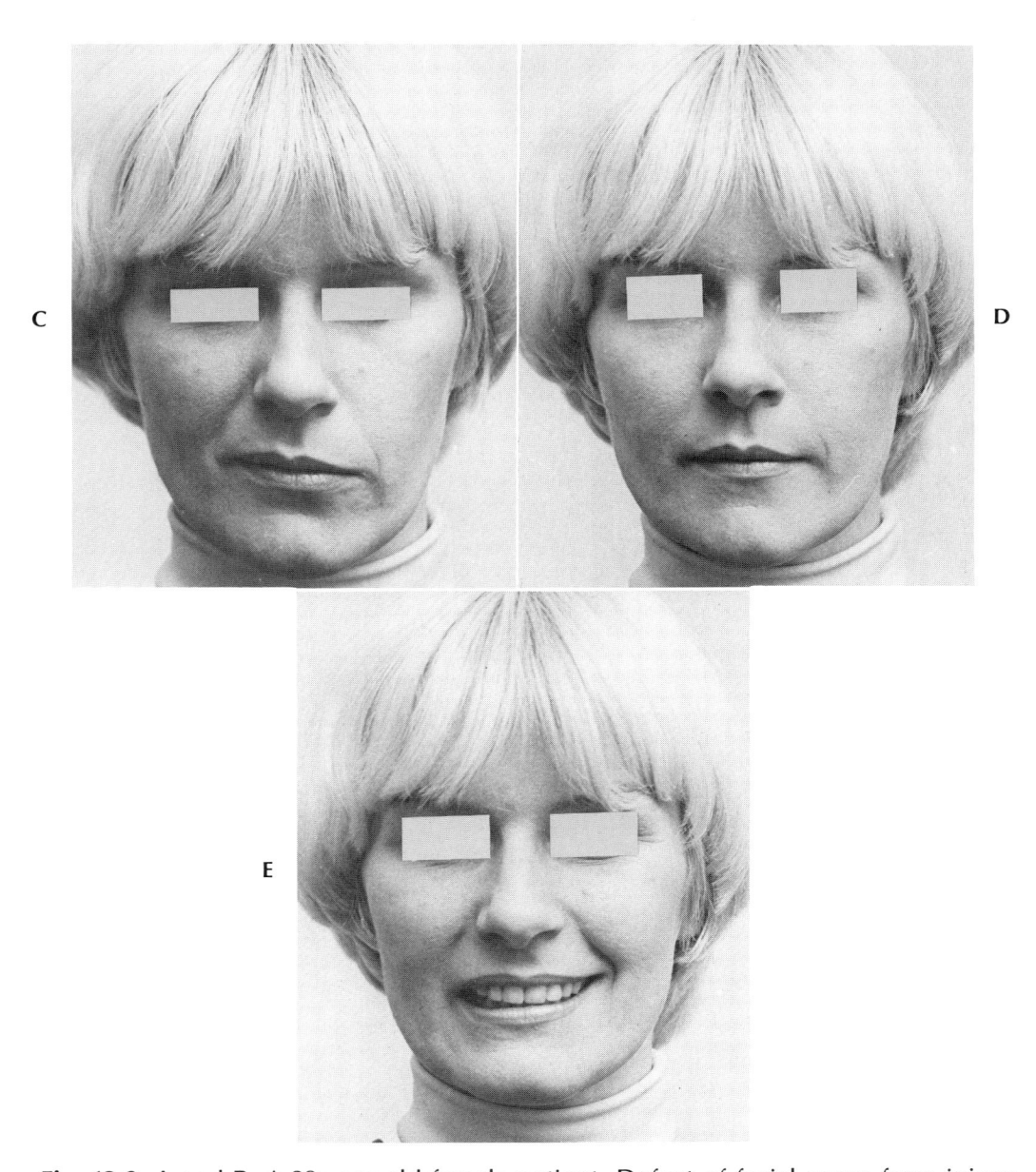

Fig. 12-6. **A** and **B,** A 29-year-old female patient. Defect of facial nerve from injury of parotid area (traffic accident). Only branch to lower lip was preserved. Six nerve grafts of 6 cm length were used to reestablish continuity. **C** to **E,** Result after 1 year.

Contemporary concepts in free nerve and muscle grafting

or with the segment at the cross section where there is a predominance of the corresponding fibers (Fig. 12-6).

Within the temporal bone, this problem is not so acute because one graft is sufficient to bridge a defect, but it is important to prevent malrotation.

Provision of nerve grafts

Different nerves are suitable as donor nerves. A donor nerve must be easily accessible and its resection should cause a negligible functional loss. It should be situated in an area where irritation by neuroma formation is minimal.

The sural nerve meets this condition very well. It is easily found behind the lateral ankle. Using several transverse incisions, one can obtain a long segment. In the proximal half of the calf the nerve is situated in the subfacial space and possible neuroma formation is not a problem. The nerve consists of several fascicles: at its distal portion it separates into several branches, each of different size. By microsurgical longitudinal splitting, grafts of any diameter can be obtained. The functional loss, namely, hypoesthesia along the outer margin of the foot, is minimal. Another suitable source of nerve grafts for the facial nerves are the branches of the cervical plexus. They are found at the posterior margin of the sternocleidomastoid muscle in the region of its upper and middle third. Other suitable donor nerves are the cutaneus antebrachii medialis and the cutaneus femoris lateralis nerve.

The donor nerve is transected into sections longer than the distance between the proximal and the distal stump. Transection is performed by a sharp microscissor. At first, the epineurium is cut. By a small lateral movement the epineurium is shifted away to prevent it from overlapping the cross section; then the transection is completed.

In theory it may happen that after nerve grafting the distal suture line is blocked by scar tissue, preventing ingress of arriving sprouts. In this case, resection of the distal suture site with a new neurorrhaphy has to be carried out. This problem is seen more often in long defects of peripheral nerves but not so in facial surgery because grafts are usually rather short.

Application of nerve grafts in facial nerve surgery

During the last years the confidence in the results of nerve grafts has increased very much. Nerve grafting has been used for restoration of the continuity of the facial nerve (Fig. 12-6). An important new technique is the transfer of axons from one facial nerve to the other across the face. Grafts can be used to connect individual branches of the same facial nerve if partial destruction has occurred.

A wide field for nerve grafting has been opened by the new techniques of muscle transposition and muscle transplantation. After a free muscle grafting was developed, it was believed that a free grafted muscle survives only if grafted into another muscle.[6] In the meantime, we learned that free grafted muscles can be reinnervated by nerve grafts without any muscle contact.[20] Reinnervation of transposed muscles, deprived of their original nerve supply, is another possibility.[7] Nerve grafts can be used to lengthen the motor nerve of a muscle whose transplantation is planned. For example, if we want to transplant a normal platysma of the one side to a paralyzed side, it is useful to lengthen the motor branch to this muscle by a sufficiently long nerve graft in a first step. In the second step the muscle can be transplanted without loss of its nerve supply. We applied this technique successfully in one patient.

Looking forward

The new technique of muscle grafting by microvascular anastomosis will open new indications for nerve grafting. Restoration of the continuity of the hypoglossus nerve is indicated if this important nerve has been destroyed. Not only is motor function important, but also restoration of sensory nerves is essential in central lesions of the trigeminus nerve in order to prevent exulceration of the cornea. This can be achieved by a nerve graft connecting the major occipital nerve across the cranial cavity with the distal stump of the ophthalmic nerve.[20] After resection of the inferior alveolar nerve by cancer surgery, the sensibility of the lower nerve can be restored by a long nerve graft.

Careful observation and attention to technique will enable us to graft areas heretofore impossible. Examples of this can be found in the restoration of motor nerve function as in the hypoglossus nerve, sensory functions as in the inferior alveolar nerve, and restoration sensation to the cornea by grafting of the major occipital nerve across the cranial cavity with the distal stump of the ophthalmic nerve.

REFERENCES

1. Ballance, C., and Duel, A. B.: The operative treatment of facial palsy by introduction of nerve grafts into the fallopian canal and by other intratemporal methods, Arch. Otolaryngol. **15:**1, 1932; Trans. Am. Otolaryngol. Soc. **21:**288, 1931.
2. Bunnel, S.: Suture of facial nerve within the temporal bone with report of the first successful case, Surg. Gynecol. Obstet. **45:**7, 1927.
3. Conley, J. J.: Facial nerve grafting in treatment of parotid gland tumors; new techniques, Arch. Surg. **70:**359, 1955.
4. Conley, J. J.: Facial nerve grafting, Arch. Otolaryngol. **73:**332, 1961.
5. Duel, A. B.: The operative treatment of facial palsy, Br. Med. J. **2:**1027, 1934.
6. Freilinger, G.: Diskussionsbemerkung an der 4. Tagung der Deutschen Plastischen Chirurgie, Frankfurt am Main, 5.-8. Sept. 1973.
7. Freilinger, G.: A new technique to correct facial paralysis, Plast. Reconstr. Surg. **56:**44-48, 1975.
8. Kreutzberg, G. W.: Physiology and pathology dendrites. Adv. Neurol., vol. 12, New York, 1975, Raven Press.
9. Lathrop, F. D.: Facial nerve grafting, Trans. Am. Acad. Ophthalmol. Otolaryngol. **68:**1060, 1964.
10. May, M.: Anatomy of the facial nerve, Laryngoscope **83:**1311-1320, 1973.
11. Maxwell, J. H.: Repair of the facial nerve after facial lacerations, Trans. Am. Acad. Ophthalmol. Otolaryngol. **58:**733, 1954.
12. Meissl, G.: Third International Symposium on Facial Nerve Surgery, 9-12 August 1976, Zurich, Switzerland.
13. Miehlke, A.: Über den chirurgischen Wiederaufbau des Gesichtsnerven nach extratemporalen Läsionen, Dtsch. Med. Wochenschr. **85:**506, 1960.
14. Miehlke, A.: Extratemporalis facialis Chirurgie, Z. Laryngol. Rhinol. Otolaryngol. **40:**338, 1961.
15. Miehlke, A.: Surgery of the facial nerve, ed. 2, Munich, 1973, Urban & Schwarzenberg.
16. Millesi, H., Berger, A., and Meissl, G.: Experimentelle Untersuchungen zur Heilung durchtrennter peripherer Nerven, Chir. Plast. **1:**174-206, 1972.
17. Millesi, H., Ganglberger, J., and Berger, A.: Erfahrungen mit der Mikrochirurgie peripherer Nerven, Chir. Plast. Reconstr. **3:**47-55, 1967.
18. Millesi, H.: Zum Problem der Überbruckung von Defekten peripherer Nerven, Wien. Med. Wochenschr. **118:**182-187, 1968.
19. Millesi, H.: Microsurgery of peripheral nerves, Hand **5**(2):157-160, 1973.
20. Millesi, H., and Samii, M.: Erfahrungen mit verschiedenen Wiederherstellungsoperationen am Nervus facialis. In Hohler, H., editor: Planung und Wiederherstellungs-Chirurgie aus Klinik und Forschung, Stuttgart & New York, 1975, F. K. Schattauer Verlag.

13 Free whole muscle grafting: a survey

LARS HAKELIUS

The background of free muscle grafting is described. Denervation of striated muscle approximately 2 weeks before transplanting will initiate changes in metabolism and enzymatic activity to create a so-called plastic state. This condition is optimal for free grafting. In the recipient site, the grafted muscle must be placed against a living muscle denuded from its surrounding fascia. The graft will survive by ingrowth of blood vessels and will create a biochemical attraction to stimulate outsprouting of nerves from the immediate area. Once innervated by surrounding nerves, the muscle will take on its desired function.

The first attempt to transplant striated muscle was made in 1874 by Zielonko.[48] He placed free muscle grafts into the lymph sac of frogs. The transplants shrunk and after 1 month were replaced by fibrous tissue. In 1881 Gluck[17] reported survival of free muscle grafts taken from rabbits and transplanted to the tensor fasciae latae muscle of hens. In 1890 Magnus[27] tried to reproduce these experiments, without success. In 1893 Volkman[46] emphatically stated that Gluck's report was false and that grafted pieces of muscle never survive. The graft is replaced by scar tissue, which will be penetrated by only a few regenerating muscle fibers from the recipient muscle. In 1882 Helferich[18] removed a fibrosarcoma of the triceps brachii muscle of a man and filled the defect with a piece of muscle, 70 grams of weight, from a dog. The transplant was rejected.

Several succeeding reports have described unsuccessful muscle grafting.[34,38]

In the early 1950s a Russian group led by Studitsky devised a technique whereby an entire muscle could be regenerated from minced muscle fragments.[40] He considered that the regenerated muscle fibers originate from surviving myogenic nuclei of the minced graft. This group has also reported successful grafting of whole muscle bellies in young rats.[47] They considered that denervation of the transplant about 2 weeks prior to grafting might be of benefit for graft survival.

Thompson, in a series of reports, described free transplantations of whole muscle bellies, initially in dogs[42] and later in patients with facial palsy.[43,44] A prerequisite for survival was motor denervation of the graft 2 to 3 weeks before transplantation. The muscle was transplanted onto a normal muscle from which it was revascularized and reinnervated. In the patients with facial palsy the muscles of the healthy side were used as the source of reinnervation for the graft. It was placed partly or totally on the

---

This chapter is built on the following papers:

Hakelius, L., Nyström, B., and Stålberg, E.: Histochemical and neurophysiological studies of autotransplanted cat muscle, Scand. J. Plast. Reconstr. Surg. **9:**15, 1975.

Hakelius, L., and Nyström, B.: Histochemical studies of end-plate formation in free autologous muscle transplants in cats, Scand. J. Plast. Reconstr. Surg. **9:**9, 1975.

Hakelius, L., and Nyström, B.: Blood vessels and connective tissue in autotransplanted free muscle grafts of the cat, Scand. J. Plast. Reconstr. Surg. **9:**87, 1975.

Contemporary concepts in free nerve and muscle grafting

muscle of the healthy side corresponding to the paralyzed one, which was to have its function improved. The part of the graft not in contact with healthy muscle or the tendon of the graft was then positioned on the paralyzed side in such a way that the contraction of the graft would reproduce the normal action of the paralyzed muscle. In this way some restoration of the dynamic function of the paralyzed side of the face could be accomplished.

Histochemistry and reinnervation of striated mammalian muscle

Differences of enzyme constitution have been shown with histochemical staining methods in fibers of mammalian muscle.[32] The differences reflect the different metabolic pathways used by the fibers. Fibers rich in oxidative enzymes, such as succinic dehydrogenase and NADH-tetrazolium reductase favor an oxidative metabolic pathway, whereas fibers rich in phosphorylase mainly use glycolytic metabolism. Ogata[32] named fibers rich in oxidative enzymes "red fibers" and those with small amounts of these enzymes "white fibers." This parallels the myoglobin content.[8] Engel[12] showed that the staining properties for myofibrillar ATPase were approximately inverse to that of oxidative enzymes. In addition, the red fibers stain strongly for fat and the white for glycogen.

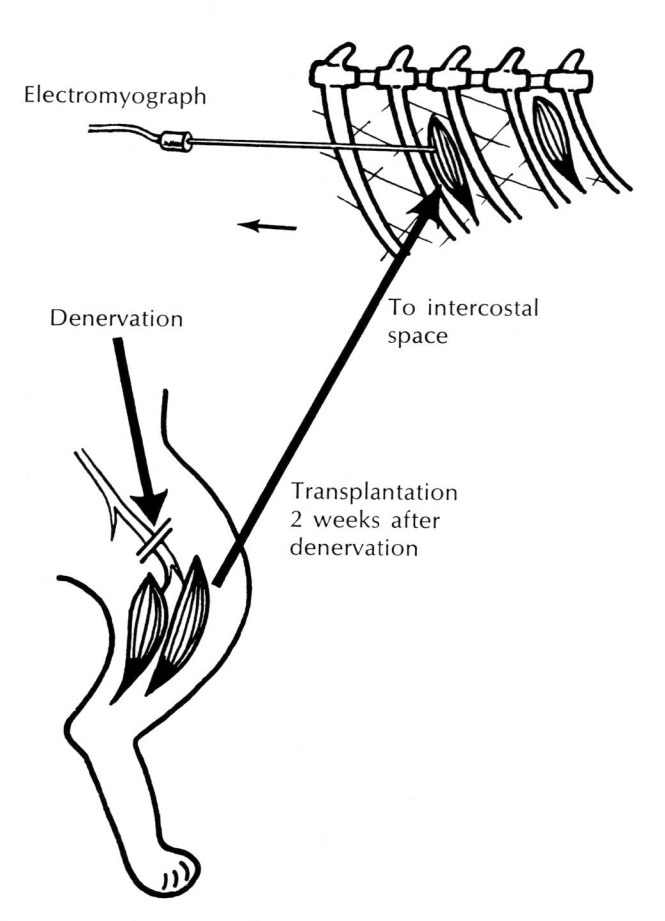

Fig. 13-1. Schematic illustration of experimental model.

Different muscle bellies contain different proportions of red and white fibers.[31] The muscles with a high percentage of red fibers contract slowly, and those with mainly white fibers contract fast.[2] The red, slow twitch muscles can work continually for long periods and the fast, white ones are rapidly exhausted.[35] This difference has also been shown by Kugelberg and Edström[25] in motor units with red and white fibers respectively.

The anterior horn cell, its axon, and the muscle fibers innervated by this axon are called a "motor unit." One anterior horn cell of the spinal cord gives motor innervation to a varying number of muscle fibers.[16]

In a motor unit, all the muscle fibers are of the same histochemical type.[11] In cross-innervation experiments, where a motor nerve to a red muscle has been sutured to the sectioned distal end of a nerve to a white muscle, this muscle has shown an increased percentage of red fibers after reinnervation has taken place, a finding that means that the nerve reinnervating the muscle fiber determines its histochemical profile.[37]

After denervation, changes in muscle metabolism and enzyme activity have been found both with biochemical and histochemical techniques. There is a reduction of anaerobic glycolytic enzymes in the white fibers and a decrease in aerobic enzymes in the red fibers, resulting in less differentiation of their enzymatic patterns.[20]

After reinnervation the histochemical properties of different fiber types again are developed, but the normal checkerboard pattern is replaced by scattered groups of fibers of the same type, so-called type grouping.[23]

If partial denervation of a muscle occurs, the denervated fibers are reinnervated by collateral sprouting of nerve twigs from neighboring normal nerve fibers.[9,19]

In reinnervated muscle, the boundaries of the motor unit coincide to a large extent with the fascicles, indicating that collateral sprouting may be hindered by the interfascicular connective tissue.[26] Collateral sprouting does not normally take place between two muscle bellies, probably because of the perimuscular fascia. However, Erlacher[14] in guinea pigs obtained reinnervation of a paralyzed muscle from a pedicle flap based on an adjacent muscle.

Experimental studies of histochemistry and reinnervation of whole muscle grafts

For study of revascularization and reinnervation of free muscle transplants, the peroneus longus and tertius muscles of adult cats were used as grafts. The cats were anesthetized with sodium pentobarbital (Nembutal). Denervation of the muscles intended as grafts was performed by excision of a 1 cm segment of the common peroneal nerve above the fibular head. Two weeks later the peroneus longus and tertius muscles were transplanted to two intercostal spaces (Fig. 13-1). Before grafting the perimuscular fascia of the grafts was removed. The grafts were then placed under the intercostal fascia in direct contact with the fibers of the intercostal muscle. Both ends of the grafts were sutured to the intercostal fascia under slight tension.

For histological and histochemical studies of the change of enzyme-constitution in transplanted muscle fibers, 24 muscles were denervated 2 weeks before transplantation and two muscles were transplanted without previous denervation. The grafts were then removed at intervals from 5 days to 44 weeks after transplantation. In the study of end-plate formation, seven previously denervated grafts were examined at intervals from 5 to 44 weeks. Normal and denervated muscles left in situ were also examined.

In 16 grafts, electromyograph (EMG) recordings were made at the time of extirpation (5 days to 44 weeks after grafting).

HISTOLOGICAL AND HISTOCHEMICAL METHODS

Specimens used for muscle histology or histochemistry were processed into 6 to 7 mm long pieces and rapidly frozen in liquid propane. The specimens not immediately used were stored at $-70°$ C. Serial sections, at right angles to the fiber direction, were made 16 μm thick in a cryostat at $-25°$ C.

Sections were stained for myofibrillar adenosine triphosphatase (ATPase) according to Padykula and Herman.[33] The two oxidative enzymes NADH-tetrazolium reductase (NADH-TR) and succinic dehydrogenase (SDH) were demonstrated by the methods of Scarpelli, Hess, and Pearse[39] and Nachlas, Tsou, de Souza, Cheng, and Seligman,[30] respectively, with some modifications.[31] Phosphorylase activity was demonstrated by the method of Takeuchi and Kuriaki[41] as modified by Eränkö and Palkama.[15] Lipids were visualized by use of Sudan black B according to Baker's method[3] and glycogen was demonstrated by the periodic acid–Schiff (PAS) reaction.[29]

Connective tissue was visualized by two staining methods (van Gieson and Azan). The larger vessels could also be examined with this technique, whereas smaller vessels and capillaries had to be studied in sections stained for ATPase, since blood vessels and capillaries are rich in alkaline phosphatase.[22]

For investigation of the end-plate structure, fresh specimens were fixed in 10% formalin for 4 hours before sectioning and incubation. Sections were cut on a freezing microtome. The Couteaux[6] modification of the Koelle-Friedenwald[24] staining was used with acetylthiocholine as the substrate. Sections were incubated at 37° C for 10 to 135 minutes. The structures visualized by this technique are the cholinesterase-containing subneural apparatuses or the postsynaptic structures.[5]

ELECTROMYOGRAPHICAL METHODS

At the time of extirpation the grafts were first carefully exposed in order to leave the innervation to the graft intact. Before recordings from the grafts were made, the EMG activity of a normal intercostal muscle was recorded to determine if the level of anesthesia was superficial enough to retain intercostal breathing. Concentric EMG needle electrodes connected to a one-channel EMG apparatus were used in this test. The EMG was recorded on analog tape for later analysis on a storage oscilloscope. The recordings were made from at least two sites of the transplant at different depths and from the normal underlying intercostal muscle.

Results

The transplants, when removed, showed a decrease in volume from 0 to 50% compared to the time of grafting. There was no sign of infection, inflammatory reaction, or scar tissue formation around them at any time. Generally the grafts had the color of healthy muscle.

In the normal muscles studied there was no obvious difference between the proportions of red and white muscle fibers in the peroneus longus and tertius muscles. The cross-sectional areas of red and white muscle fibers were estimated to be of the same proportion in both muscles.

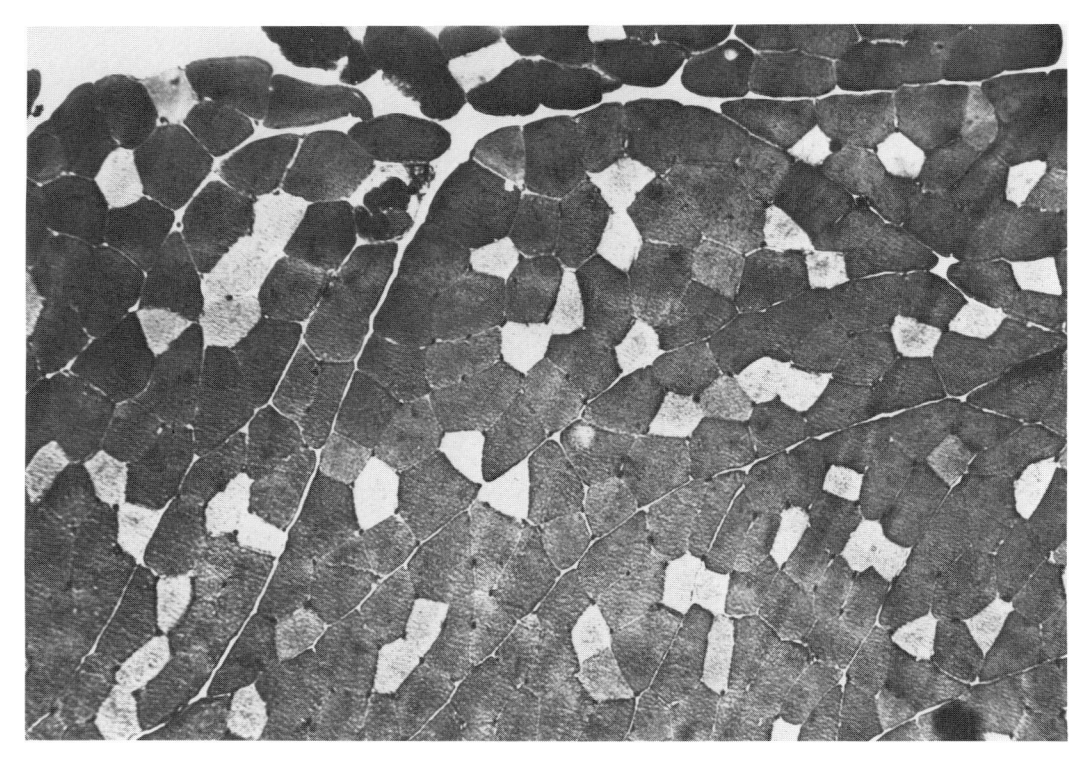

Fig. 13-2. Cross section of normal peroneus longus muscle, stained for myofibrillar ATPase. Note muscle spindle above to the left. (160×.)

MUSCLE HISTOCHEMISTRY

In sections from normal muscle the checkerboard pattern of red and white muscle fibers was seen (Fig. 13-2). Red fibers showed a strong staining for oxidative enzymes and fat but a weak one for phosphorylase, glycogen, and ATPase. In white fibers the opposite staining pattern occurred. At the time of transplantation, 2 weeks after denervation, the histochemical appearance was fairly normal and only insignificant atrophy was seen. In muscles denervated and left in situ for 7 weeks, muscle fiber atrophy was evident and histochemically the red and white fibers stained nearly alike for oxidative enzymes. Five days after transplantation a cross section of the grafts showed three zones. In the outer zone, the red and white fibers could be distinguished by staining both for oxidative enzymes and ATPase. In the middle zone, no normal muscle fibers could be seen. This zone appeared to consist of necrotic remnants of fibers, but it stained well for NADH-TR and SDH and not at all for ATPase. The inner zone consisted of structurally intact muscle fibers, slightly smaller and rounder than in the outer zone. In sections stained for ATPase, red and white fibers could be separated in this zone, but they showed little or no reaction when stained for oxidative enzymes and they could not be distinguished in these stainings.

In the 10-day-old graft the entire cross-sectional area showed fibers of uniform characteristics in stainings both for ATPase and oxidative enzymes, and the muscle fibers were smaller than in the 5-day-old grafts. At both 5 and 10 days, the fibers showed no reactions for phosphorylase, glycogen, or fat.

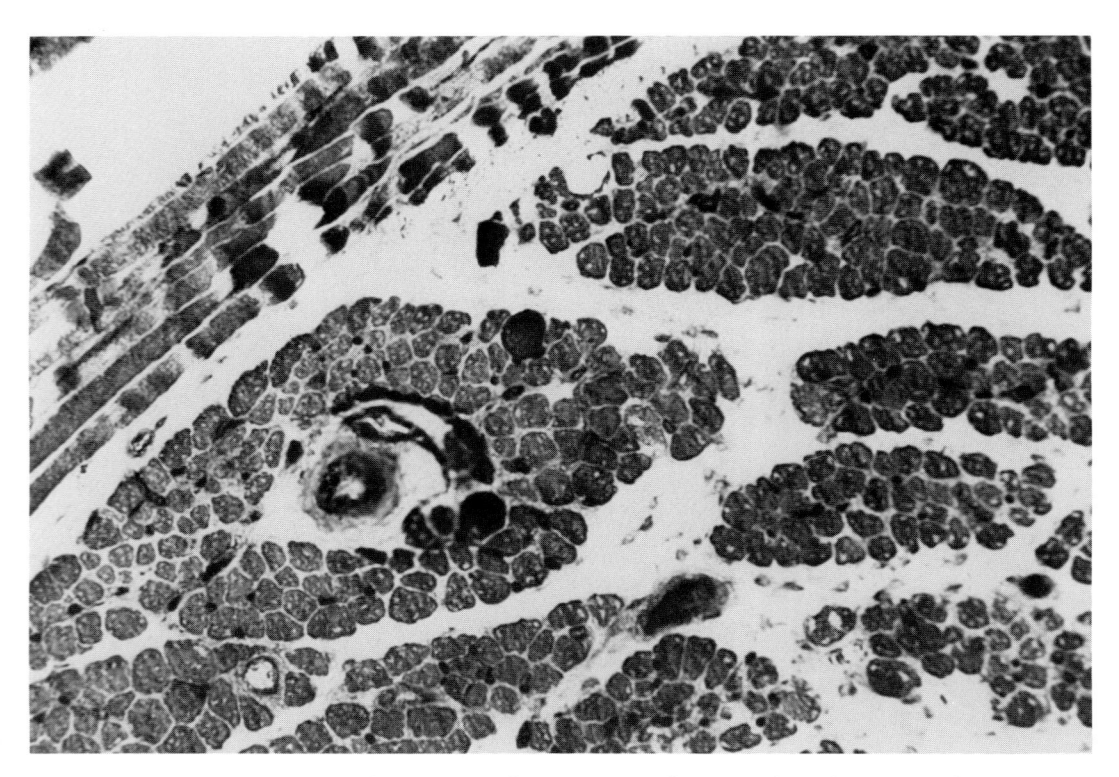

Fig. 13-3. Cross section of peroneus longus muscle 2 weeks after transplantation, stained for myofibrillar ATPase. The fibers have uniform staining intensity, comparable to that of intercostal fibers (above to the left). (160×.)

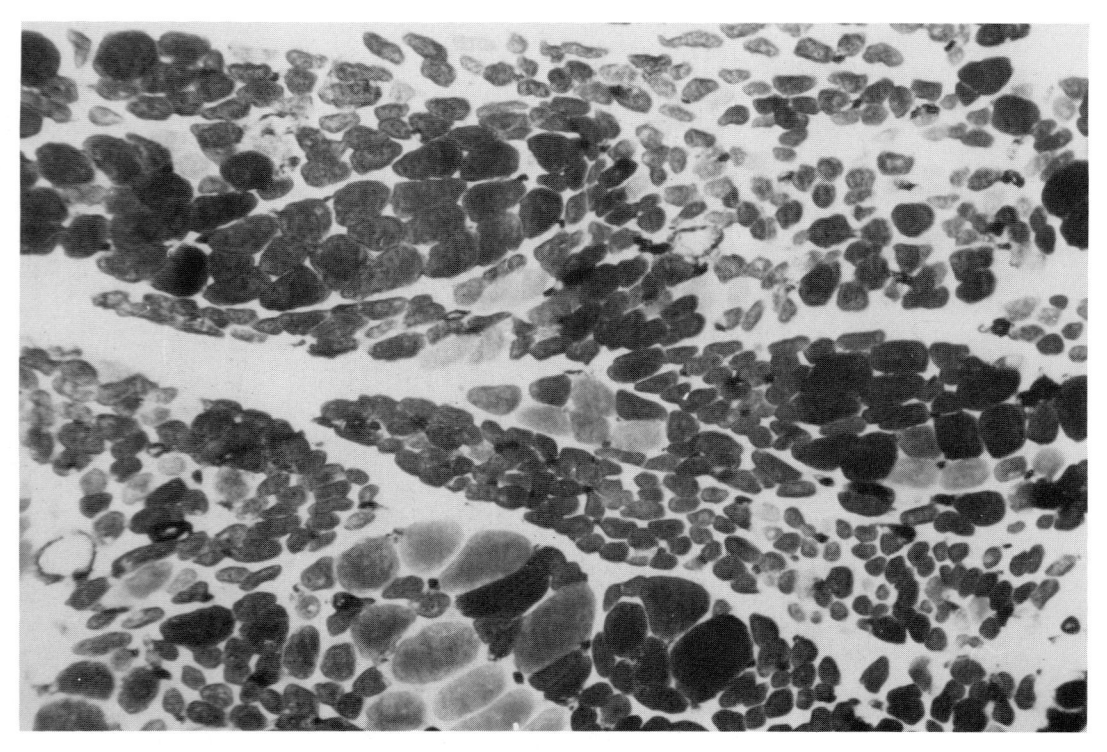

Fig. 13-4. Cross section of previously denervated peroneus tertius muscle 8 weeks after transplantation, stained for myofibrillar ATPase. (160×.)

The transplants examined after 2, 4, and 6 weeks showed muscle fibers of uniform size. The staining characteristics were the same as in the 10-day-old transplant (Fig. 13-3).

In the transplants removed after 8, 10, and 12 weeks, there was a tendency toward redifferentiation of the fibers into red and white ones (Fig. 13-4). A pronounced difference in size between some large fibers in scattered groups and the general fiber population existed.

During the period from 14 to 18 weeks most of the muscle fibers in the grafts were reinnervated as demonstrated by the histochemical staining reactions. There was obvious type grouping, which varied in different muscles. The fibers at this time also stained well for fat.

In the transplants examined from 19 to 26 weeks after grafting, most fibers were of normal size, but some, especially of the white ones, were evidently larger than normal.

In the oldest grafts, investigated 40 to 44 weeks after transplantation, there was a varying degree of type grouping (Fig. 13-5). Most fibers were of the red or white types, but groups of intermediate fibers were also found. Generally the white fibers were larger than the red ones, and it appeared that the difference in size between the two types was increased compared to normal muscle. In some of the grafts of this age and in those 19 to 26 weeks old, there was a dominance of white fibers over red ones.

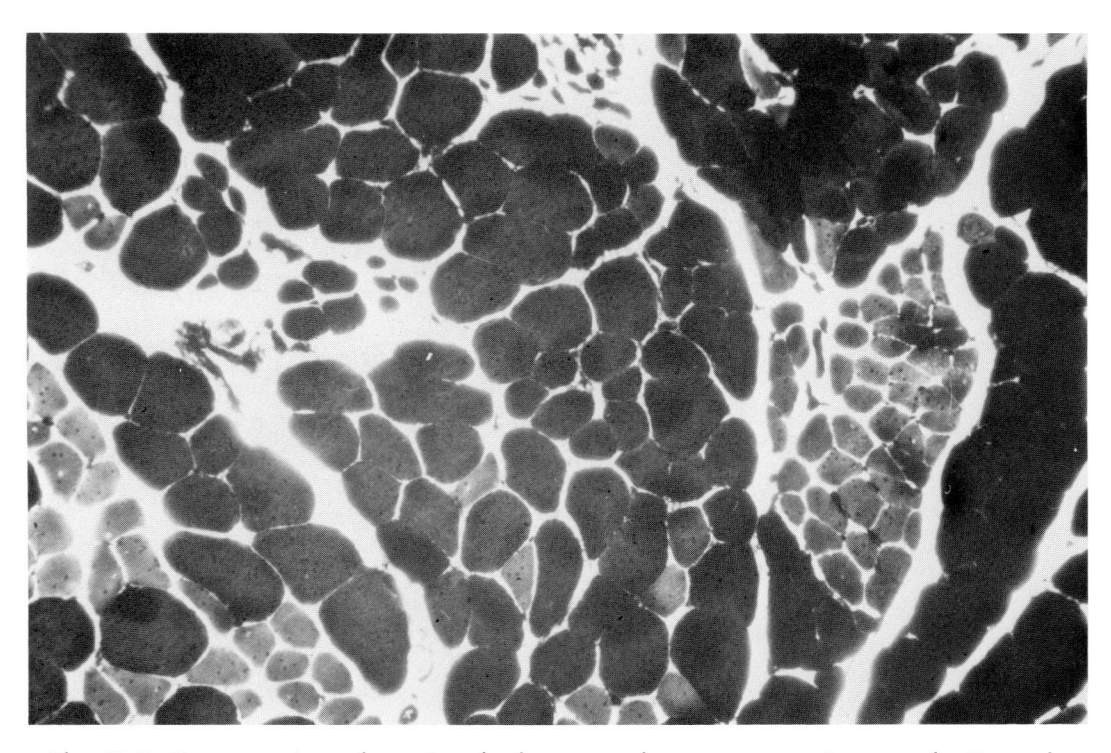

Fig. 13-5. Cross section of previously denervated peroneus tertius muscle 40 weeks after grafting, stained for myofibrillar ATPase. Note the type grouping. (160×.)

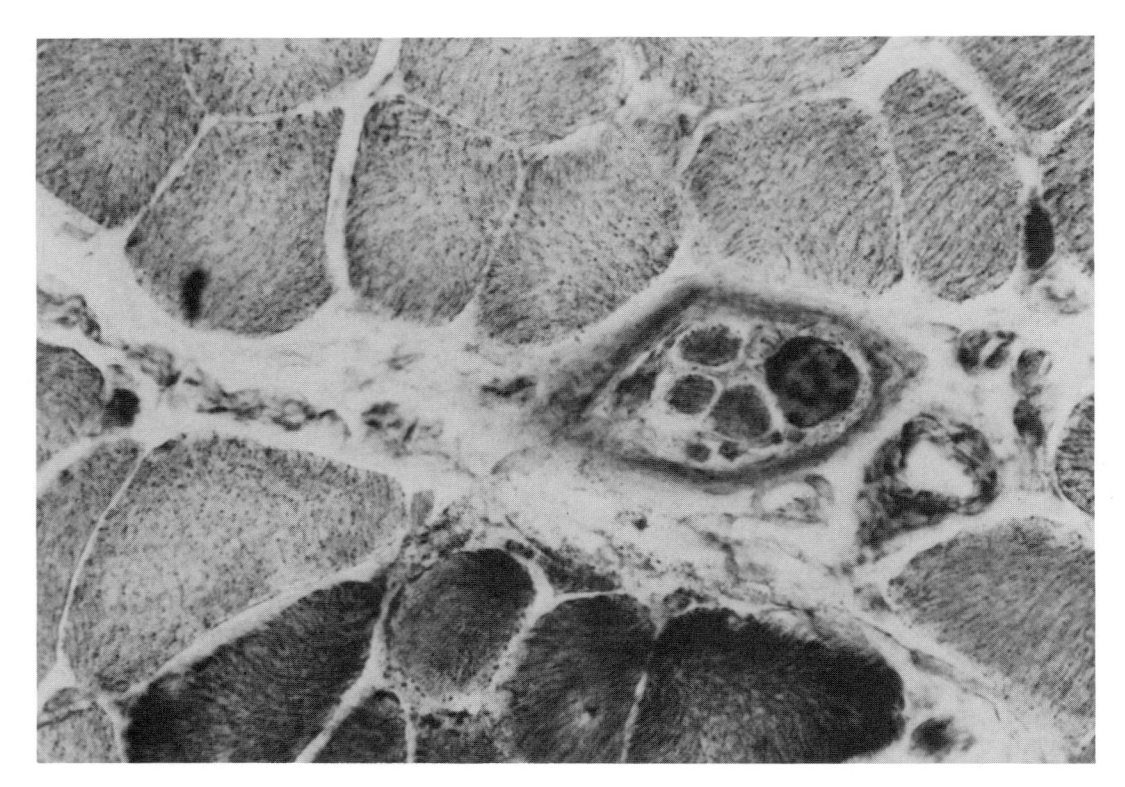

Fig. 13-6. Cross section of transplant of peroneus tertius muscle 40 weeks after grafting, stained for NADH-TR. Red and white extrafusal muscle fibers are seen and an apparently normal muscle spindle. (650×.)

In the whole series of grafts, no remnants of old muscle spindles occurred. Two apparently newly formed spindles were seen at 12 and 40 weeks, respectively (Fig. 13-6).

In the two transplantations made without previous denervation strong fibrosis was seen at the removal after 24 weeks, and the existing muscle fibers were less mature than in the transplants of the same age denervated beforehand.

END-PLATE FORMATION

In the normal fan-shaped peroneal muscles of the cat the end plates were found in a narrow zone at the middle portion of the fibers as previously described for muscles of this type[4] (Fig. 13-7). The normal end plates were generally ramified, with the ramifications separated from each other (Fig. 13-8). After 2 weeks of denervation, such as at the time of transplantation, the end plates appeared normal. In denervated muscles left in situ, the end plates were smaller after 7 weeks than were normal ones and showed a less distinct border of their ramifications.

Five weeks after grafting very few end plates were seen. They were small and stained weakly even after long incubation periods (135 minutes compared to 10 minutes in the normals). The end plates appeared in short and narrow zones both in the deep and in the superficial part of the graft. Ramifications were still visible in

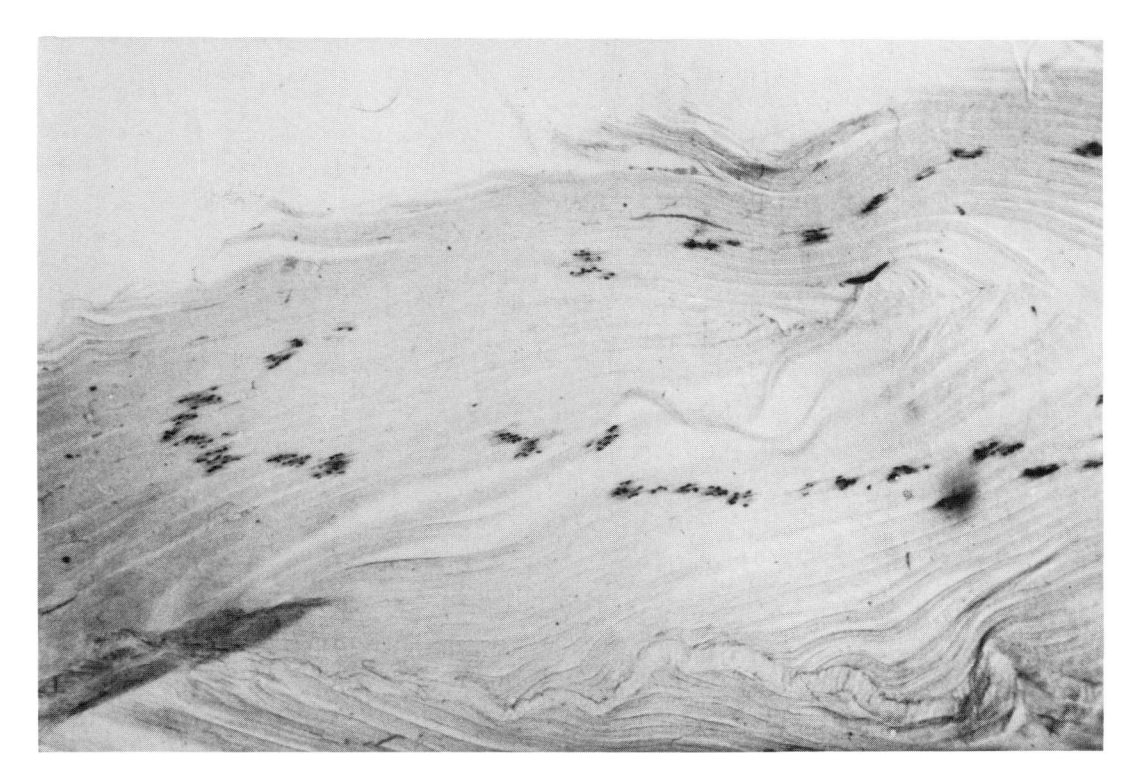

Fig. 13-7. Longitudinal section of long peroneal muscle showing fan-shaped arrangement of muscle fibers and narrow zone of end plates stained for cholinesterase. (16×.)

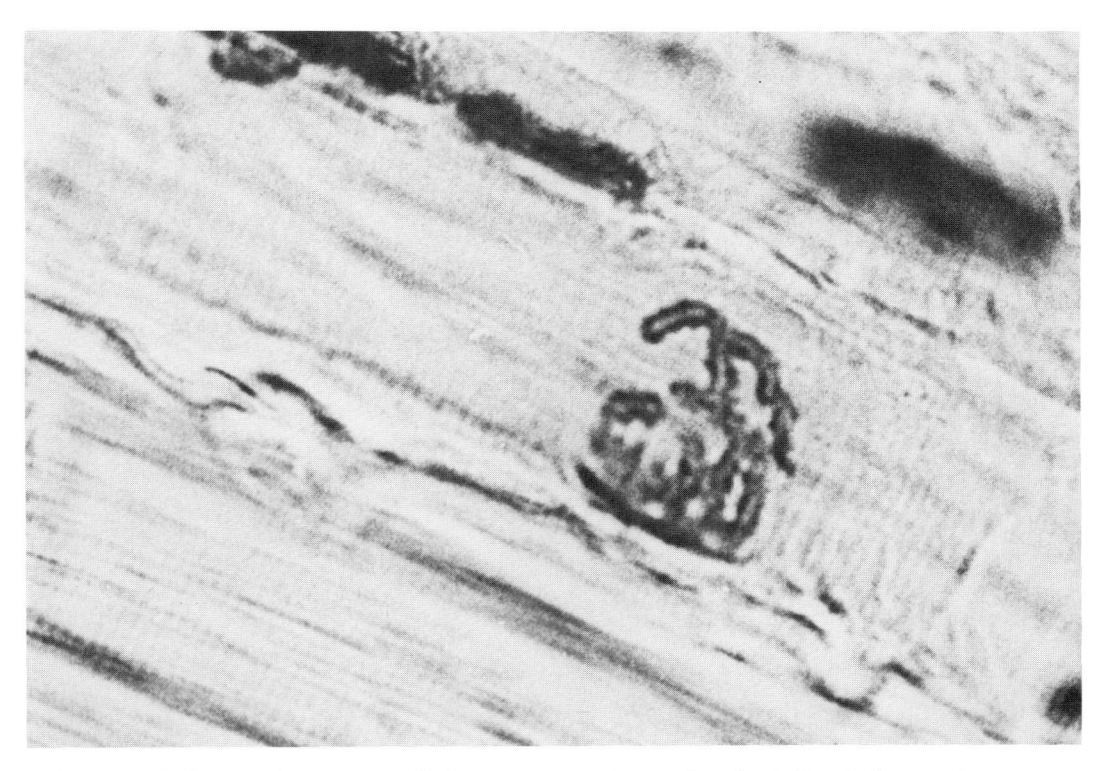

Fig. 13-8. Subneural apparatus in long peroneal muscle of adult cat. Apparatuses are ramified with unbroken ramifications. (1100×.)

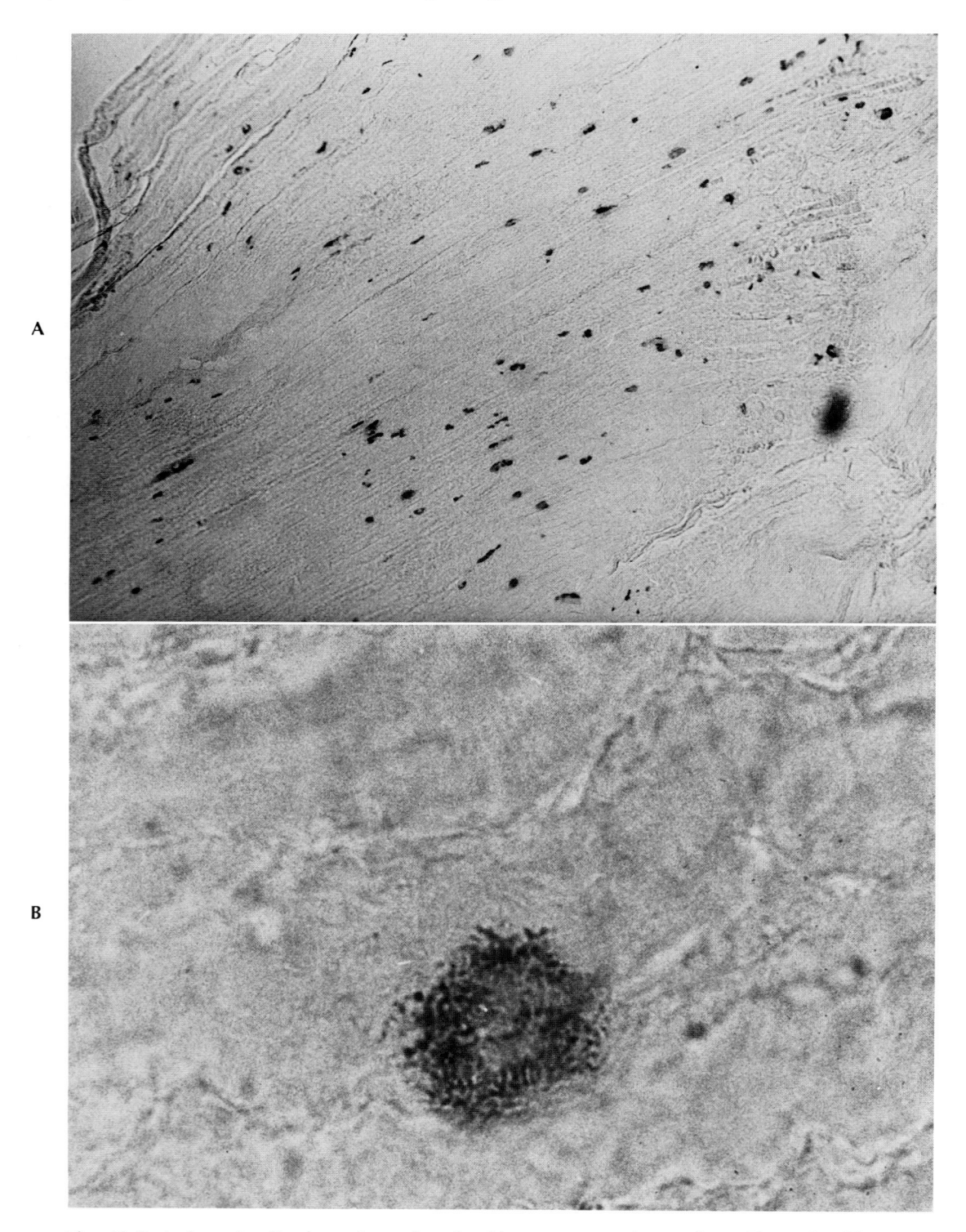

Fig. 13-9. A, Longitudinal section of graft of long peroneal muscle at 12 weeks. There are many small, rounded cholinesterase-positive plaques distributed throughout muscle. **B,** Subneural apparatus from long peroneal muscle of adult cat 7 weeks after denervation. Apparatus is smaller than in normal cats, and outline is irregular. (**A,** 60×; **B,** 1400×.)

Free whole muscle grafting: a survey

these apparently disintegrating end plates. In the same graft a few small rounded lightly stained plaques were seen.

In the 7- and 9-week-old grafts, the original end plates were fragmented and small. Rounded, lightly stained plaques were more numerous than in the 5-week-old graft and were scattered throughout the sections.

In the 12-week-old graft, no old fragmented end plates were found, but an exceptional number of small rounded cholinesterase-positive plaques were stained throughout the muscle (Fig. 13-9). Because of the great mass of these immature end plates, it was likely that there was more than one end plate on each muscle fiber (Fig. 13-10).

In the specimens examined 20, 24, and 40 weeks after grafting, this massive scattering of end plates was not seen. Instead, the end plates occurred in groups or short bands along the muscle length, and only some scattering remained in parts of the grafts. The end plates were now more mature, and ramifications were seen.

REVASCULARIZATION AND FIBROSIS

In cross sections of normal muscles large vessels are found in the interfascicular connective tissue. The distribution of the capillaries is regular, and they are generally situated at the angles of the polygonal fibers. Around the red muscle fibers there usually is one capillary at each angle, whereas white muscle fibers have fewer capillaries than angles (Fig. 13-11). In muscles denervated for 2 weeks and left in situ, a slight

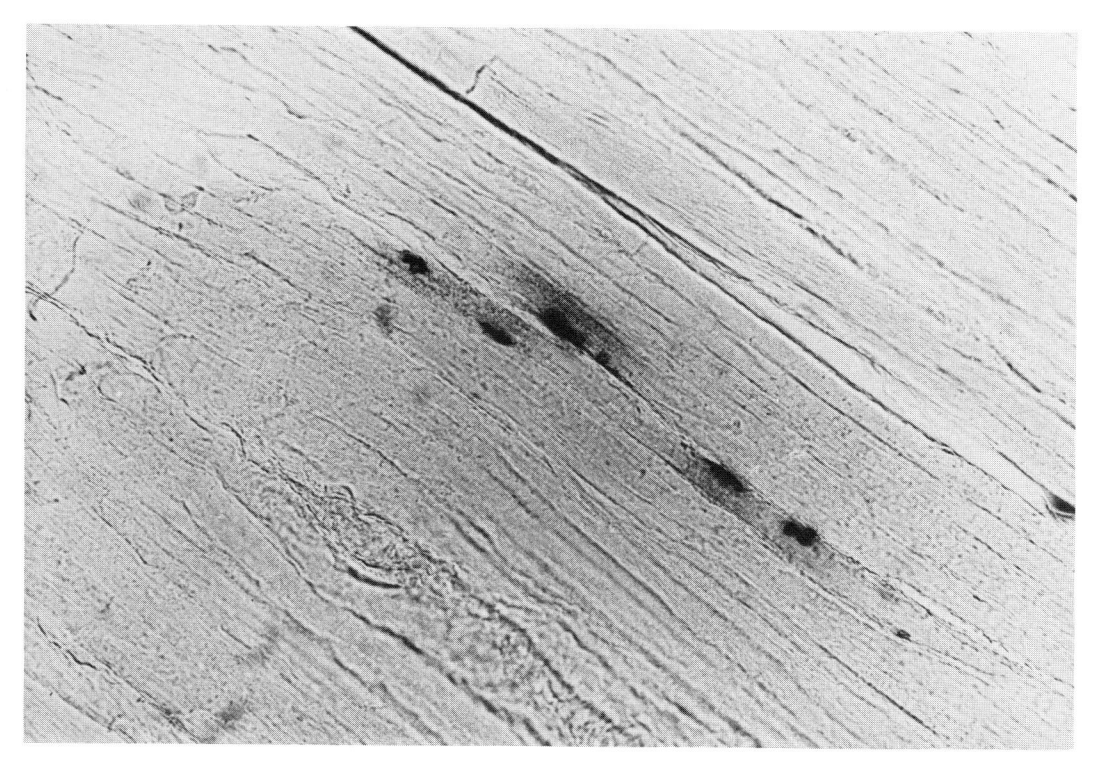

Fig. 13-10. Longitudinal section through graft of peroneus tertius muscle at 20 weeks, showing four subneural apparatuses on same muscle fiber. (190×.)

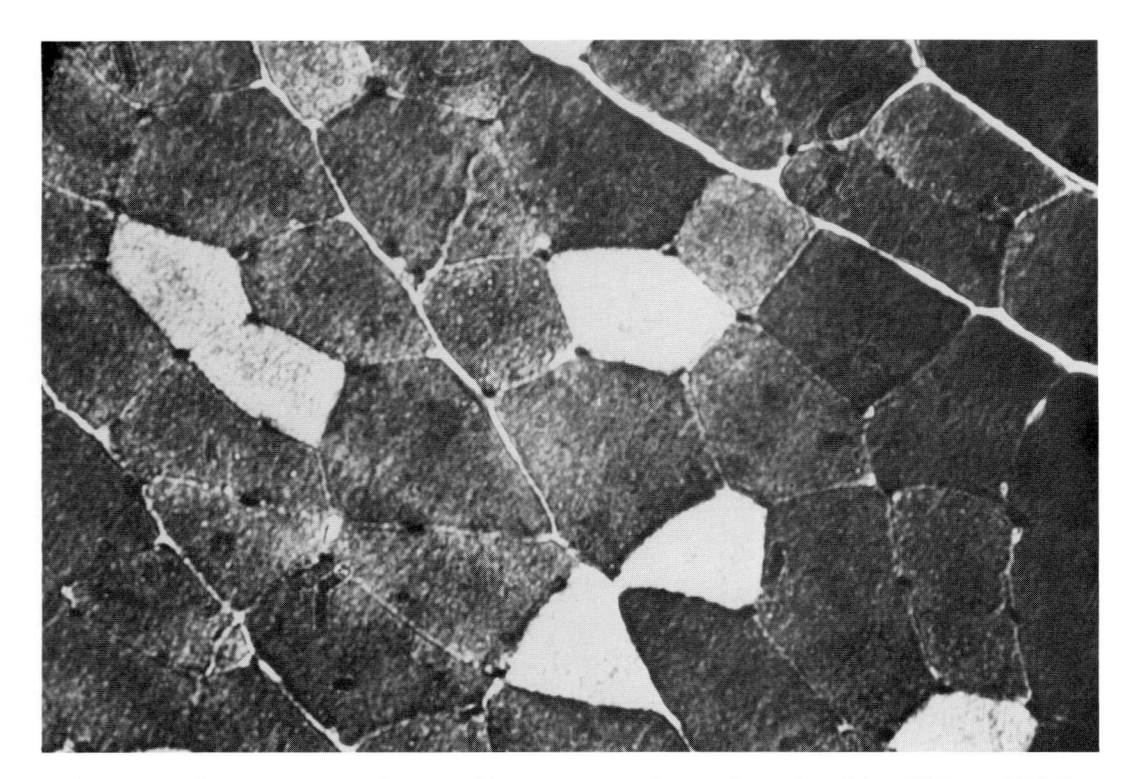

Fig. 13-11. Cross section of normal long peroneal muscle stained for ATPase. Lightly stained red muscle fibers are supplied by dark capillaries lying at fiber angles. Darkly stained white muscle fibers are less supplied with capillaries. (400×.)

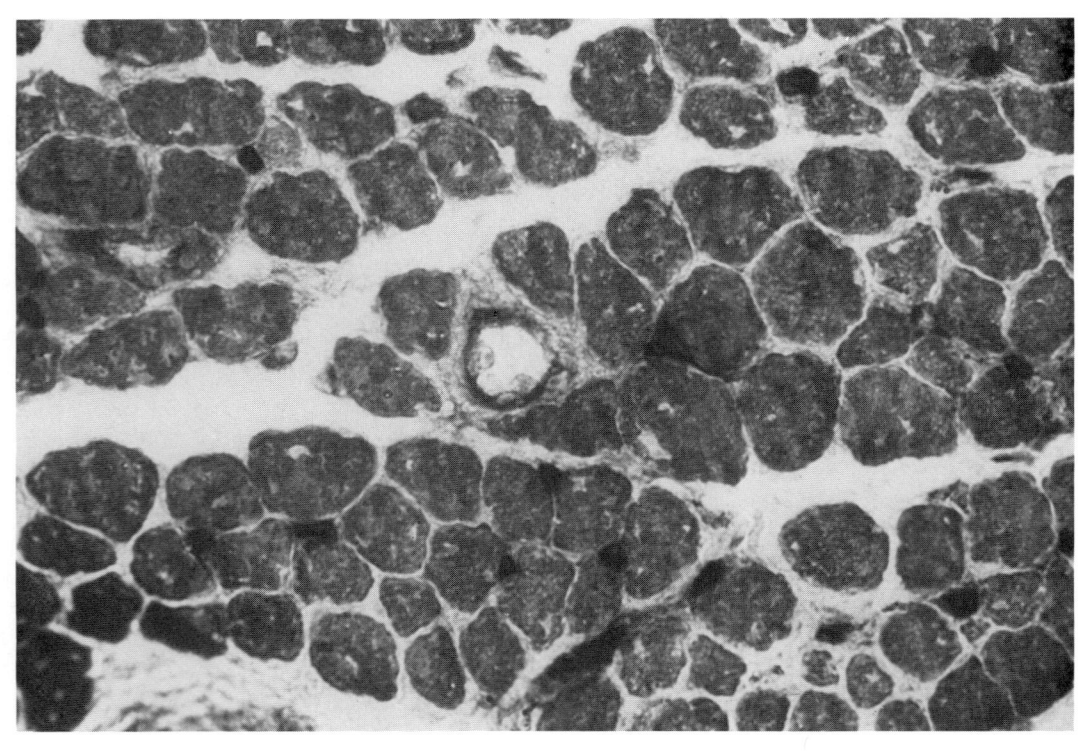

Fig. 13-12. Cross section of graft of long peroneal muscle 2 weeks after transplantation. Scattered thick-walled capillaries are seen. No regular capillary network exists, and many fibers are not in contact with a capillary. (ATPase stain, 400×.)

Free whole muscle grafting: a survey

increase in capillary density occurred. After 7 weeks the capillary network had become irregular in the muscles left in situ. Most muscle fibers were in relation to only one or two capillaries, and the capillary walls were thicker than in the normal muscle.

In 5-day-old grafts large vessels were observed in the periphery of the graft but very few capillaries were seen. After 10 days, thick-walled irregularly shaped capillaries were noted at distances of at least five muscle fiber diameters from each other (Fig. 13-12). This sparse population of capillaries remained until the grafts were 8 to 12 weeks old, when reinnervation occurred. The capillary density then increased, and the walls appeared more delicate. In transplants older than 15 to 18 weeks the capillary network had regained a nearly normal appearance (Fig. 13-13).

In cross sections of normal muscles interfascicular strands of connective tissue are seen but not the endomysial lining of the individual muscle fibers with the methods used (Fig. 13-14). At the early stages after grafting a sharp increase in perimysial and endomysial connective tissue took place. With increasing reinnervation a gradual disappearance of the perimysial and endomysial connective tissue occurred (Fig. 13-15). In the most mature grafts, only a minimal increase of perimysial connective tissue remained (Fig. 13-16). In muscles transplanted without previous denervation extensive fibrosis took place.

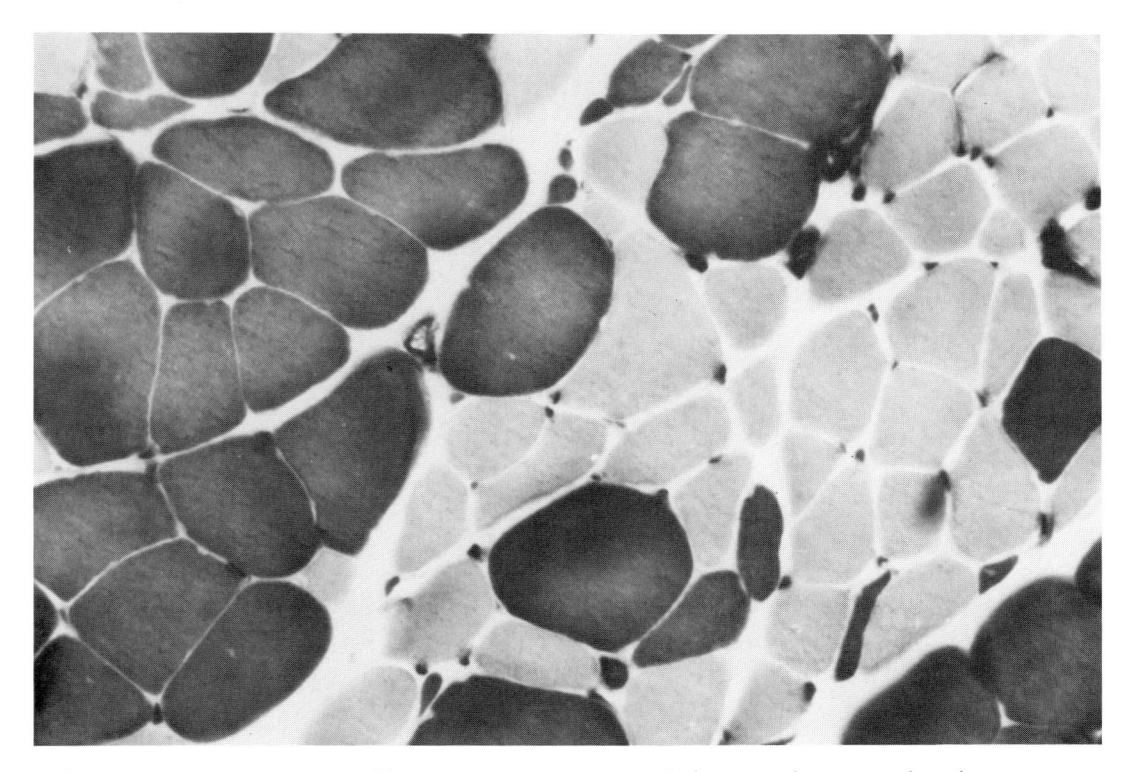

Fig. 13-13. Cross section of long extensor carpi radialis muscle 18 weeks after transplantation. Fairly regular capillary network is formed in type group of red muscle fibers (lightly stained). Among white fibers (darkly stained) there are few capillaries. At this stage, capillaries have a normal appearance (compare Fig. 13-12). (ATPase stain, 400×.)

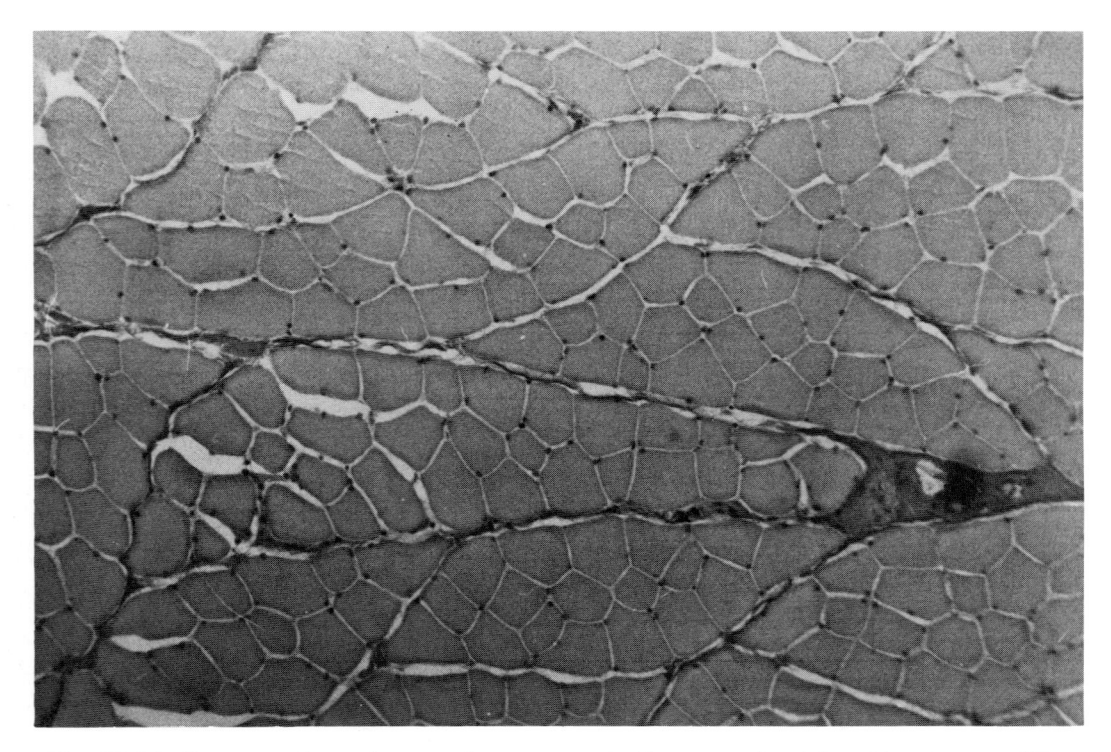

Fig. 13-14. Cross section of normal peroneus tertius muscle stained by the van Gieson technique. Perimysial strands of connective tissue encircle the muscle fascicles, but there is no visible endomysium. (160×.)

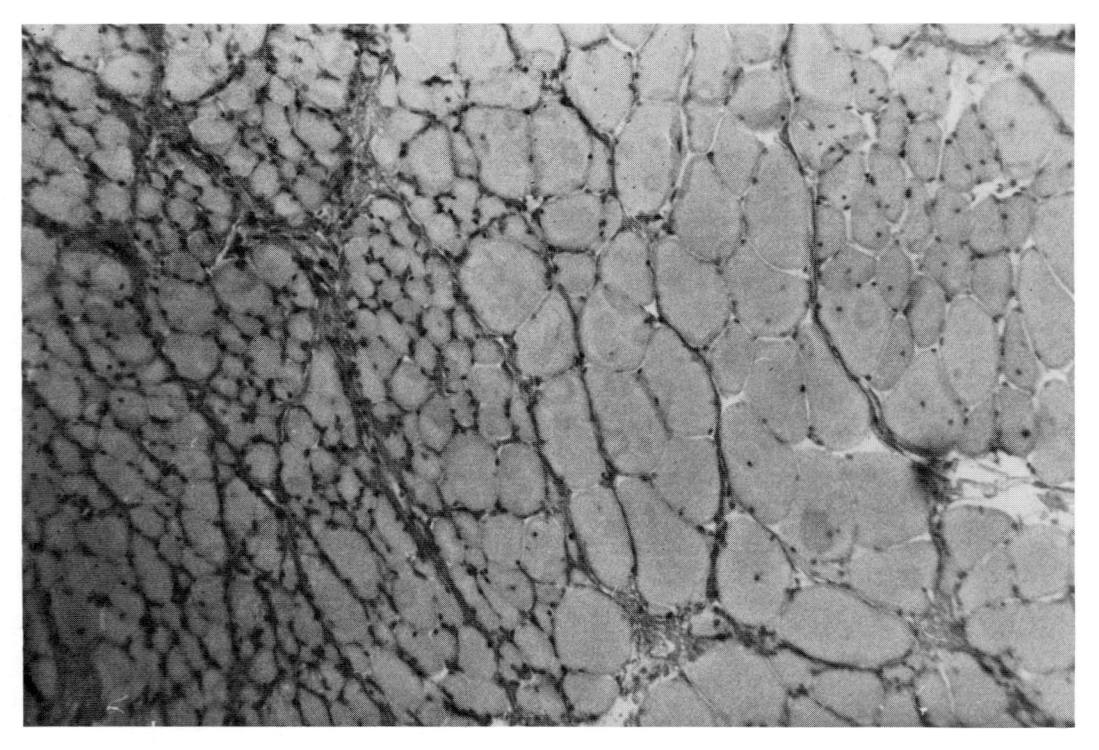

Fig. 13-15. Cross section of peroneus tertius muscle 16 weeks after transplantation. In right half, reinnervation is prominent. Interfascicular strands of connective tissue are thin, and a small amount of endomysial connective tissue is seen around fibers. In left half, most muscle fibers are still denervated. In this part, interfascicular strands of connective tissue are thicker and each fiber is surrounded by thickened endomysium. (Van Gieson's stain, 160×.)

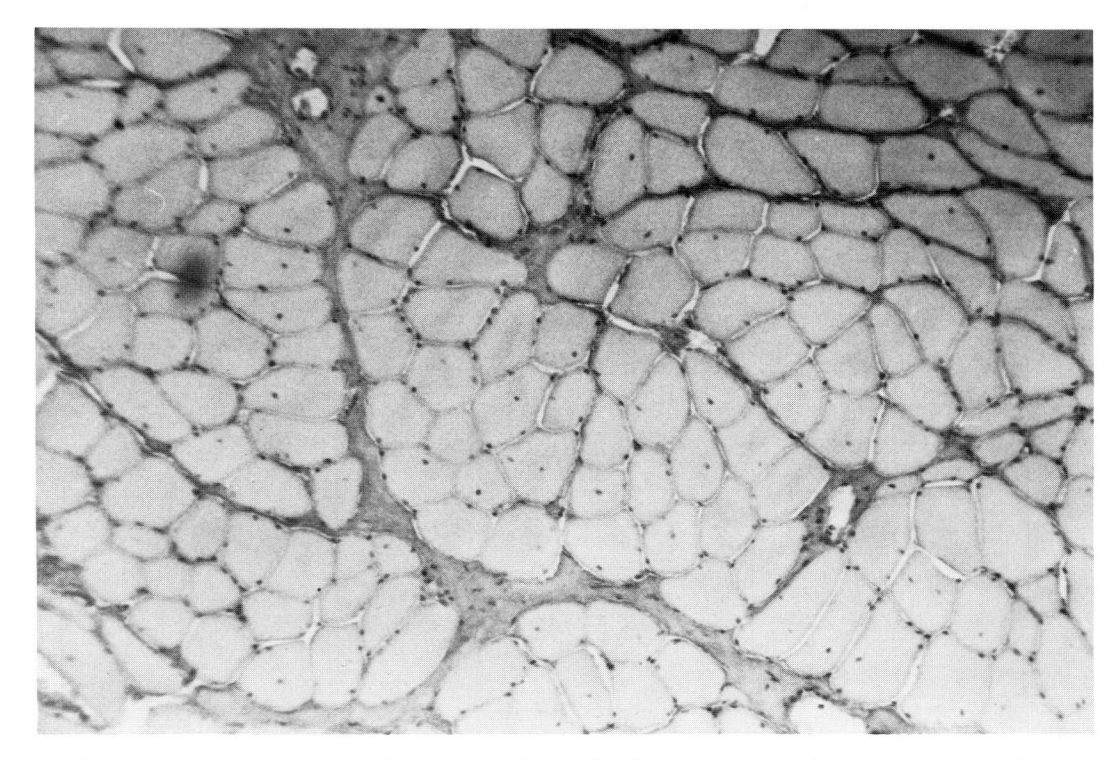

Fig. 13-16. Cross section of 40-week-old graft of peroneus tertius muscle. Interfascicular connective tissue is thicker than in normal muscle (compare Fig. 13-14), but most fibers do not show thickening of endomysium. (Van Gieson's stain, 160×.)

ELECTROMYOGRAPHY

Fibrillation potentials and occasionally positive sharp waves were seen in all examined transplants up to 14 weeks as a sign of denervated muscle fibers in the grafts.

Voluntary activity, defined as activity synchronous to the EMG of the underlying intercostal muscle, was observed as early as 4 weeks after grafting, and in the graft examined 6 weeks after reinnervation, action-potential complexes were more frequent. The older transplants demonstrated a relatively full interference EMG pattern (Fig. 13-17), but a quantitation was difficult because maximal innervation is dependent on the depth of the anesthesia. The reinnervated action potentials generally consisted of 2 to 5 phases.

Discussion

In the present study the histochemical, histological, and electromyographical findings strongly suggest that whole muscle bellies transplanted 2 to 3 weeks after denervation will survive and become reinnervated. Why transplants prepared in this way do survive when primarily transplanted muscles do not, is not fully understood. Several factors probably play a role in the outcome of grafting after denervation.

After denervation, changes in the muscle metabolism and enzyme activity have been found by biochemical and histochemical techniques. There is a reduction of anaerobic, glycolytic enzymes in the white fibers and a decrease in aerobic enzymes in the red fibers, resulting in less differentiation of the enzymatic patterns.[20] In pre-

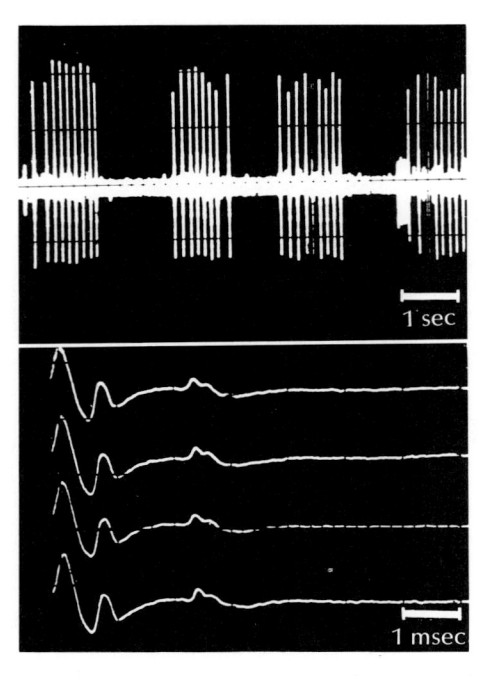

Contemporary concepts in free nerve and muscle grafting

Fig. 13-17. EMG activity from peroneus tertius muscle 40 weeks after transplantation. Upper trace shows motor unit activity synchronous with breathing. Lower trace demonstrates one action potential, corresponding to one spike in upper trace, generated by at least four different muscle fibers. Oscilloscope sweep is moved downward with each discharge.

dominantly white muscles there is also an increase of the capillary bed.[45,36,21] These changes, as Thompson[42,43] stated, may possibly explain the good results of muscle transplantation after denervation.

In the present experimental study, at the time of grafting, 2 weeks after denervation minimal changes were found with qualitative histochemical methods. These results are similar to those noted after denervation of muscles in the rat.[20] On the other hand, an increase in the capillary supply was noted at this time. In muscles denervated for 7 weeks, the dedifferentiation of red and white fibers was quite apparent, probably indicating a decrease of metabolic activity. A decrease of capillary density paralleled this metabolic change.

In free grafts of full-thickness skin, anastomoses between the larger vessels of the recipient and the original vessels of the graft have been demonstrated.[1] In fat grafts, a large proportion of the original vascular system also survives transplantation.[34] Large, probably original vessels were found in the 5-day-old muscle grafts, and it seems possible that outgrowing vessels from the recipient tissue have anastomosed with these large vessels and reestablished a graft circulation in a manner similar to that found in free skin grafts. The fact that few capillaries were seen in the grafts at 5 and 10 days in the ATPase preparations implies that much of the capillary network was lost. In the older grafts the normal pattern of capillaries was gradually restored, with a pronounced increase in capillary density in grafts 8 to 12 weeks old. This development was paralleled by reinnervation of the fibers. The increased vascularity was probably related to higher metabolic demands of the reinnervated muscle fibers. Because of the gradual reappearance of the capillaries, it seems that most of the capillary network was newly formed after grafting, whereas the larger vessels survived transplantation.

Signs of reinnervation of the grafts when tested by EMG techniques were first recorded in the 4-week-old specimen. In the 5-week-old graft examined for motor end plates a few, small, immature end plates appeared. The earliest signs of histochemical change indicating reinnervation were found at 6 weeks, and at 9 to 12 weeks fairly normal red and white fibers were found. The time gap between the first signs of reinnervation demonstrated by EMG and the histochemical redifferentiation is probably explained by the trophic influence of the motor neuron on the muscle fiber. The muscle must be active for a certain period of time before histochemically detectable signs of reinnervation can be demonstrated by changed staining characteristics or increased size of the muscle fibers.

In the present study, large type-groups were not seen in the reinnervated grafts, although minor grouping was prominent corresponding to the EMG recordings showing action-potential complexes with a moderately increased number of phases. The nerve sprouts invading the graft encounter a mass of denervated muscle fibers. If there is a sufficient number of sprouts, competition will ensue between them for reinnervation of the muscle fibers. Therefore, fiber type grouping should not be so pronounced as it would be if reinnervation took place through the original motor nerve, where a single axon may reach the muscle long before others and cause very large type-groups to form.[23,26]

The great difference in size between white and red fibers in the older grafts may reflect the nonphysiological position of the graft. The ends of the graft were sutured to the intercostal fascia and with contraction of the graft the sutured ends of the graft could not approach each other, a state similar to immobilization or tenotomization. Under such circumstances the muscle will atrophy, especially the red fibers, whereas the white ones may enlarge.[13,10]

The reinnervation of the muscle fibers in the grafts took place through formation of new end plates, partly in earlier end-plate free zones. Csillik and Savay[7] showed that in reinnervation through the motor nerve after crush the new end plates were formed at or about the old ones. New end-plate sites have, however, been found at end-plate free zones of denervated frog muscle, when a nerve was implanted into the muscle.[28]

REFERENCES

1. Bellman, S., and Velander, E.: Vascular reaction following experimental transplantation of free full thickness skin grafts. In Transactions of the International Society of Plastic Surgeons, first congress, Baltimore, 1957, The Williams & Wilkins Co., pp. 493-496.
2. Buller, A. J., Eccles, J. C., and Eccles, R. M.: Differentiation of fast and slow muscles in the cat hind limb, J. Physiol. (London) 150:399, 1960.
3. Charleton, H. M., and Drury, R. A. B.: Histological technique, ed. 3, London, 1957, Oxford University Press.
4. Coers, C.: Contribution a l'étude de la jonction neuromusculaire. II. Topographie zonale de l'innervation motrice terminale dans les muscles striés, Arch. Biol. Paris 64:495, 1953.
5. Couteaux, R.: Contribution à l'étude de la synapse myoneurale, Rev. Can. Biol. 6:563, 1947.
6. Couteaux, R.: Remarques sur les méthodes actuelles de détection histochimique des activités cholinestérasiques, Arch. Intern. Physiol. 59:526, 1951.
7. Csillik, B., and Sávay, G.: Die Regeneration

der subneuralen Apparate der motorischen Endplatten, Acta Neurovegetat. **19:**41, 1959.
8. Drews, G. A., and Engel, W. K.: An attempt at histochemical localization of myoglobin in skeletal muscle by the benzidine-peroxidase reaction, J. Histochem. Cytochem. **9:**206, 1961.
9. Edds, M.: Collateral regeneration of residual motor axons in partially denervated muscles, J. Exp. Zool. **113:**517, 1950.
10. Edström, L.: Selective atrophy of red muscle fibres in the quadriceps in long-standing knee-joint dysfunction, J. Neurol. Sci. **11:**551, 1970.
11. Edström, L., and Kugelberg, E.: Properties of motor units in the rat anterior tibial muscle, Acta Physiol. Scand. **73:**543, 1968.
12. Engel, W. K.: The essentiality of histo- and cytochemical studies in the investigation of neuromuscular disease, Neurology **12:**778, 1962.
13. Engel, W. K., Brooke, M. H., and Nelson, P. G.: Histochemical studies of denervated or tenotomized cat muscle: illustrating difficulties in relating experimental animal conditions to human neuromuscular disease, N.Y. Acad. Sci. **138:**160, 1966.
14. Erlacher, P.: Direct and muscular neurotization of paralyzed muscles. Experimental research, Am. J. Orthop. Surg. **13:**22, 1915.
15. Eränkö, O., and Palkama, A.: Improved localization of phosphorylase by the use of polyvinyl pyrrolidone and high substrate concentration, J. Histochem. Cytochem. **9:**585, 1961.
16. Feinstein, B., Lindegård, B., Nyman, E., and Wohlfart, G.: Morphologic studies of motor units in normal human muscles after various period of atrophy, J. Anat. **78:**15, 1955.
17. Gluck, T.: Ueber Muskel- und Sehnenplastik, Langenbecks Arch. Klin. Chir. **26:**61, 1881.
18. Helferich, 1882. Quoted by R. Magnus; see reference 27.
19. Hoffman, H.: Local reinnervation in partially denervated muscle: a histophysiological study, Aust. J. Exp. Biol. Med. Sci. **28:**383, 1950.
20. Hogan, E. L., Dawson, D., and Romanul, F. C. A.: Enzymatic changes in denervated muscle. II. Biochemical studies, Arch. Neurol. **13:**274, 1965.
21. Hogenhuis, L. E. H., and Engel, W. K.: Histochemistry and cytochemistry of experimentally denervated guinea pig muscle, Acta Anat. **60:**39, 1965.
22. Kabat, E. A., and Furth, J.: Histochemical study of distribution of alkaline phosphates in various normal and neoplastic tissues, Amer. J. Pathol. **17:**303, 1941.
23. Karpati, G., and Engel, W. K.: "Type grouping" in skeletal muscles after experimental reinnervation, Neurology **18:**447, 1968.
24. Koelle, G. B., and Friedenwald, J. S.: A histochemical method for localizing cholinesterase activity, Proc. Soc. Exp. Med. **70:**617, 1949.
25. Kugelberg, E., and Edström, L.: Differential histochemical effects of muscle contractions on phosphorylase and glycogen in various types of fibres: relation to fatigue, J. Neurol. Neurosurg. Psychiatry **31:**415, 1968.
26. Kugelberg, E., Edström, L., and Abbruzzese, M.: Mapping of motor units in experimentally reinnervated rat muscle, J. Neurol. Neurosurg. Psychiatry **33:**319, 1970.
27. Magnus, R.: Ueber Muskeltransplantation, Münch. Med. Wochensch. **37:**515, 1890.
28. Miledi, R.: Induced innervation of end-plate free muscle segments, Nature **193:**281, 1962.
29. Mowry, R. W., and Millican, R. C.: A histochemical study of the distribution and fate of dextran in tissues of the mouse, Am. J. Pathol. **28:**522, 1952.
30. Nachlas, M. M., Tsou, K.-C., De Souza, E., Cheng, C.-S., and Seligman, A. M.: Cytochemical demonstration of succinic dehydrogenase by the use of a new p-nitrophenyl substituted ditetrazole, J. Histochem. Cytochem. **5:**420, 1957.
31. Nyström, B.: Histochemistry of developing cat muscles, Acta Neurol. Scand. **44:**405, 1968.
32. Ogata, T.: A histochemical study of the red and white muscle fibres, Acta Med. Okayama **12:**216, 1958.
33. Padykula, H. A., and Herman, E.: The specificity of the histochemical method for adenosine triphosphatase, J. Histochem. Cytochem. **3:**170, 1955.
34. Peer, L. A., and Walker, J. C.: The behavior of autogenous human tissue grafts, Plast. Reconstr. Surg. **7:**73, 1951.
35. del Pozo, E. C.: Transmission fatigue and contraction fatigue, Am. J. Physiol. **135:**763, 1942.
36. Romanul, F. C. A., and Hogan, E. L.: Enzymatic changes in denervated muscle. I. Histochemical studies, Arch. Neurol. **13:**263, 1965.
37. Romanul, F. C. A., and Van der Meulen, J.: Slow and fast muscles after cross innervation, Arch. Neurol. **17:**387, 1967.

38. Roy, P. R.: Behaviour of free autogenous muscle graft into the skeletal muscle of dog, J. Exp. Med. Sci. **9:**78, 1966.
39. Scarpelli, D. G., Hess, R., and Pearse, A. G. E.: The cytochemical localization of oxidative enzymes, J. Biophys. Biochem. Cytol. **4:**747, 1958.
40. Studitsky, A. N.: Free auto- and homografts of muscle tissue in experiments on animals, Ann. N.Y. Acad. Sci. **120:**789, 1964.
41. Takeuchi, T., and Kuriaki, H.: Histochemical detection of phosphorylase in animal tissue, J. Histochem. Cytochem. **3:**153, 1955.
42. Thompson, N.: Investigation of autogenous skeletal muscle free grafts in the dog, Transplantation **12:**353, 1971.
43. Thompson, N.: Autogenous free grafts of skeletal muscle, Plast. Reconstr. Surg. **48:**11, 1971.
44. Thompson, N.: Treatment of facial paralysis by free skeletal muscle grafts. In Transactions of Fifth World Congress of Plastic and Reconstructive Surgery, London, 1972, Butterworth & Co. (Publishers), Ltd., p. 66.
45. Tower, S. S.: Atrophy and degeneration in skeletal muscle, Am. J. Anat. **56:**1, 1935.
46. Volkmann, R.: Ueber die Regeneration des quergestreiften Muskelgewebes beim Menschen und Säugethier, Beitr. Pathol. Anat. **12:**235, 1893.
47. Zhenevskaya, R. P., Rumyantseva, O. N., Novosylova, I. L., and Proshlyakova, E. V.: Regeneration process in the transplant of intact muscle of young rats, Zh. Obshch. Biol. **26:**569, 1965. (In Russian.)
48. Zielonko, J.: Ueber die Entwicklung und Proliferation von Epithelien und Endothelien, Arch. Mikrosk. Anat. **10:**351, 1874.

14 Free minced-muscle grafting

LEWIS BERGER
LEONARD R. RUBIN

The concept of free grafting of mouse minced striated muscle has been described by Studitsky. We have used dogs to investigate the feasibility of grafting the minced muscle in higher animals and to create a larger and stronger muscle by inbedding of the minced mass in the belly of a long muscle. The fragments regenerate to form a whole solid muscle. The host enveloping muscle supplies outsprouting of nerve axons that innervate the graft muscle mass to form new myoneural junctions.

The results of the experiment verifies minced-muscle grafting in dogs to create a whole living muscle within a host muscle that is stronger and has greater contractility than did the original host muscle.

In 1952, Studitsky[54] published his early experience with free grafting of minced autogenous and homologous striated muscle in mice. Since that time, Carlson and others[14-21] have elaborated on his work and have speculated on the mechanism of survival and regeneration of the minced pieces into a homogenous contracting muscle. However, despite voluminous reports, experimentation has failed to present any clinical application for this phenomenon. This lack of purpose has stimulated us to perform ongoing experimentation that has the possibility of widespread practical uses.

Principle of minced-muscle grafting

Studitsky has emphasized that the success of minced-muscle grafting was dependent on reduction of the muscle to a "plastic stage."[60] This plastic state is characterized by a change to anaerobic metabolism, nuclear proliferation, and increased RNA content. This would prepare for the activating of myoblasts and the production of myotubes. A rapid ingrowth of blood vessels and nerve fibers would then ensue. A similar plastic state could be obtained by denervation of striated muscle approximately 2 weeks prior to grafting with a resulting increase in survival.[59]

After grafting, the reformation of the minced muscles into a whole muscle mass is accomplished by active regeneration of myotubes from myoblasts. Three origins of the monocytes have been suggested. Mauro[41,42] described an undifferentiated mononuclear cell located below the basement membrane of the muscle fiber as the origin of the myoblast. He called it a "satellite cell." Another school advocates that some myonuclei, surrounded by a thin membrane of sarcoplasm, survive as the remaining sarcoplasm degenerates to commence regeneration. This process was designated "dedifferentiation of muscle" by Carlson.[20] A third, and the least supported theory, is the presence of a circulating cell that becomes a source of myoblasts.[10,52] These cells enter the field of damaged muscle to become the precursors of myoblasts, which eventually form myotubes.

Historic background of striated muscle grafting

During the past century, many physiologists believed that damaged striated muscle could not regenerate, let alone have the ability to survive free grafting. Indeed, Peer[45] in his volume on grafting made a reference supporting this viewpoint. After World War II, interest in skeletal muscle regeneration was stimulated by workers such as LeGros Clark,[22,23] Albrook,[3-5] Lash,[36] Mauro,[41,42] and others.[50] The published works by Studitsky was challenged by workers in the U.S.S.R. and other Eastern Block countries where the papers were readily available.[20] In 1972, Carlson published his monograph[20] where he consolidated all of his experience with minced-muscle grafting as well as that of others. This overall investigation of minced-muscle regeneration confirmed the basic findings of Studitsky and co-workers[54-60] and further elucidated mechanisms of muscle regeneration.

Favorable ambiance for successful minced-muscle grafting

Muscle must first be minced into 1 mm pieces and then placed directly on contact with functioning striated muscle. Either white (fast) or red (slow) muscle may be used interchangeably, as it is the motor nerve that will ultimately determine the muscle type.[13,27,35,40] The immediate effect is to produce myoblasts, which then form myotubes and subsequently form muscle fibers. The early stages of regeneration occur independently of neurovascular supply. For the process of regeneration to continue, motor innervation is essential.[30,51,52,58,60,65-69] Observations of the progressive stages of regeneration reveal that the vascular supply develops first, on a random basis, followed by tendon regeneration and lastly by neurotization, which proceeds from proximal to distal. Should neurotization fail, the neurotrophic and functional effects will not take place and the muscle mass would degenerate.

One can demonstrate three basic zones of regeneration. The peripheral is the most mature and demonstrates the earliest myotube and fibroblast formation. Tendon attachment occurs early in this region. Fibroblastic activity is pronounced here. The second zone is known as the "intermediate zone." It is rather narrow and is of a more immature state. The central zone contains the minced-muscle cells, which have not started to change. It is void of vasculature. The peripheral zone increases in size and maturity with time as the central zone diminishes.[20]

While regeneration is proceeding in the anticipated fashion, it is also undergoing molding. This molding process is controlled predominantly by physical forces. The pressures exerted by the surrounding tissues result in the gross shape of the regenerate. As the tendons regenerate and establish attachments, they exert needed longitudinal tension on the muscle, which is probably responsible for the longitudinal orientation of the muscle fibers.[49] This explains why if two muscles are minced and replaced together, only one muscle will result.[20]

There appears to be a constant race between the formation of scar by fibroblasts and the formation of new muscle fibers by the myotubes. The success of muscle grafting will be altered by excessive fibrosis. Under most conditions, there exists a longer latent period for muscle regeneration and then for fibroblastic growth. As stated by Carlson[20] in discussing the problem of scarring, "the problem of intense competition between collagen and muscle development is decided usually in favor of the connective tissue under normal circumstances." To minimize scarring, we have placed minced muscle directly into a pocket of a functioning muscle through a small incision. This would accomplish the desired goal of increased functional muscle survival. This would indeed permit an increase in bulk (size) of an existing muscle and could be used clinically to improve the function of an underdeveloped or atrophied or traumatized muscle, or give cosmetically more appealing contours.

The regenerated tendons in minced-muscle regeneration are not optimal.[31] Placing minced muscle into the pocket of a functional muscle, which may or may not be totally active, would obviate the need to form new tendon attachments. The plastic state has had a chemotactic effect on the surrounding nerves and blood vessels, which invade the minced-muscle mass quickly and provide needed nutrition and neurotization. Thus the race between fibroplasia and muscle regeneration would be in favor of the latter. With these objectives in mind, the following experiment was undertaken.

The minced-muscle experiment

The experimental animals were eight adult beagle dogs, which were anesthesized with general endotracheal anesthesia. A paramedian abdominal incision extending across the inguinal ligament was carried proximal to the ipsilateral knee. The right and left sides of the abdomen and legs were used at random in alternating dogs. A portion of the external oblique muscle was excised, and all visible fascia and connective tissue bands were removed by sharp dissection. The donor site was then sutured with 3-0 chromic suture. The muscle was minced on a small glass dish with a small scissor into pieces measuring approximately 1 cubic millimeter. This muscle was then weighed. The gracilis muscle was carefully exposed so as not to create any additional trauma. It was not mobilized. A small longitudinal incision measuring approximately 1.5 to 2 cm was made with a scalpel on the anterior surface of the muscle. With use of Steven's scissors, a pocket was created within the muscle by dissection proximally and distally. The minced muscle fragments were then placed into the pocket and the fascia was closed with a continuous suture of 4-0 Prolene. The remaining minced muscle was weighed, and the amount that had been implanted was calculated. The wound was closed in the usual fashion. At time intervals ranging from 10 to 19 weeks, the skin incisions were reopened, with similar incisions being created on the opposite side to expose the normal gracilis muscle. The muscles were then mobilized to expose the neurovascular supply. Each muscle was stimulated by 0.5 milliampere. Both mucles were then excised from their origins along the pubis and the pubic rami and from their insertions on the proximal tibia. All loose connective tissue was then excised. The nerve supply was identified with a 7-0 nylon suture. Specimens were stimulated directly through the nerve supply, with use of various stimulating forces and with the muscle under varying tensions. Specimens were preserved in 10% neutral formalin and stained.

Results

BULK (SIZE) OF MUSCLE GRAFT SURVIVAL

Two dogs expired of probable pneumonia. Observations of the remaining six dogs resulted in surprising minimal amount of surrounding scar tissue except for one dog. Five muscles demonstrated an obvious increase in mass compared to the contralateral controls. These observations were supported during weighing of the surgically controlled specimens. There was an average 19% increase in weight of the recipient muscle with an apparent 88% survival of the transplanted mass. The average weight of the controls was 3.93 grams as compared to 4.56 grams for the experimental specimen with an average of 0.7 grams being implanted.

One animal showed no clinical increase in size of the experimental muscle as compared to its control. There was only an insignificant 0.1-gram difference in weight between the controlled and the experimental muscle. Microscopic examination of this specimen revealed a large amount of scar tissue, mostly external to the muscle. This scarring supports the probability that extrusion of the minced muscle from its pocket occurred before any regeneration could have occurred.

In two instances, the weight of the experimental muscle exceeded that of the control plus the minced muscle implanted. This could be accounted for in three ways:

1. The possibility that there may have been differences in the weight of the contralateral muscles. This was unlikely but statistically possible.
2. Persistent edema of the experimental limbs in early regenerates 2 to 4 weeks old accounts for one third of the mass.[20] It may be that this edema exists for a longer period of time in some instances.
3. Technical differences in harvesting the specimen by either incomplete excision of the entire contralateral control muscle or leaving an excessive amount of connective tissue on the experimental muscle.

Microscopic findings were supportive of our clinical impression of the increase in mass. They also demonstrated a surprising paucity of fibroblastic activity. The microscope clearly showed that the implanted surviving muscle had oriented itself in the longitudinal fashion of the existing muscle.

MUSCLE-STRENGTH OBSERVATION

We believe that our results in determining muscle strengths of the grafted muscle to be unreliable. It was found that in all our cases, two nerves innervated the muscles; a larger proximal and a smaller distal. With our instrumentation we were unable to simultaneously stimulate both. We were also unable to control temperature, humidity, and the effects of anaerobic metabolism. It was, however, our distinct impression that the experimental muscle strength was at least equal to or greater than the control in all instances.

Microscopic examination constantly demonstrated similar findings. Distinguishing preexisting muscle from regenerated muscle was very difficult (Figs. 14-1 to 14-3). In many areas the regenerate appeared to merge imperceptively with the normal muscle. The regenerated muscles were in general smaller, mean 28.7 μm versus 47.9 μm, and showed a much wider range of size, 44.2 μm versus 24.6 μm, than the normal muscle. The experimental muscles demonstrated considerably more connective tissue than did the control. The regenerated muscle was arranged in clusters separated by connective tissue, with some specimens revealing individual muscle fibers enveloped in scanty connective tissue. The nuclei of the muscle regenerates were peripheral as in a normal muscle and were otherwise unremarkable. Multinucleated giant cells, of foreign body type, were seen in areas of regenerating muscle in all specimens. Muscle spindles appeared more frequently than in the control. The spindles appeared generally normal except for possible edema-like fluid surrounding the intrafusal myofibers. Nerves could be easily identified within, or in the vicinity of, the regenerates, and these appeared normal. At least two specimens revealed probable partial tendon formation. There was no evidence of any bone or cartilage formation. One specimen showed little if any evidence of muscle regeneration and was the same specimen that clinically appeared to

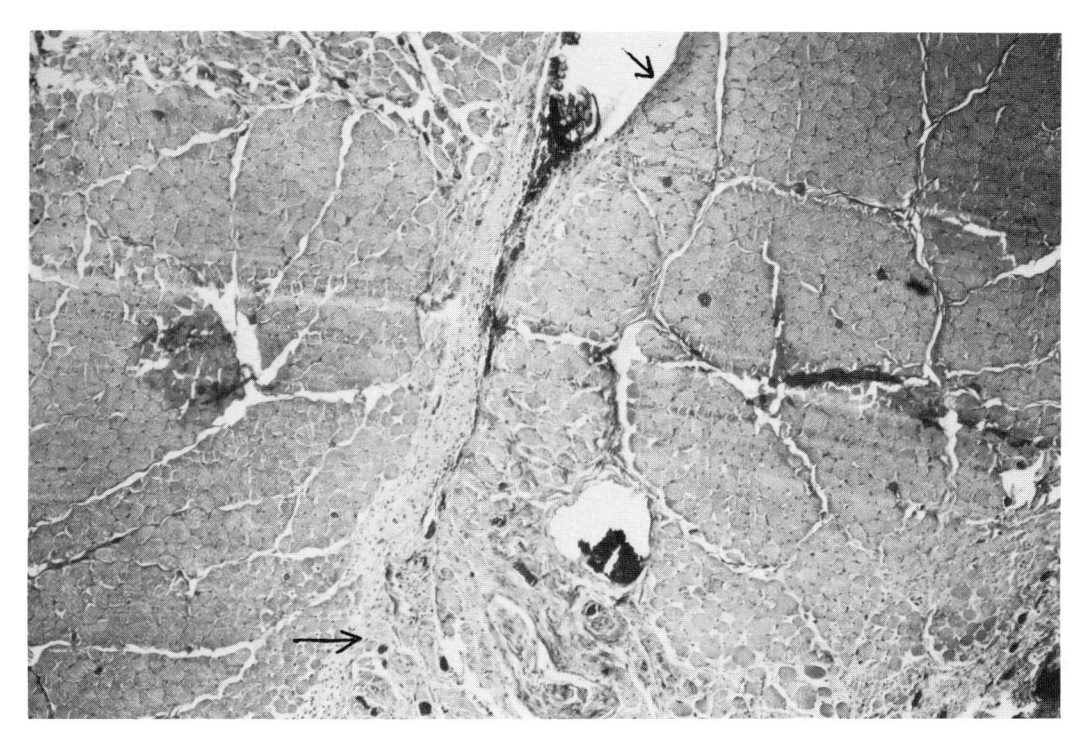

Fig. 14-1. Figs. 14-1 to 14-3 demonstrate range of variation. This section shows imperceptible merging of normal and regenerated muscle. *Arrows,* Minced-muscle regenerates. Regenerated muscle in lower right shows larger variation in fiber size and increased connective tissue. (Hematoxylin and eosin, 10×.)

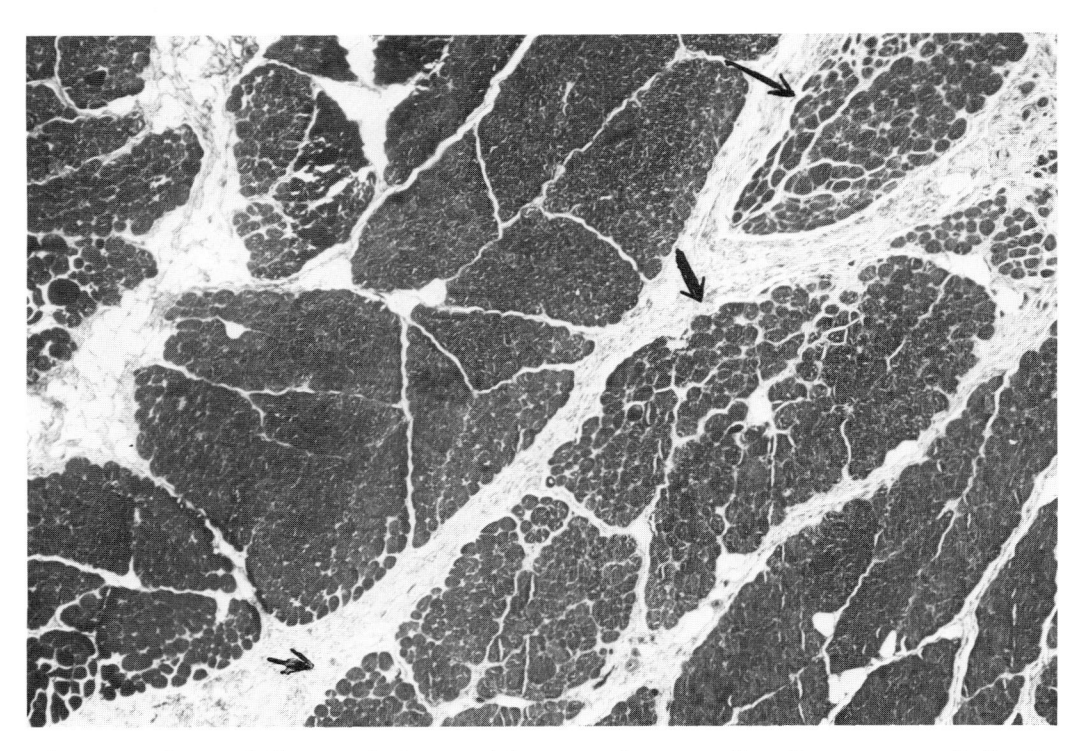

Fig. 14-2. Area of fiber variation and increased connective tissue more distinctly separated from normal. *Arrows,* Grafted muscle. (Trichrome, 10×.)

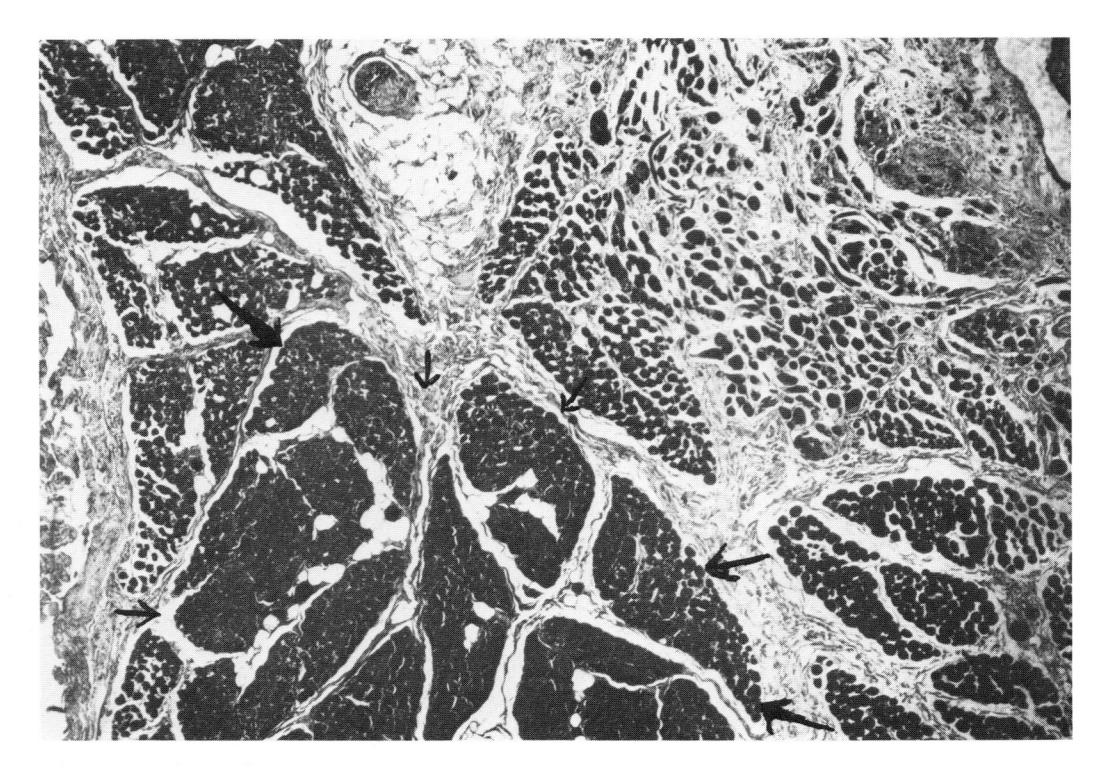

Contemporary concepts in free nerve and muscle grafting

Fig. 14-3. The only preexisting muscle is within *arrows*. Remaining areas clearly demonstrate noticeable fiber variation, a generally smaller muscle fiber, and the most significant amount of connective tissue seen in any of the specimens. (Trichrome, 10×.)

have extruded the minced muscle. The remaining specimens were characterized by apparent muscle regeneration in the anticipated areas.

Discussion

Regeneration is defined as the renewal, regrowth, or restoration of a body or bodily part, tissue, or substance after injury or as a normal body process. Regeneration of parts is a process most limited to lower animals. However, in higher animals there are examples of the appendage regeneration, such as the antlers of a deer. Nevertheless, regeneration is constantly occurring at a cellular level as in the epidermis and nerves and can occur to a great extent, as we now see, in muscles given the proper circumstances. The critical aspects of regeneration are the following:

1. Loss of substance
2. Cell population with a capability to respond to the loss
3. Ability to organize and orient the new cell population into an anatomical and functional unit
4. Limitation and repression of the reparative process by scar formations, which would inhibit functional ability.

The stimulus to the regenerative process is almost universally a mechanical loss because of trauma. Loss from infection and tumor probably rarely results in regeneration. Functional loss alone, from atrophy, scar formation, and so on does not result in regeneration. The usual response to functional loss, as seen in higher animals, is hypertrophy of the remaining tissue. This is seen in varying degrees in mammalian liver, intestine, thyroid, kidney, and so forth. Apparently, however, some functional loss must be present, in addition to the mechanical or physical loss, for regeneration to occur. This observation is probably teleologically more significant than it is biologically.

Traumatic loss of tissue, and in the instance of consideration here, muscle, is a frequent occurrence. Since clinical muscle regeneration does not appear to occur, one might conclude that either the higher life forms do not have a cell population capable of regeneration or so much scar is produced as to obstruct anatomical regeneration.[1,11,22,28,29,46] It appears that the latter occurrence may be responsible.

Now that free grafting of striated muscle has been shown to be possible, the use of minced muscle as described by Studitsky offers some interesting observations with far-reaching clinical applications. It becomes apparent that the survival of free muscle grafts, dependent on the grafts being in contact with a functioning striated muscle, is qualified by the rapid ingrowth of blood vessels and nerves, which facilitate myotube formation and muscle fibrils before the overgrowth of fibroblasts and fibrous scar. The use of minced grafts placed into pockets of functioning or partially functioning muscles appear to favor the race for graft survival.

The regenerated minced muscle assumes the shape of the pocket into which it was placed, regardless of its original shape.[20,47] It takes on tension forces through its recipient host and secondarily receives tendon attachments needed for survival.

With minced-muscle grafts that survive, clinical applications become apparent. We could gain an increase in bulk (size) of an existing muscle functionally impaired by trauma or disuse, or partially atrophied by delayed reinnervation after nerve injury. The bulk could increase the muscle strength functionally or be cosmetically important by filling contour defects. Clinically, minced-muscle grafting could be used to reanimate the paralytic face in the human when the degenerative process had gone too far and too long. A new horizon appears for the treatment of individuals with various muscular disorders. An interesting clinical application might be the grafting of minced muscles into the pharynx and soft palate when velopharyngeal insufficiency exists.

Summary

A dog model has been used to demonstrate the consistency of survival of free minced-muscle grafts placed in a pocket of an existing functioning muscle. There is a documented increase in bulk (size) and an observed but not documented increase in contractile strength. Clinicial application appears to be possible.

REFERENCES

1. Adams, R. D., Denny-Brown, D., and Pearson, C. M.: Diseases of muscle, New York, 1953, Paul B. Hoeber, Inc., Medical Book Department of Harper & Row, Publishers.
2. Adams, R. D., Denny-Brown, D., and Pearson, C. M.: Diseases of muscle, a study in pathology, ed. 2, New York, 1962, Harper & Row, Publishers.
3. Allbrook, D.: An electron microscopic study of regenerating skeletal muscle, J. Anat. **96:**137, 1962.
4. Allbrook, D. B., and Aitken, J. T.: Reinnervation of striated muscle after acute ischaemia, J. Anat. **85:**376, 1951.
5. Allbrook, D., Baker, W. De C., and Kirkaldy-Willis, W. H.: Muscle regeneration in experimental animals and in man, J. Bone Joint Surg. **48B**(1):153, 1966.

6. Aloisi, M., Mussini, I., and Schiaffino, S.: Activation of muscle nuclei in denervation and hypertrophy. In Kakulas, B. A., editor: Basic research in myology, Amsterdam, 1971, Excerpta Medica Foundation (ICS 294, p. 338).
7. Altschul, R.: On nuclear division in damaged skeletal muscle, Rev. Can. Biol. **6:**485, 1947.
8. Altschul, R.: Nuclear proliferation ("nucleosis") in damaged skeletal muscle. A critical review, Z. Zellforsch. **56:**425, 1962.
9. Altschul, R.: Nucleosis of skeletal muscle: Its value as a biological test, Science **103:** 566, 1962.
10. Bateson, R. G., Woodrow, D. F., and Sloper, J. C.: Circulating cell as a source of myoblasts in regenerating injured mammalian skeletal muscle, Nature **213:**1035, March 1967.
11. Betz, H.: Contribution a l'étude de la dégénérescence et de la régénération musculaire I and II. Arch. Anat. Microsc. Morphol. Exp. **40:**46, 1951.
12. Bintliff, S., and Walker, B. E.: Radioautographic study of skeletal muscle regeneration, Am. J. Anat. **106:**233, 1960.
13. Buller, A. J., Eccles, J. C., and Eccles, R. M.: Interactions between motoneurones and muscles in respect of the characteristic speeds of their responses, J. Physiol. **150:**417, 1960.
14. Carlson, B. M.: Regeneration of the completely excised gastrocnemius muscle in the frog and rat from minced muscle fragments, J. Morphol. **125:**447, 1968.
15. Carlson, B. M.: Regeneration of the rat gastrocnemius muscle from sibling and nonsibling muscle fragments, Am. J. Anat. **128:** 21, 1970.
16. Carlson, B. M.: Relationship between the tissue and epimorphic regeneration of muscles, Am. Zool. **10:**175, 1970.
17. Carlson, B. M.: The regeneration of a limb muscle in the axolotl from minced fragments, Anat. Rec. **166:**423, 1970.
18. Carlson, B. M.: The regeneration of entire muscles from minced fragments. In Mauro, A., Shafig, S. A., and Milhorat, A. T., editors: Regeneration of skeletal muscle and myogenesis, Amsterdam, 1970, Excerpta Medica Foundation (ICS 218, p. 25).
19. Carlson, B. M.: Muscle morphogenesis in limb regenerates following removal of stump musculature, Anat. Rec. **169:**289, 1971.
20. Carlson, B. M.: The regeneration of minced muscles, Monogr. Dev. Biol. **4:**3, 1972.
21. Carlson, B. M., and Gutmann, E.: Contractile and histochemical properties of sliced muscle grafts regenerating in normal and denervated rat limbs, Exp. Neurol. **50:**319-329, 1976.
22. Clark, W. E. LeGros: An experimental study of the regeneration of mammalian striped muscle, J. Anat. **80:**24, 1946.
23. Clark, W. E. LeGros, and Wajda, H. S.: The growth and maturation of regenerating striated muscle fibers, J. Anat. **81:**56, 1946.
24. Coleman, J. R., and Coleman, A. W.: Muscle differentiation and macromolecular synthesis, J. Cell Physiol., suppl. **1:**19, 1972.
25. Cosmos, E.: Muscle-nerve transplants, Physiologist **16**(2):167, May 1973.
26. Dawson, J. W.: Changes in cross-striped muscle in the healing of incised wounds, J. Pathol. Bacteriol. **13:**174, 1909.
27. Dubowitz, V.: Cross-innervated mammalian skeletal muscle: histochemical, physiological and biochemical studies, J. Physiol. **193:** 481, 1967.
28. Forbus, W.: Pathologic changes in voluntary muscle Arch. Pathol. **2:**318, 1926.
29. Goodman, G. C.: On the regeneration and redifferentiation of mammalian striated muscle, J. Morphol. **100:**27, 1957.
30. Guth, L.: "Trophic" influences of nerve on muscle, Physiol. Rev. **48:**645, 1968.
31. Gutmann, E., and Hasek, M.: Fate of syngeneic and allogeneic homografts of minced muscles in the rat, Physiol. Bohemoslov. **23:**321, 1974.
32. Hay, E. D.: Electron microscopic observations of muscle dedifferentiation in regenerating amblystoma limbs, Dev. Biol. **1:**555, 1959.
33. Hay, E. D.: Regeneration of muscle in the amputated amphibian limb. In Mauro, A., Shafig, S. A., and Milhorat, A. T., editors: Regeneration of striated muscle and myogenesis, Amsterdam, 1970, Excerpta Medica Foundation (ICS 218, p. 3).
34. Hess, A., and Rosner, S.: The satellite cell bud and myoblast in denervated mammalian muscle fibers, Am. J. Anat. **129:**21, 1970.
35. Hikida, R. S., and Lombardo, J. A.: Regeneration of pigeon fast and slow muscle fiber types after partial excision and mincing, J. Cell Biol. **61:**414, 1974.
36. Lash, J. W., Holtzer, H., and Swift, H.: Regeneration of mature skeletal muscle, Anat. Rec. **128:**679, 1957.
37. Lee, J. C.: Electron microscope observations on myogenic free cells of denervated skeletal muscle, Exp. Neurol. **12:**123, 1965.
38. Lentz, T. L.: Cytological studies of muscle dedifferentiation during limb regeneration of the newt *Triturus,* Am. J. Anat. **124:**447, 1969.

39. Levender, G.: Ueber die Regeneration der quergestreiften Muskulatur, Arch. Klin. Chir. **202:**677, 1941.
40. Margreth, A., Salviati, G., and Carraro, U.: Neural control on the activity of the calcium-transport system in sarcoplasmic reticulum of rat skeletal muscle, Nature **241:**285, 1973.
41. Mauro, A.: Satellite cell of skeletal muscle fibers, J. Biophys. Biochem. Cytol. **9:**493, 1961.
42. Mauro, A., Shafiq, S. A., and Milhorat, A. T.: Regeneration of striated muscles and myogenesis, Amsterdam, 1970, Excerpta Medica Foundation (ICS 218).
43. Muir, A. R., Kanji, A. A. M., and Allbrook, D.: The structure of the satellite cells in skeletal muscles, J. Anat. **99:**435, 1965.
44. Murray, M. R.: Skeletal muscle tissue in culture. In Bourne, G. H., editor: The structure and function of muscle, New York, 1960, Academic Press, Inc., p. 111.
45. Peer, L. A.: Transplantation of tissues, Baltimore, 1959, The Williams and Wilkins Co., vol. 1, p. 337.
46. Pogogeff, I. A., and Murray, M. R.: Form and behavior of adult mammalian skeletal muscle in vitro, Anat. Rec. **95:**321, 1946.
47. Reznik, M.: Origin of myoblasts during skeletal muscle regeneration, Lab. Invest. **20:**253, 1969.
48. Reznik, M.: Satellite cells, myoblasts and skeletal muscle regeneration. In Mauro, A., Shafig, S. A., and Milhorat, A. T., editors: Regeneration of striated muscle and myogenesis, Amsterdam, 1970, Excerpta Medica Foundation (ICS 218, p. 133).
49. Rumyantseva, O. N.: New data on the role of tension on the differentiation of myogenous tissue, Arkh. Anat. Gistol. Embriol. **39**(12):51, 1960. (In Russian.)
50. Samsonenko, R. V.: Development of muscular tissue in implanted minced-muscle tissue in the site of completely removed muscular organs in frogs, Arkh. Anat. Gistol. Embriol. **33**(2):56, 1956. (In Russian.)
51. Singer, M.: The influence of the nerve in regeneration of the amphibian extremity, Q. Rev. Biol. **27:**169, 1952.
52. Singer, M.: The trophic quality of the neuron: some theoretical considerations, Prog. Brain Res. **13:**228, 1964.
53. Speidel, C. C.: Studies of living muscles, Am. J. Anat. **62**(2):179, Jan. 1938.
54. Studitsky, A. N.: Restoration of muscle by means of transplantation of minced-muscle tissue, Dokl. Akad. Nauk S.S.S.R. **84**(2):389, 1952. (In Russian.)
55. Studitsky, A. N.: Principles of restoration of muscle in higher vertebrates, Trudy Inst. Morphol. Zhivot. **11:**225, 1954. (In Russian.)
56. Studitsky, A. N.: Experimental surgery of muscles, Moscow, 1959, Izdatelstvo 'Nauka,' p. 338. (In Russian.)
57. Studitsky, A. N.: Free auto- and homografts of muscle tissue in experiments on animals, Ann. N.Y. Acad. Sci. **120:**789, 1964.
58. Studitsky, A. N.: The neural factor in the development of transplanted muscles. Exploratory concepts in muscular dystrophy II, Amsterdam, 1973, Excerpta Medica Foundation, p. 351.
59. Studitsky, A. N., and Zhenevskaya, R. P.: Theory and practice of the auto- and homotransplantation of muscles, Moscow, 1967, Izdatelstvo 'Nauka.'
60. Studitsky, A. N., Zhenevskaya, R. P., and Rumyantseva, O. N.: The role of neurotrophic influences upon the restitution of structure and function of regenerating muscles. In Gutmann, E., and Hnik, P.: The effect of use and disuse on neuromuscular functions, Prague, 1963, Publishing House of the Czechoslovak Academy of Sciences, p. 71.
61. Volkmann, R.: Ueber die Regeneration des quergestreiften Muskelgewebes beim Menschen und Säugetier, Beitr. Pathol. Anat. Allgem. Pathol. **12:**233, 1893.
62. Walker, B. E.: A radioautographic study of muscle regeneration in dystrophic mice, Am. J. Pathol. **41:**41, 1962.
63. Walker, B. E.: The origin of myoblasts and the problem of dedifferentiation, Exp. Cell Res. **30:**80, 1963.
64. Walker, B. E.: Skeletal muscle regeneration in young rats, Am. J. Anat. **133:**369, 1972.
65. Zhenevskaya, R. P.: The role of nervous connections on the early stages of muscle regeneration, Doklady Akad. Nauk S.S.S.R. **121:**182, 1958. (In Russian.)
66. Zhenevskaya, R. P.: The influence of de-efferentation on the regeneration of skeletal muscle, Arkh. Anat. Gistol. Embriol. **39**(12):42, 1960. (In Russian.)
67. Zhenevskaya, R. P.: Restoration of muscle by the method of transplantation of minced-muscle tissue under conditions of sensory deprivation, Arkh. Anat. Gistol. Embriol. **40**(6):46, 1961. (In Russian.)
68. Zhenevskaya, R. P.: Experimental histologic investigation of striated muscle tissue, Rev. Can. Biol. **21**(3 & 4):457, 1962.
69. Zhenevskaya, R. P.: The significance of sensory neurons for the structure and regeneration of skeletal musculature, Arkh. Anat. Gistol. Embriol. **44**(5):57, 1963. (In Russian.)

15 Nerve-end implantation into a denervated muscle

WILLIAM H. McCOY, III
LEONARD R. RUBIN

Since 1913 the literature has had several papers describing the implantation of a free nerve ending into the substance of a denervated muscle. However, experience in humans has demonstrated uncertain results. This paper has utilized 15 dogs in a controlled experiment where a denervated muscle was innervated with a free nerve end. The controlled result shows that axons do sprout from the nerve end to form new neuromuscular anastomoses, resulting in normal muscular contraction.

Cessation of adequate function of the facial nerve inevitably produces dire physiological and psychological consequences. The delicate balance of facial muscle movement that visually communicates each moment's thought process to the environment is absent, and even the rudimentary control necessary for eating and drinking is compromised. Moreover, the obvious asymmetry contributes to, at best, mediocre social interaction. The dilemma then is reconstruction of the mechanism of transferring all of the myriad central nervous system impulses, whether conscious or subconscious, to the corresponding and appropriate normal facial movements.

One of the dynamic approaches to this problem has concerned itself with the direct implantation of motor nerves into previously denervated striated muscle. This technique, if consistently successful, would be an invaluable alternative in those cases unsuitable for direct nerve suture, interposition of autogenous nerve grafts, transfer of masticatory muscles, or free muscle grafts, and a useful adjunct in others. However, lack of consistent objective scientific evidence to substantiate this phenomenon has necessitated its further study in animal models before its implementation as a clinical tool.

This report describes this phenomenon and the results obtained in our laboratory from a canine animal model, followed by a discussion of its proposed use as a alternative treatment in selected cases of facial paralysis.

Historical review

One of the first attempts at direct neurotization of paralyzed muscles was performed by Steindler[23] in 1914 and 1915, although this had previously been suggested by Heineke who conducted experiments involving direct nerve implantation into paralyzed muscles (with rabbits as the experimental model) and reportedly succeeded in obtaining satisfactory contractions of the muscles by faradic stimulation after 2 to 8 weeks. Erlacher had previously claimed the so-called hyperneurotization of healthy muscle by direct implantation with positive clinical contraction after 4 weeks. Steindler claimed success in both experimental dog models and clinical cases; however, by his own admission, these results were preliminary and inconclusive. Later, in 1916, using dogs and cats with direct implantation of sciatic nerves into the vastus lateralis, he noted contraction after stimulation to weak faradic current and he surmised that, indeed, direct neural neurotization was possible.

In 1950, H. Hoffman[9] investigated work previously performed by Hines, Wehrmacher, and Thompson (1945), van Harreveld (1945), and Weiss and Edds (1945) to show, indirectly, complete reinnervation of skeletal muscle by axon sprouting of those motor nerves remaining after partial denervation. The histological evidence seemed to suggest that the increased force of contraction in these muscles (rat) was not attributable to hypertrophy but rather to reinnervation of existing fibers, thus some credence was given to the theory of "neural neurotization."

In 1950, J. T. Aitken[1] had undertaken a study to show hyperneurotization of a previously denervated muscle and to dispute the previous work, which failed to show a direct correlation between clinical impression and histological evidence. The results of his work (in rabbits) failed to confirm significant reinnervation with clinical contraction unless supernormal stimulus was used. However, he showed by comparison that the histological picture of implantation of nerve fibers differs in the previously denervated muscle by irregular branching and the formation of new end plates (these differed in size and shape from normal, and several were occasionally seen on one muscle fiber and in ectopic locations). He concluded, therefore, that new end plates were formed, albeit irregularly, and did function to a limited degree.

Clinical electromyographic investigation of Abbe lip flaps by A. T. DePalma (1958)[3] and I. Isaksson (1961)[12] revealed reinnervation of the transposed muscle correlated with functional recovery. Further evidence of this phenomenon was obtained in the histological and histochemical investigations by N. Thompson (1961)[24] to support motor reinnervation whether by existing myoneural end plates or the formation of new ones. (All of which would seem to corroborate earlier studies of muscular reinnervation—"muscular neurotization.")

Later, in 1971, Thompson attacked the problem more directly after discovering that autogenous free muscle grafts (denervated 2 to 3 weeks previously) could be transferred with 80% viability, both in experimental animals (dogs) and in human subjects. He further established by electromyographic, histological, and histochemical techniques that these free grafts were innervated by the motor neurons of nearby, normal muscle (that is, "muscular neurotization") and this could be used in the treatment of facial paralysis. Accordingly, he transplanted free muscle grafts (palmaris longus, extensor digitorum brevis, among others) to the face directly in contact with normally innervated muscles (whether by the fifth or seventh cranial nerve) and reported encouraging results to substantiate his earlier work. Hakelius and Stålberg (1974, 1975)[6-8] conducted a similar study, with the additional parameter of single fiber electromyography, with these two similar conclusions: (1) previously denervated free muscle grafts remain viable and are innervated by adjacent normal muscle, and (2) free muscle grafts can be employed in the treatment of facial paralysis with some improvement of the affected side whether by active or passive mode.

Advances in microsurgical technique reported by J. W. Smith (1972)[20] and Anderl (1973)[2] as applied to direct fascicular suturing and transfacial nerve grafting seemed to obviate the necessity for pursuing investigation of "neural neurotization." J. W.

Smith (1972)[20] claimed some improvement in voluntary muscle movement after transfacial nerve grafting but recognized the necessity for consideration of all the dynamic (and static) techniques in dealing with such cases. Anderl too realized that in especially difficult cases (such as with children and trauma) the alternative of "neural neurotization" (which he assumed to be fact) would be a great asset and used this technique accordingly based on "experimental, clinical observation, and personal experience"[2] reporting partial success. Freilinger[5] also reported two clinical cases of nerve implantation; however, supramaximal stimuli were necessary to evoke electromyographic potentials, and the potential for a spontaneous recovery of facial nerve paralysis in his two selected cases again left in doubt the explanation (perhaps "neural neurotization") for his results.

Since the validity of "neural neurotization" might produce a useful adjustment to the treatment of facial paralysis, an experiment was designed to investigate this phenomenon. This preliminary study reports the results of implanting a mixed motor nerve (median) of the canine pectoral limb directly into a previously denervated muscle (biceps brachii), and discusses its proposed clinical application.

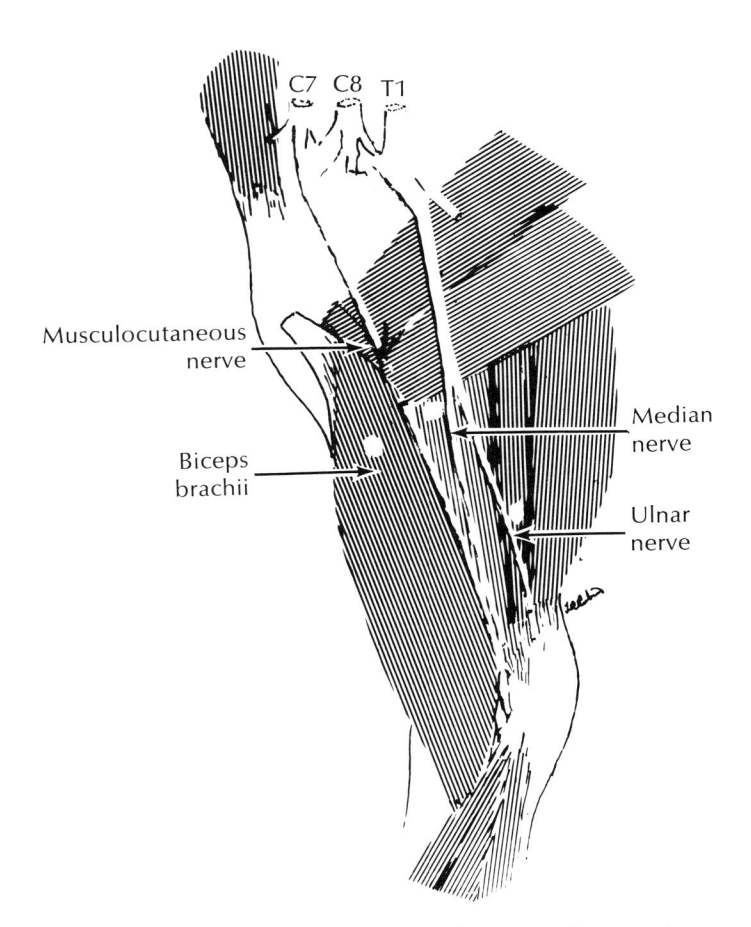

Fig. 15-1. Canine pectoral limb with complete division of musculocutaneous nerve. *Arrow,* Suture for identification at proximal portion.

Contemporary concepts in free nerve and muscle grafting

Materials and methods

Fifteen 12 to 14 kg. beagles (mixed sex) were used as experimental animals. Under general anesthesia (methoxyflurane, Penthrane) complete denervation of the biceps brachii of the right pectoral limb was performed by complete transection of the musculocutaneous nerve in the axilla, the nerve was subsequently tagged with a permanent suture of 4-0 Prolene for future identification (Fig. 15-1), and testing for complete denervation with a standard (Weck portable) nerve stimulator was performed routinely.

Three to 4 weeks postoperatively, the median nerve of the same pectoral limb was sectioned at the level of the midpoint of the biceps brachii and inserted into a pocket in the midbelly of the muscle by securing it with two 6-0 Ethilon sutures (epineurium to fascia) (Figs. 15-2 and 15-3).

Animals were reexplored on the operated site (right pectoral limb) and the control side (left pectoral limb) at 2- and 3-month intervals. Examinations were made by comparison of size of involved muscles, evidence of atrophy of fibrosis, response to standard nerve stimulation by the (Weck portable) nerve stimulator, and stimulation EMG pattern.

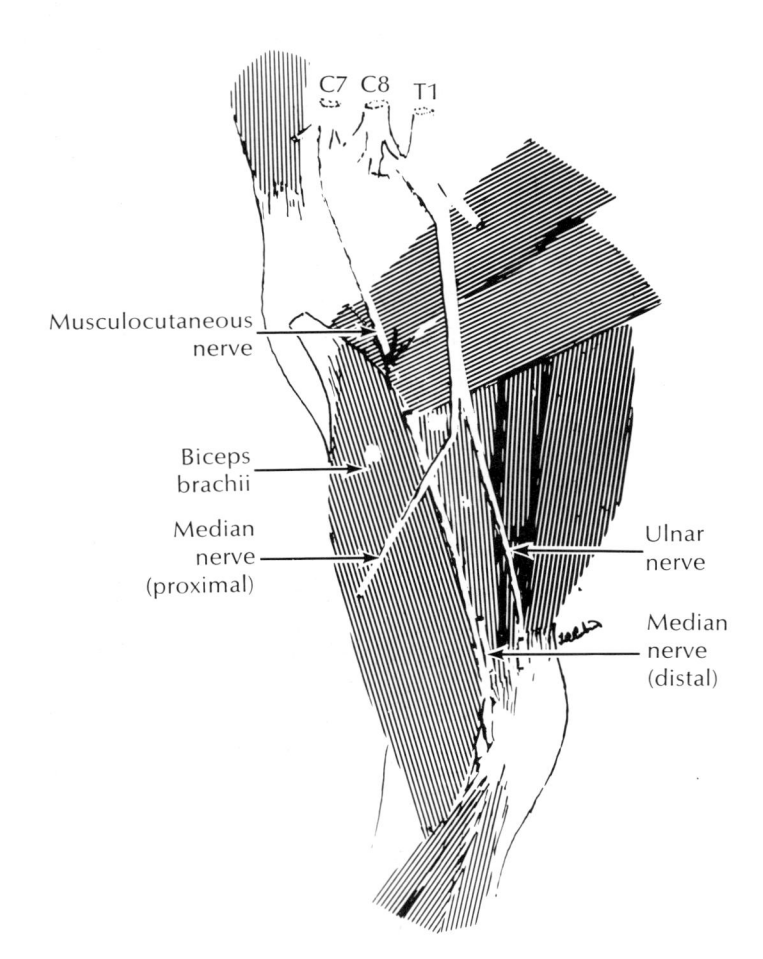

Fig. 15-2. Canine pectoral limb with median nerve implant in place (after division at level of midpoint of biceps brachii).

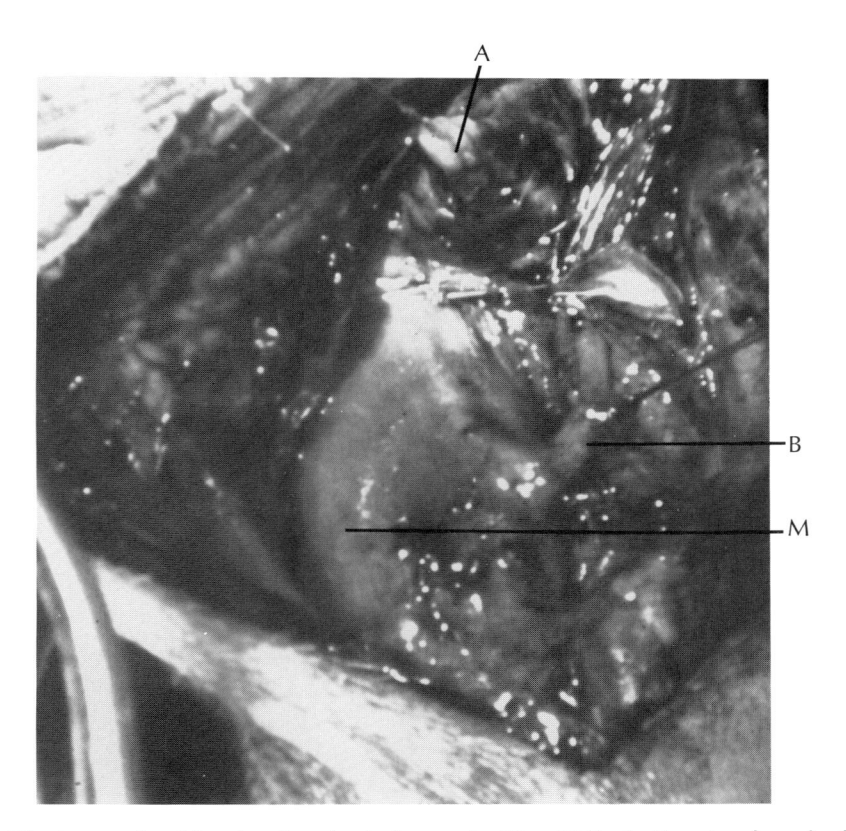

Nerve-end implantation into a denervated muscle

Fig. 15-3. Photograph of in vivo implant shown in Fig. 15-2. **A,** Proximal end of musculocutaneous nerve (with suture for identification). **B,** Implanted median nerve. **M,** Biceps brachii.

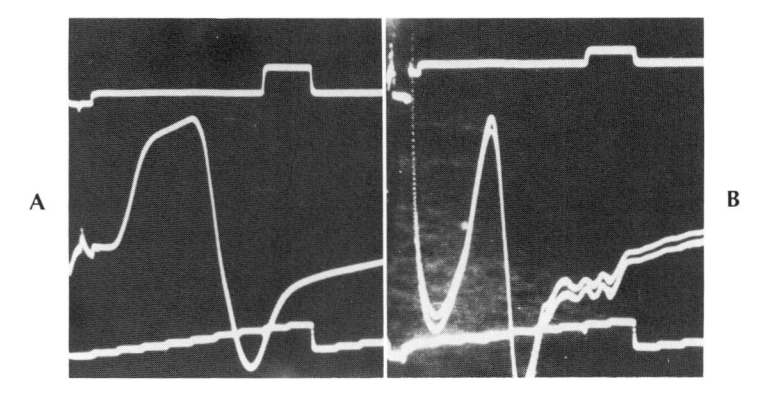

Fig. 15-4. Patterns of stimulation by electromyograph (strength of 0.5 milliamperes with duration of 0.5 milliseconds). **A,** Control (stimulation of musculocutaneous nerve). **B,** Experimental (stimulation of median nerve implant). General configuration and amplitude are similar to the control.

171

Results

Serial examinations of the biceps brachii on experimental versus control sides revealed no significant evidence of atrophy or fibrosis on inspection of all these muscles with nerves implanted. (Three became dislodged during the postoperative period and showed considerable atrophy, fibrosis, and no response to stimulation.)

Stimulation of the implanted median nerve on the experimental side after its isolation at a proximal site (with a Weck portable nerve stimulator) and stimulation of the musculocutaneous nerve on the control side resulted in active contraction with no discernible clinical difference. In addition, electromyographic patterns (stimulation electromyograph) were similar upon rheobasic stimulation (Fig. 15-4). Additional testing by stimulation of all nerves of the brachial plexus and surrounding tissues, even with supernormal stimuli, failed to result in any clinical contraction of the involved muscle or similar electromyographic pattern.

Discussion

The results of this study indicate that, indeed, a muscle can be reinnervated by direct nerve implantation ("neural neurotization"). The explanation for this phenomenon may involve axon sprouting at the end of the implanted nerve and its subsequent contact with new or previously existing myoneural end plates. Whatever the mechanism of establishing the neuromuscular unit, the experimental evidence (including clinical response to stimulation) suggests that this technique may be useful in those cases of facial nerve disruption in which the affected muscles remain viable without significant atrophy, but identification of the distal portions of motor nerves is difficult.

The technical ease of inserting the proximal portion of the facial nerve (or interposed nerve graft) into viable facial muscles in the acute cases or facial muscle substitutes (that is, muscle transfers or free muscle grafts) in the chronic cases would seem to provide many alternatives to the present static and dynamic approaches to dynamic synchronous and symmetrical facial reanimation while the progress in microneurovascular anastomosis proceeds.

REFERENCES

1. Aitken, J. T.: Growth of nerve implants in voluntary muscle, J. Anat. **84**:38-39, 1950.
2. Anderl, H.: Reconstruction of the face through cross-face nerve transplantation in facial paralysis, Chir. Plastica (Berlin) **2**:17-46, 1973.
3. DePalma, A. T., Leavitt, L. A., and Hardy, S. B.: Electromyography in full thickness flaps rotated between upper and lower lips, Plast. Reconstr. Surg. **21**(6):448-452, 1958.
4. Edds, M. V.: Collateral regeneration of residual motor axons in partially denervated muscles, J. Exp. Zool. **113**:517-547, 1950.
5. Freilinger, G.: A new technique to correct facial paralysis, Plast. Reconstr. Surg. **56**(1):44-48, 1975.
6. Hakelius, L., and Stålberg, E.: Electromyographic studies of free autogenous muscle graphs in man, Scand. J. Plast. Reconstr. Surg. **8**:211-219, 1974.
7. Hakelius, L.: Transplantation of free autogenous muscle in the treatment of facial paralysis, Scand. J. Plast. Reconstr. Surg. **8**:220-230, 1974.
8. Hakelius, L., Nyström, B., and Stålberg, E.: Histochemical and neurophysiological studies of autotransplanted cut muscles, Scand. J. Plast. Reconstr. Surg. **9**:15-24, 1975.
9. Hoffman, H.: Local re-innervation in partially denervated muscle. A histophysiological study, Aust. J. Exp. Biol. Med. Sci. **28**:383-397, 1950.
10. Hogan, E. L., Dawson, D. M., and Romanul, F. C. A.: Enzymatic changes in denervated muscle, Arch. Neurol. **13**:274-281, 1965.

11. Hogenhuis, L. A. A., and Engel, W. K.: Histochemistry and cytochemistry of experimentally denervated Guinea pig muscle, Acta. Anat. 60:39-65, 1965.
12. Isaksson, I., Johanson, B., Petersen, I., and Sellden, E.: Electromyographic study of the Abbe and fan flaps, Acta. Chir. Scand. 123:343-350, 1950.
13. Karpati, G., and Engel, W. K.: Type grouping in skeletal muscles after experimental reinnervation, Neurology 18:447-455, 1968.
14. Kugelberg, E., Edström, L., and Abbruzzese, M.: Mapping of motor units in experimentally reinnervated rat muscle, J. Neurol. Neurosurg. Psychiatry 33:319-329, 1970.
15. Pollock, L. J., et al.: Reaction of degeneration in electrodiagnosis of experimental peripheral nerve lesions, War Med. 7(5):275-283, 1945.
16. Rees, T. D., Rhodes, R. D., and Converse, J. M.: Pelliation of facial paralysis, Am. J. Surg. 120:82-87, 1970.
17. Romanul, F. C.: Enzymes in muscle, Arch. Neurol. 11:355-368, 1964.
18. Romanul, F. C., and Van Der Meulen, J. P.: Slow and fast muscles after cross innervation, Arch. Neurol. 17:387-402, 1967.
19. Roy, P. R.: Behavior of free autogenous muscle graft into the skeletal muscle of dog, J. Exp. Med. Sci. 9:78-83, 1966.
20. Smith, J. W.: Advances in facial nerve repair. Surg. Clin. North Am. 52(5):1287-1304, 1972.
21. Stålberg, E., and Ekstedt J.: Single fibre EMG and microphysiology of the motor unit in normal and diseased human muscle. New Dev. Electromyogr. Neurophysiol. 1:113-129, 1973.
22. Steindler, A.: The method of direct neurotization of paralyzed muscles, Am. J. Orthoped. Surg. 13:33-45, 1915.
23. Steindler, A.: Direct neurotization of paralyzed muscles: further study of the question of direct nerve implantation, Am. J. Orthoped. Surg. 14:707-718, 1916.
24. Thompson, N., and Polland, A. C.: Motor function in Abbe flaps, Br. J. Plast. Surg. 14:66-75, 1961.
25. Thompson, N.: Treatment of facial paralysis by free skeletal muscle grafts, Transactions of the Fifth International Congress of Plastic and Reconstructive Surgery, Chatswood, NSW, Aust., 1971, Butterworths Pty. Ltd., pp. 66-82.
26. Thompson, N.: Investigation of autogenous skeletal muscle free grafts in the dogs, Transplantation 12(5):353-363, 1971.
27. Thompson, N.: Autogenous free grafts of skeletal muscle, Plast. Reconstr. Surg. 48:11-27, 1971.
28. Tower, S.: Atrophy and degeneration in skeletal muscle, Am. J. Anat. 56(1):1-43, 1935.
29. Wohlfart, G.: Collateral regeneration in partially denervated muscles, Neurology 18:175-180, 1958.

16 Fundamentals of microvascular suturing

KIYONORI HARII
KITARO OHMORI

The acknowledged masters in free muscle and tissue grafting describe in detail their techniques for obtaining successful microvascular grafting results.

Fundamentals of microvascular suturing

In 1960, Jacobson and Suarez became the first persons to attempt anastomosis of vessels less than 3 mm in diameter under an operating microscope, which is essentially an instrument used in otologic surgery.

Since then, with improvements in operating microscopes, the availability of instruments for anastomosis of small vessels, and advances in suturing materials and methods, microvascular technique has developed to the point where it is possible to successfully anastomose vessels less than 1 mm in diameter.

This technique has added an epoch-making dimension to the field of plastic reconstructive surgery, that is, the feasibility of transplanting various composite tissues nourished by a small vessel pedicle by means of microsurgical revascularization.

The fundamental technique of microvascular anastomosis is described herein, together with an outline of some of the available instruments and suture materials.

Implements

OPERATING MICROSCOPE

Binocular surgical loupes and classical simple operating microscopes may provide some useful magnification. However, the modern, sophisticated operating microscope with electrically controlled zoom optics and focus adjustment has increased the accuracy of microvascular technique.

Furthermore, various equipment such as a binocular stereoscopic assistant scope, an observation tube, cinecamera, and videorecorder can additionally be attached in accordance with the surgeon's requirements.

We recommend the Zeiss operating microscope (OPMi-6) for microvascular anastomosis in plastic surgery because this multipurpose microscope has a bright field of view, its magnification and focus are controlled by a foot pedal, and its head can easily be tilted in the direction of the vessels to be anastomosed (Fig. 16-1).

MICROINSTRUMENTS

Various instruments for microsurgery are now commercially available, but only a few are essential for microvascular surgery.

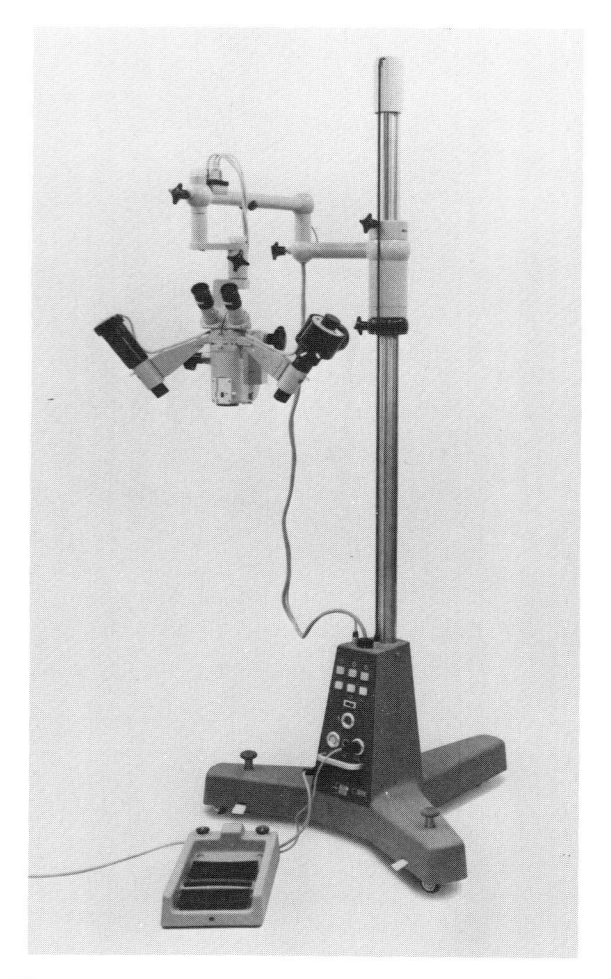

Contemporary concepts in free nerve and muscle grafting

Fig. 16-1. Zeiss operating microscope (OPMi-6).

1. Spring-handled needle driver. The standard Barraquer and Castroviejo ophthalmic needle drivers are available. We use a needle driver with a lock or a ratchet. The selection of a needle driver is closely related to the anastomosis technique (p. 178).
2. Spring-handled microscissors. Various types of scissors are available, but comparatively long-handled (more than 10 cm) scissors with either straight or curved thin and sharp blades are preferable. The straight-bladed scissors are used to cut the vessels and the curved-blade scissors to cut suture threads and connective tissue surrounding the vessels.
3. Microforceps. Several pairs of jeweller's forceps are used. Two pairs of No. 5 forceps are essential in the anastomosis of vessels, whereas two pairs of No. 2 forceps are used in the dissection of vessels. Sometimes No. 7 forceps (curved tip) are useful as microdissectors or counterpressors.
4. Microvascular clamps. Various types of single and double clamps have now been devised. We do not routinely use such double clamps as those devised by O'Brien, Ikuta, Kleinert, Acland, and Tamai. The reason is then even though

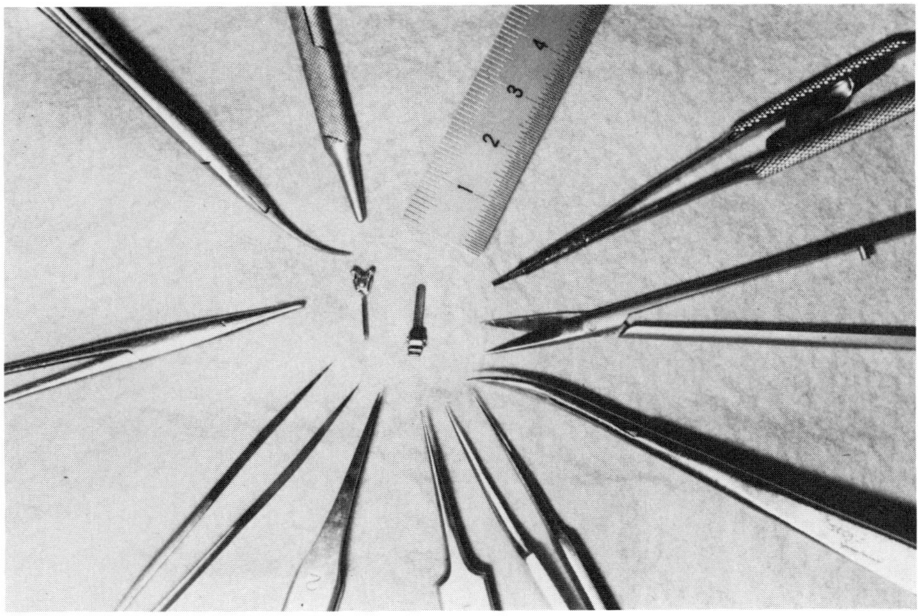

Fundamentals of microvascular suturing

Fig. 16-2. Instruments for microsurgery; their tips are enlarged.

double clamps facilitate approximation of severed vascular stumps, the actual tension and twist of the anastomosed vessels could be masked after the use of double clamps. We usually find Heifetz's neurosurgical clips satisfactory in the anastomosis of small vessels more than 0.8 mm in diameter. For even smaller vessels (especially in experimental surgery) the weakly sprung Heifetz's clips or Acland's clips are available, and they do not cause damage to the intima.

The above described are the essential microinstruments for small vessel anastomosis, but if one's funds permit, it is advisable to obtain other instruments such as a bipolar coagulator with microforceps attached and counterpressor (Fig. 16-2).

SUTURE MATERIALS

Nonreactive tensile suture threads with atraumatic needles are suitable. Buncke and Schulz developed metal-coated nylon thread in 1966, and later O'Brien and others also developed thread of the same type.

At present, ultrafine caliber monofilament nylon is advocated as the best suture material for microvascular anastomosis.

Ethicon (U.S.A.), Davis and Geck (U.S.A.), S & T (Germany), Microfine (Australia), and Crown (Japan) are representative suture materials now commercially available.

We prefer to use the 10-0 monofilament nylon suture with a ⅜ circle, tapered-point fine needle of less than 100 μm caliber (such as Crown 10-0 DY and S & T 10V43). These sutures are quite satisfactory for anastomosis of vessels with diameters of 0.8 mm or more. For vessels of lesser diameter, 11-0 sutures may be required (Fig. 16-3).

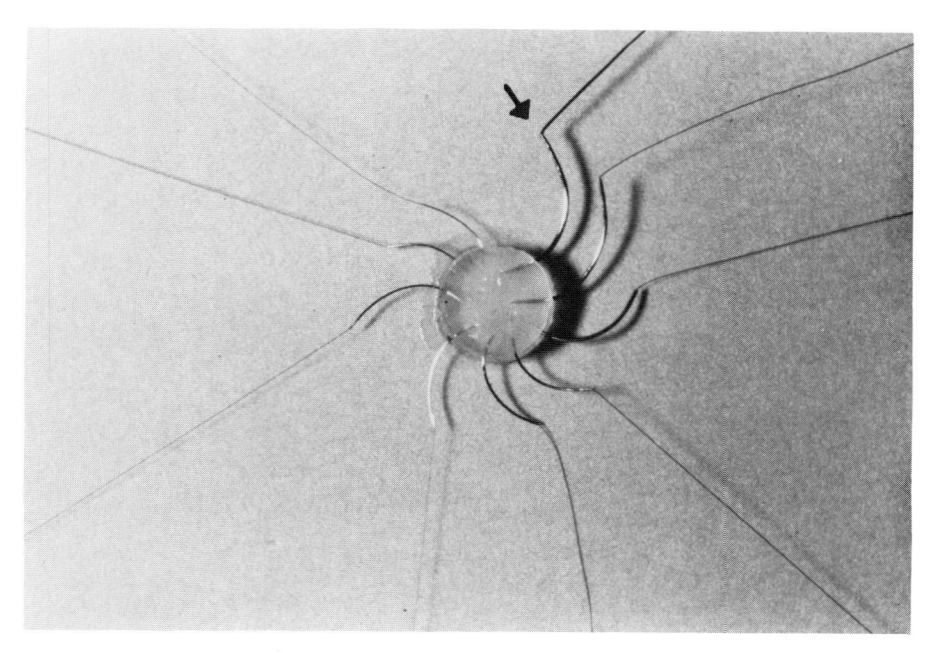

Contemporary concepts in free nerve and muscle grafting

Fig. 16-3. Various available sutures. *Arrow* indicates 8-0 monofilament nylon suture; then *clockwise* various 10-0 monofilament nylon sutures and 11-0 sutures are shown.

Techniques of microvascular anastomosis
SURGEON'S POSITION AND HANDLING OF TOOLS

Surgeons who are anxious to perform microvascular surgery clinically must first be prepared to spend many tiring hours in the laboratory learning the fundamental techniques.

The surgeon must first become accustomed to handling the sophisticated equipment and controls of the microscope and study draping, lighting, adjusting the focus, etc.

He must then learn to maintain a suitable operating stance, supporting his elbows and wrists on a stable table. Under magnification, it is difficult for even a surgeon well-experienced in normal macrosurgery to immediately acquire accurate eye-hand coordination.

One also must learn to manipulate the fine microinstruments atraumatically with no hand tremor. Supporting the elbows and wrists in position, one should hold instruments with thumb and index and middle fingers, as in gripping a pencil. The middle finger supports the instrument, while gentle manipulation with thumb and index finger opens and closes the spring-handled instrument. Such preliminary techniques can be mastered by cutting and suturing a soft Silastic tube under various magnifications. After a small piece of Silastic tube is fixed to a small board with sticky tape, it is placed at the center of the field of vision. The tube is then cut transversely with sharp microscissors.

Once the divided ends of the Silastic tube are approximated, the surgeon is ready for anastomosis. Now the suture thread is removed from its package, with care taken not to damage the needle-thread junction (8-0 monofilament nylon is easier to handle at first than 10-0 nylon).

The needle should be held at a point half its length from the tapered point for good

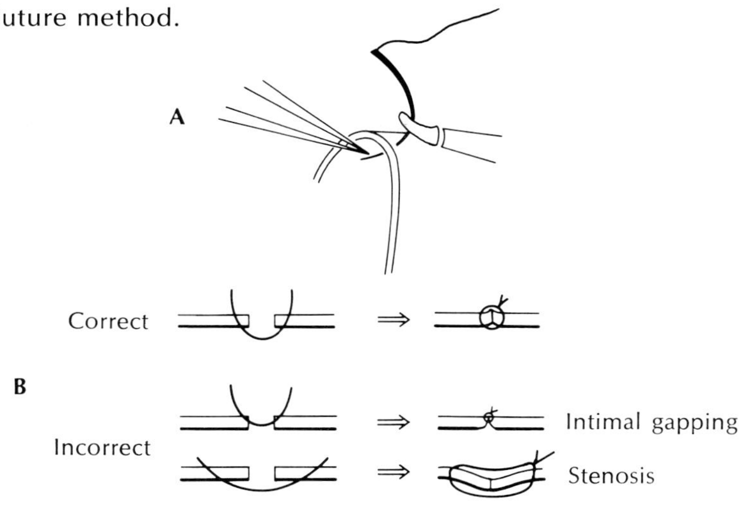

Fundamentals of microvascular suturing

Fig. 16-4. Suture method.

A

B

Correct

Incorrect — Intimal gapping

Stenosis

control in driving the tip of the needle. When the surgeon is a right-handed individual, the needle driver is held in his right hand and No. 5 microforceps in his left hand (and vice versa if he is left handed).

The Silastic tube should be kept in a horizontal position parallel to the surgeon so that the divided segments can be referred to as the left segment and right segment (permitting simple explanation of the anastomosis technique).

Magnification is adjusted after the instruments held in both hands are visible in the field of vision.

The needle, grasped by the jaws of the needle driver held in the right hand, is placed in a position twice wall thickness from the edge of the right segment and driven through the full thickness of the wall. The No. 5 forceps held in the left hand are inserted into the lumen of the right segment as a counterpressor while the needle is passing through the wall (Fig. 16-4).

After the needle has passed through the wall, it is again grasped with the needle driver and passed through the full thickness of the wall of the left segment from inside to outside with a bite of equal size. After passing through both ends of the tube, the needle is pulled slowly until the tail of the thread is visible in the field of vision. The thread usually is tied with two knots, but several knots are made initially for training purposes (p. 178).

In the initial stage, low magnification permits easier handling of the instruments and thread, but one must later train under a magnification greater than 15.

SUTURE TECHNIQUE

There is a close relationship between suture technique and the needle driver used. There are two types of needle driver available, one without a lock or a ratchet and the other with a lock or a ratchet.

When one uses the former type, he must keep the needle in a position easy to pick up again while tying the suture with the needle driver and the forceps held in the other hand. In this case, there are two representative ways of positioning and managing the barely visible needle.

Fig. 16-5. Tying knots.

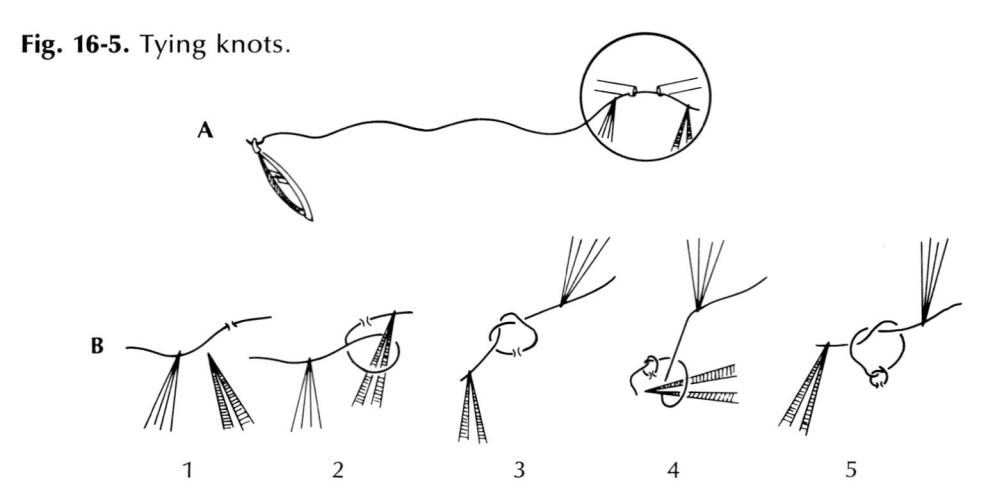

One way is that in which the needle is positioned in a particular spot outside the field of vision after it has been passed through the vascular walls. Then, after the knot has been tied, the distal end of the thread is pulled back so that the needle automatically comes back into view. This would be one of the simple suture methods, but in clinical cases there is the possibility of the needle's being lost because of hemorrhaging, swabbing of the operation field with gauzes, etc.

The other way is that in which one keeps the needle in the field of vision by attaching it to tissue beside the vessels to be anastomosed. After the thread is tied, the needle can again be picked up by the needle driver. However, the working field of vision under a microscope is so limited that the needle easily could interfere in tying of the thread and causes problems.

Some microsurgeons like to use the No. 2 forceps instead of a needle driver without a lock, but these forceps are not strong enough to drive a needle through thick vascular walls of vessels with diameters greater than 2 mm.

On the other hand, if a needle driver with a lock (or a ratchet) is used, the needle can be held without locking a ratchet when it is passed through the vascular wall. After it has passed through the walls of both vascular stumps, the needle is held by the needle driver and the thread is slowly pulled until the tail appears in the field of vision. The ratchet of the needle driver is then locked, and the needle driver is placed in position. Thus one can always keep the needle in the same position. Tying of the thread is accomplished with two pairs of No. 5 forceps, each pair being held in each hand.

In this way, one can continually keep the needle thread in the same position and not lose it in the complicated operative field. Many microsurgeons hesitate to use the needle driver with a lock because they are afraid of hand tremor when the lock is in action. However, we always use a lock outside the field of vision, and hazardous tremor is thus avoided (Fig. 16-5).

TECHNIQUE OF ANASTOMOSIS

The technique of microvascular anastomosis is based on conventional vascular anastomosis technique. For vessels less than 3 mm in external diameter, single interrupted suture anastomosis is adopted. The continuous suture or mattress suture would make the anastomosed orifice stenotic.

Fundamentals of microvascular suturing

Mastery of this technique can only be acquired by daily practice with experimental animals for at least 2 months. Although various animals are available for this purpose, rats are the most ideal for such practice as they are not expensive and are easy to anesthetize and house. Furthermore, the vessels of rats show the least spasms among experimental animals and are easy to prepare.

After the vessels to be anastomosed have been exposed, both stumps of vessels are placed in position under minimal tension. Now the operating microscope is brought into working position.

MICROSURGICAL DISSECTION OF SMALL VESSELS

Before proceeding to the anastomosis of small vessels themselves, one should first learn how to dissect them under magnification. One can, through this procedure, be-

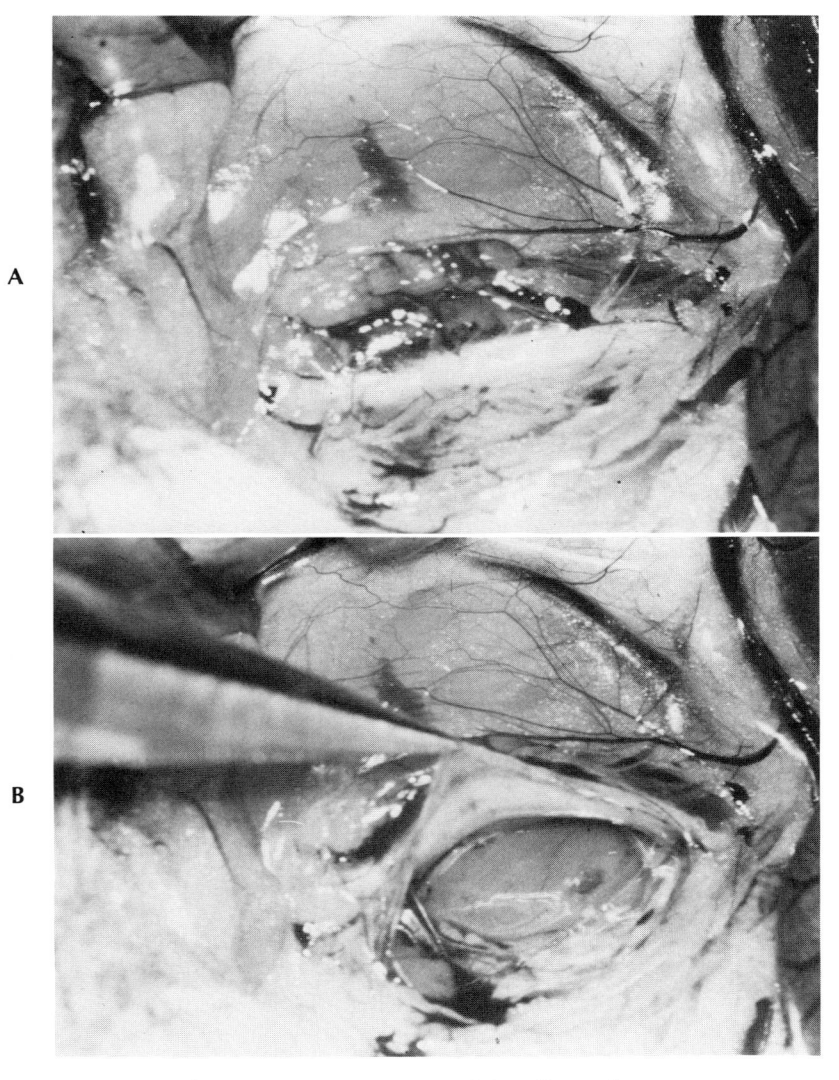

Fig. 16-6. Rat's aorta and its dissection.

come familiar with the microinstruments and operating microscope, and it is the simplest method of mastering the fundamental technique of microsurgery.

The most suitable material for this purpose is the abdominal aorta of rats. It is attached with the vena cava inferior, and one will find that it is quite difficult to separate them atraumatically under magnification.

A rat is initially anesthetized by the open ether-drop method, and then anesthesia is maintained with sodium pentobarbital (Nembutal) administered intraperitoneally (the Nembutal dosage is 3 to 5 mg per 100 grams of body weight).

After complete removal of abdomen hair, the rat is laid on a cork operating board in a dorsum-down position and fixed to the board with disposable syringe needles piercing its legs.

Laparotomy is performed through a lower abdomen incision, and all bowels are retracted to one side so that the aorta in the retroperitoneum is easily exposed. Now the operating microscope is swung into position and fine adjustments are made.

Dissection proceeds into the connective tissue between the aorta and the vena cava inferior by use of two pairs of No. 2 microforceps and curved microscissors, with care taken not to damage the thin and fragile venous wall. The aorta should be dissected from the point of branching of the renal artery to the point of bifurcation into the common iliac arteries. Several small branches should be ligated or coagulated with a bipolar coagulator (Fig. 16-6).

After mastering microdissection of the abdominal aorta of rats, one should become further experienced in the dissection of smaller vessels, such as the carotid artery, common iliac artery, and femoral artery. One will find that, despite their smaller size, the latter arteries are easier to dissect than is the aorta.

ARTERIAL ANASTOMOSIS

The first step in practicing anastomosis is repair of a rat's abdominal aorta. After the aorta has been completely dissected from the vena cava inferior over a length of 2 cm, a rubber sheet made from a thin surgeon's glove is placed under the dissected aorta to isolate it from the surrounding tissues.

After the size of the aorta is measured, the first microclamp is placed on the aorta

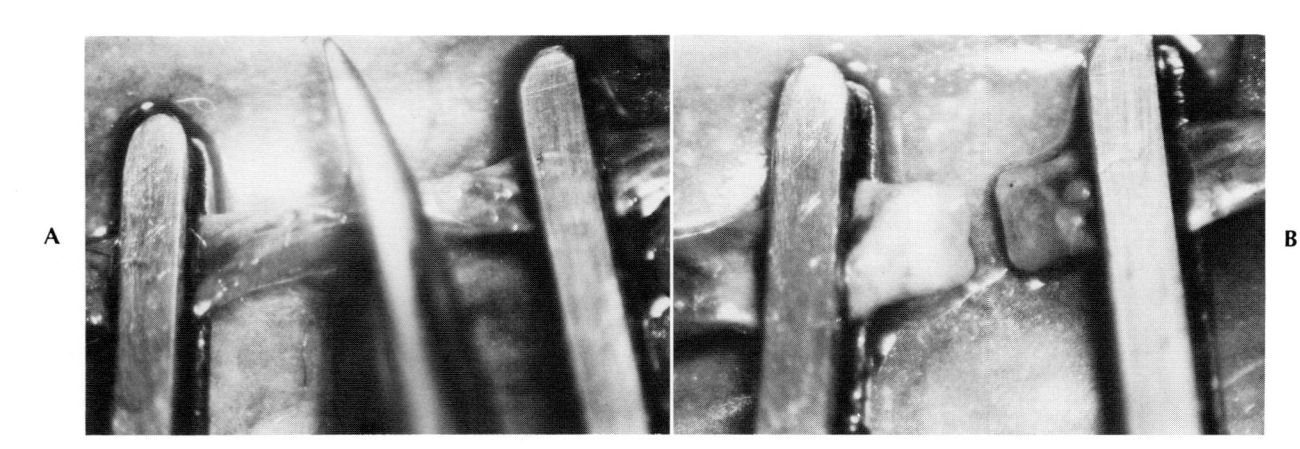

Fig. 16-7. Cutting isolated aorta.

Fundamentals of microvascular suturing

slightly distal to the point of branching of the renal artery, and the second clamp slightly proximal to the point of bifurcation of the iliac arteries.

The aorta is then severed transversely with the straight microscissors. For accurate cutting, the jaws of the scissors should be held perpendicular to the main axis of the aorta (Fig. 16-7).

Immediately after severance of the aorta, both stumps should be irrigated with a heparinized saline solution (20 I.U. per milliliter of saline) to remove blood clots. Irrigation is accomplished through a 26-gauge hypodermic needle whose tip is bent and connected to a disposable syringe. Frequent irrigation is necessary during anastomosis to avoid drying of the vessel wall.

Adventitectomy

Stripping of the adventia of vessels to be anastomosed is dependent on the properties of the vessels themselves. These properties vary with the kind of animals, location of vessels (subcutaneous, intra-abdominal, intracranial, and muscular), age, and so forth. In thin wall vessels, such as veins, intracranial small arteries, and small arteries less than 1 mm in diameter, excessive trimming of the adventitia makes the walls fragile and difficult to anastomose. In such case, only loose strands of collagen fibers drooping into the lumen should be trimmed.

It is usual in clinical cases for the fine fibrous strands drooping into the lumen from the vascular stump to be gently pulled along the long axis of the vessel with No. 5 forceps, and for the adventitia extending over the stump to be resected with fine microscissors (Fig. 16-8).

After cleanly cut ends of both stumps are obtained, the tips of No. 5 forceps are gently inserted into the lumen to enlarge the collapsed vascular lumen. If strong spasms of the vessels are noticed, a 2% lidocaine (Xylocaine) solution may be dropped to relieve the spasming. The vessel stumps are then again irrigated with a heparinized saline solution and arranged for anastomosis.

The initial two stay sutures are usually placed slightly anterior to the equator of the vessels, approximately 150 degrees apart, with one end of each suture being left long for temporary traction. This allows the posterior edges to fall away from the needle point and avoids the error of picking up the opposite intima when the needle is passed through the anterior intima (Cobbett's eccentric biangulation) (Fig. 16-9).

The needle is passed through the full thickness of the vascular wall (including the adventitia, media, and intima of vessels) with a needle bite about twice wall thickness in vessels less than 2 mm in diameter.

When there is tension between the two vascular stumps, the needle bite is a little larger, and so the suture should be tied with a surgical knot.

Each stitch is cut with one end left long for traction while the next stitch is being formed (Fig. 16-10).

Our histological examinations have shown that these threads appearing in the vascular lumen do not lead to thrombus formation (Fig. 16-11), while poor coaptation of the intima easily leads to thrombus formation (Fig. 16-12).

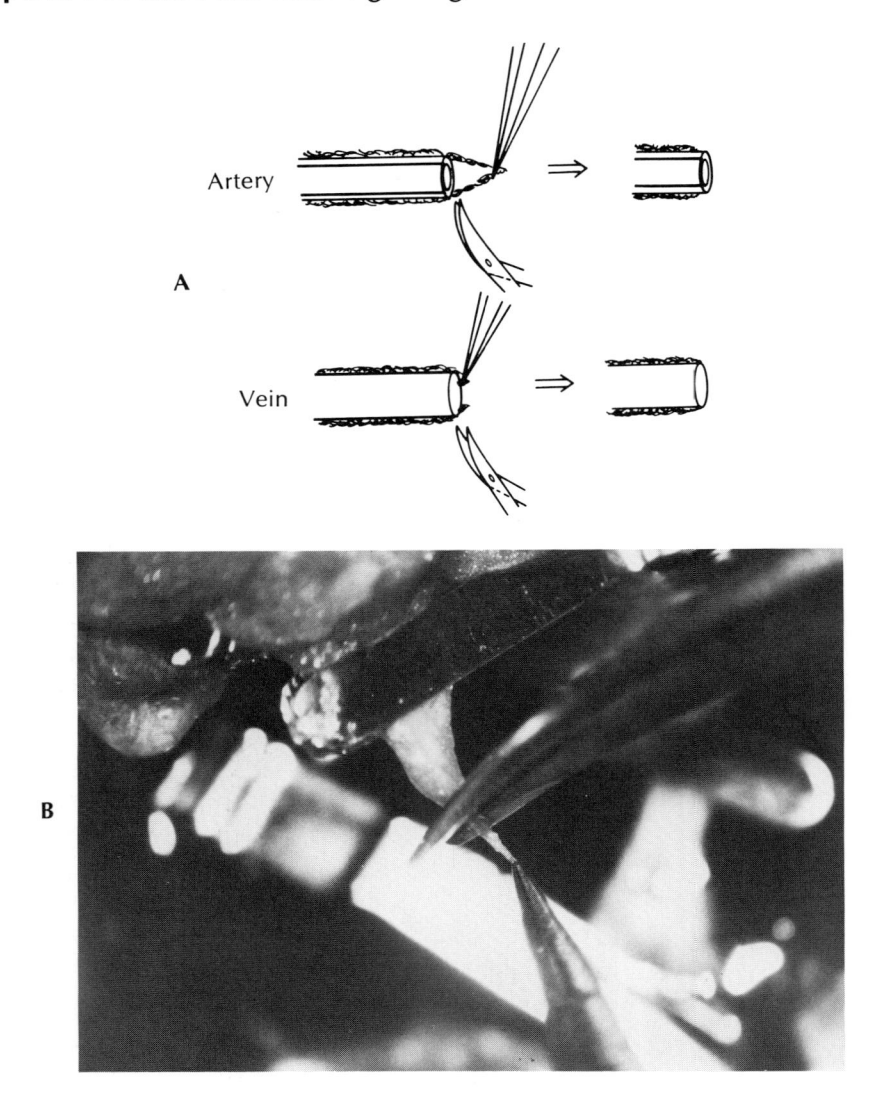

Contemporary concepts in free nerve and muscle grafting

Fig. 16-8. Adventitectomy in schema and clinical adventitectomy.

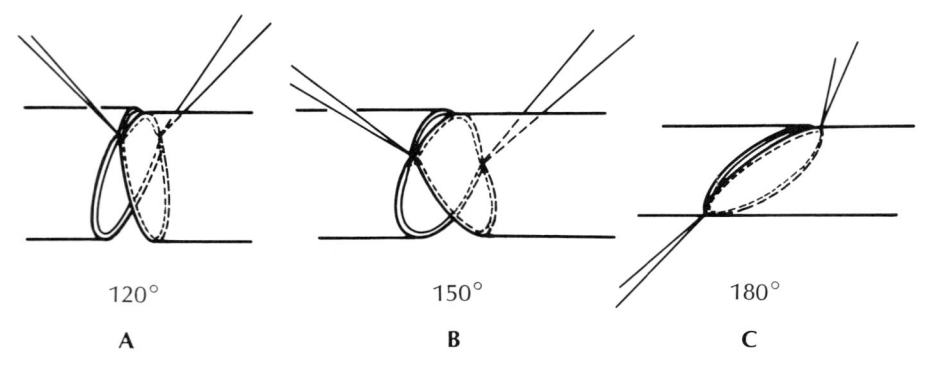

Fig. 16-9. Various types of stay sutures. **A**, Cobbett's asymmetric biangulation. **B**, Modified asymmetric biangulation. **C**, Conventional biangulation.

Fundamentals of microvascular suturing

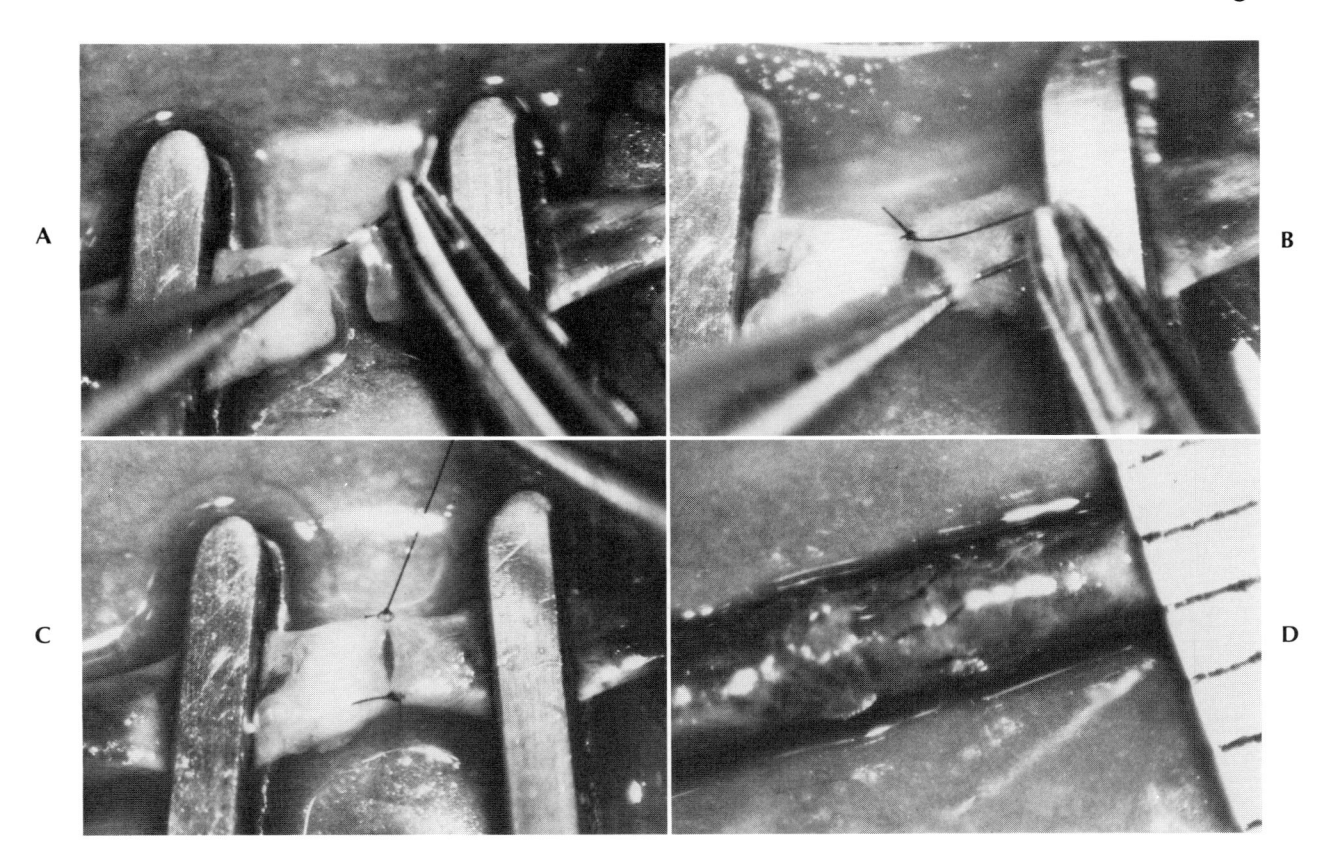

Fig. 16-10. Anastomosis of rat's aorta.

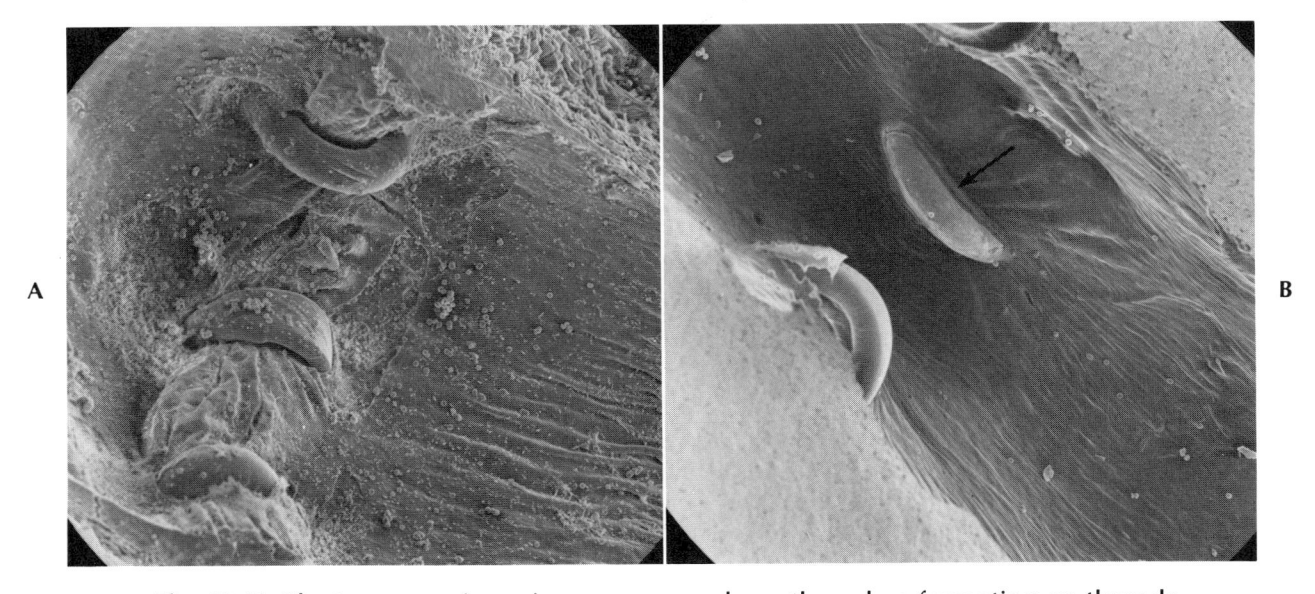

Fig. 16-11. Electron scanning microscope reveals no thrombus formation on threads appearing in lumen. **A,** One hour after anastomosis of rat's femoral artery. **B,** 28 days after anastomosis, the exposed thread *(arrow)* is covered by thin end.

185

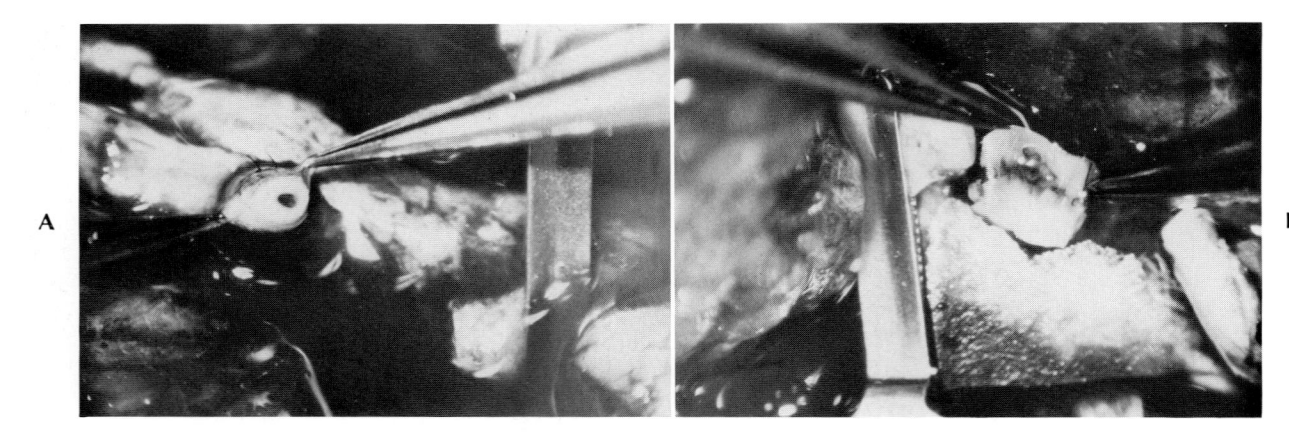

Contemporary concepts in free nerve and muscle grafting

Fig. 16-12. Acute thrombosis caused by poor coaptation of intima in anastomosis of human superficial temporal artery.

After placement of the two stay sutures, two or three interrupted sutures are placed on the anterior surface, with the number depending on the external diameter of the arteries (for example, two stitches for a 1 mm artery and three for a 1.5 mm artery).

The number of stitches could be reduced if one could place the stitches in accurate apposition.

After completion of anterior wall repair, the clamps are rotated and one stay suture is passed beneath the vessels to expose the posterior wall.

After irrigation of the vascular lumen, parts of several stitches placed on the anterior wall can be seen inside the lumen.

The posterior wall gap is then repaired with several interrupted sutures placed in succession in accordance with the illustration.

Approximately eight sutures are required for repair of a 1 mm artery, and 10 sutures for a 1.5 mm artery. Prior to removal of clamps, the rubber sheet used as a base is wrapped around the anastomosis to minimize blood leakage after unclamping.

The distal clamp is opened first, and a sudden burgeoning of blood is observed flowing back proximally beyond the anastomosis. When this backflow is slow, constricture of the anastomosis is suggested.

After checking of this backflow, the proximal clamp is removed. If the anastomosis is satisfactory, the blood flow through the anastomosis is vigorous and accompanied by good pulsation. Leakage can be controlled by temporary (5 to 10 minutes) application of a rubber cuff.

Radical patency test

To clarify the patency of the anastomosis, a No. 2 forceps is used to close the vessel at a point immediately distal (downstream) to the anastomosis line while another forceps is used to squeeze the blood from out of the downstream segment. Then, while the forceps on the downstream side are kept closed, the forceps on the proximal side are opened. With a patent anastomosis, the empty space is quickly filled with blood flowing through the anastomosis (Fig. 16-13).

Fundamentals of microvascular suturing

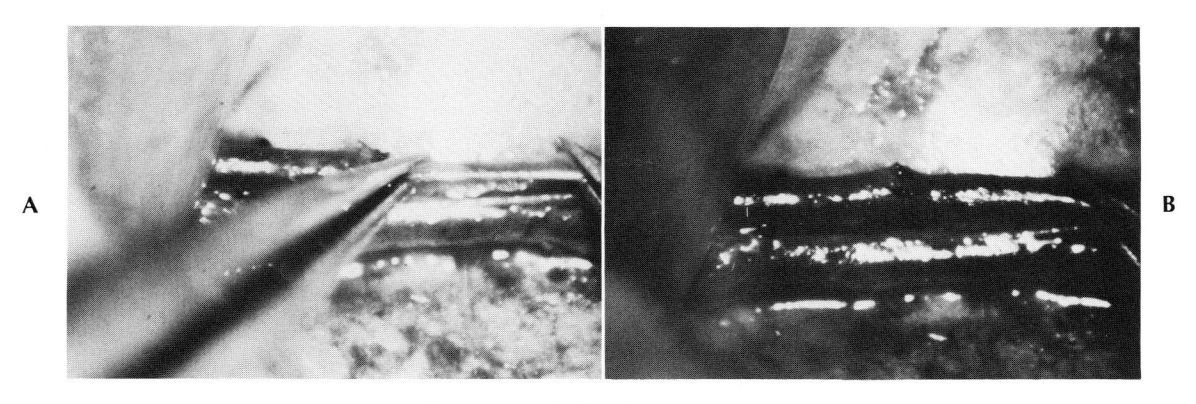

Fig. 16-13. Radical patency test.

After 100% patency of anastomosis of the aorta has been obtained, the next step is repair of the common iliac artery or common carotid artery in rats. These arteries are 1 to 1.2 mm in external diameter, and the aorta is 1.3 to 1.5 mm in external diameter.

The final step in anastomosis of the artery is repair of the femoral artery of a rat. Through a longitudinal incision on the medial thigh, the femoral sheath is exposed macroscopically. The final dissection to separate the femoral artery from the femoral vein and nerve should be performed under low magnification ($3\times$ to $5\times$). The small branches, such as the inferior epigastric vessels, are ligated or coagulated. After the femoral artery and vein, respectively, are separated for lengths of about 2 cm, a few drops of 2% Xylocaine are dropped onto the vessels to relieve spasms.

Prior to anastomosis, a thin rubber sheet is placed beneath the artery, and vascular clamps are placed in position (Acland's clip may be suitable here as it will not damage the tiny vessels).

Vascular anastomosis is carried out in the same manner as in the case of the aorta, but the number of stitches is reduced because of the smaller diameter (0.8 to 1 mm in external diameter) (Fig. 16-14).

VENOUS ANASTOMOSIS

The essential venous anastomosis technique is the same as that in the case of an artery. However, because the wall is thin and fragile, the needle bite should be about three to four times wall thickness.

The initial two stay sutures are placed about 180 degrees apart, and the number of stitches used in about two thirds that for an artery.

Continuous irrigation with a heparinized saline solution could enlarge the lumen and facilitate anastomosis Because the blood pressure is low, there is minimal leaking from a venous anastomosis after unclamping, and so the rubber sheet cuff is not necessary.

The final step in training is the challenging anastomosis of a rat's femoral vein, one of the most difficult operations and suitable for polishing a surgeon's mastery of the technique. Fortunately, the wall of a small vein in a human is thicker than that in an experimental animal, and so there is no need for disappointment in anastomosing small veins (Fig. 16-15).

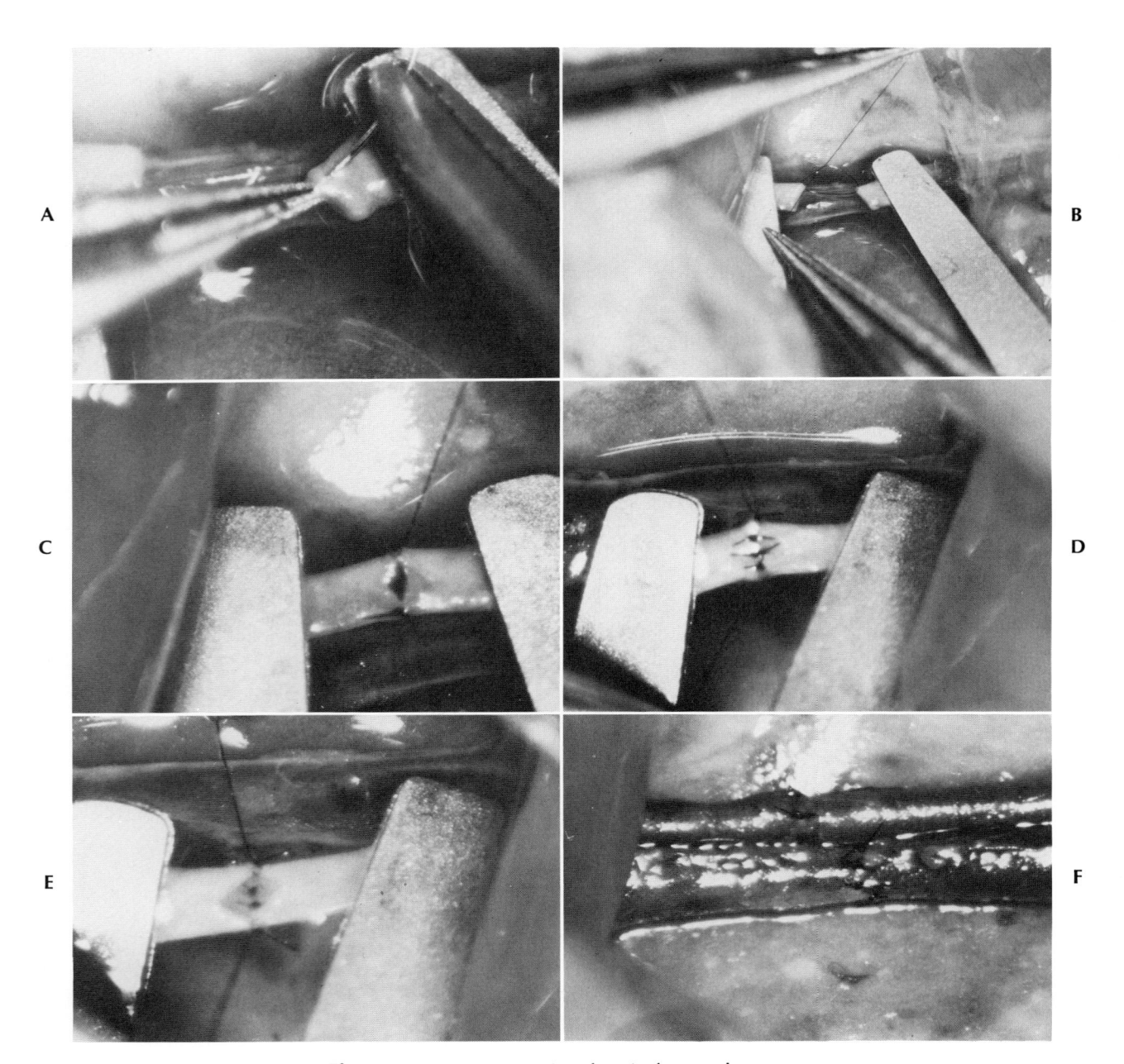

Contemporary concepts in free nerve and muscle grafting

Fig. 16-14. Anastomosis of rat's femoral artery.

Fundamentals of microvascular suturing

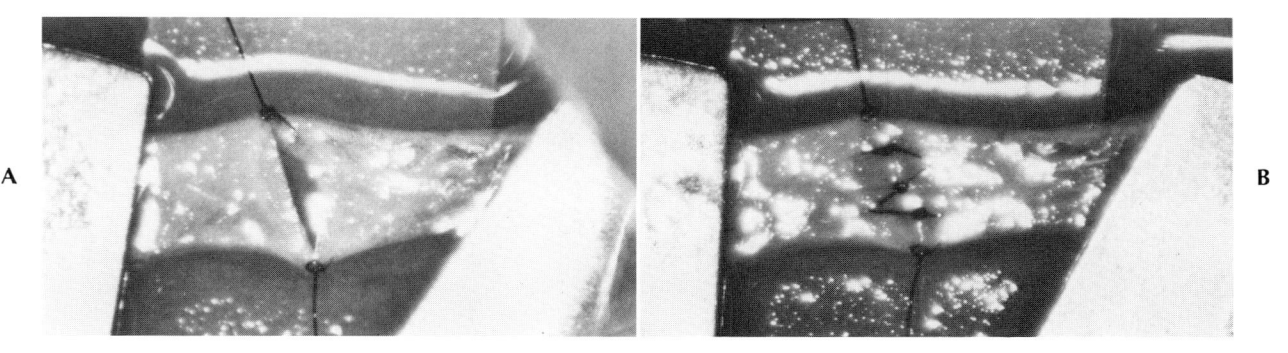

Fig. 16-15. Anastomosis of rat's femoral vein.

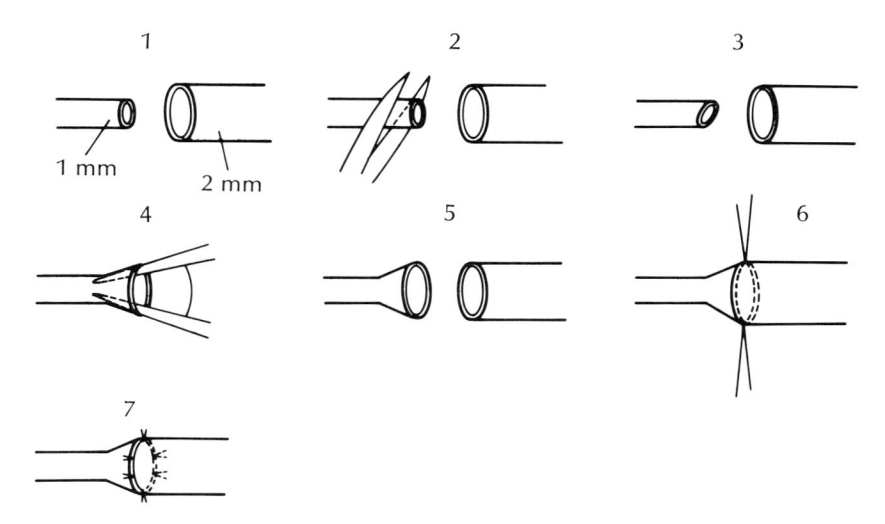

Fig. 16-16. Anastomosis between vessels of different diameters.

ANASTOMOSIS OF VESSELS OF DIFFERENT DIAMETERS

When one begins to experience actual clinical operations, one will soon encounter discrepancies in size between the two vessels to be anastomosed. Such discrepancies should be accommodated by end-to-end anastomosis with oblique transection of the smaller vessel in order to accomplish approximation of the circumferences of the two vessels, interposition of a vein graft, and end-to-side anastomosis. We prefer end-to-end anastomosis because it is considered to secure the best blood flow.

The smaller vessel is transected obliquely and then gently spread out with fine No. 5 forceps inserted into the lumen in order to obtain a larger circumference. In this way, the circumference of the smaller vessel can be made to approximate that of the larger vessel (Fig. 16-16).

END-TO-SIDE ANASTOMOSIS

We believe end-to-end anastomosis to be the safest and simplest in clinical microvascular surgery. However, end-to-side anastomosis may be applied in such special cases as those in which a blood flow distal to the anastomosis should be secured. The technique of end-to-side anastomosis is only a modification of that of end-to-end anastomosis.

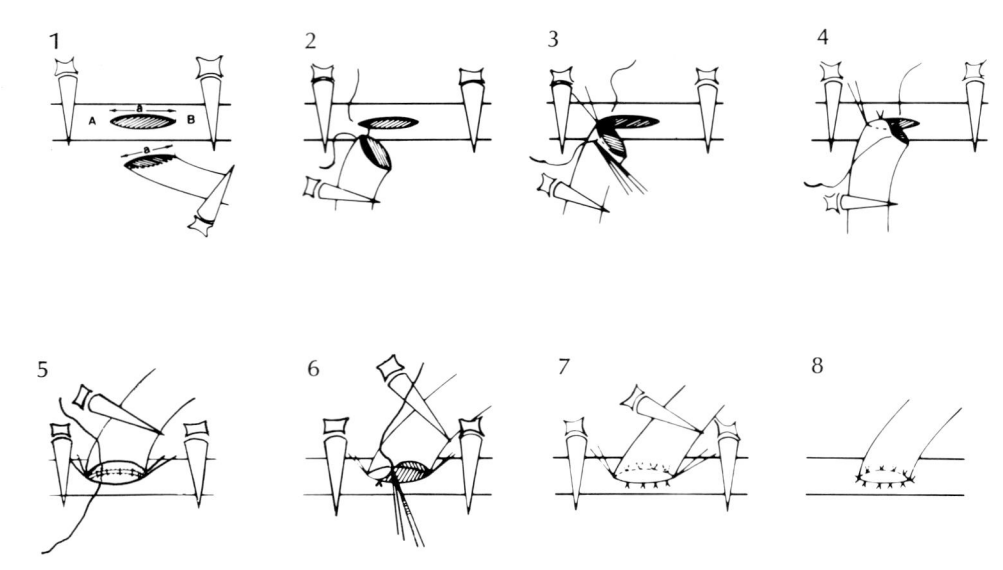

Contemporary concepts in free nerve and muscle grafting

Fig. 16-17. Schema of end-to-side anastomosis (by Harii).

Comment

The technique of microvascular anastomosis has been described in detail herein. In clinical practice, there are several points that differ from those in animal experiments, namely, thickness of the vessel wall, spasming, and a tendency toward thrombus formation. In experimental animals (especially rats), frequently no thrombus is formed because of poor coaptation of the intima, whereas in a human, poor coaptation of the intima is one of the greatest incidental causes of thrombus formation. Other causes of thrombus formation are kinking and torsion of the anastomosed vessels, and a reduced blood flow through stenotic anastomosis. Particularly in venous anastomosis, tension of the anastomosis site is likely to cause thrombosis.

Several anticoagulants have been used, but no surgeon has been able to use them effectively without side effects. We believe that there is no requirement in a satisfactory anastomosis for systemic administration of an anticoagulant during or after an operation.

REFERENCES

1. Acland, R. D.: Thrombus formation in microvascular surgery: an experimental study of the effects of surgical trauma, Surgery **73:** 766, 1973.
2. Acland, R. D.: Prevention of thrombosis in microvascular surgery by the use of magnesium sulphate, Br. J. Plast. Surg. **25:**292, 1972.
3. Buncke, H. J., and Schulz, W. P.: Total ear reimplantation in the rabbit utilizing microminiature vascular anastomosis, Br. J. Plast. Surg. **19:**15, 1966.
4. Cobbett, J.: Small vessel anastomosis: a comparison of suture techniques, Br. J. Plast. Surg. **22:**16, 1967.
5. Daniel, R. K., and Taylor, G. I.: Distant transfer of an island flap by microvascular anastomosis, Plast. Reconstr. Surg. **52:**111, 1973.
6. Harii, K., Ohmori, K., and Ohmori, S.: Successful clinical transfers of ten free flaps by microvascular anastomoses, Plast. Reconstr. Surg. **53:**259-270, 1974. Discussion by Goldwyn, **53:**469, 1974.
7. Harii, K., and Ohmori, K.: Direct transfer of large free groin skin flaps to the lower extremity using microvascular anastomoses, Chir. Plastica (Berlin) **3:**1, 1975.
8. Harii, K., Ohmori, K., and Torii, S.: Free gracilis muscle transplantation with micro-

neurovascular anastomoses for the treatment of facial paralysis, Plast. Reconstr. Surg. **57:** 133, 1976.
9. Jacobson, J. H., and Suarez, E. L.: Microsurgery in anastomosis of small vessel, Surg. Forum **2:**243, 1960.
10. Östrup, L. T., and Fredrickson, J. M.: Distinct transfer of a free, living bone graft by microvascular anastomoses, Plast. Reconstr. Surg. **54:**274, 1974.
11. Tamai, S., Sasauchi, N., Hori, Y., Tatsumi, Y., and Okuda, H.: Microvascular surgery in orthopaedics and traumatology, J. Bone Joint Surg. **54B:**637, 1972.
12. Taylor, G. I., Miller, G. D. H., and Ham, F. J.: The free vascularized bone graft: a clinical extension of microvascular techniques, Plast. Reconstr. Surg. **55:**533, 1975.

PART IV

REANIMATION OF THE PARALYZED FACE

SECTION ONE
Immediate or early treatment, 194

SECTION TWO
Intermediate surgical treatment for facial paresis—4 months to one year, 241

SECTION THREE
Late surgical treatment for facial paresis—after 12 months, 278

SECTION ONE

Immediate or early treatment

17 Value of galvanic muscle stimulation immediately after paresis

BERNARD S. POST

Despite the usual teaching that galvanic stimulation to a paretic muscle does not delay degeneration, evidence is cited that the stimulation maintains biochemical activity and prolongs the maintenance of normal structure. Degeneration may eventually occur if nerve continuity is not restored within a reasonable time. However, bidding for time, one may use the therapy because it is valuable and indicated.

How does one decide whether or not surgical intervention is called for in a particular case?

The necessity for surgical treatment is almost generally accepted in a number of cases of facial paralysis. There is no doubt about the immediate necessity for surgery in a palsy of the facial nerve complicating chronic otitis media. On the other hand, nobody would consider decompressing in the case of a central facial palsy.

In the case of Bell's palsy or other endotemporal facial paralysis, there is mixed opinion about whether to intervene, since many of these cases generally tend to recover spontaneously. This palsy begins without apparent cause and without pain, in many instances. The pathological condition is commonly in the vertical part of the nerve, which becomes red and swollen, with its trunk tightly constricted by the nerve sheath and bony wall of the fallopian canal. Both Jonkees[14] and Hunt, independently, as well as many others, have reported this.

There are numerous investigators who take up the opposite point of view, insisting that surgery for Bell's palsy should not be done. The main basis of their arguments lies in the fact that it is hard to judge the effect of treatment of any type in this condition. First of all, nearly three fourths of the patients heal spontaneously. Verjaal[8] compared results when aspirin and galvanic stimulation were used alone, with those when no treatment was given at all. The percentage of recovery was identical when judged by the same standards. Taverner[25] reported nearly the same results. Cortisone has also proved to be equally ineffective over a large series of patients. Because of this, even the people that believe in decompression are afraid to make claims since there has not been a large enough series beyond that of Jonkees,[14] who reported a series of a few more than 180 patients (1965).

Jonkees has presented a number of arguments in favor of surgery in cases of Bell's palsy, as follows:

1. In the first 6 to 8 weeks the nerve is swollen and there is strong vascular injection. This has been substantiated during surgery when after the sheath has been opened, the nerve protrudes, being expelled by strong edema. The central end of the edematous nerve is nearly always clearly delineated from the normal position of the nerve. If one operates after more than 8 weeks from the onset,

other changes are also seen. It has been reported that the sheath and nerve can grow together and after the incision the nerve does not bulge as much as in the earlier cases, thereby still being subject to the pressure. If the surgeon waits still longer after the onset of the paralysis to operate, he may find no edema or vascular injection at all. Instead there is atrophy. In this case the surgeon does not usually have the impression that the patient has been decompressed once the canal is opened.

2. The results of decompression in patients who were operated on within 2 weeks of onset are usually excellent. Complete recovery is very common in them. Before 3 months after onset, some favorable results can be possible, though this is dependent on the length of the existence of the paralysis before the surgery. After more than 3 months the results are so disappointing that Jonkees does not proceed with any measures for them.

3. Janssen[13] has reported that in his series of 183 decompressions, all on patients within 6 weeks of onset of paralysis, there was recovery of function by 1 week after surgery in 10% of the group. This suggests that the function of a number of nerve fibers can recover very quickly as long as the damage is limited to neurapraxia. Janssen[13] believes that decompression seems to have a double function. It not only takes away the pressure upon the degenerating fibers and offers those in a condition of neurapraxia the possibility to recover, but it also accelerates the regrowth of completely degenerated fibers by creating good conditions and better vascularization and by preventing the ingrowth of connective tissues.

4. Jonkees[14] has also set forth a serendipitous benefit from decompression surgery in patients in whom the basic diagnosis has been wrong. He reports a few cases in which a tumor of the middle ear was found, and in three cases where a masked mastoiditis was uncovered. This is not the ideal way to determine indications for surgery but because there must be a percentage of error in diagnosis, such a procedure could bring benefits.

5. Another strong argument is that patients do not suffer much during decompression surgery. There is an average of about 1 week's stay in the hospital. Most people can leave the hospital after 5 days. Infections, which might prolong stay, are not too frequent. Jonkees[14] reports one case of postoperative tinnitus in 180 cases. Careful selection of cases with reasonable indications and promptness of intervention are important factors in the surgical form of therapy.

There is no reason to assume that the damaging influence on the facial nerve in Bell's palsy is essentially different from that in a facial paralysis secondary to a chronic otitis media. In the later case it is considered an urgent indication for surgery. Yet how difficult it can be to dare to operate on a patient who has a 4-to-1 chance of a spontaneous recovery.

The new forms of diagnostic investigation today, as described in this chapter, has made it a bit easier to decide. Laumans[17] has pointed out from his examinations of a large number of fresh facial palsies that a paralysis that is complete after 2 weeks will never recover completely. This is especially true if the tone of the facial muscle is bad and if the electromyography shows the presence of fibrillations. In those cases there is no question of 80% recovery. The figure will probably be a lot less. Nerve excitability tests can tell us after 1 week what the prognosis will be. We also know that when the facial nerve can be stimulated to function at its exit from the stylomastoid foramen, every lesion proximal to the foramen is nondegenerative or only slightly so. Collier[1] and Richardson and Wynn Parry[22] demonstrated that if normal conduction is maintained for 3 days after onset of paralysis, the prognosis is good, and if it is for more than a week, the prognosis is excellent, with expected recovery. Laumans[18] has stated that a difference in excitability needing more than 3.5 milliamperes of stimulating current between the normal and affected sides may be the indication for surgery.

Further serial tests may show changes for the worse after the first 2 weeks, which could then make consideration of decompression necessary. One of the great problems in getting the best time to intervene with surgery lies in the fact that we see only a few of the patients shortly after the onset of paralysis. They see the doctor who tells them to do nothing more since 80% get better by themselves. Bell's palsy should be treated and considered as an emergency and hospitalized on the same day so that discriminating tests can be started at once. In this way proper surgical data can be accumulated and really evaluated in its true light. In selected cases under conservative treatment, nearly 100% of results are unsatisfactory. The method that will probably yield the greatest amount of discrimination would involve the use of nerve excitability measurements and electromyography in the early stages after onset, followed in later stages by intensity and duration curves and further electromyography. This must be done in a large group of patients so that we may not only judge the surgical results but also the conservative treatment, which has claimed large percentages of cures that might not have been so.

Value of galvanic muscle stimulation immediately after paresis

The importance of galvanic stimulation in maintaining the nutrition of a muscle deprived of its nervous influence was first reported by Reid[21] in 1841, who then proceeded to use galvanism in certain cases of paralysis. By World War I many patients with denervated muscles were being treated with electricity and were under close scrutiny because its value was seriously challenged for the first time.

Langley and Kato[15] (1915) concluded that electrical stimulation had no effect on muscles that had been denervated experimentally. Their findings caused them to conclude that the atrophy that developed in denervated muscle was a fatigue phenomenon caused by the fibrillation that follows denervation. The question was raised as to whether further activity caused by electrical stimulation would be beneficial or harmful. Langley and Hashimoto[16] (1918) claimed that there were too many variables present to permit accurate evaluation of the effect of electrical stimulation. Hartman and Blatz[7] (1920) concluded that neither massage nor galvanic electrostimulation were beneficial to denervated muscle.

Roberts[23] (1916) reported favorably on the beneficial effects of electrostimulation in the treatment of nerve injuries from World War I. In 1918 there was a symposium on the subject that produced many arguments pro and con. Conflicting views were presented, and even those investigators who were in favor of using electrotherapy disagreed with each other as to the type of current to be used, when treatment should be started, and for how long it should be continued. After the end of World War I electrotherapy came into favor again, mainly because it was believed that it was a harmless procedure and therefore no patient should be deprived of the possible benefits that might be derived from its application.

World War II started the dilemma again. At that period in time with a new crop of severe war injuries involving muscle and nerve, all the old controversies were rekindled and the conflicting attitudes returned once again. Electrotherapy was now, once more, an open question. Many claimed that the treatments were uncomfortable, time consuming and inconvenient for the patient, as well as expensive to employ in terms of time and personnel involved. These controversies started a series of experiments by an impressive array of scientists who showed that under certain conditions, galvanic treatment of denervated muscle slows and diminishes the atrophy of individual muscle fibers and keeps fibrosis to a minimum. It was also claimed that more recovery was present in the treated muscles than in those that were untreated. Names such as Solandt and Magladery,[24] Eccles,[2] Gutmann,[6] and Hines and Wehrmacher[8] were involved in studying all phases of the therapy.

In the experimental studies of those who had claimed that electrical stimulation had no benefit, review of the studies seemed to indicate that treatment was inadequate and was applied under conditions that were complicated by skeletal immobilization which in itself can produce atrophy.[14] Pollock et al.[20] (1951) concluded that electrotherapy produced bad effects in the form of contractures in antagonist muscles. They reported that greater contractures in greater severity occurred in the antagonist gastrocnemius muscle when an extremity, after peroneal nerve section and suture, was treated by electrical stimuli. This was also found in an experiment upon the sciatic nerve.

Clinically, Jackson,[12] as well as Jackson and Seddon,[11] showed that the volume of the hand in ulnar nerve paralysis was better maintained when the affected muscles received regular galvanic stimulation, which also reduced the time between the reappearance of motor unit activity and the onset of voluntary contractions as evaluated by electromyographic studies. More recent studies have taken most of these factors into consideration, and although many factors involved have as yet been unexplained, much progress has been made toward resolving many of the outstanding questions. Electrotherapy could produce beneficial effects in a combination of three ways. The first is by retardation of the rate and influencing of the nature of muscle fiber atrophy. The second might be by shortening of the time interval between injury and onset of recovery. The third may be reflected by reduction of the period required to restore muscles to full power after reinnervation. Despite individual variations in the rate and extent of muscle wasting, there is now good evidence that electrical stimulation retards and diminishes the progress of muscle fiber atrophy so that less atrophied muscle fibers await innervation than would otherwise be the case.[9]

It has been clearly shown that electrical stimulation has no effect on the regeneration of axons and the connections that they have established with denervated muscle. However, Gutmann and Gutmann[4,5] reported a higher degree of recovery in treated muscles in their experimental studies.

There are numerous factors to be considered in order to properly apply electrotherapy so that as much as possible can be gained from its exhibition. The strength of the stimulus is exceedingly important since weak stimuli cause only feeble contractions and are ineffective in retarding atrophy. Strong contractions, on the other hand can easily fatigue atrophied or denervated muscle, and this may be a bad effect. The particular muscles that require to be treated predispose to success or failure, in that those more superficial and readily accessible have the best opportunity to heal. Muscles that are difficult to reach cannot have the proper stimulation applied. Another important factor is the size of the muscle, since smaller muscles respond better to treatment than do massive antigravity muscles. The effectiveness of electrotherapy is proportional to the frequency of treatment; thus treatment given two times daily is more effective than that given once a day, which, in turn, is better than once every 3 or 4 days. The duration of each treatment is also important, and it must be judged on the basis of the patient's general condition, muscular status, and degree of atrophy. Gutmann and Gutmann[4,5] believe that galvanic exercise improves metabolic conditions in the denervated muscles though how this is achieved is unknown. They suggest that it might be ascribed to beneficial effects on the circulation, on the grounds that muscle activity increases circulation and that electrotherapy is less effective when there is an associated injury to a major blood vessel. Ziemssen[27] in 1885 reported that circulation through the denervated muscles is increased during and after galvanic stimulation. Electrical stimulation, in addition to retarding weight loss in denervated muscle, is said to slow the deterioration of muscle protein.[3] Hines and Wertheimer[8] reported in 1944 that electrical stimulation reduces the loss of glycogen and retards the reduction in adenosine triphosphatase, which is associated with denervation activity. All patients do not have the conditions required for beneficial effects from electrotherapy. Treatment therefore must be modified and tailored to meet the particular needs of each individual patient. Some investigators believe that electrical stimulation has little effect if applied after the onset of motor recovery. They believe that nothing is to be gained by continuing the electrical treatment beyond this point, since at this stage the patient can help himself by exercising. Gutmann and Gutmann[4,5] claim that galvanic exercise accelerated the return of the volume of the muscle to its predenervated state and that stimulation in the later stages of recovery was still effective in improving the quality of muscle function though the effects were greatly reduced. For this reason they advocated continuation of electrical treatment until motor recovery was well advanced.

Conclusion

Let us sum up the facts discussed above with the following four statements: (1) Electrical stimulation has no effect on axon growth; it therefore does not speed up the onset of recovery. (2) Electrical stimulation retards the denervation atrophy of striated muscle. Therefore it has value in maintaining denervated muscles in satisfactory condition of volume and tone until reinnervation commences. (3) The effectiveness of electrical stimulation in retarding denervation and atrophy depends on such factors as strength of the stimulus, site and size of the muscle, the frequency and duration of each treatment, and the state of the denervated muscle. (4) After the onset of motor recovery active exercise by voluntary effort is more effective than contractions induced electrically. However, if exercise is not visible, it might be wise to continue with electrical stimulation until clinical observation of improvement and exercise is seen.

REFERENCES

1. Collier, J.: Proc. Roy. Soc. Med. **48:**253, 1955.
2. Eccles, J. C.: Disuse atrophy of skeletal muscle, Med. J. Aust. **11:**160, 1941.
3. Fischer, E., and Ramsey, V. W.: The effect of daily electrical stimulation of normal and denervated muscles upon their protein content and upon some of the physiochemical properties of the protein, Am. J. Physiol. **145:**583, 1946.
4. Gutmann, E., and Guttmann, L.: Effect of electrotherapy on denervated muscles in rabbits, Lancet **1:**169, 1942.
5. Gutmann, E., and Guttmann, L.: The effect of galvanic exercise on denervated and reinnervated muscles in the rabbit, J. Neurol. Neurosurg. Psychiatry **7:**7, 1944.
6. Gutmann, E.: Metabolic reactability of the denervated muscle. In Gutmann, E., editor: The denervated muscle, Prague, 1962, Publishing House of the Czechoslovak Academy of Sciences, chap. 11.
7. Hartman, F. A., and Blatz, W. E.: Studies in the regeneration of denervated mammalian muscle. Effects of massage and electrical treatment, J. Physiol. (London) **53:**290, 1920.
8. Hines, H. M., and Wehrmacher, W. H.: Physiologic factors involved in atrophy and regeneration of skeletal muscle, J. Iowa State Med. Soc. **34:**142, 1944.
9. Hoffman, A., and Wertheimer, E.: Stoffwechselregulationen; Glykogenansatz beim kunstlich gereizten entnervten Muskel, Pfluegers Arch. Gesam. Physiol. **216:**337, 1927.
10. Hines, H. W., Melville, E., and Wehrmacher, W. H.: The effect of electrical stimulation on neuromuscular regeneration, Am. J. Physiol. **144:**278, 1945.
11. Jackson, E. C. S., and Seddon, H. J.: Influence of galvanic stimulation on muscle atrophy resulting from denervation, Br. Med. J. **2:**485, 1945.
12. Jackson, S.: The role of galvanism in the treatment of denervated voluntary muscle in man, Brain **68:**300, 1945.
13. Janssen, F. P.: Ober de postoperatieve facialisverlamming, thesis, Amsterdam, 1963.
14. Jonkees, L. B. W.: Arch. Otolaryngol. **81:**497, May 1965.
15. Langley, J. N., and Kato, T.: The rate of loss of weight in skeletal muscle after nerve section with some observations on the effect of stimulation and other treatment, J. Physiol. (London) **49:**432, 1915.
16. Langley, J. N., and Hashimoto, M.: Observations on the atrophy of denervated muscles: J. Physiol. (London) **52:**15, 1918.
17. Laumans, E. P. J.: On the prognosis of peripheral facial paralysis of endotemporal origin, thesis, Amsterdam, 1962.
18. Laumans, E. P. J.: Arch. Otolaryngol. **81:**478, May 1965.
19. Molander, C. O., and Steinitz, F. S.: Effect of galvanic current on paralyzed muscle: experimental study on dog, Arch. Physiol. Ther. **22:**154, 1941.
20. Pollock, L. J., et al.: Electrotherapy in experimentally produced lesions of peripheral nerves, Arch. Physiol. Med. **32:**377, 1951.
21. Reid, J.: On the relation between muscular contractility and the nervous system, London Edinburgh Monthly Journal of Medical Science **1:**320, 1841.
22. Richardson, A. T., and Wynn Parry, C. B.: Theory and practice of electrodiagnosis, Ann. Phys. Med. **4:**41, Feb.-May 1957.
23. Roberts, F.: Degeneration of muscle following nerve injury, Brain **39:**297, 1916.
24. Solandt, D. Y., and Magladery, J. W.: The relation of atrophy to fibrillation in denervated muscle, Brain **63:**255, 1940.
25. Taverner, D.: Lancet **2:**1052, 1954.
26. Verjaal, A.: Ned. Tijdschr. Geneeskd. **98:**671, 1954.
27. Ziemssen, H. W. von: Die Elektrizitaet in der Medicin, ed. 4, part II: Diagnostisch-therapeutischer Theil, Berlin, 1885.

18 Medical treatment for Bell's palsy

SYDNEY LOUIS

Approximately three fourths of all patients afflicted with Bell's palsy, treated or untreated, recover completely; the remainder have some residual defect of function. Corticosteroids seem to be of some limited value. No large controlled series of cases have shown any one treatment to be of great value.

Any claims for successful therapy of Bell's palsy need to be viewed against the background of the natural history of the disorder. It is clear from many sources that the majority of patients with Bell's palsy, treated or untreated, recover in periods of weeks to a few months. Generally quoted figures are that two thirds to three fourths recover completely, with the remainder having some residual defect of function, either paralysis, contracture, or involuntary movements. The data on natural history become still more vague because in most series, many of the patients have been subjected to multiple different therapies, each unproved or controversial.

Generally, it is clear that recovery occurs in 80% to 90% of patients, so far as the patient or a casual observer is concerned. Depending on the care with which patients are examined, subtle residual abnormalities, including mild synkinesis, may be seen in as many as 76% of patients. Although not absolute, one may say that improvement is more probable in younger than in older patients, in those in whom weakness is incomplete or partial, and in those in whom neither salivation nor taste defect nor hyperacusis are present. Early commencement of recovery also correlates better with a more favorable outlook for complete recovery. The amount, severity, and distribution of pain seems to bear little relationship to the outlook. Other prognostic indicators are related to electrodiagnostic studies and are dealt with elsewhere in this volume.

A further point needs to be stressed, before treatment is to be considered. Andrashke and Frick,[2] among others, have reported that 90% of patients with incomplete paresis, recovered fully, whereas only 25% of those with complete paralysis cleared completely. This means that any small series is inevitably biased, and this may explain much of the conflicting data in the literature.

Following are the general and specific therapies that have been suggested:
1. *General therapy*
    a. Reassurance and discussion of the illness

  b. Care for the affected eye
  c. Splinting, massage, and exercises
  d. Electrical stimulation
 2. *Specific therapy*
  a. Steroids
  b. Antihistamines and cervical sympathectomy
  c. Dehydrating agents

General therapy

Discussion with the patient. It is clearly of the utmost importance that the patient be reassured as to the benign nature of the condition. Bell's palsy occurs in patients of all ages and for many is the first occurrence of a neurological defect. It gives rise in many circumstances to great panic and the assumption of a "stroke" by the patients and their families. Reassurance and explanation of the benign nonprogressive nature of the disorder, as well as acquainting the patient with the probability of complete recovery, are critical.

Care for the affected eye. Because the eyelid on the affected side may not close and blinking is suppressed, one must exercise care in protecting the cornea from foreign bodies or from drying. This involves alerting the patient to the possibility of injury to the eye when outdoors. The patient should always wear either an eye shield or glasses to prevent foreign objects from entering the eye whenever he or she is outdoors or in a windy environment. Frequent use of artificial tears in the form of eye drops is recommended.

Splinting, massage, and exercises. Massage has been recommended along with exercises in front of the mirror to try to speed up the recovery process. No good evidence has been presented to show that this makes any great difference to the rate or degree of recovery. It may be of some value in the patient who is already recovering and who exercises to strengthen the muscles. It has been held that, in patients who are not recovering rapidly after the first few weeks of complete paralysis, the face should be splinted, and particularly the corner of the mouth should be elevated toward the ear to prevent traction injury to the muscles. There is again no convincing evidence that this is beneficial. Most of these patients will develop facial contracture on that side, whether splinted or not.

Electrical stimulation. The value of this procedure is based upon some studies done in 1944 on rabbit muscle. On the basis of this data electrical stimulation to facial muscles is recommended in those patients who show no restoration of function after the third or fourth week. The large study of Parke and Watkins[7] in 1949 and that of Mosforth and Taverner[6] in 1958 both found it to be ineffective in changing the course of Bell's palsy.

Specific therapy

Many European authorities tend to be more aggressive in their attitude to the treatment of facial palsy and to the use of drugs, in combination. In the United States, on the other hand, conservative therapy has largely related to the use of steroids. The European use of drugs is based upon pathophysiological considerations; thus in the early stages an effort is made to reduce edema through the use of low molecular weight dextrans and other dehydrating agents (such as urea); steroids are recommended in large dosages as well as ergotamines (such as the mixture called Hydergine) for their sympatholytic functions. After the fifth day of the illness the regime is supplemented with vasodilators such as nicotinic acid or histamine to offset any ischemia. Regimes such as these are dictated by the clinical experience of these authors, for there is little data to support either the supposed pathophysiologic mechanisms or the efficacy of these therapies against such mechanisms.

The data in favor of stellate block, ergotamine preparations, procaine infusions, or dehydrating agents are certainly not impressive enough to justify their risks in what is essentially a benign disorder. The study of Kime[5] demonstrated an impressive recovery rate with the use of nicotinic acid, but it was uncontrolled, as were similar supporting studies.

Corticosteroids, on the other hand, appear to have been universally accepted and have been subjected to several major studies. Unfortunately the definitive controlled study has yet to be performed. Taverner and co-workers' study[8] compares prednisone against a controlled group receiving corticotrophin. Adour and associates[1] failed to complete a controlled trial because the treated patients were easily identified by being rendered free of pain within the first few hours of the study. They abandoned their control group and treated all patients, comparing them to a previously seen, untreated group. They noted benefit in the treated group who had received prednisone 40 mg per day for 4 days, tapered over an additional 4 days. The benefits of such steroid usage appeared to be a more rapid recovery, in a somewhat shortened time, for a larger proportion of patients. Adour and his group suggested that when steroid treatment was not contraindicated, all patients with Bell's palsy should receive a short course of 60 mg of prednisone daily for 4 days, tapered over an additional 6 days. I do not believe that a conclusive case has been proved for the universal administration of corticosteroids in Bell's palsy.

The medical therapy of Bell's palsy, therefore, is largely symptomatic and depends, in the main, upon the favorable natural history of the disorder in the majority of patients.

REFERENCES

1. Adour, K. K., Wingerd, J., Bell, D. N., Manning, J. J., and Hurley, J. P.: Prednisone treatment for idiopathic facial paralysis (Bell's palsy), N. Engl. J. Med. **287:**1268, 1972.
2. Andrashke, H., and Frick, E.: Idiopathische Fazialis-parese, Prognose and Therapie, Munch. Med. Wochensch. **109:**1650, 1967.
3. Hanser, W. A., Karnes, W. E., Annis, J., and Kurland, L. T.: Incidence and prognosis of Bell's palsy in the population of Rochester, Minnesota, Mayo Clin. Proc. **46:**258, 1971.
4. Karnes, W. E.: Diseases of the seventh cranial nerves. In Dyck, P. J., Thomas, P. K., and Lambert, E. H., 1975, editors: Peripheral neuropathy; Philadelphia, W. B. Saunders Co., vol. 1, p. 570.
5. Kime, C. E.: Bell's palsy: a new syndrome associated with treatment by nicotinic acid: a guide to adequate medical management, Arch. Otolaryngol. **68:**28, 1958.
6. Mosforth, J., and Taverner, D.: Physiotherapy for Bell's palsy, Br. Med. J. **2:**675, 1958.
7. Park, H. W., and Watkins, A. L.: Facial paralysis: analysis of 500 cases, Arch. Phys. Med. **30:**749, 1949.
8. Taverner, D., Cohen, S. B., and Hutchinson, B. C.: Comparison of corticotrophin and prednisolone in treatment of idiopathic facial paralysis (Bell's palsy), Br. Med. J. **4:**20, 1971.
9. Zülch, K. J.: Idiopathic facial paresis. In Vinken, P. J., and Bruyn, G. W., editors: Handbook of clinical neurology, Amsterdam, 1970, North-Holland Publishing Co., vol. 8, p. 205.

19 Present-day concepts of surgical treatment for Bell's palsy

BLOYCE HILL BRITTON

Surgery is only necessary in a small percentage of total Bell's palsy cases; however, it is in these cases that considerable controversy remains. A well-controlled series of surgery versus nonsurgery in Bell's palsy is sorely needed. The principle of surgical intervention is to allow the edematous facial nerve to expand from its constricted temporal canal. Several techniques are described.

Present-day concepts of surgical treatment for Bell's palsy

Very few benign maladies cause as much distress and concern in a patient's mind as facial paralysis. Indeed the same concern is manifested by the physician called upon to evaluate and advise such a patient. The discussion in this chapter deals with current surgical concepts in the management of idiopathic peripheral facial paralysis (Bell's palsy) but is limited to those cases manifesting complete or total paralysis. It is well known that those with partial or incomplete paralysis of the Bell's type will all regain normal or near normal facial function with or without therapy. Today it is commonly accepted that Bell's palsy is a diagnosis of exclusion, whereby all known causes of peripheral facial paralysis are ruled out before this diagnosis is made.

Thoughts of surgical treatment in this condition date back to 1932 when Balance and Duel[2] discussed the theories and possibilities of surgical procedures upon the facial nerve. Refinements in surgical approaches and techniques since that time allow total exploration and exposure of the facial nerve from its brainstem origin into the parotid gland.[6] Many otologists today believe that there are certain indications for surgical decompression of the facial nerve in selected cases of Bell's palsy and that there are benefits from the surgery.

Many forms of medical treatment have been advised in the past including the use of galvanic stimulation, vasodilation medications, and sympathetic block. Recently there has been a large treatment series reported that seems to show the efficacy of corticosteroid treatment of this condition.[1] There has also been a recent report of a well-controlled series refuting any advantage to treatment with corticosteroids.[7] Unfortunately at the time of this writing, there is no reported controlled series relating surgical to nonsurgical treatment. This most certainly will need to be done before a definitive answer can be given on this topic.

Rationale of surgical management

The basic purpose of surgical decompression of the facial nerve is to regain maximum return of function and to avoid or minimize complications of degeneration and regeneration such as synkinesis, contractures, twitching, and crocodile tears. This, of course, is the basic purpose of medical or surgical treatment. The basic premise of surgical decompression is based upon release of pressure within the facial canal ascribed to primary or secondary ischemia of the facial nerve with associated edema.

To analyze this situation, however, we must ask ourselves several questions. How many patients with this condition obtain satisfactory recovery? At this point we are faced with the dilemma of how return of function is reported in the literature. Terms such as good, fair, poor, patient satisfied, patient unhappy, etc. have been utilized. Some very complicated percentage scales have been developed, unfortunately all different. The one recovery state that there is no question about is total or complete recovery without residua. The majority of studies that have been reported indicate highly variable figures. Hauser[4] in 1971 reported 24% recovered normal function. Taverner[10] in 1968 reported a 60% normal recovery rate. Peitersen and Anderson[8] in 1967 showed an 81% normal recovery. Generally, the degree of return of function, the rapidity of return of function, and presence or absence of late complications are felt to be related to whether there has been a physiologic block to nerve function (neurapraxia) or whether there has been partial or total denervation (axonotmesis). Any form of treatment, therefore, is directed at improving the prognosis of those patients who will not get complete return. These are the patients who will not obtain a satisfactory return of function without treatment and are in general the same group of patients for which surgical therapy may be considered.

Are there any methods of determining prognosis in the individual patient? This question is extremely critical. The important time period for this assessment is within the first 2 to 3 weeks. At this point I would like to exclude those patients who demonstrate clinical evidence of return of function within the first 2 to 3 weeks, that is, visible return of motion or muscle tone. These patients usually will go on to obtain a quite satisfactory recovery of function. However, within the first 2 to 3 weeks there is a group of patients who will not show clinical evidence of return and will not go on to total recovery. It is in this group that the use of electrical testing has been of help. Electromyographic examination has not been helpful as an early prognostic indicator since typically the changes seen on the study are 10 to 14 days after changes have already occurred within the nerve itself. The earliest electrical indication of partial denervation or total denervation is the facial nerve excitability test.[5] This is the most common test used today. The degree of denervation demonstrated with this test is fairly well correlated with the degree of functional return and the presence or absence of complications. With this test percutaneous stimulation using a negative square wave is applied to the normal and abnormal facial nerve. This stimulus measures 600 microseconds of duration with 6 pulses per second. The current intensity (milliamperes) is increased to the point where visible muscular contraction of the facial muscles is noted. This electrical test show changes that have occurred 2 to 3 days prior to the test. In other words, if the facial nerve is totally severed, then the first indication of denervation may be detected 2 to 3 days later. It is believed that a difference between the normal and abnormal stimulus values of 2.5 milliamperes or greater is an indication of partial denervation. Total loss of ability to stimulate the involved nerve is considered evidence of denervation, total or near total. The common method of testing is to sequentially test the patient with the facial nerve stimulation test on a daily basis until clinical evidence of functional return is noted. If over the span of testing partial denervation or total denervation is detected, it is believed that these are the cases with the poorest outlook for spontaneous recovery and are considered to be the most likely candidates for surgical decompression.

In these selected cases, does surgical treatment have a place? The answer to this question has many facets. First, in the hands of an experienced otologic surgeon, there should be extremely little risk to the patient in regard to impairment of his middle or inner ear function, or further damage to the facial nerve by facial nerve decompression surgery. This has been well documented in the past. Second, even though the facial nerve excitability test is considered to be 2 to 3 days late in its information, we cannot accept this test without reservation. This test does not indicate an all-or-none status of the facial nerve fibers. The controversy here has been that if there is partial denervation or total denervation, surgery cannot reverse denervation. There have, however, been cases reported[9] and numerous cases unreported where the facial nerve excitability test showed severe or total denervation and yet the patient with surgery noted immediate partial return of function or return of function within a short period of time inconsistent with degeneration and regeneration time intervals. This must mean that in these cases the electrical test was not truly reflecting severe degeneration of all the nerve fibers. Another surgical finding seen by all surgeons performing facial nerve surgery is the noticeable edema of certain segments of the facial nerve when the nerve is decompressed and the sheath is opened. Many times this edema can produce visible enlargement of a segment of the facial nerve to two or three times the normal diameter. A nerve normally will show some bulging through the sheath whenever the sheath is incised; however, the swelling previously described is most certainly more than seen with a normal nerve. This fact has been clinically verified by incision or removal of the sheath from the facial nerve in other conditions in the ear.

In summary, the patient with a total Bell's palsy is observed closely for clinical evidence of return of movement or muscle tone. Simultaneously a series of electrical tests, performed with the facial nerve excitability test, are done up to the time of clinical evidence of return of function. If before the patient shows evidence of clinical return of function, the facial nerve excitability values change to a difference of 2.5 milliamperes or more compared to the normal side then this patient is suspected of having partial denervation and is considered a surgical candidate. The same holds true if the patient suddenly loses all facial nerve excitability response. These are the cases that have the poorest prognosis, and these are the cases that are advised to have facial nerve decompression.

The single most important topognostic or localizing study that can be done concerning the facial nerve is the test of reflex tearing (Schirmer's test).[3] This determination localizes the area of the disorder to the infrageniculate or suprageniculate areas. This is quite important in order to determine the extent of surgical exposure if surgery is indicated. A significant decrease in reflex tear production is considered indicative of suprageniculate involvement of the facial nerve. It is in these cases, therefore, that the facial nerve is exposed from its exit point in the internal auditory canal to its exit point distally at the stylomastoid foramen. If the patient, however, has normal reflex tearing, then the disorder is localized to the segments of the facial nerve distal to the geniculate ganglion.

Surgical approaches and technique in facial nerve decompression
TRANSMASTOID APPROACH

The transmastoid approach is the most commonly used approach to identify and decompress the horizontal (tympanic) and vertical (mastoid) segments of the facial nerve. This approach allows decompression of the facial nerve from an area immediately distal to the geniculate ganglion through the stylomastoid foramen ordinarily without the need for disruption of the middle ear ossicles. The posterior bony canal wall is preserved in this approach, and the tympanic membrane remains intact throughout the procedure. The technical points in this procedure can be enumerated as follows:

1. The mastoid cortex is exposed through a full postauricular incision.
2. A complete mastoidectomy is then performed by use of constant suction irrigation and multiple cutting and diamond burrs. Particular attention is placed on obtaining adequate bone removal posteriorly over the sigmoid sinus so that the operator can obtain a proper anteroposterior plane of view to see the horizontal segment of the facial nerve through the facial recess and posterior epitympanum. The posterior and midepitympanum is opened as wide as possible in order to gain direct view of the horizontal segment of the facial nerve from above and posterior. Often one is able to see anterior to the malleus head once this attic bone has been removed. Particular care, of course, must be taken not to contact the malleus or incus heads with the burrs.
3. The facial recess area is opened widely so that the surgeon can see the long process of the incus and the stapes, and again the horizontal segment of the facial nerve from another angle.
4. The bone overlying the vertical or descending portion of the facial nerve is then carefully removed until a thin eggshell thickness of bone remains over the nerve. In the vertical segment, this bone removal encompasses approximately 40% to 50% of the diameter of the nerve. This exposure is carried through the bone of the stylomastoid foramen.
5. A small angulated instrument is then used to remove the remaining bone overlying the nerve. Ordinarily it is not necessary to drill away any bone over the horizontal portion of the facial nerve. Anatomically this bone is quite thin and can be removed with various straight and angulated instruments working through the facial recess and through the medial aspect of the posterior epitympanum underneath the heads of the malleus and incus. In the horizontal segment, approximately 30% of this surrounding bone is removed. Bone removal in the horizontal segment continues past the cochleariform process to a point immediately distal to the geniculate ganglion.
6. This is the point where some surgeons terminate the procedure. Other surgeons at this point use an extremely sharp microknife to longitudinally incise the facial nerve sheath in all the areas of exposure. Most commonly there is edema involving the entire course of the nerve in Bell's palsy. The most prominent edema seems to be in the vertical segment; however, at times, it may be most prominently noted in the horizontal segment.

COMBINED MIDDLE FOSSA–TRANSMASTOID APPROACH

This combined middle fossa–transmastoid approach is used if there is evidence of a significant reduction of tearing on the involved side indicating suprageniculate involvement of the facial nerve. The initial steps are exactly as outlined in the transmastoid procedure with the exception that a small opening is placed through the bone overlying the anterior epitympanum. This opening is quite helpful as it gives one an immediate landmark for identification during the second portion of the procedure from the middle fossa approach. Following are the important technical points with the addition of the middle fossa approach:

1. A curvilinear incision is made starting in the preauricular area above the zygoma and curving superiorly and posteriorly. This incision is carried through the temporalis muscle and fascia, with care being taken to ligate the temporal artery.
2. A rather square-shaped bone flap of approximately 8 × 10 cm. in dimension is then outlined. This is done with constant suction irrigation and multiple cutting and diamond burrs, with care being taken not to injure the underlying dura.
3. The bone flap is then removed and saved, and the middle fossa dura is carefully elevated from the floor of the middle fossa. A self-retaining middle fossa retractor is then inserted and the dura further retracted and held in place.
4. The small opening in the tegmen that has been created from the transmastoid approach is then identified. This lies immediately posterior to the area of the geniculate ganglion and the greater superficial petrosal nerve. Bone overlying the greater superficial petrosal nerve and the geniculate ganglion is removed, and the facial nerve is traced into the internal auditory canal (the labyrinthine segment). It is at this point again that some surgeons will split the sheath of the facial nerve or leave the sheath intact.
5. The middle fossa retractor is then removed and the dura is allowed to expand. The bone flap is replaced and the skin incision is closed with subcutaneous and skin sutures.

The surgical morbidity associated with either the transmastoid or the combined transmastoid and middle fossa approach is minimal. Possible complications include cerebrospinal-fluid otorrhea or infection. Both of these complications are unusual. A possible complication is hearing loss either of a sensorineural type or possibly a conductive type if the middle ear ossicles have been partially dislocated during the procedure. This complication again, however, is seldom seen.

Summary

The brief review of the surgical treatment of Bell's palsy as it is currently practiced today has been presented. Fortunately, surgery is only necessary in a small percentage of total Bell's palsy cases; however, it is in these cases that considerable controversy remains. The basic aim of surgery is twofold: (1) to prevent further progressive degenerative involvement of additional nerve fibers within the facial nerve and (2) perhaps to create a better milieu for regeneration of fibers that have already gone on to degeneration. If these aims are accomplished, they offer the patient the most rapid and complete return of function possible with a minimum of complications from the paralysis. There seems little question that a well-controlled series of surgery versus nonsurgery in Bell's palsy is sorely needed. Until that time however, many otologists believe that surgery has a definite place in the management of certain selected cases of Bell's palsy.

REFERENCES

1. Adour, K. K., Wingerd, J., Bell, D. N., Manning, J. J., and Hurley, J. P.: Prednisone treatment for idiopathic facial paralysis (Bell's palsy), N. Engl. J. Med. **287**:1268, 1972.
2. Balance, C., and Duel, A. B.: The operative treatment of facial palsy by the introduction of nerve grafts into the fallopian canal and by other intratemporal methods, Arch. Otolaryngol. **15**:1, 1932.

3. Britton, B. H.: Surgery in Bell's palsy, Otolaryngol. Clin. North Am. **7:**511, 1974.
4. Hauser, W. A., et al.: Incidence and prognosis of Bell's palsy in the population of Rochester, Minnesota, Mayo Clin. Proc. **46:**258, 1971.
5. Hilger, J. A.: Facial nerve stimulator, Trans. Am. Acad. Ophthalmol. Otolaryngol. **68:**74, 1964.
6. House, W. F., and Crabtree, J. A.: Surgical exposure of petrous portion of seventh nerve, Arch. Otolaryngol. **81:**506, 1965.
7. May, M., Wette, R., and Sullivan, J.: The use of steroids in Bell's palsy: a prospective controlled study, Laryngoscope **86:**1111, 1976.
8. Peitersen, E., and Andersen, P.: Spontaneous course of 220 peripheral non-traumatic facial palsies, Acta Otolaryngol. Suppl. **224:**296, 1967.
9. Sheehy, J. L.: Facial nerve decompression, two interesting cases, Arch. Otolaryngol. **87:**39, 1968.
10. Taverner, D.: The management of facial palsy, Br. J. Laryngol. Otol. **82:**585, 1968.

20 Nerve grafting by microscope in the cranium

LEONARD MALIS

The facial nerve is severed or destroyed in 20% of microsurgically totally removed acoustic neuromas. Some seventh nerve ends in the area can be sutured end to end, whereas others require bridging grafts, with a sural nerve being used. It takes about 2 years after suturing for the face to function. The results show that facial function is better than 50% in all patients and eventually clearly superior to the results of the spinofacial or hypoglossal facial anastomosis.

The facial nerve has been severed or destroyed in 20% of our microsurgically totally removed acoustic neuromas. The causes of the destruction have been discussed in Chapter 6. In a few cases, the nerve was lost directly at the brainstem with no proximal fibers being left for any intracranial anastomosis. In a number of other cases, the nerve has been lost distally in the internal auditory canal or even in the facial canal. The rest of the sacrificed facial nerves have been cut in the area where they traverse the cerebellopontine angle, most often either at the apex of the anterior part of the tumor where the nerve often is thinned to an almost membranous layer or directly at the anterior edge of the internal auditory meatus where the nerve, tightly pressed against the petrous pyramid dura by the tumor, makes a sharp angulation into the internal auditory meatus. The facial nerve may be thinned out and adherent at that point so that even under magnification I have been unable to free it. Additional patients after having what has been otherwise a clean removal have demonstrated wide separation of facial nerve fibrils with tumor between them, which would guarantee a recurrence of the tumor if this portion is left in place. After prolonged intrafascicular dissection some of these nerves have been destroyed and others have been deliberately cut in order to remove what appeared to be a significant amount of tumor tissue infiltrating the facial fibers.

Generally, when the nerve has been destroyed at the apex of its curve, the amount of increased length produced by the long stretch of time of these larger tumors leaves sufficient redundancy to permit end-to-end anastomosis. Unfortunately, the oppor-

Reanimation of the paralyzed face

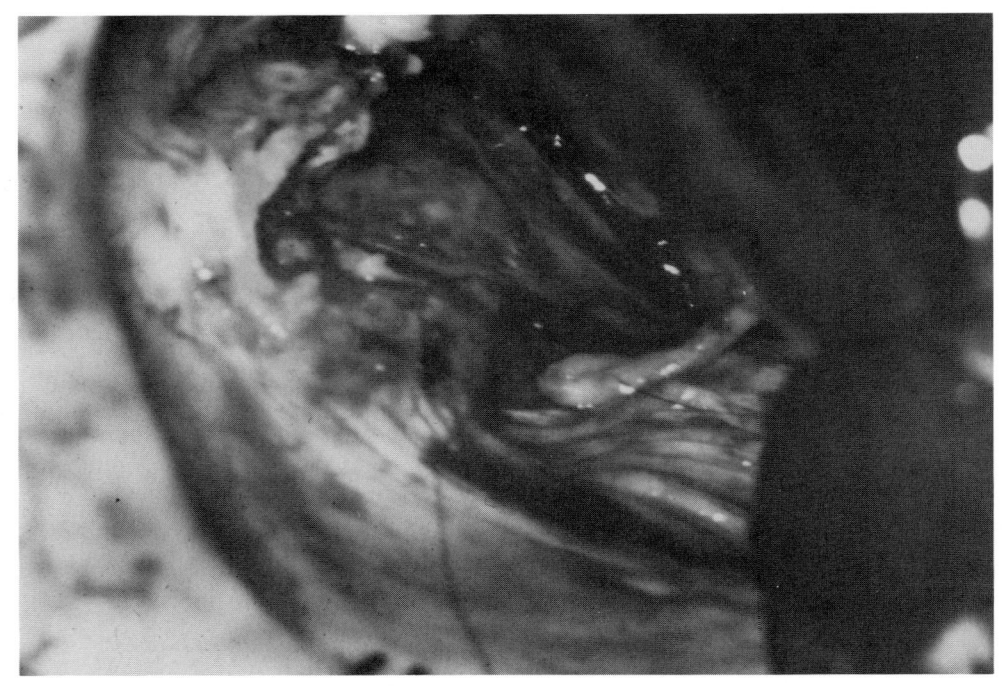

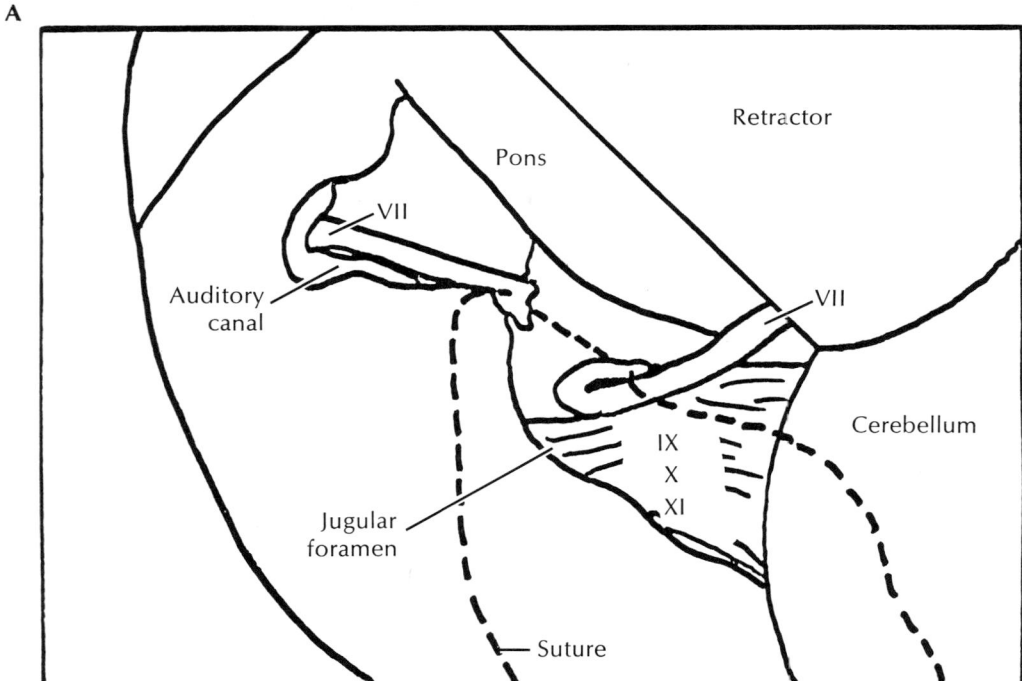

Fig. 20-1. A, Left retrolabyrinthine suboccipital craniectomy. A 4 cm acoustic neuroma has been removed, including the drilling out of posterior wall of internal auditory canal. Facial nerve was cut just medial to anterior rim of meatus. Proximal end of facial nerve that had been tremendously stretched by tumor has been trimmed, and a 10-0 monofilament suture has been passed through the cut ends of proximal and distal portions of nerve.

Nerve grafting by microscope in the cranium

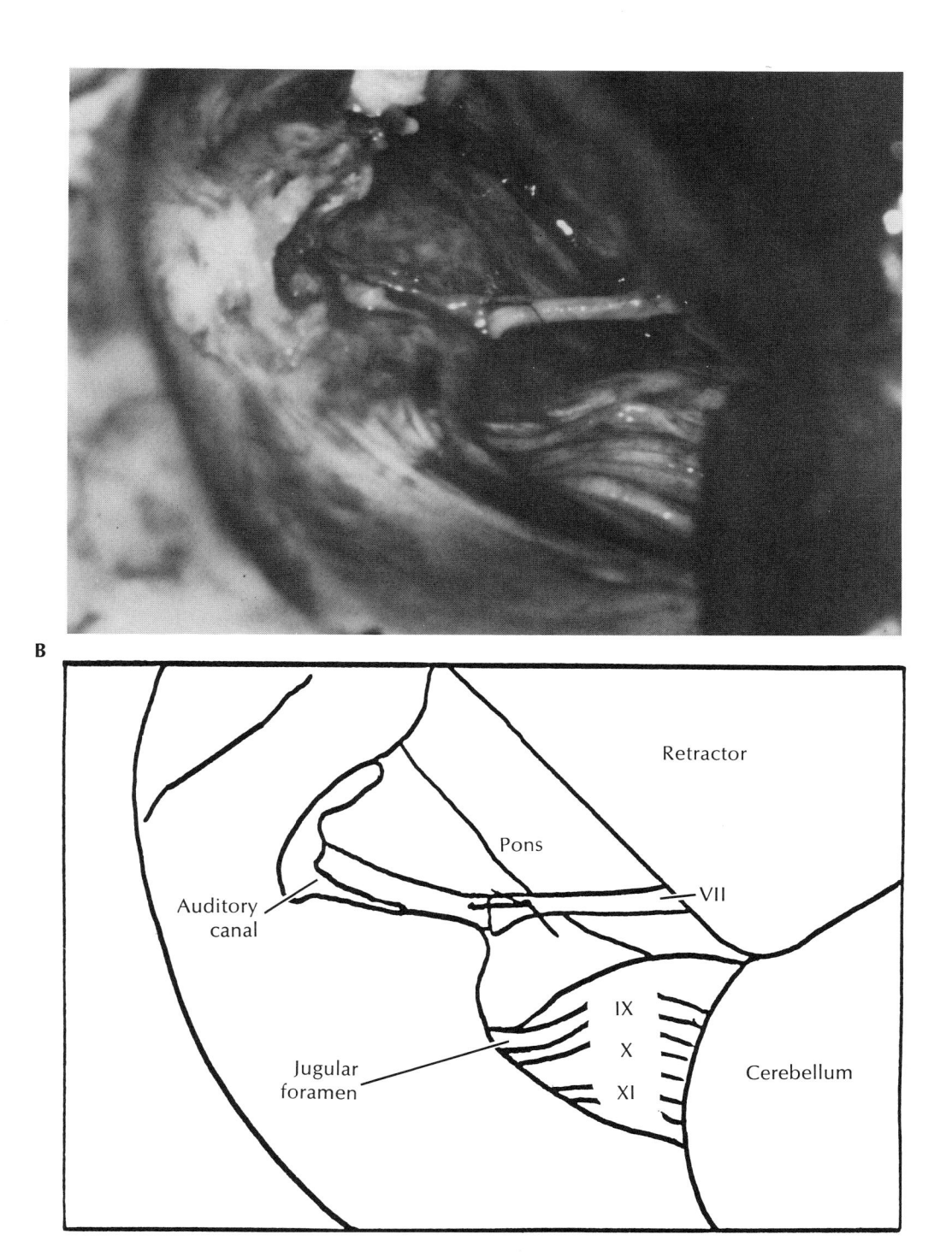

Fig. 20-1, cont'd. B, Same case as that in **A.** Left retrolabyrinthine suboccipital craniectomy. Facial nerve ends had been approximated by tying of the sling suture with microforceps. Patient has satisfactory facial function 2½ years after repair.

tunity to carry this out is at the end of what usually has been a particularly long operative procedure with its accompanying fatigue for the surgeon. The difficulty is compounded by limited space, since we work with rarely more than 1.5 cm of cerebellar retraction even for the largest tumors. Because the nerve is going to be suspended across the cavity, not resting on anything, and because the nerve itself scarcely resembles a normal neural structure but is in these cases a thinned out and ragtag distorted band of fibers, clean anastomosis is rarely possible. On the other hand, sometimes the very presence of shreds of the archnoid layer and some thickening probably of epineurial tissue as a result of the long-standing tumor gives a little more purchase for the suture.

The use of a sharp blade and a small block upon which to trim the ends of the nerve has rarely been adequate, and I have had to gently trim the nerve as best as feasible with a sharp microscissors to reach a reasonably squared-off end. I have then sutured the two ends together using a 10-0 monofilament nylon suture through and through as a sling suture (Fig. 20-1, *A*). After even the minimal trimming, however, it is frequently necessary, while the suture is being tied with the tying microforceps, to release the cerebellar retractor down to the least space through which the forceps can be manipulated to take the remaining tension off the nerve. This may well preclude the placing of precise epineurial sutures let alone an intrafascicular anastomosis (Fig. 20-1, *B*). Despite these limitations, a remarkable degree of neural function has returned in these patients.

The delay in reinnervation is so great that I find it most difficult to explain. Entirely unlike that of external grafting or internal-external grafting where the usual rule of approximately a millimeter a day does apply, after internal anastomosis end to end in the actual facial nerve it has generally taken about 2 years for the face to begin functioning. This, of course, violates the principle that muscle tissue will probably have little useful function if more than a year passes by before reinnervation takes place and that after 2 years there will generally be no satisfactory reinnervation. It would appear that the facial nerve is indeed an exception to this rule, which otherwise appears to apply to most peripheral nerves. Facial function has been better than 50% in all these patients and has eventually been clearly superior to the results of the spinofacial or hypoglossofacial anastomosis though in no case has there been significant function in less than 20 months.

When the nerve has been lost at the entrance to the internal auditory meatus, the same considerations and technique are applied to the repair. However, here greater drilling out of the posterior wall of the canal may be necessary simply in order to get room enough to do the anastomosis. At the lateral end of the canal, I have been unable to suture the neural stump but in one case in a young man the proximal nerve was brought up to the point of the entrance to the facial canal at the crista and was held there by a drop of tissue adhesive applied to the nerve more medially in the canal. A strip of gelatin foam was then placed to help maintain the distal approximation, and facial function in this patient returned at the same rate as in the sutured group. Unfortunately, in the other cases where the nerve was lost this far distally, there was not enough proximal nerve to permit this technique without the use of grafting. As stated earlier, no technique of anastomosis or graft has been feasible if the nerve was lost directly at the brainstem.

Nerve grafting

Dott, in 1958,[2,6] published his results in four cases in which he used sural nerve grafts to the proximal end of the facial nerve in the posterior fossa. The graft was then brought out through the craniectomy and tunneled under the muscle layer to an area close to the parotid gland for later suture to the distal facial nerve. Working without microscopy or microsurgical suture material, he designed his own 7 mm straight needles and microneedle holder just for the intracranial anastomosis, using fine silk suture. He used a predegenerated sural graft 15 cm in length. After a delay of 90 days after the proximal anastomosis to permit neural growth down the graft, he exposed the distal end of the graft, cut the facial nerve extracranially at the stylomastoid foramen and anastomosed it to the graft at that point. He apparently had first carried out this procedure in 1935 in a patient who had an acoustic neuroma removed. His other cases were secondary to petrous bone injury. In 1963 Dott[3] reported that he had had no failures but that the best result had not exceeded an 80% reinnervation.

Drake[4], in 1960, published four cases of internal-external graft by essentially the same technique, except that he did not use predegenerated grafts nor did he delay the external anastomosis. His results were good, and the photographs showed even more strikingly balanced facial movement than those in Dott's publication. Drake also described a case of direct intracranial facial end-to-end anastomosis with a good result, without the advantage and benefit of the microtechnique I had available for my first case 10 years later.

Bentley and Hill[1] had shown that predegeneration of a graft made no difference in the end results of experimental grafts, which, of course, would go along with Drake's successes. Dott's hypothesis of delayed distal anastomosis to permit axonal regrowth to reach the distal end of the graft by the time of the eventual secondary procedure seems logical enough and should provide a clean junction zone without occlusive scar. The empirical evidence does suggest that equal results are achieved without the delay.

Present-day usage of the extra–petrous nerve graft should carry with it at least as high a success rate and as good a set of results as what Dott and Drake reported. There now arise two special objections to a relatively routine use of the procedure. When Dott was doing the procedure, there was no significant possibility of sparing the facial nerve and so the preparation and removal of the sural nerve could have been carried out at the time of the craniotomy on a rather regular basis. Today it would be much more awkward, with only 10% of patients where the facial nerve has been cut and the proximal but not the distal end preserved, to then stop, find a way to enter the popliteal space, and dissect a sufficient portion of sural nerve to carry out the anastomosis. It would appear hardly justified to take the sural nerve routinely when it would only be used in perhaps 10% of the patients. In the same manner, it seems to involve more procedure than one prefers to reopen the posterior fossa a week or two later after the patient is recovering from craniotomy in order to then attach a nerve graft in this tender area, though this is what Drake did in his first case. However, in another patient, Drake[5] described the inadvertent aspiration of the graft by the sucker during closure, and apparently he did not reopen to replace the graft. The combination of these two restricting conditions has prevented me from carrying out Dott's grafting procedure in those patients in whom end-to-end anastomosis intracranially is not feasible and yet there remains only a proximal stump for suture of the graft.

For those patients in whom neither preservation of the facial nerve nor end-to-end primary intracranial anastomosis has been possible, I prefer instead to have a purely external grafting and anastomosis carried out, preferably facial-facial nerve graft, as originally described by Smith.[7]

REFERENCES

1. Bentley, F. H., and Hill, M.: Experimental surgery: nerve grafting, Br. J. Surg. **24:**368-387, 1936.
2. Dott, N. M.: Facial paralysis—restitution by extra-petrous nerve graft, Proc. Roy. Soc. Med. **51:**900-902, 1958.
3. Dott, N. M.: Facial nerve reconstruction by graft bypassing the petrous bone, Arch. Otolaryngol. **78:**426-428, 1963.
4. Drake, C. G.: Acoustic neuroma: repair of facial nerve with autogenous graft, J. Neurosurg. **17:**836-842, 1960.
5. Drake, C. G.: Intracranial facial nerve reconstruction, Arch. Otolaryngol. **78:**456-460, 1963.
6. Kettel, K.: Repair of the facial nerve in traumatic facial palsies, Arch. Otolaryngol. **67:** 65-66, 1958.
7. Smith, J. W.: A new technique of facial animation. Transaction of the Fifth International Congress of Plastic Surgeons, Chatswood, NSW, Aust., 1971, Butterworths Pty, Ltd., pp. 83-84.

21 Establishing facial nerve continuity in the temporal canal

BRIAN F. McCABE
LEE A. HARKER

Immediate nerve repair often leads to extensive neuroma formation. This has been verified by clinical and animal experimentation. The optimal time to repair a neural defect is 21 days after injury. The use of the microscope allows for meticulous removal of damaged nerve and scar and for careful suturing. Use of sleeves of plastic and paper tape is condemned.

In foregoing chapters there have been many descriptions of substitutions for the function of the facial nerve. There can be no argument that there is no adequate substitution for connecting the facial musculature to the facial nucleus. Anything less than this, including crossover transfers, must be termed second choice. The facial neurosurgeon then must have at his command the full knowledge of pathophysiology of peripheral nerve surgery including the deficits of substitution anastomosis, or he does not serve his patient optimally. But simply a knowledge of the technique of facial neurorrhaphy and grafting is not adequate to this end. Since the facial nerve is a unique nerve in the body, it is thus out of the exclusive province of the neurosurgeon. Most neurosurgeons today admit that the recent advances in facial nerve surgery have been contributed by nonneurosurgeons. The principles of facial nerve grafting are a combination of the clinical appreciation of the results of various plans and techniques of neurorrhaphy and an understanding of the basic processes that go on in degeneration and regeneration of neural tissue. The following is an attempt to provide these. Special attention is paid to repair within the temporal bone.

Processes that continue after nerve interruption

Upon the interruption of a peripheral myelinated motor nerve there are both degenerative and regenerative process that continue and overlap each other in time. A knowledge of these processes as they occur over time is important in the timing of the neurorrhapy to maximize regeneration and optimize the result.

There are various degenerative processes that occur. The earliest changes occur in the nerve cell body itself. In a matter of hours after the nerve cell body no longer has

Reanimation of the paralyzed face

control of its motor end plate, the Nissl bodies enlarge and then fade and apparently break up, to distribute themselves near the nerve cell membrane. This begins in a matter of a few hours after the injury. After an axon is cut, the axoplasmic membrane loses its sodium-pump capability. This occurs at 24 to 72 hours. When that occurs, the nerve is no longer stimulable percutaneously. This has been termed the "reaction of degeneration." After this the axoplasmic membrane and axoplasm begin to break up and are carried away by macrophages. It takes 5 to 10 days for this process to be complete. When the integrity of the axoplasmic membrane is lost, the myelin coat begins to break up and is also carted away by macrophages. This process takes approximately 14 to 20 days to be complete. A late degenerative change is shrinkage of the now empty distal Schwann cell tubule, which begins at about 2 months and is maximal at about 2 years. Finally, at about 6 months there begins actual nerve cell body loss in the facial nucleus, which continues for at least a year.

At the same time, there are various regenerative processes that go on. The most sensitive structure to the injury is the nerve cell body itself. As the Nissl substance distributes through the cytoplasm, the cell slowly enlarges to about twice its normal size. The cytoplasm becomes packed with masses of RNA in preparation for massive manufacture of axoplasm. This begins in the first few hours after the injury and reaches a peak at 3 weeks (Fig. 21-1). The next activity occurs in the distal Schwann sheath and also to some degree in the proximal Schwann sheath, both of which begin to proliferate after the first day. The next activity is connective tissue proliferation. This begins at 3 days and continues over the next 2 months. Fibroblasts invade from outside the cut nerve and also from inside, from that connective tissue between nerve fascicles and also from endoneurium. This connective tissue spreads the nerve fascicles by invading the proximal cut end (Fig. 21-2) and at the same time diverting and becoming intertwined with axoplasmic filaments trying to cross the nerve gap. This produces the proximal neuroma. Connective tissue also invades the distal cut end, spreading it and becoming intertwined with proliferating Schwann sheath tubules. This admixture of tissues is termed the distal glioma. The most self-defeating event of all however is invasion of connective tissue of the distal tubules themselves, to the exclusion of axoplasmic filaments attempting to fill them (Figs. 21-2 to 21-4).

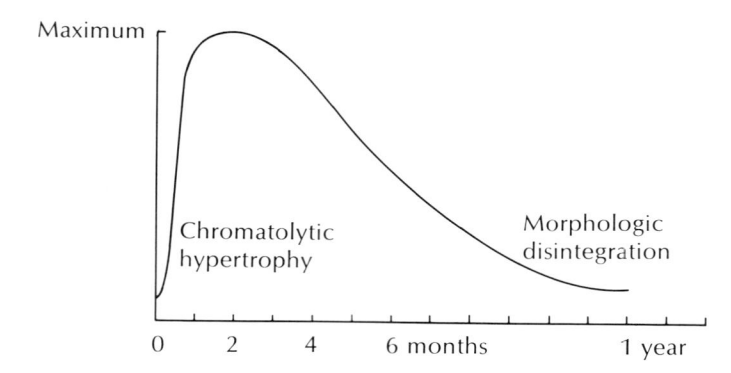

Fig. 21-1. Curve represents ability of nerve cell to manufacture axoplasm over time (proteosynthetic ability).

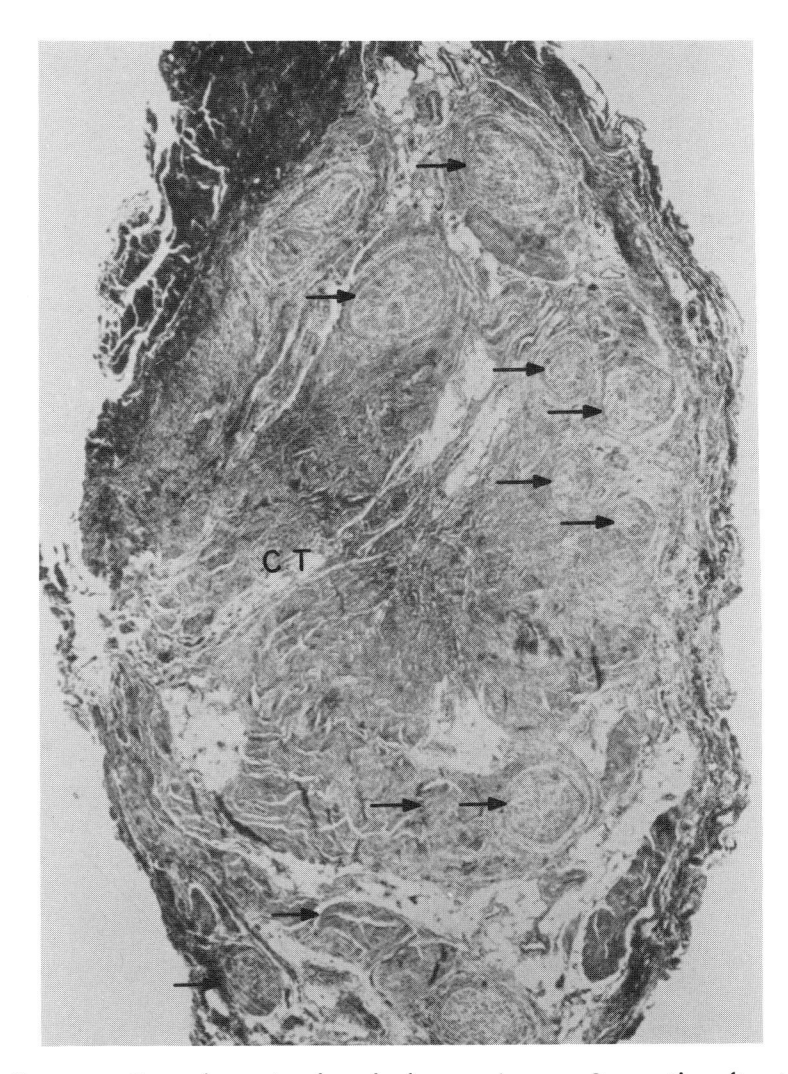

Fig. 21-2. Cross section of proximal end of nerve in man 3 months after transection of nerve. Nerve fascicles, *arrows*, are widely spread by invading connective tissue, **CT.**

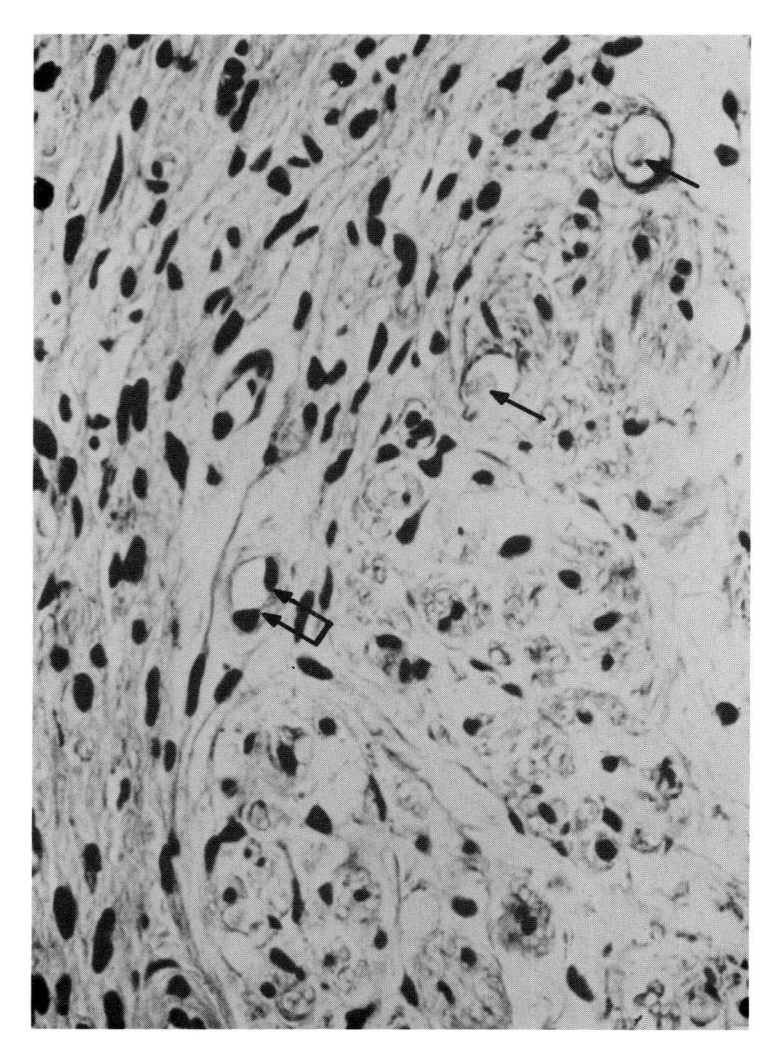

Fig. 21-3. Connective tissue invasion of distal tubules, excluding axoplasmic filaments attempting to fill them. *Double arrow,* Distal tubule that is still open. *Single arrows,* Two tubules, each containing a fibroblast.

Timing of the operation

The optimum time to repair the neural defect is 21 days after the injury. There are a number of reasons for this. First, it is at this point that the nerve cell body is at peak metabolism and ready to push axoplasm across the nerve gap in the greatest quantity. At this time the connective tissue that has invaded each end of the nerve stump can be cut away to take some of the advantage away from the interfering connective tissue. This really does not shorten the nerve ends or widen the gap significantly over what would be if immediate repair were done because most injuries are lacerations, wherein the surgeon has to trim back the nerve ends to uninjured nerve and also to obtain a good square-cut nerve ending. The signal advantage of this timing is that *the neural elements and the connective tissue will be on equal footing in the race to fill the distal*

Establishing facial nerve continuity in the temporal canal

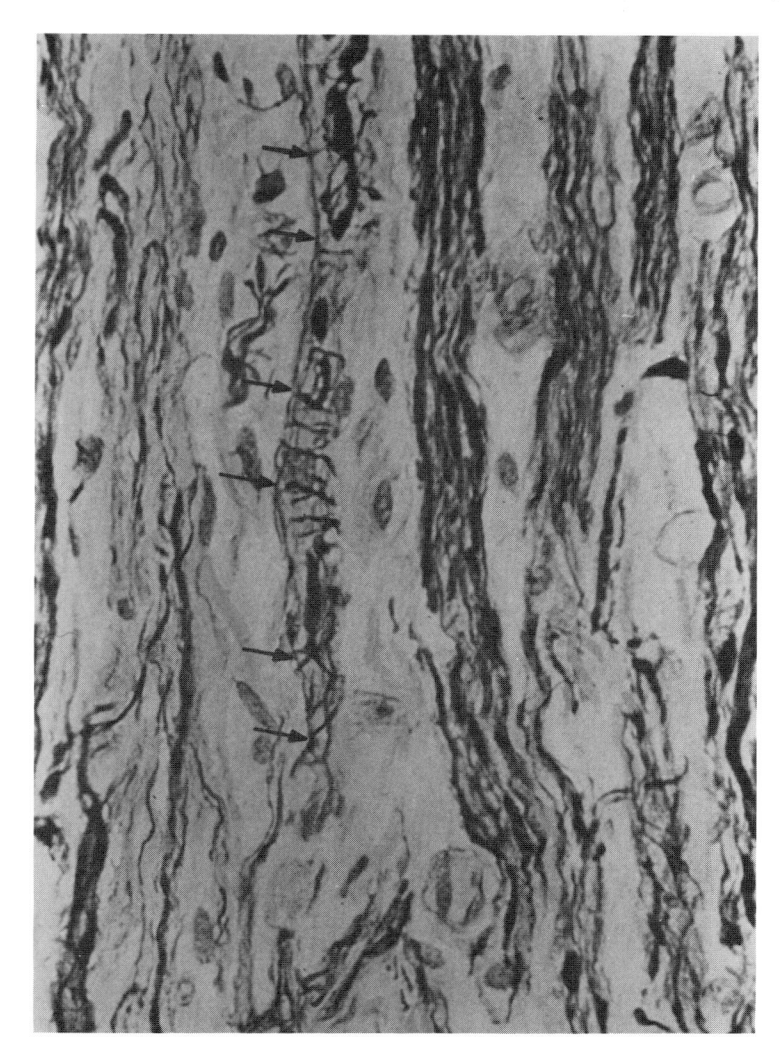

Fig. 21-4. Even though a tubule may be filled, an axoplasmic filament goes to great effort in attempt to enter it. *Arrows* point to filament going around and around distal tubule.

tubules. Delayed repair is not only physiologically sound but has been borne out by practical experience. A considerable experience in neural repair was accumulated during World War II. It was found that during reexploration of closed wounds for various reasons in which an immediate neurorrhaphy had been performed, as a rule, an intraneural neuroma had formed at the repair site with the nerve diameter four to five times normal at this site. These neuromas were excised and the nerve was rejoined. The pathological picture was typical of an amputation neuroma. It then became the practice in many war injury centers to apply the "2- to 3-week rule." The superior results stimulated considerable animal experimentation that elucidated the mechanisms described above.

If the repair cannot be done on the twenty-first day, it should be done as soon after that as possible. The reasons for this are numerous. First, the chromatolytic hypertrophy of the nerve cell body slowly decreases after 3 weeks and reaches an asymptote at about 1 year. This may be at a point even below resting activity of the cell. Second, the distal tubule starts shrinking at about 2 months and at some period thereafter will no longer receive an axoplasmic filament. Third, the longer a nerve cell body is prevented from regenerating its motor end plate in its denervated muscle, the greater the chance for the nerve cell to disappear from the facial nucleus.

Appropriate action according to location of the injury

If the lesion is within the temporal bone, such as that in a temporal bone fracture, the mastoidectomy and opening of the fallopian canal for repair should be delayed until the twenty-first day. If the lesion is in the soft tissues of the face or neck injuring the main trunk or the upper or lower main division of the nerve, such as that in a penetrating injury, at the closure of the laceration the nerve ends should be identified and tagged with colored suture. The nerve ends can even be brought roughly together to make their identification even more easy. Then definitive neurorrhaphy should be delayed until the twenty-first day after injury. If the injury is to one of the named important branches of the nerve such as the ramus zygomaticus, the ramus buccalis, or the ramus mandibularis, immediate repair can be performed with expectation of good result because the closer the injury is to the denervated muscle the more regeneration there will be over the vertically disposed anastomosing fibers.

After 1½ years there would appear to be nothing to be gained by facial neurorrhaphy and some other method of facial rehabilitation should be utilized.

Methods of repair

The first principle of facial neurorrhaphy is that there is no substitute for meticulous epineural approximation. This will not completely exclude connective tissue invasion of tubules within the nerve because endoneurium is connective tissue, but at least it will provide a dam against external invasion and, by the law of mass action, benefit the repair. The procedure is entirely microsurgical. The main trunk should receive at least six sutures, and the upper or lower main division at least four. Use of sleeves of plastic and paper tape, and particularly paper taping to the exclusion of suturing, should be mentioned only to be condemned. Within the temporal bone where the nerve ends cannot be mobilized, a gap will be necessarily created, necessitating a cable graft. This will produce a superior result to rerouting across the middle ear, because the segmented blood supply of the nerve is undisturbed. Since the nerve is not subject to motion in the fallopian canal, suturing is unnecessary and the nerve ends should be meticulously opposed and then covered with gelatin sponge or gelatin film. Our experiments have shown that the best instrument to cut off the proximal neuroma and distal glioma is a Teflon-coated stainless steel razor blade. This is superior to either a Weck surgical blade, a Bard-Parker surgical blade, or a new iris scissors. The author prefers 8-0 monofilament nylon for neurorrhaphy. It has high visibility in the wound, and its slickness is an advantage in minimal tissue drag of the following segment after the needle is passed through the epineurium.

Final note

This chapter constitutes a revision of a prior report by one of us (B.F.M.) wherein it was promulgated that there were a number of situations where immediate repair was deemed advantageous over delayed repair.

SUGGESTED READINGS

1. Crabtree, J. A.: Tympanoplastic technique in congenital atresia, Arch. Otolaryngol. **88**:63, 1968.
2. Ducker, T. B., et al.: Metabolic background for peripheral nerve surgery, J. Neurosurg. **30**:270-280, 1969.
3. McCabe, B. F.: Facial nerve grafting, J. Plast. Reconstr. Surg. **45**:70-75, 1970.
4. McHugh, H. E.: Surgical treatment of facial paralysis and traumatic conductive deafness in fractures of the temporal bone, Ann. Otolaryngol. **68**:855-889, 1959.
5. Sheehy, J. L.: Surgery of chronic ototis media in otolaryngology, Hagerstown, Md., 1972, Harper & Row, Publishers, vol. 2, chap. 10.

22 Management of facial nerve paresis in malignant tumors of the parotid gland

JOHN CONLEY

In a series of 278 malignant tumors of the parotid gland, 60% required some type of radical ablation, with one third being left with some permanent deficit in facial movement. The most efficient method of rehabilitation is by free autogenous nerve grafting, with use of the microscope for the suturing. When the proximal segment is not available, the hypoglossal nerve crossover was used in 122 cases to rehabilitate the paralyzed face. Cross-face nerve grafting, muscle interdigitation, and muscle transposition are alternate and supplementary methods.

Management of facial nerve paresis in malignant tumors of the parotid gland

An understanding of the relations of the facial nerve in malignant tumors of the parotid gland has added significantly to the management and prognosis of these serious problems. This has evolved from a better understanding of the biology of these tumors, the surgical anatomy of this region, and the development of surgical techniques to comply with these factors. One of the most significant developments in the rehabilitation of radical ablations on this gland has been the incorporation of the various methods of facial rehabilitation.

It is important to appreciate the relative proportion of partial and total nerve resections, and the various possibilities for rehabilitation. In a review[2] of 278 malignant tumors of the parotid gland, I found the following percentages:

32%   All or part of nerve intact
42%   Not grafted
26%   Facial nerve grafts

In the first group, 32% of the patients had all or part of the nerve intact at the end of the operation and did not require rehabilitation. These patients had primarily smaller low-grade neoplasms of the lateral lobe that had been diagnosed at the time of surgery by frozen-section examination, and they underwent total parotidectomy at that time. In the second group, 42% of the patients had radical ablations of the facial nerve and were not grafted because the size of the wound or the quality of the tissue bed made the procedure unrealistic. These resections usually included the ear, the adjacent skin, parotid gland, mandible, neck, and a portion of the temporal bone. Flap transplantation was necessary to rehabilitate most of these wounds. These patients had extensive high-grade neoplasms, previous and successful treatment, or extension beyond the parotid gland itself. Twenty-six percent underwent facial nerve grafting. This group consisted of a total nerve graft following radical parotidectomy with a regional cuff of normal tissue or in association with radical neck dissection.

In regard to extent of surgery of the 278 malignant parotid tumors, the following was also found:

68%   Radical ablation
32%   Some variety of conservation surgery

Reanimation of the paralyzed face

These data indicate the gravity of the case load in that review. Approximately one third of these undergoing partial resection of the nerve had some permanent deficit in facial movement.

It is obvious from this data that there are circumstances in the treatment of malignant parotid tumors (1) where it is justified to save all or part of the facial nerve, (2) when nerve grafting is unrealistic, and (3) when the paralyzed face can be immediately rehabilitated by a variety of nerve and muscle substitutions.

Free nerve grafting

The most efficient method of rehabilitation in the classical radical parotidectomy is free autogenous nerve grafting (Fig. 22-1). This graft is procured from the sensory branches of the cervical plexus (C3 or C4). In most instances, the ipsilateral side is used. If there is gross metastasis in the neck, the contralateral cervical plexus, iliofemoral, or sural nerves are available. It is desirable to have a main trunk with three or four branches. This graft bridges the gap between the proximal segment of the facial nerve and the multiple cut ends in the cheek (Fig. 22-2). It is approximated with 8-0 atraumatic monofilament suture material. However, a variety of suture material, ranging from 6-0 to 10-0, has been used. Magnifying loops or the dissecting microscope may be used to gain precise placement of the suture. There should be no tension whatsoever at the suture line. The site of approximation is encased in a soft silicone tube 1 cm in length that is nonconstrictive. The flaps are carefully approximated over this delicate repair, and the wound is drained, either by Penrose drain or with a hemovac system.

When the tumor has approached the stylomastoid foramen or when it has invaded the main trunk, it may be desirable to remove the tip of the mastoid to engage the

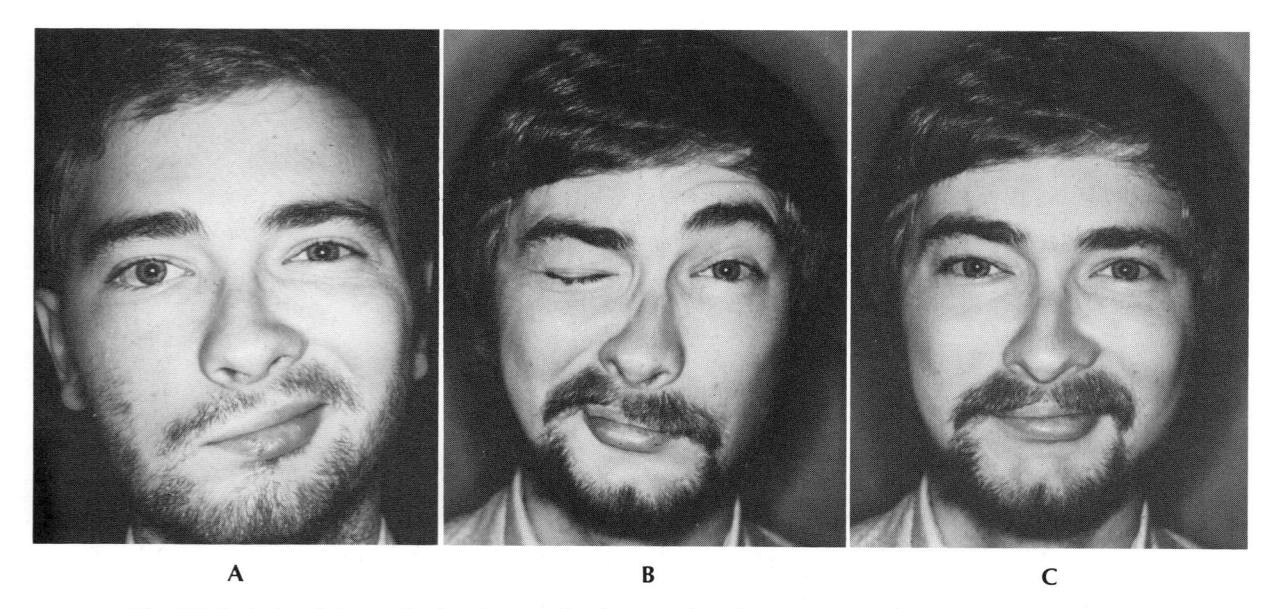

Fig. 22-1. A, Facial paralysis after radical resection for mucoepidermoid carcinoma of right parotid gland. **B,** Free autogenous facial nerve graft functioning after 10 months. **C,** Controlled smile.

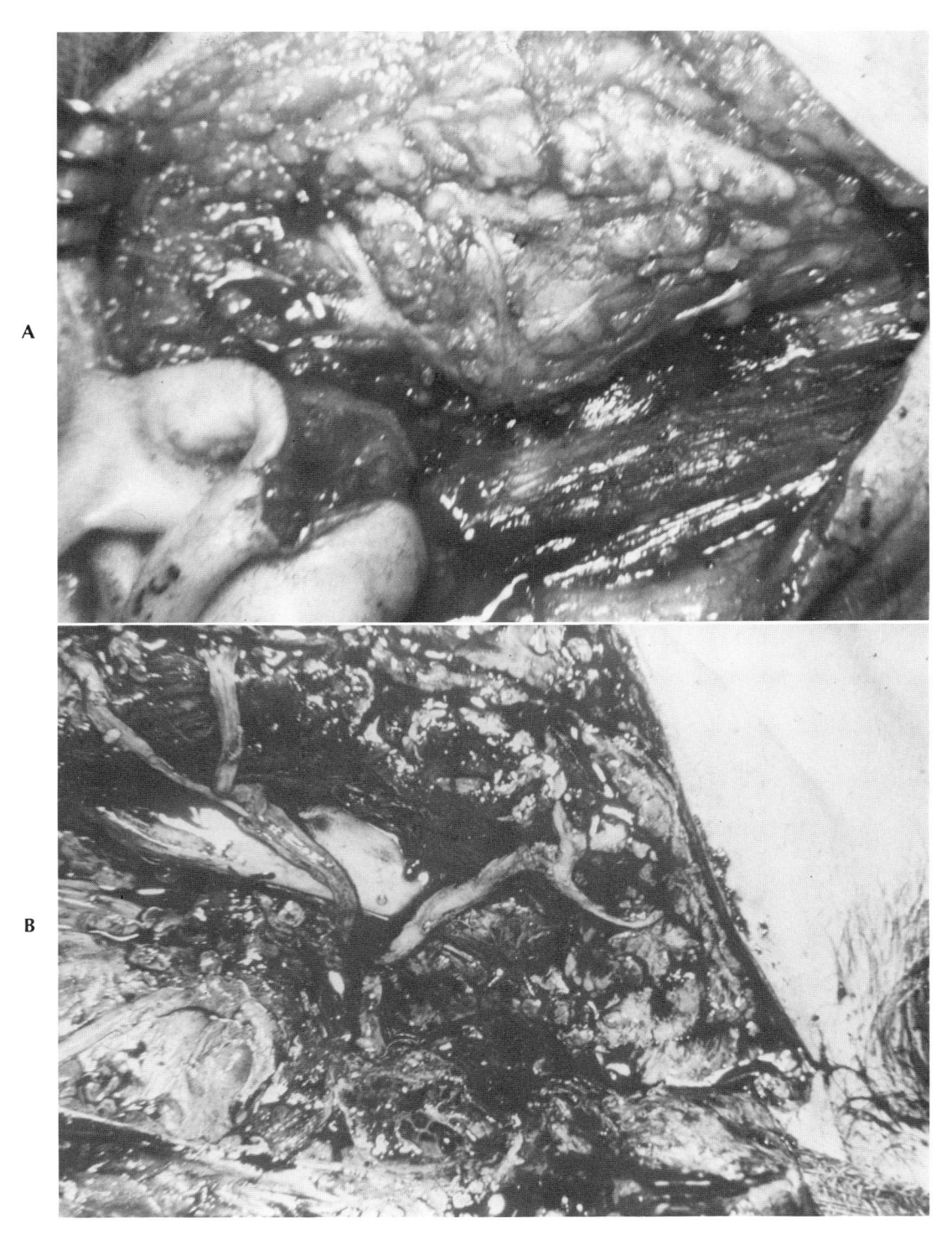

Fig. 22-2. A, Intact facial nerve system. **B,** Grafted facial nerve system. Cut masseter muscle used in muscle interdigitation is close to mimetic muscles.

fallopian canal. The facial nerve is usually smaller in size in the mastoid bone than in the parotid gland, and this size differential with the graft is, to some degree, compensated by oblique cutting of the proximal segment. It is important to control the margins of the proximal nerve stump by frozen-section analysis.

Free autogenous nerve grafting has been carried out in over 150 cases. When the criteria relative to the technique and the tissue bed are met, one can expect some degree of movement of the face in 95% of the cases. The earlier signs of return of movement occur about the commissure of the mouth after an interval of 6 to 12 months, depending on the length of the graft and the volume of regenerating axons. Tone may appear 1 or 2 months prior to this. It is a curious and unexplained fact that when the anastomosis is accurate there is often good tone in the face immediately and in these cases a tarsorrhaphy is not necessary. This is more striking in the young. Could it be possible that a subliminal quantity of neural energy passes through the approximated nerves immediately, and this gives some tone to the face? As the movements spread throughout the face, the patient is able to close the eyes and move the middle third of the face upon intention to a very satisfactory degree. Movement of the forehead and platysma muscle return in only approximately 15% of the cases. Movement of the face continues to improve for an interval extending over 2 years. These movements are basically mass movements; they are weaker than the normal size, exhibit varying degrees of dyskinesia, and only partially respond to emotional expression. With consistent training and concentration, approximately 5% of the patients can attain 80% to 90% function, but the majority range between 50% to 70% function.

Transfacial crossover

Transfacial nerve grafting may be considered in radical ablations of the facial nerve when the proximal segment is not available for anastomosis. This would occur in association with radical temporal bone resections, or in any degenerative condition affecting the central portion of the main stump of the facial nerve (severe Bell's palsy, stroke, neoplasms, central neoplasms of the nerves or of the intracranial cavity). We have done 10 of these operations and have modified the original technique of Scaramella,[4] Anderl,[1] and Millesi[3] by using 25 to 28 cm of the complete thickness of the sural nerve and grafting it to the proximal and distal segments of the cut ends of the main trunk of the cervical division on the normal side. The graft is tunneled through the cheek and upper lip to the paralyzed side and is approximated to the cut distal segments of that facial nerve. The most important branch is always the zygomatic division. The deficit on the normal side is never more than 10% and is usually limited to a weakness of the lateral portion of the lower lip. This is not conspicuous as it is in partial balance with the paralyzed side. The small contralateral deficit, the use of the two segments of the lower cervical division, and the full thickness of the sural nerve establish the optimal conditions for maximum input from the opposite side. Theoretically, this should have significant advantages over the approximation of a second or third division branch to a cable graft. In this latter instance the intrinsic capacity for a large volume of axonal regrowth and migration is restricted, and the attrition on the axons that are regrowing is increased. The results were understandably weaker than total ipsilateral nerve grafting but were of the same quality as far as mass movement, dyskinesia, and weakness of emotional expression were concerned.

Hypoglossal crossover

In my experience, hypoglossal crossover is superior to spinal accessory crossover to reactivate movement in the paralyzed face. This is explained on the fact that the hypoglossal nerve is associated with physiological functions of talking, chewing, and swallowing, whereas the spinal accessory is associated with the elevation of the shoulder. The face receives such a high input of neural energy from the hypoglossal nerve that it may have more tone than the normal side (Fig. 22-3). It may also have an excessive amount of movement upon eating, and talking, and swallowing, and in this respect, it may be grossly overactive. This quality of excessive movement diminishes spontaneously over 10 or 20 years, however, and can be controlled to a certain degree by restricting the tongue movements. Movement begins to return in 4 to 6 months and is basically mass movement. The commissure and the middle third of the face are the first to respond, and then this improves and spreads throughout the face over the following 12 months. In long-standing facial paralysis, tone and movement may not be apparent for an interval of 18 to 24 months (Fig. 22-4).

There have been 16 cases of hypoglossal crossover, using either the entire nerve or a split segment of it, in rehabilitation after radical parotid gland surgery. These cases represent instances where the proximal segment of the facial nerve was deficient or as part of the study program. A self-limiting technical factor in parotid ablation is the available length of the hypoglossal nerve to the distal secondary or tertiary division of the cut facial nerve. Approximation under tension will result in failure or reduce the axonal regrowth.

A total of 122 hypoglossal crossovers have been performed for various types of facial paralysis, and the results have been very gratifying. In an ideal case, the chances of obtaining movement are over 95%. The complaints of the types of patients who undergo radical ablation for a malignant process in this area are minimal. This may be

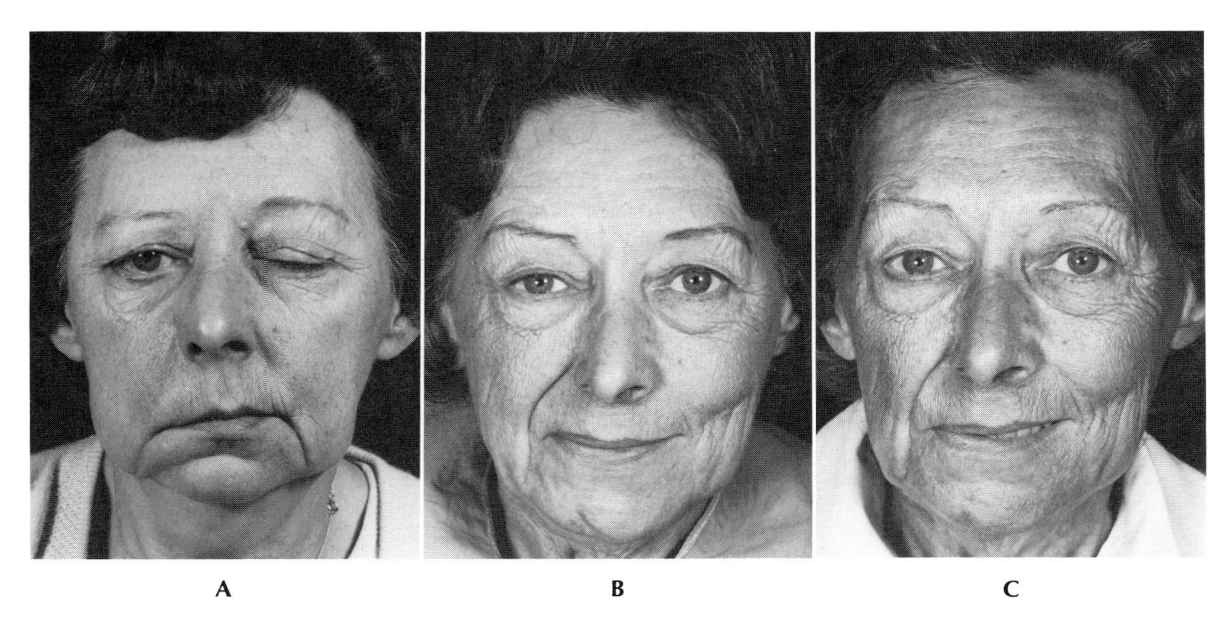

Fig. 22-3. A, Complete, long-standing facial nerve paralysis on right. **B,** Excellent return of movement from hypoglossal crossover. **C,** Six years later.

Reanimation of the paralyzed face

attributable to the fact that the emphasis is placed on the treatment of the cancer, and the crossover is considered a plus in the immediate rehabilitative process. Individuals who have had a facial paralysis for over 2 years have a somewhat different psychological attitude. They are frequently conditioned by a physician who has had disappointing experience with facial rehabilitation, and this is understandably reflected in their counseling. In our series, 22% of the patients had minimal atrophy of the ipsilateral side of the tongue, 53% moderate atrophy, and 25% severe atrophy. Three percent of the patients with immediate hypoglossal crossovers complained of postoperative difficulty in swallowing. All those with long-standing facial paralysis complained of food sticking in the cheek preoperatively, and 10% complained postoperatively. Two percent of those who had immediate rehabilitations complained of difficulty in swallowing. None of the long-standing cases complained of this preoperatively, and 12% complained of it postoperatively. Two percent of those who had immediate rehabilitations complained of slurring of speech postoperatively. Sixteen percent of the long-standing cases complained of slurring of speech preoperatively and 10% postoperatively. There was no intention in this review to try to insinuate that the incidence of deficit should be

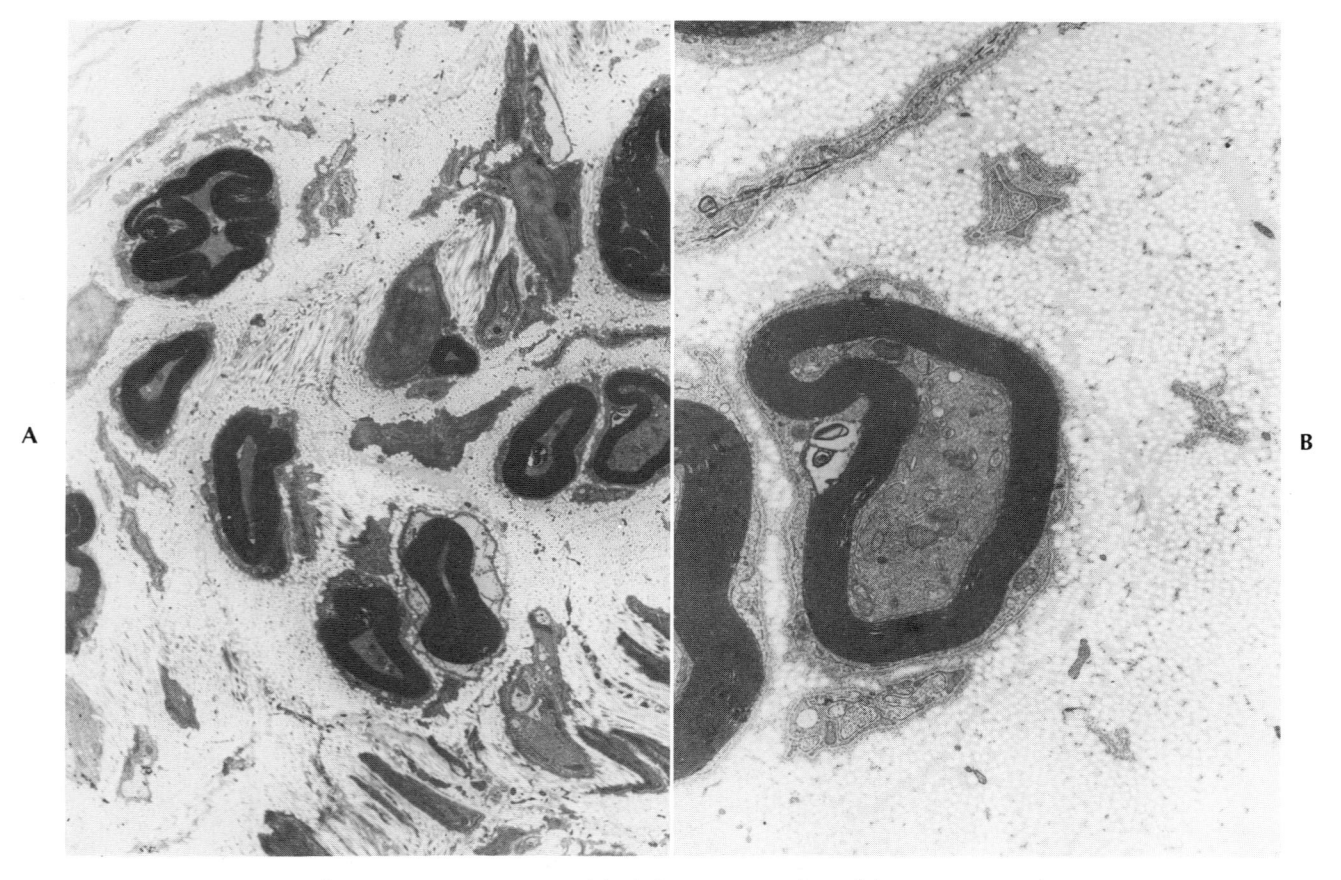

Fig. 22-4. A, Electron microscopy of facial nerve paralyzed for 33 years, showing various stages of fibrosis and myelin degeneration. This nerve system will accept rehabilitation. **B,** Higher magnification of same nerve.

Management of facial nerve paresis in malignant tumors of the parotid gland

more than they had adapted to. Some surgeons have emphasized what to them are overwhelming handicaps in dysfunction, and this is reflected in the patient's attitude. Head and neck surgeons treating cancer are routinely involved in crippling techniques and, perhaps, adapt to these situations with a more optimistic response than the uncompromising standards of perfection in other specialties. This is naturally reflected in their attitude on priorities.

Muscle interdigitation

Muscle interdigitation has become a routine part of the radical ablation, when it is realistic (Fig. 22-5). It is, perhaps, the most significant factor in "spontaneous return" of movement of the face when the nerve graft is not performed. There is no question that it is also operative in some instances, even when not employed as a specific technique, because of the surgical proximity of these two groups of muscles. It is highly probable that it contributes to tone and movement of the face in many of the cases of free autogenous nerve grafting.

The cut surfaces of the masseter (or pterygoid, or temporal muscles) are spliced into the cut surface of the mimetic muscles. Their approximate positions sometimes make this a very simple technique of transposition and suture. The axons from the cut surface of the masticatory muscles promptly begin to grow into the degenerating axons of the mimetic muscles. This invasion has only a few millimeters or centimeters to cover

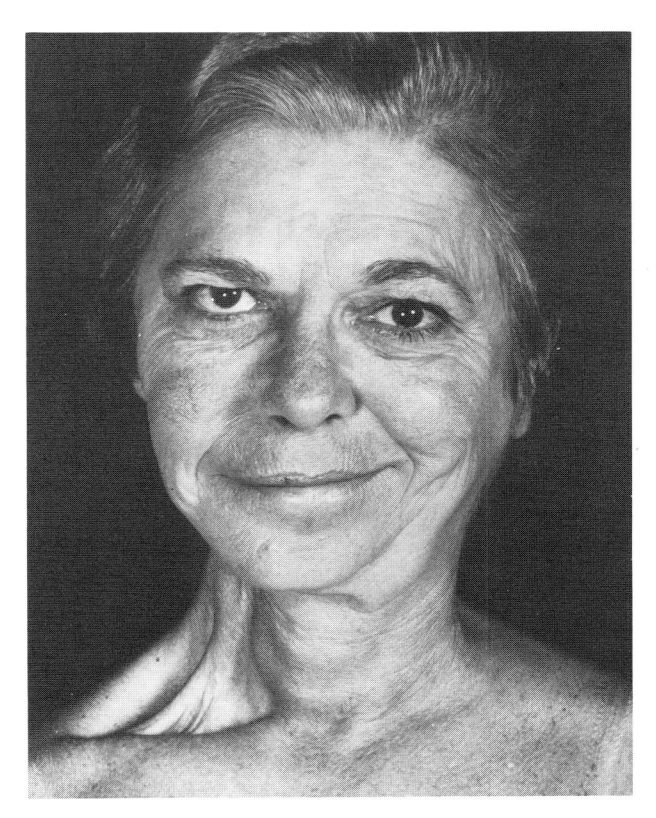

Fig. 22-5. "Spontaneous return" of movements of face because of muscle interdigitation.

Reanimation of the paralyzed face

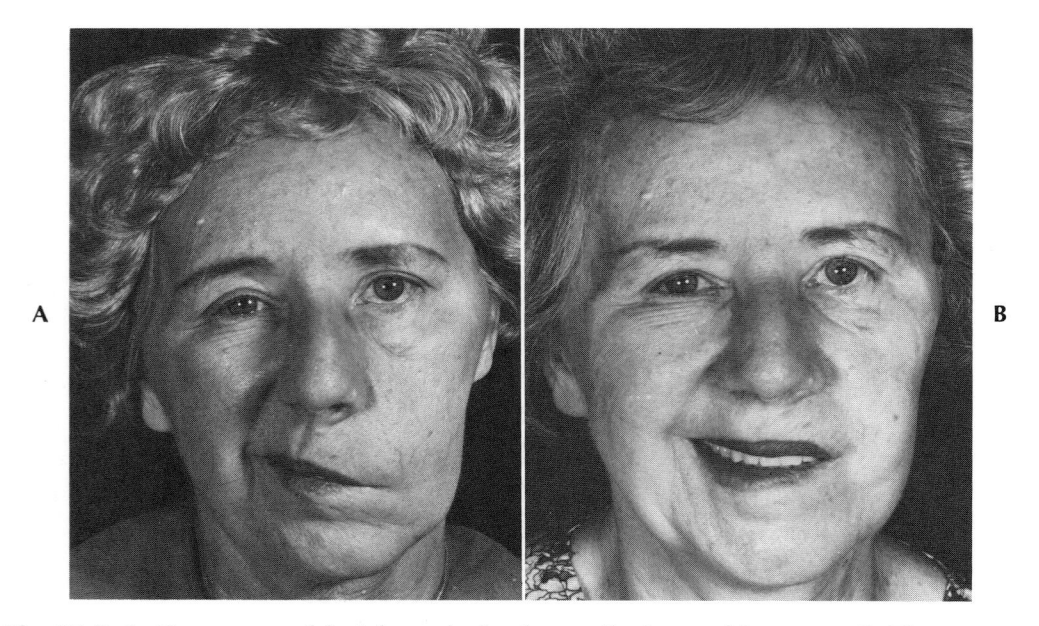

Fig. 22-6. A, Two years of facial paralysis after radical parotidectomy. **B,** Three years after nerve implantation.

and supplies the new system of neural energy to the face. It is not surprising to see movement within 3 months. It appears first about the commissure and middle third of the face and then spreads peripherally. It is basically mass movement and is produced by tightening of the masticatory muscles. It is usually devoid of excessive tightness and dyskinesia and is often smoother in response than nerve grafting or nerve crossover. It is a technique that should be considered as complementary in every radical ablation on the parotid gland and, also, as one of the methods of facial rehabilitation in long-standing cases of paralysis where there are only islands of muscle surviving in the mimetic system. In this latter instance, the masticatory muscles are used to refertilize the face with active muscle substance, thus supplying the essential ingredient for rehabilitation once muscle fibrosis has developed. In these extreme circumstances, one may wish also to supplement muscle transposition with a direct implant of a nerve graft from the proximal stump or a nerve crossover (Fig. 22-6).

Muscle transfer

These techniques are useful to regain some support and movement to the face when the peripheral nerve system has been obliterated and when the mimetic muscle system is atrophic or resected. This substitution of masticatory muscle augments, supports, and moves the face to varying degrees.

These muscles may be moved simultaneously with a radical parotidectomy or an extended resection of the area. Although they are not a substitute for nerve rehabilitation, they may, advertently or inadvertently, complement the return of movement. The temporal and masseter muscles are the ones most commonly used (Fig. 22-7). The external and internal pterygoid muscles may be interdigitated to the adjacent facial muscles after a major ablation of the mandible, parotid, and adjacent tissues. When

Management of facial nerve paresis in malignant tumors of the parotid gland

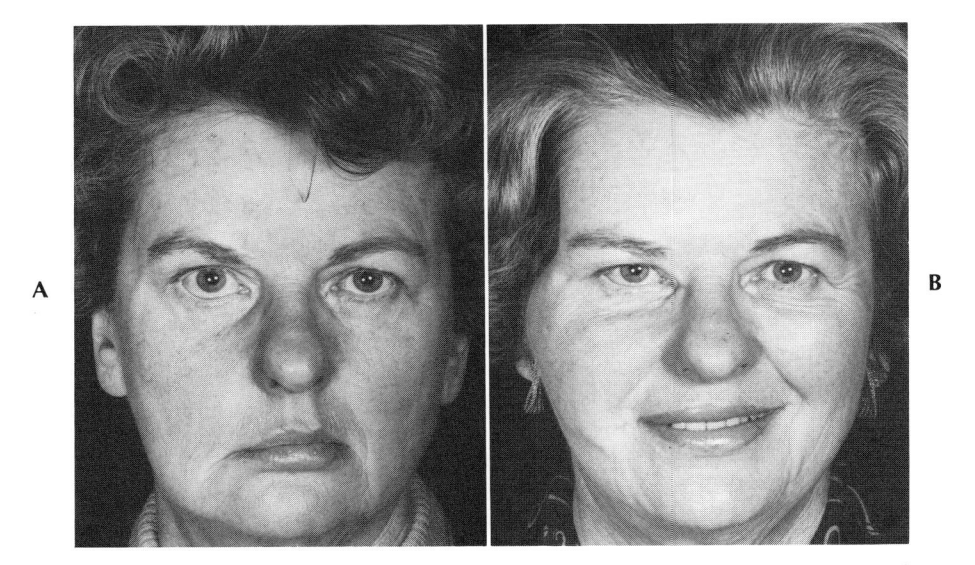

Fig. 22-7. A, Long-standing right facial paralysis. **B,** Six months after hypoglossal crossover and temporal muscle transfer.

these muscles are not available, the sternocleidomastoid muscle may be considered. The muscles are placed in proximity with the cut mimetic muscles after overcorrection of the face. It is important that their nerve and blood supply remain intact. When this concept is specifically applied, an excellent return of movement can be expected in the majority of cases. It is mass movement and can be trained to comply with human emotion to a slight degree. The face always moves upon mastication. Overcorrection may not be realistic at the time of the primary ablation, and this may result in drooping about the commissure. This weakness can be improved in a year or two by localized fascial stripping.

Muscle transposition or interdigitation may be employed in long-standing facial paralysis. It is, indeed, essential when there is severe end-stage muscle fibrosis. The temporal and masseter muscles are the most commonly used. The masseter muscle is in good position for transfer to the commissure, upper and lower lips and cheek. The temporal muscle can be transferred about the orbit, cheek, commissure, and upper and lower lips. These muscles can be used for regional paresis or as a total muscle unit. The temporal muscle will extend to the commissure by overcorrection of the face, and there is no need to gain length by incorporating the epicranium or the temporal fascia. Movement is gross and not so forceful as in the primary muscle transfers. These are precisely the cases where one would consider nerve grafting, nerve crossover, or nerve implantation to augment the muscle transfer. Fascial stripping may eventually add to the basic support.

Free muscle transplantation supported by nerve and blood vessel anastomosis may find a place in this program when regional muscles are not available, when augmentation is desirable, and when the tissue bed is heavily scarred.

Free muscle-tendon onlay grafts are ingenious and serve a highly specific purpose in improving regional and localized paresis about the eye and mouth. These segmental weaknesses in the partially paralyzed face have been one of the most challenging and elusive problems. The mechanical principles of the muscle-tendon unit grafts have contributed to alleviate this enigma. The limitations placed on the volume of a free muscle transplant without a functional nerve or blood vessel system will, hopefully, be overcome by microsurgical anastomosis. These techniques are more adaptable as secondary procedures because of their sophisticated and individual nature.

REFERENCES

1. Anderl, H.: Cross face nerve transplantation in facial palsy, Transactions of the Sixth International Congress for Plastic and reconstructive Surgery, Paris, 1975, Manson.
2. Conley, J.: Salivary glands and facial nerve, Stuttgart, 1975, Georg Thieme Verlag.
3. Millesi, H., Berger, A., and Meissl, G.: Fascicular nerve grafting using microsurgical technique, Transactions of the Fifth International Congress for Plastic and Reconstructive Surgery, Chatswood, NSW, Aust., 1971, Butterworths Pty, Ltd., pp. 586-592.
4. Scaramella, L.: L'anastomosi tra i due nervi facciali, Arch. Otologia **82**:209-215, 1971.

23 Primary nerve suturing of severed motor nerves in facial trauma

NAHUM BEN-HUR

The severely traumatized face first requires general lifesaving measures such as possible tracheostomy and blood transfusions. When the wounds are cleansed and the severed facial nerve ends are found, the traumatic ends must be cut back and sutured without tension by use of a loop to place 10-0 nylon sutures. If a gap of tension occurs, free nerve grafting using the greater auricular nerve is the method of choice.

This volume and the effort, energies, and time that went into its publication are a testimony to the devastating effects of the unanimated human face. The facial countenance is the major respresentative feature of man from the functional, emotional, and esthetic viewpoint. The best hope of restoration of animation in traumatic transection of the facial nerve lies in the initial and perhaps definitive care at the time of injury or soon thereafter.

This section shall direct its attention to immediate emergency care of the patient as a whole, evaluation of the facial injury in particular, minimal initial diagnostic testing, and definitive treatment of the traumatized facial nerve as indicated.

In evaluating a patient injured severely with facial nerve transection, one must, of course, initially ensure that other possible life-threatening injuries are first stabilized. Release of respiratory impingement, establishment of adequate airway, control of major bleeding, and treatment of hypovolemia always takes precedence. In all of these considerations, a multidisciplinary approach is mandatory. Attention can next be turned to evaluation of the facial injury. Since the face is rich in vascular supply, alarming bleeding can occur readily. Almost all acute hemorrhage can be controlled with pressure dressings, or by direct digital pressure. The temptation to blindly clamp major pumping bleeding vessels must be resisted if further injury to vital structures, such as the facial nerve or parotid duct, are to be avoided.

After stabilizing acute clinical problems, one can now direct his attention to an orderly evaluation of the facial injury. The examination should include a thorough consideration of all local tissues: skin, subcutaneous tissue, muscle, vessels, glands,

Reanimation of the paralyzed face

ducts, cartilage, bone, teeth, and nerves. Obviously, an accurate knowledge of the anatomy involved is a necessity. Assessment of motor, sensory, secretory, and reflex function of the seventh nerve is now made.

Evaluation of the bony substructure is made by palpation, superficially and intraorally, supplemented with radiograms of the skull, facial bones, and cervical spine. A high index of suspicion for a cervical spine injury must be maintained in treatment of all facial injuries, especially roadway accidents. A Water's view and orbital tomograms are especially valuable in a thorough examination of the facial skeleton. Ophthalmological consultation is critical in complete evaluation of orbital and maxillary fractures. When available, photographs can be helpful in evaluating the preinjury appearance. Type- and cross-matching for blood replacement may be a wise precaution.

A multidisciplinary approach for definitive treatment of a severely injured patient in the operating room is usually necessary. The order of priority is (1) lifesaving procedures, (2) restoration of function, and (3) esthetic considerations. The type of anesthesia is the next valid consideration, that is, local versus general anesthesia and oral endotracheal versus nasal endotracheal intubation. This question is of more than academic consideration as at times interdental wiring is required for facial skeletal stabilization.

Pathophysiology of nerve injury

If a deficit of facial nerve function is demonstrated clinically, an obligatory controlled surgical exploration of the wound is indicated. In a *complete transection* (neurotmesis) of a nerve, classic wallerian degeneration of the distal segment occurs and the proximal segment degenerates to the first node of Ranvier. Repair in complete transection is accomplished by direct reanastomosis by epineural repair or by nerve grafting by use of segments of the greater auricular nerve as cable grafts.

Partial transection presents a more difficult clinical problem. The severed part behaves like a complete transection with ultimate proximal and distal swellings (a double hump—camel swelling)[1]. The part in continuity may suffer axonotmesis or such violent intraneural disruption that ensuing reparative scarring precludes spontaneous regeneration of function. Thus, a partial transection presents an awkward clinical problem that can only be resolved by evaluation of the apparent direct damage to the nerve, knowledge of the vector of injury, and estimation of the extent of surrounding tissue injury; all tempered by the surgeon's experience and available resources.

Exploration of the facial nerve in the face of a clinical deficit may reveal local injury with a grossly intact facial nerve. In this case *axonotmesis* or *neurapraxia* is said to be the cause of the apparent clinical paralysis. *Axonotmesis* is characterized by maintenance of the supportive stromal elements of the nerve and by total interruption of the axons. Excellent clinical regeneration occurs because intact endoneural elements serve as a scaffolding guide for regenerating axons. The rate of recovery is as in a standard repair, that is, 1 to 2 mm per day. *Neurapraxia,* on the other hand, implies limited localized demyelinization. Initially, complete paralysis occurs. However, the nerve recovers function rapidly in a matter of days to weeks. Thus the clinical difference between axonotmesis and neurapraxia is one of rates of recovery.

Surgical techniques

Once a diagnosis of seventh nerve dysfunction is made in an open wound, an immediate exploration should be undertaken. Copious irrigation and meticulous débridement are the initial steps. We have found repeated irrigations with saline solution by use of an irrigating device to be particularly helpful. Careful débridement of the minimal amount of devitalized tissue and all foreign material is essential. If a complete or partial transection of the facial nerve is discovered, one should commence wound closure with neurorrhaphy. Identification of the proximal nerve stump is not always easy. The laceration may have to be incised into normal tissue along the known anatomical course of the nerve until positive identification of the nerve is made. The distal end of the transected nerve may be sought in a retrograde or anterograde fashion with a nerve stimulator. Restraint must be used with nerve stimulators as rapid fatigue of the distal stump occurs quickly. The neurorrhaphy is performed either with loops at a magnification of 4 to 6 or preferably under an operating microscope. The proximal and distal ends are cut sharply with a double-edged razor blade through a normal-appearing segment of the nerve. Two 10-0 monofilament nylon sutures are placed through the perineurium of each funiculus at 180 degrees and the epineurium is sutured at each 90-degree angle. If there is undue tension at the neurorrhaphy site, a segmental funicular cable graft of greater auricular nerve must be interposed. Careful hemostasis and proper wound closure in layers complete any good anatomical would repair. Although extensive experimental work has been done with nerve sheathing at the time of neurorraphy, I believe this is not necessary.

Recovery of nerve function

Evaluation of nerve regeneration is obtained by electrical means, surgeon observation, and patient impression. The affected side is continuously compared with the noninvolved side. Results are variable. A good result consists of normal resting tonus, facial symmetry, normal voluntary and spontaneous motor activity, and complete closure of the eyelids. The recovery times vary with the type of damage and the anatomical location of the injury.

Clinical cases

Our clinical series consists of the following 29 cases of injury to the facial nerve where primary immediate nerve repair was attempted:
1. 7 involving the main trunk
2. 8 involving the frontal branch
3. 6 involving the mandibular branch
4. 2 involving the zygomatic and labial branch
5. 2 involving the zygomatic and frontal branch
6. 4 involving the labial and mandibular branch

The patients ages ranged from 4 to 67 years of age.
The causes of the facial nerve injuries were as follows:
1. 26 war injuries caused by
   a. High-velocity missile bullets
   b. Low-velocity missile hand grenades
   c. Mortar shelling
   d. Mine explosions
2. 2 road accidents

Reanimation of the paralyzed face

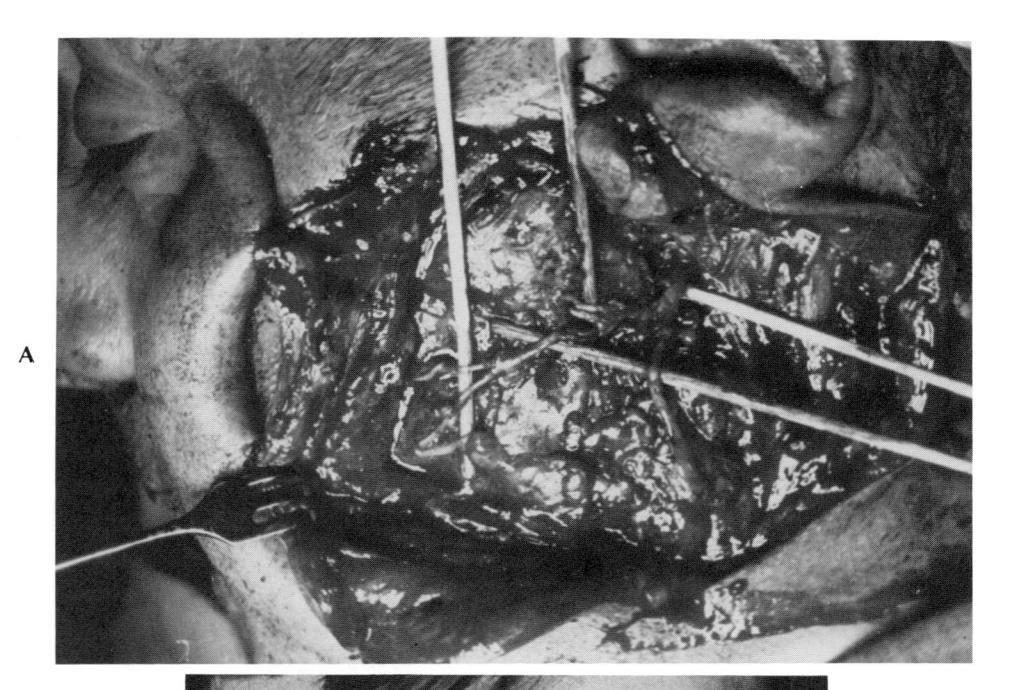

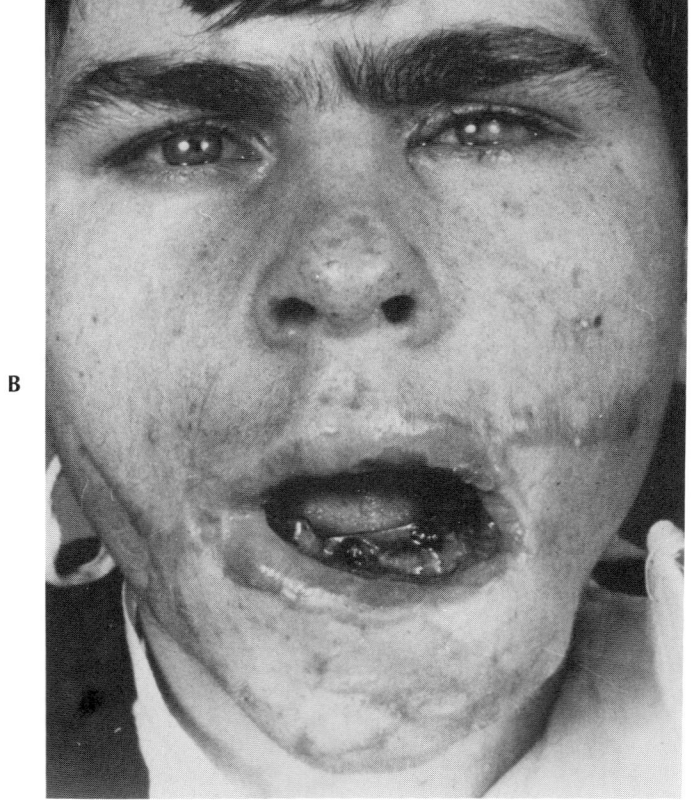

Fig. 23-1

238

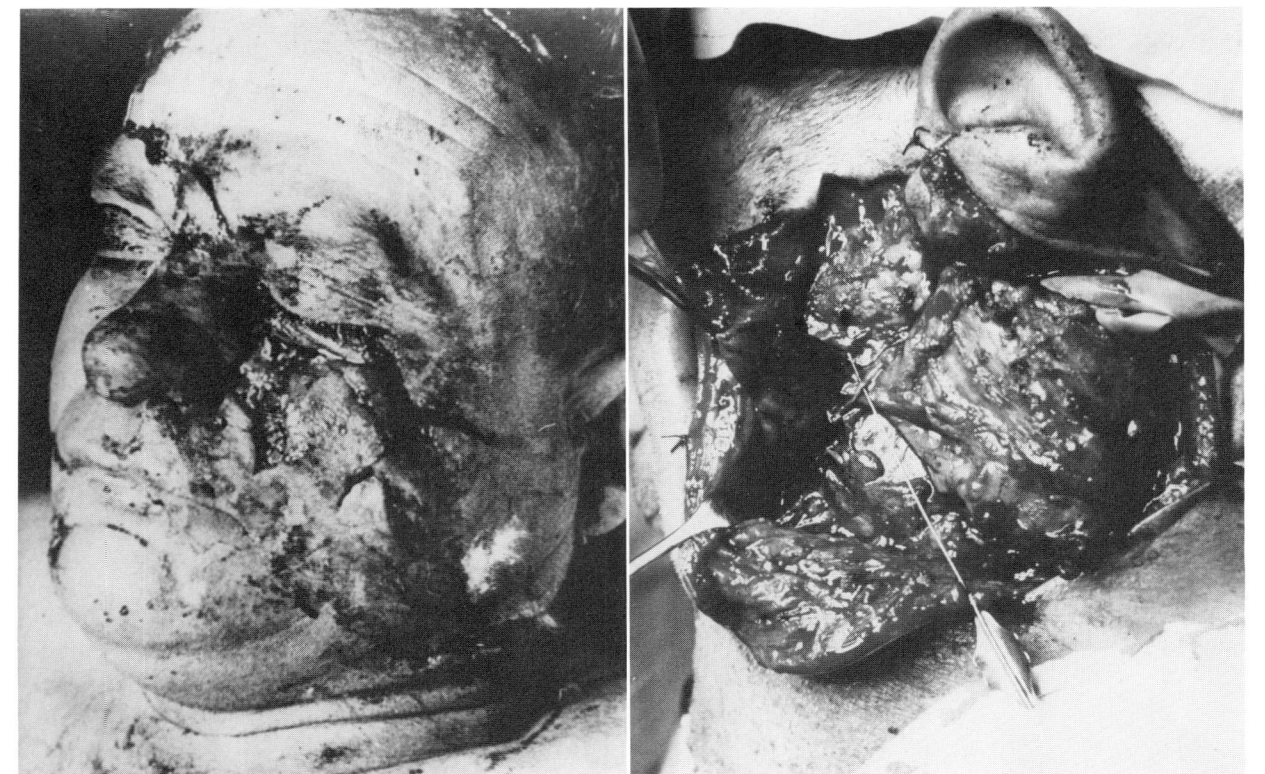

Primary nerve suturing of severed motor nerves in facial trauma

Fig. 23-2

CASE 1—MINE EXPLOSION

A 19-year-old male sustained multiple injuries while disarming a field mine. In addition to other injuries, he sustained multiple lacerations of the face, especially to the left side, destruction of the left eye, and fracture of the left mandibular ramus. At surgical exploration under general anesthesia by tracheostomy, the disrupted frontal, zygomatic, and labial branches of the facial nerve were sutured with 10-0 monofilament nylon under an operating microscope at a magnification of 10 (Fig. 23-1, *A*). At 9 months postoperatively, he regained facial symmetry and active movements of the mouth and forehead (Fig. 23-1, *B*).

CASE 2—ROAD ACCIDENT

A 52-year-old white male (Fig. 23-2, *A*) sustained multiple windshield lacerations of the left side of the face in a road accident. Examination revealed paralysis of the left zygomatic and labial branches. Nerve stimulator examination confirmed the transections. At exploration, the transected branches were sutured with 10-0 monofilament nylon under operating microscope at a magnification of 20 (Fig. 23-2, *B*). Active movements returned after 3 months.

Summary

I believe that primary repair of transections of the facial nerve should be considered initially in any clinical setting where an extensive microsurgical procedure would not prove detrimental to the patient's ultimate survival. Primary repair, when feasible, tends to obviate secondary procedures, delayed recovery, and atrophy of distal musculature and may perhaps obviate other more elaborate nerve transpositions or muscle transfers. Primary repair by microsurgical techniques has proved successful in our hands.

REFERENCE

1. Sedden-Sedden, H.: Surgical disorders of peripheral nerves, ed. 2, Edinburgh, 1975, Churchill Livingston.

SECTION TWO

Intermediate surgical treatment for facial paresis—4 months to 1 year

24 Cross-face nerve grafting—up to 12 months of seventh nerve disruption

H. ANDERL

A detailed description of the technique of cross-face nerve grafting is given for restoration of balanced function to the paralyzed face. The sural nerve from one or two legs is used as the graft. We in the clinic believe that early grafting, preferably within 2 to 3 months, is imperative, since success of the operation depends on the time from paralysis to grafting. Facial muscle degeneration, although slower than other muscles, does not regenerate totally to recover complete function.

The reconstruction of mimic muscular function and of harmony in the expression of the human face may only be brought about through a successful nerve suture or, in case of a defect, through a nerve transplantation of the damaged facial nerve (nervus facialis). In the course of the last years, the endeavors to bring about reconstruction of that nerve, especially in its intracranial and intratemporal course[8,14,23,28,30,41,50,79] have made great progress, supported by microsurgical suture[4,39,47,52–54,65,66,70,71] and techniques of nerve transplantation.[10,55,61a,64] They have prevented the grave consequences of facial paralysis in many patients.

Despite these good results it is not possible to have positive results in all cases, either because the roots of the facial nerve have been destroyed intracranially, or because a healthy proximal nerve stump cannot be found, or further because regeneration of nerves and muscles after a reconstructive intervention fails to set in, or because operations on the most proximal nerve section cannot be performed as yet for want of experience and facilities. To regenerate such an irreparably damaged facial nerve, spinofacial anastomoses[21,31,51] with the nervus hypoglossus, the nervus accessorius, and the nervus phrenicus have been successful ever since Faure, 1898.[27]

Reanimation of the paralyzed face

With these predominantly motor nerve crossovers, the results are excellent concerning tone and facial symmetry, and often enough astonishing activity by volition is brought about through exercise. It is impossible, however, to restore to the patient natural emotional expression of the face. The relatively high functional gain is deteriorated by mass movements and uncontrollable muscle twitches caused by unconscious innervation of the formerly successful organ.

Although by numerous older and more recent static or dynamic substitute operations, individual paralyzed sections of the face can be corrected, a natural synchronization of the numerous muscle groups cannot be brought about. Based upon clinical as well as electromyographical observations in patients with facial palsy, a reinnervation of the paralyzed paramedian muscles starting from the contralateral side[13,21] was noted, a phenomenon caused by the dense peripheral ramification of the facial nerve and its special aptitude of regeneration. This spontaneous restitution from the healthy side, however, is not sufficient to regenerate useful muscle function; yet it may be responsible for keeping up a certain tone and thus a longer survival of the muscles. The excellent regenerating qualities of this nerve[19,45,48] are observed time and again in the treatment of facial spasm[17,30] or in the facial tic where often up to two thirds of the nerve branches have to be severed in order to obtain success and where relapses nevertheless are frequent. Even in extensive extratemporal peripheral injuries major

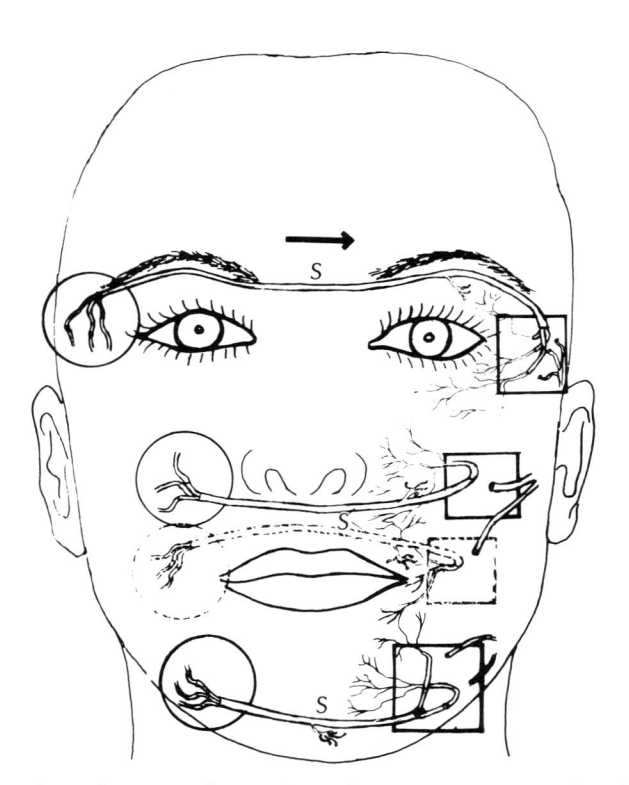

Fig. 24-1. Position of single transplants, **S,** with anastomoses on healthy side *(circles)* and on paralyzed side *(squares)* of face. One graft *(dotted line)* in lip can be exchanged with graft in chin.

losses of function are rare. As observed in Bell's palsy no considerable losses are noted with a partial restitution of as little as 30% to 50% of the nerve fibers.[26]

These special qualities of the facial nerve have encouraged us to use part of the peripheral facial nerve of the healthy side of the face for the restitution of the paralyzed face muscles. As a principle, several nerve sections of the healthy facial nerve are selected and severed, and after anastomosis the nerve impulse is routed over one or several nerve transplants to the paralyzed half of the face where reinnervation of the muscles is effectuated by coupling to the paralyzed peripheral facial nerve (Fig. 24-1). This method appears even more reasonable in regard to the selective severance of facial branches of the healthy side to establish the balance and the removal of considerable muscle preponderance in cases of facial paralyses, and if these nerve sections are not lost, they can again take up their function.[18]

History

In 1970, Scaramella[62] presented one case in which he performed an anastomosis to the intact buccal ramus on one side of the face and transmitted the nerve impulse by a sural graft positioned submental to the paralyzed stem of the facial nerve of the opposite side of the face. The girl gained symmetry, some active movement, and exact lid closure after 1 year.

In 1971 James Smith[67] presented three cases with anastomoses of two fascicles from the buccal zygomatic plexus of the healthy side to one sural graft and connection of that to the main portion of the paralyzed facial nerve. Three to 6 months later he could observe improvement in terms of facial symmetry.

Independent from these methods, we at the clinic tried initially to restore the most inportant functional zones of the face: the orbital, the buccal, and the mandibular areas. The nerves leading to these muscle groups, the rami zygomatici, rami buccales, and the ramus marginalis were connected with the corresponding main branches of the facial nerve of the opposite side of the face by way of sural nerve grafts. The operation is done in two stages. In 1972 we presented four cases of what are called selective cross-face nerve transplantation. In a follow-up from 4 to 18 months in three cases a good-to-satisfactory result in the eye and mouth region could be achieved.[3-6] During the last years many other surgeons have performed such cross-face nerve transplantations or faciofacial anastomoses as they are called.

The field of application primarily only covering the innervation of paralyzed muscles has been enlarged in the meantime. Results of a combination of the cross-face principle with free muscle transplantation and muscle transposition are known.

Special anatomical consideration
HEALTHY SIDE

For the procedure three areas of the extratemporal nervus facialis[37,46] are of importance, the ramus zygomaticus, rami buccales, and ramus marginalis.

The peripheral ramifications of the ramus zygomaticus, rami buccales, and ramus marginalis, which mostly supply the various muscle groups, form a sort of plexus formation. In anatomical nomenclature the singular expressions "ramus zygomaticus"

Reanimation of the paralyzed face

and "ramus marginalis" are often used. As a matter of fact there are several main branches as in the rami buccales.

For the ramus zygomaticus the area suitable for the nerve connection lies somewhat outside of the lateral orbital edge. The small facial fascicles branch off partly below the subcutis and lie on the lateral muscles of the orbicularis oculi. The fascicles used for the innervation of the upper lid closure run in a somewhat deeper layer, often in or under the muscles to the lateral eye region.

For the *rami buccales* two sections are of interest, both lying about 1 cm behind the nasolabial fold. One is to be found about 1 cm, the other 2.5 cm below the foramen intraorbitale. In the cranial section nerve fibers, some thin and some thick, run in a sort of plexus in the direction of the upper lip on the one hand, supplying the muscles for the pursing of the mouth and the lifting of the lip. On the other hand, some other thicker branches run in the direction of the medial lower lid supplying the quadratus labii superior and part of the lower lid muscles themselves. This anastomosis with the ramus zygomaticus can be found in 80% of the cases.[22,46] The second area of the peripheral rami buccales that is important lies about 2.5 cm below the foramen infraorbitalis, comprising nerve fibers running to the upper and lower lips, as well as supplying bigger nerves for the buccinator muscle in the proximal area.

In many cases the existence of anastomoses with the ramus marginalis can easily be shown by stimulation. The nerves running in the buccal area conduct a large percentage of all the nerve fibers of the facial nerve. They possess an extensive interfascicular fiber exchange. Therefore especially in this area even larger fascicles can be sacrificed for the connection without risk.

The *ramus marginalis* will be taken into consideration for a connection only when not enough fascicles in the buccal area are available. At the level of the foramen mentale two thicker nerves run at a distance of 1 cm from each other above the mandibular edge in the direction of chin and lower lip. From these two nerves the fascicles then branch off to the muscles, and it is possible here as well to select three such fascicles for the connection.

Of a certain importance are communications of the peripheral facial branches with branches of the trigeminal nerve existing above all in the infraorbital area and in the area of the foramen mentale. Especially in the extreme distal area of the facial nerve the sensory fibers run along with the facial fascicle to the innervated organs; here a differentiation is very difficult. Thus, from the point of view of operational technique, it is important not to get too far into the periphery and, above all, to perform an exact selection of the facial fascicles by means of electrostimulation, which will be described below. These sensory branches are unsuited for innervation; they reduce the volume of motor fibers that are to be supplied for the paralyzed muscles. There is no escaping the connection of a small part of sensory fibers. In axon budding in the transplant to the paralyzed side this fact can be also observed by touching and by releasing of sensory sensations as in the Tinell-Hoffmann sign.

PARALYZED SIDE

The anatomy in the paralyzed half of the face concerns especially the main branches of the facial nerve distributed predominantly within the parotid. Whereas in the healthy side it is possible to detect nerve fibers by means of electrostimulation and ensuing muscle twitches, this aid of exploration does not exist here as a consequence of nerve degeneration. Only anatomical facts can be relied upon. There are, however, no absolutely patent signs where the various facial branches can be detected with exactitude, since variability is too great. Yet we know certain directional lines and structures that make location possible.

For primary exploration the frontal parotid margin is an important landmark. From there the rami zygomatici run across the arcus zygomaticus in two to three thin nerves in the direction of the orbita. One or the other nerve may lie rather superficially near the subcutis; the thicker nerves, however, are embedded somewhat deeper, immediately over the periosteum in light connective tissue. Anteriorly, several connections with the rami buccales exist immediately behind emergence from the parotid gland. Posteriorly, small nerve branches run to the ramus temporofrontalis.

The *rami buccales* emerge from the parotid gland in the area of its entire frontal margin, with three, four, or even more, thicker nerves being prominent, connecting right away in branches with one another. An essential directional structure is Stenson's duct. In its proximity there is always a larger buccal branch to be found. After insertion of a probe into Stenson's duct of the parotid from the mouth, the probe can be touched and in its immediate vicinity a ramus buccalis can be identified. They lie embedded in fat and connective tissue directly on the fascia masseterica.

The proximal *ramus marginalis*, in the form of mostly two, thicker parallel branches, runs in the posterior third of the mandible, usually along and above the bone margin and farther and then runs across the facial artery and vein. One may best demonstrate it by locating the vessels where they reach the mandible coming from the neck and pursuing them upward and downward. One can also locate the rami zygomatici and the ramus marginalis by retrograde preparation, finding them proximally from the buccal branches on the parotid margin between the lateral and medial portion in the parotid gland itself. Of additional importance in the lower parotid area are branches of the nervus auricularis magnus, a sensory nerve, which must not be anastomosed. Once the typical pattern of distribution of the facial nerve is displayed in the parotid gland a confusion is impossible.

The *ramus temporofrontalis* is not mentioned in these anatomical considerations. We know from experience that return of function in the frontal muscles is extremely uncertain. Nerve fibers for more important areas would thereby be lost.

Preoperative investigation and measures
STATE OF THE MUSCLE

If the cross-face principle for the reinnervation of the paralyzed facial muscles is to be applied, the state of the muscles is of primary importance. Therefore a thorough electrical and clinical examination must precede every operation. Advanced atrophy or, worse still, fibrosis of a part or of all muscle fibers will prevent the new budding nerve fibers to reach tissue suitable for innervation. Return of functions cannot be expected in this way. The difficulty lies in fixing the individual optimal moment for a reconstruction of the nerve. On the one hand, spontaneous reinnervation should not be interrupted; on the other hand, the result could be the more favorable if more muscle fibers could be supplied for regeneration.

Opinions are still divided on how long facial muscles can survive without nerve impulse. Experience has shown us so far that these muscle fibers perish much later than other skeleton muscles.[72] Their condition may be good even after 2 or more years, a fact that might be explained by the excellent blood circulation in the face and by the existence of a widespread net of other nerve fibers, especially of the trigeminus and limited innervations from the contralateral side.[21,71]

In a case of definite injury, a nerve transplantation will have to start as early as possible (2 to 3 months after trauma); with other paralyses, however, it should start after 6 months when there are no signs whatever of regeneration.

During *clinical* examination one can observe a bad state of the muscles from a considerable deficiency in the volume as opposed to the healthy side. Moreover, in such cases, a certain rigidity of the skin and of the underlying tissue can be felt. A definite answer, however, will be given by *electrical,* especially *electromyographical* examination.[13,59,69,73] If upon galvanic stimulation, a dull twitching of the underlying muscle appears, a good regeneration potential can still be presumed. A more accurate prognosis, however, is supplied by the EMG, which facilitates a certain quantitative statement. Control examinations spaced at intervals of several weeks show stability or a decrease of fibrillation potentials. At the same time, beginning innervation potentials, if any, can be discovered. Thus, as long as fibrillation in the muscle can be proved, the muscle is considered alive. A restoring intervention in the nerve is indicated. (See also Chapters 3 and 4.)

GENERAL CONDITION

Besides these special examinations of the paralyzed face, it is only natural to consider the general physical condition of the patient. Even if the cross-face nerve transplantation can be said to involve no special weakening of the patient, there being but little irritation by pain, the long duration of the operation of 4 to 6 hours is liable to produce certain problems, as with older patients suffering from diabetes or those patients on whom a skull operation had been performed previously. An adequate cardiological as well as general preparation is therefore necessary.

LOCAL PREOPERATIONS

All substitute surgery should be omitted before a cross-face nerve transplantation. Such surgery causes scarring and might endanger the result of this operation. We perform nothing but a dynamic and static functional amelioration of the missing lid closure, a paretic consequence especially irritating for the patient and likely to lead to permanent deterioration of the eye. For the upper lid closure we have had good results in more than 100 cases with the aid of a lid spring.[56,78] Recently lid magnets[57] were used to attain lid closure. To support the lid spring and, above all, to remove the ectropion, the implantation of a Silastic membrane into the lower lid is to be highly recommended.[2] All the corrective measures cited above are meant to be temporary and can be removed without difficulty after regeneration of muscle function. Therefore, we do not apply any more lateral tarsorrhaphy, since it constitutes a definite iatrogenic alteration.

Operation

Principally the procedure is performed in two stages: In the first stage, the healthy fascicles on the intact facial side are selected and anastomosed to sural nerve grafts.

In the second stage, 4 to 5 months later, the ends of the grafts are anastomosed with the corresponding main branches of the facial nerves of the paralyzed face. The timing in two stages is done for the following reasons:

1. Scarring between anastomoses on the paralyzed face might occur more easily when the nerve fibers are not available from the opposite face as in a one-stage operation. A revision on this area and new anastomoses would be very difficult because of its delicate structure. From experience, it is known[53,54] that the axons pass easily through the proximal and distal anastomosis of a nerve graft. However, there are cases where, after nerve transplantation, a revision at the distal anastomosis is necessary because of blockage by scar. In the extremities such a revision compared with that in the face is much less difficult.
2. As evidence of axon growth one would find a neuroma on the end of the sural graft. If there is only a small neuroma or none at all, this is a sign of bad axon budding. This fascicle should be bypassed. In case of doubt, a frozen section would show the presence of nerve fibers.
3. In a two-stage procedure, the operating time is reduced, a matter that is of value to the patient and helps the accuracy of the surgeon, despite the necessity of another intervention.
4. The two-stage procedure guarantees a further waiting time of about 4 to 5 months in case of spontaneous regeneration. If the anastomoses on the paralyzed face are performed together with anastomoses on the intact face, all big paralyzed main branches are severed, and in case of long-standing regeneration, axon growth cannot proceed into the ipsilateral facial nerve anymore. If such a late spontaneous regeneration does occur, the second stage is abandoned, and the growing of axon fibers can proceed to its normal destination without interruption.

The operations are done under general anesthesia with intubation and halothane. Because of the long procedures, special care has to be taken to position the patient on the operating table. There must be no pressure point to damage the skin or underlying nerves. The temperature of the body has to be controlled at all times, and in case of cooling, a heating blanket has to be applied. The urine output is measured with a urinary catheter. The whole face is cleaned with antiseptic solution, and the two lower legs are washed and prepared for taking the sural nerve grafts.

First operative stage

Three incisions are made on the healthy side of the face for the preparation and selection of the intact peripheral fascicles that should be the source of supply for the paralyzed side. These three areas are the peripheral distribution of the zygomatic, the buccal, and the marginal rami of the facial nerve (Figs. 24-2 and 24-3).

ORBITAL REGION

The incision is made about 0.5 cm lateral to and along the orbit for a length of about 3 cm. The dissection should be done with the help of a loop or the low magnification of the microscope immediately after the incision, since there is not much fat under the skin and one might damage the superficial nerve fibers. After lifting of the skin and subcutaneous tissue, the wound margin is fixed to both sides with several stitches (Fig. 24-3).

Reanimation of the paralyzed face

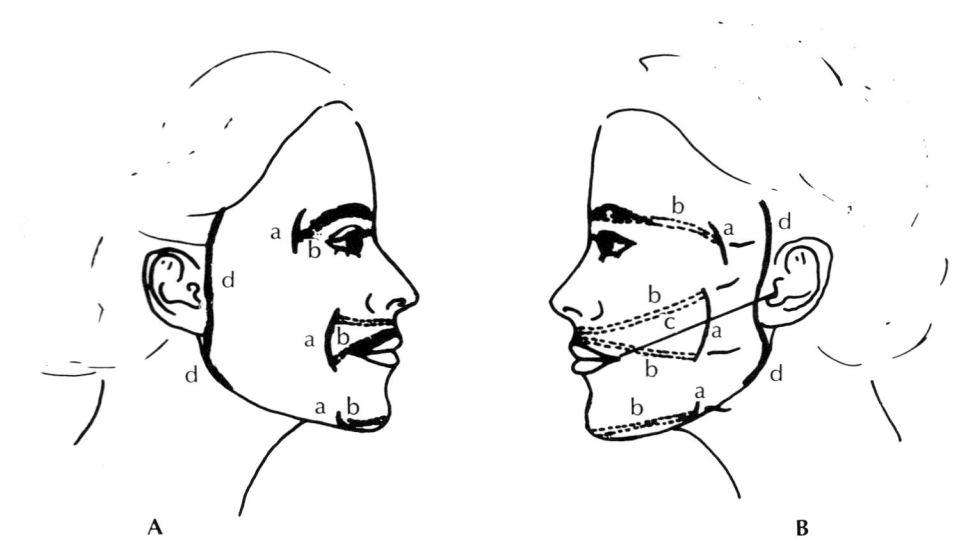

Fig. 24-2. **A,** Healthy face. **B,** Paralyzed face. *a,* Incision lines; *b,* sural grafts; *c,* position of parotid duct; *d,* face-lift incision.

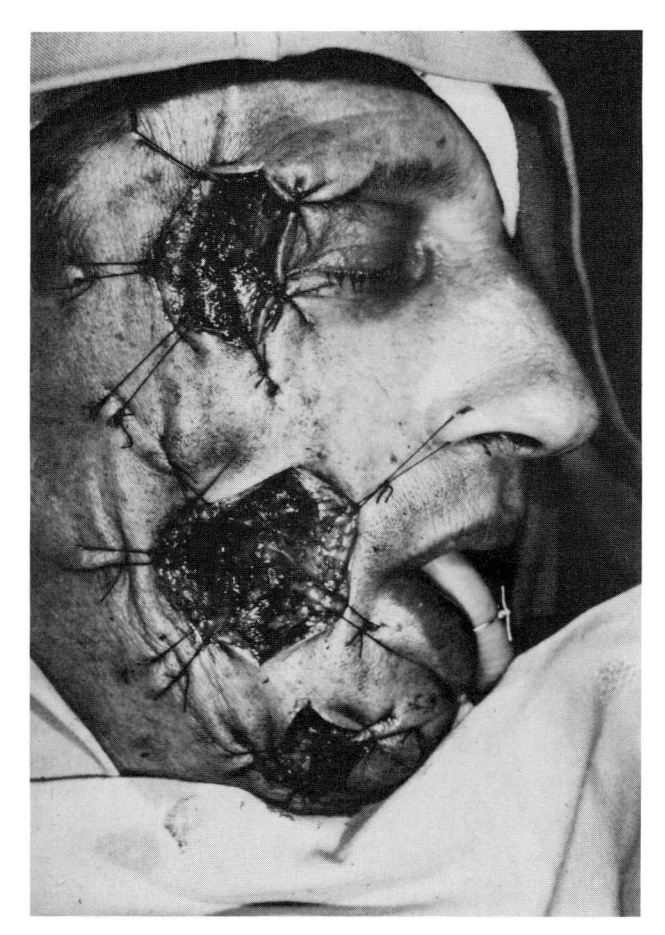

Fig. 24-3. Incision lines on healthy face with skin lifted and wound margin fixed.

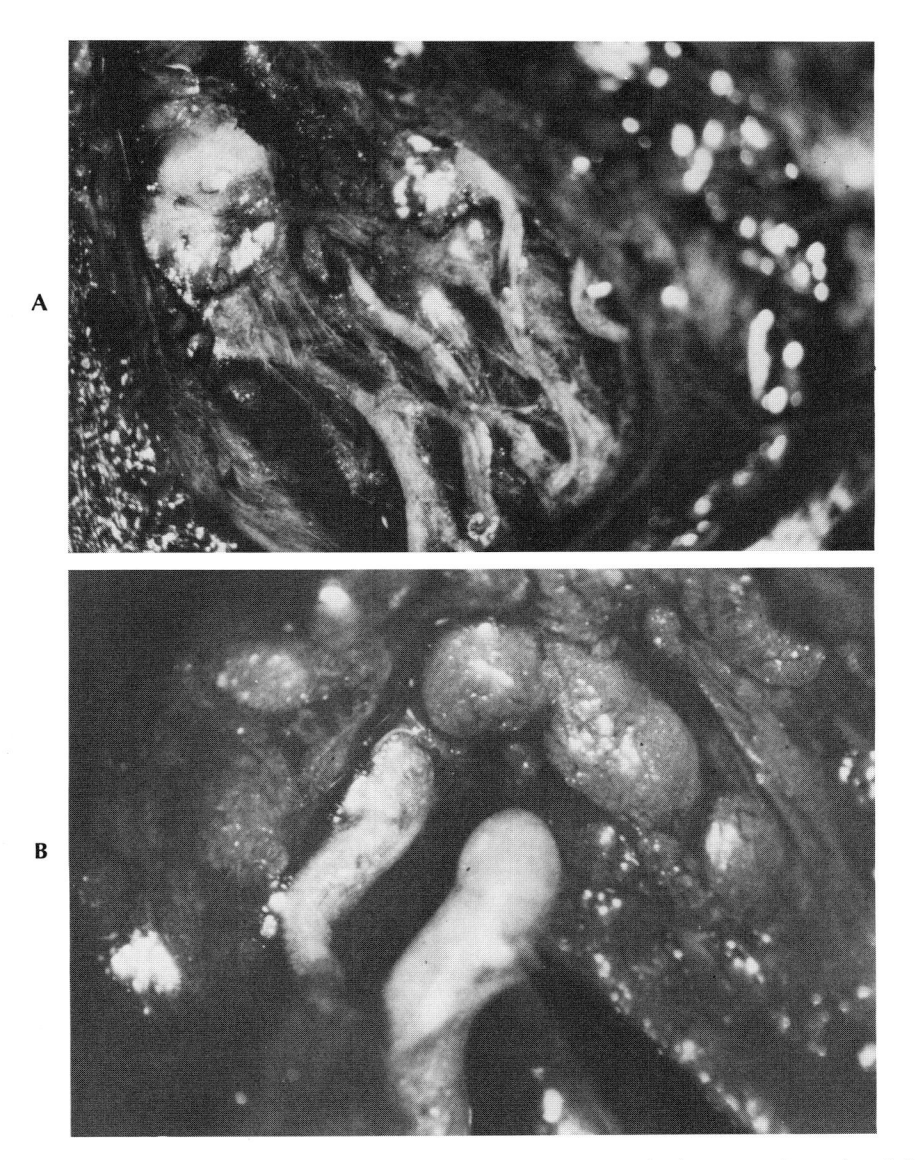

Cross-face nerve grafting—up to 12 months of seventh nerve disruption

Fig. 24-4. **A,** Part of zygomatic plexus. From this network three or four fascicles are selected for connection. **B,** Single facial nerve fascicle out of plexus of **A.** Axoplasma is protruding.

The zygomatic plexus of the facial nerve is located and demonstrated (Fig. 24-4). This plexus lies partly superficially that means on the muscles or between and beneath the fibers of the lateral orbicularis muscle. Those fibers controlling the closure of the eyelid, especially of the medial part of the lid, are situated deepest. There is a significant interfascicular exchange of nerve fibers. The selection of three or four fascicles to be divided is achieved with help of electrostimulation. The faradic current should be of low power (5 to 15 microamperes), which guarantees identification of individual fascicles and prevents a mass stimulating effect on several muscles. To ensure undisturbed function of the upper and lower lid, a drop of local anesthetic with a very fine needle can be applied to that fascicle to be severed. If there is normal

Reanimation of the paralyzed face

function of the eyelid after injection of the fascicle with the anesthetic, this nerve can be cut; thus, it is even possible to sacrifice a thicker nerve without loss of function. If there is need for more fascicles, one can go higher up toward the temporofrontal area and include fibers of this facial branch for connection. After selection, the fascicles should be marked with a very thin bank of soft yellow rubber to facilitate finding them before anastomosis with the graft.

BUCCAL REGION

The incision for preparation of healthy buccal fascicles is done about 1.5 cm behind the nasolabial fold with a length of about 4 cm. The wound margins are swung back and fixed with threads. Since the subcutaneous fat tissue here is much thicker, there is no danger of cutting fascicles by retraction of the skin. As already described in the anatomical considerations, we need the upper portion of the buccal fascicles, which ramifies to the lower lid, and the right zygomaticus, which innervates the central and contracting part of the orbicularis oris and the quadratus labii superioris. These nerves are situated mostly deep under the fat in the layer of the muscle groups. With lowest magnification of the operating microscope or a loop, these fascicles are revealed with a stronger stimulating impulse (20 to 40 microamperes). In the area of maximum muscle contraction the fat is separated until the nerve fibers are seen in the depth. These are several very thick nerves that can be dissected in a proximal and distal direction and clearly arranged before anastomosis (Fig. 24-5). Three to four fascicles are selected and identified with a colored band. In the lower part of the wound and a little bit back toward the parotid gland there are some other fascicles leading to the buccinator muscle and partly to the orbicularis muscle of the lower lip. It is most desirable to have fibers innervating these muscles because of their strong impulse. Out of these fascicles three to four should be selected also and taped. Gen-

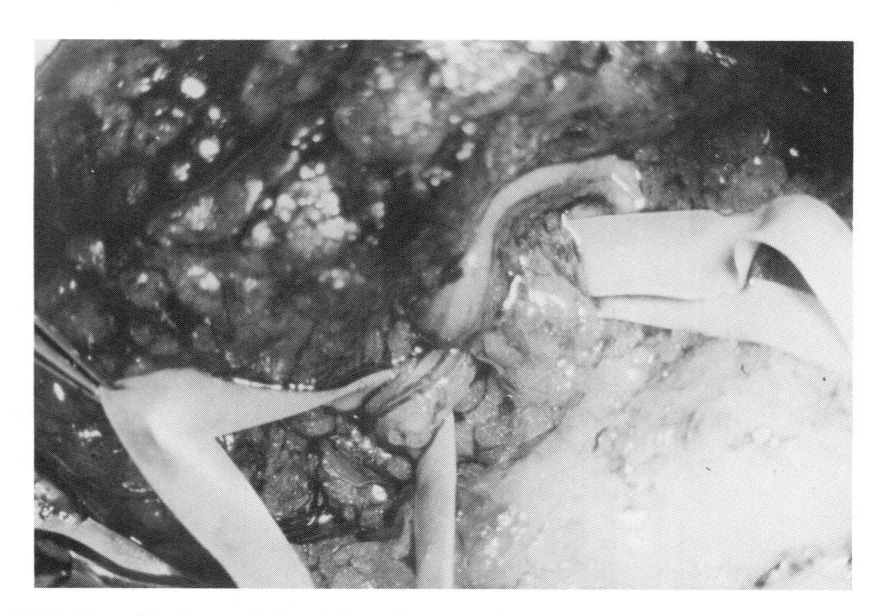

Fig. 24-5. Two big buccal fascicles slung with thin band of soft yellow rubber.

erally in this buccal area just described one is allowed to prepare as many fascicles as possible. We have never seen any visual disturbance of the facial function of the normal side. On the contrary, very often, we had the feeling that we should have sacrificed more to diminish this very strong lateral pull of the healthy angle of the mouth by using these nerves for connection to the paralyzed face.

MARGINAL REGION

The source for this connection to the healthy marginal branch is only used if enough fascicles in the buccal area cannot be found. The incision lies about 2 cm in front of the facial artery and crosses the mandible. With help of the stimulating test, the terminal branches of the ramus marginalis can be detected and two or three fascicles are available. They also have to be color banded for better identification.

PREPARATION OF NERVE GRAFTS

As has been shown up to now in clinical experience and experimental examination of animals, thin autologous nerve transplants,[10,33,54,55,63,64] because of their nutritional superiority, are far better than homologous preserved nerves or lyophilized ones. This is valid especially in the bridging of larger defects. In the autografts that are incorporated and viable, wallerian degeneration and regeneration takes place in the same way as in the appropriate distal nerve stump after trauma and consequent nerve suture. In the graft, the Schwann cells proliferate and form Büngner's bands, the important cellular unit for guiding and wrapping the outgrowing axons. Basically, there is no difference in the activity of the Schwann cells either in a graft or in the nerve stump of a disrupted nerve, since both deliver optimal guidance lines for regeneration.

Several type of nerve grafts are used: the greater auricular nerve, the lateral cutaneous femoral nerve, and the sural nerve. The first two nerves have the advantage of containing several branches that roughly correspond both in number and distribution to those of a portion of the facial nerve. Unfortunately in cross-face nerve transplantation, they are too short. The sural nerve is the best graft to use.

To obtain the sural graft, one starts the dissection behind the lateral malleolus where the saphena magna acts as a guide. After the branches of the nerve under the vein have been located, they are severed as distally as possible. The end can be armed with a suture thread. With a stripper similar to an embolectomy stripper,[7] one can free the nerve from surrounding tissue in a proximal direction until a cutaneous branch is reached and when the end of the instrument touches resistance. Here in the skin, a small transverse incision is cut, the nerve with the stripper exposed, and the small cutaneous branch cut. The same procedure is repeated upward toward the proximal calf. Generally three or four such small incisions are necessary to have the proximal end of the graft near the fossa poplitea, where the whole nerve, in a length of up to 30 to 40 cm, can be cut.

POSITIONING OF GRAFTS

In addition to the incision lines already made on the healthy face, a small auxiliary incision (1 cm) is performed in the glabella and in the middle of the upper lid and the chin (Fig. 24-6). Four additional small incisions (1 cm) are made on the paralyzed side: one in the zygomatic area, just before the hairline and a little higher than the zygomatic

Reanimation of the paralyzed face

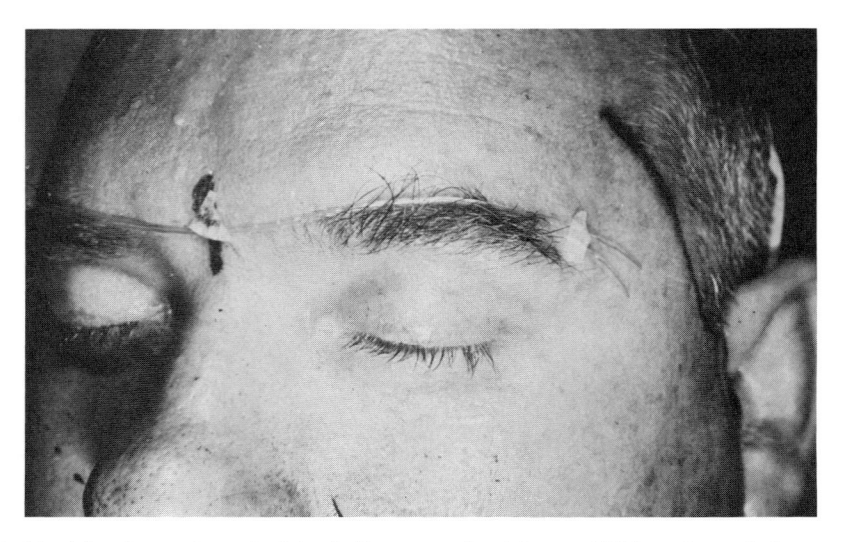

Fig. 24-6. Positioning of graft. *Black lines* are incisions. White thread demonstrates graft where it should lie under skin.

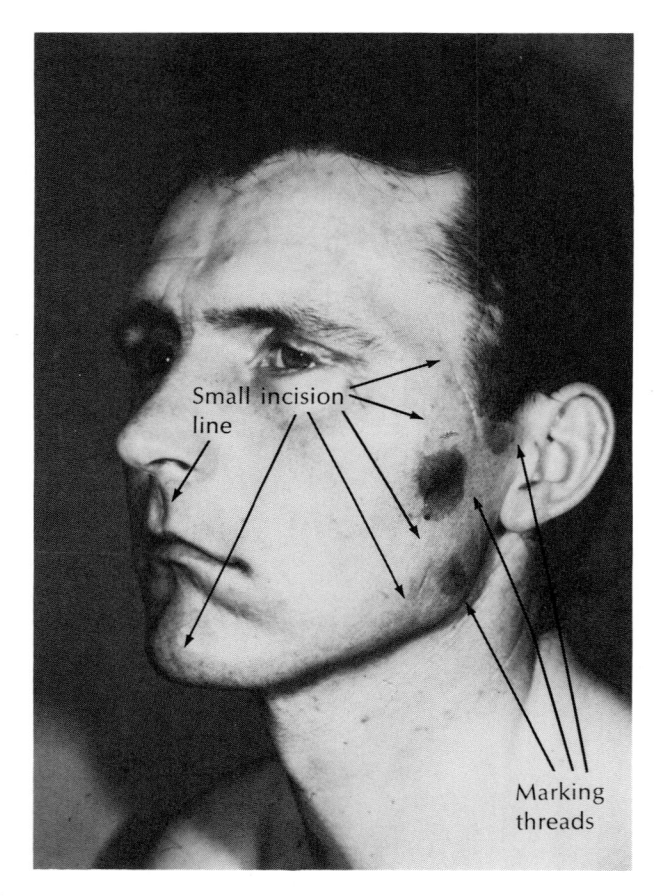

Fig. 24-7. Small incision line can be seen in front of hair border near zygomatic arch on paralyzed face. *Dark areas* represent end of marking threads under skin surface.

Cross-face nerve grafting—up to 12 months of seventh nerve disruption

arch (Fig. 24-7). This is meant not to interfere with the zygomatic branch and to have no scars in the preparation area of the second stage. The other two incisions are just over the border of the parotid gland, one of them 1 cm over and the other 1 cm under an imaginatory line from the tragus to the corner of the mouth. The last incision, if a connection to the marginal ramus is provided, lies beyond the facial artery over and near the angle of the mandible (Fig. 24-8).

For the *orbicularis oculi function* a 15 to 17 cm long piece of the sural graft is passed through the superior border of the orbicularis muscle of both sides (Fig. 24-9). This procedure can be performed after the tissue is tunneled with a blunt pricker from the small midline incision previously described toward the incision in the lateral

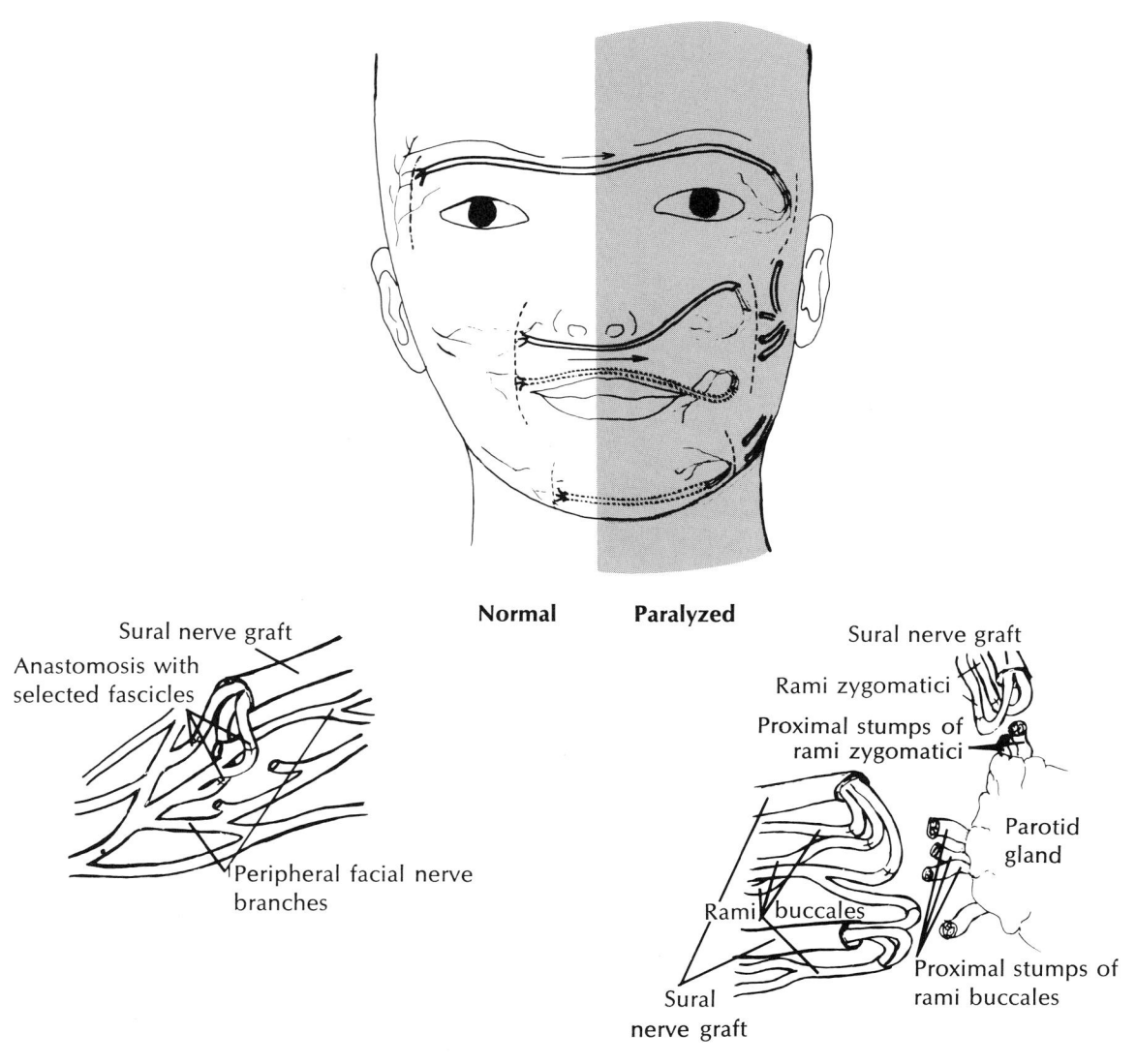

Fig. 24-8. Sketch of incision lines on healthy and paralyzed sides of face *(dashed lines)* and sural graft position. *Dotted lines* of grafts indicate possibility of exchange. Drawings outside the face demonstrate form of anastomoses.

Reanimation of the paralyzed face

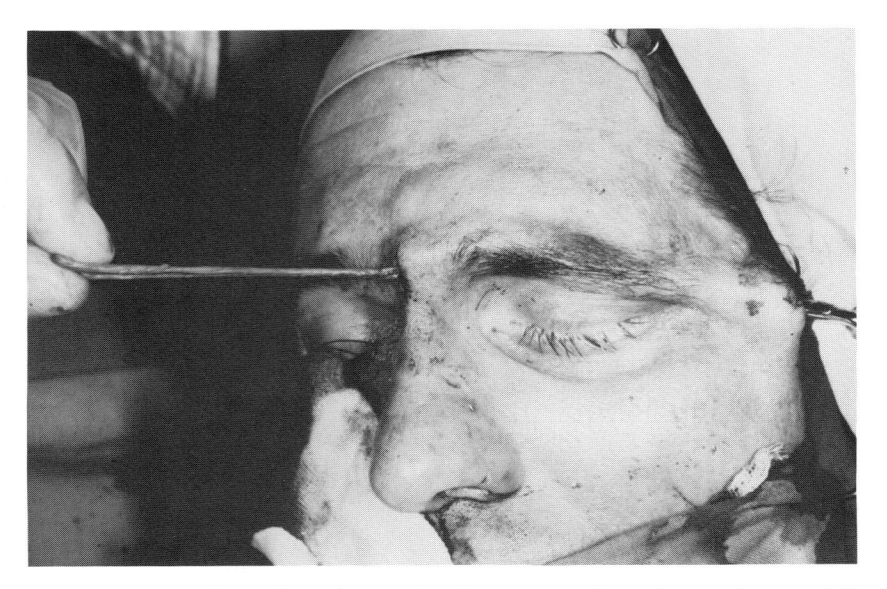

Fig. 24-9. Implanting of sural graft in orbital area. Graft is drawn from midline incision toward incision near zygomatic arch.

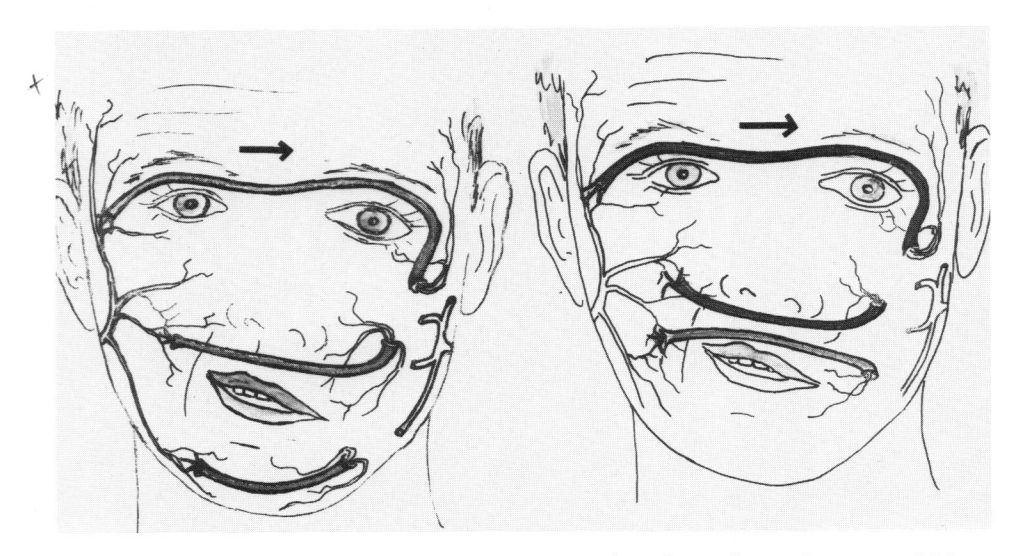

Fig. 24-10. Sketch shows variety of positioning of grafts in buccal or mandible area. *Arrow* indicates axon growth from healthy to paralyzed side of face.

healthy eye region where the prepared facial fascicles are ready for severing and anastomosis. The end of the graft is fixed on the instrument and drawn out in the midline. From here again the end of the graft is drawn through a tunnel in the direction of the incision near the zygomatic arch of the paralyzed face where the instrument was introduced. For better identification the end of the graft should be marked with a colored thread that is led out of the skin and cut neatly with the cutaneous surface (Fig. 24-7).

Cross-face nerve grafting—up to 12 months of seventh nerve disruption

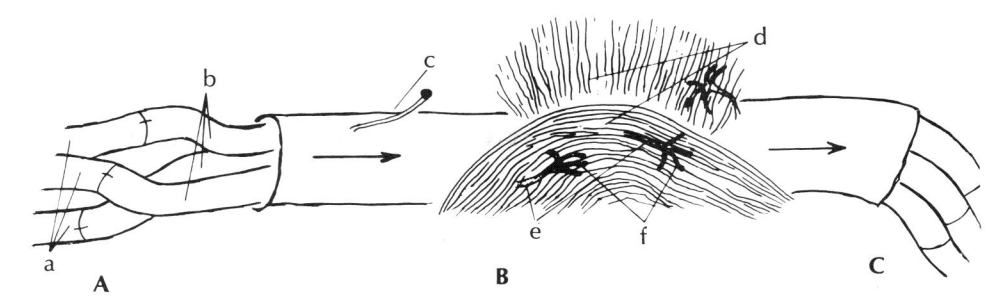

Fig. 24-11. Sketch of anatomical direction of suralis nerve, frontalis muscle, and orbicularis muscle bilaterally transplanted through face. **A,** Side of healthy anastomoses. **B,** Graft. **C,** Anastomoses on paralyzed side of face. *a,* Intact facial fascicles; *b,* fascicles of the suralis transplant; *c,* cutaneous branch of the transplant with small neuroma; *d,* frontalis and orbicularis oculi muscles; *e,* "cutaneous" branch of sural transplant ingrown in the muscles; *f,* budding axons with reinnervated and newly formed motor end plates; *g,* ramus zygomaticus → anatomical direction.

For the *lip and cheek* musculature one or two sural nerve grafts 13 to 15 cm long must be implanted. The number of grafts depends on whether there are enough facial fascicles available for anastomosis in this area and on how many and how thick the fascicles are in the sural nerve (Fig. 24-10). From the auxiliary incision in the midline the orbicularis muscle is tunneled twice (for each graft) toward the incision line in the healthy buccal area. The upper graft lies near the columella, the other near the lip margin. The ends are positioned with a little excess of length near the selected intact fascicles. From the incisions on the paralyzed buccal area the pricker is inserted twice toward the auxiliary incision in the upper lip, forming tunnels. The two ends of the grafts, already available in the midline incision, are drawn in these separate tunnels and marked with colored threads near the parotid gland. It is important that the ends of the grafts should be positioned very far back in the face and not directly in the area where the future anastomoses with the facial branches have to be performed.

If a graft is used in the *chin region,* it should be about 6 to 8 cm long and is inserted also from the midline incision across the face into the chin muscles. The procedure is similar to the one in the zygomatic and buccal region. Both ends emerge in the incision on the healthy and paralyzed side, as described previously, and are also marked with a thread.

Positioning the grafts is an important feature. They should always be transplanted in their anatomical direction: that means in the original proximal-to-distal course as in the calf (Fig. 24-11) when done so, forward—growing axons can spread from the "cutaneous branches" into the paralyzed muscle, leading to an additional neurotization, and are not lost by forming a neuroma coil. This partial neurotization in the paralyzed muscle can be observed clinically and by EMG.

The number of transplants necessary always depends on whether all sections of the face are to be reinnervated or, as in partial paralysis, only the lid region or the mouth-cheek muscles. In the former case three transplants should be used on an average (Fig. 24-10). If the sural nerve is very thin, even four sural pieces may be necessary. In any

Reanimation of the paralyzed face

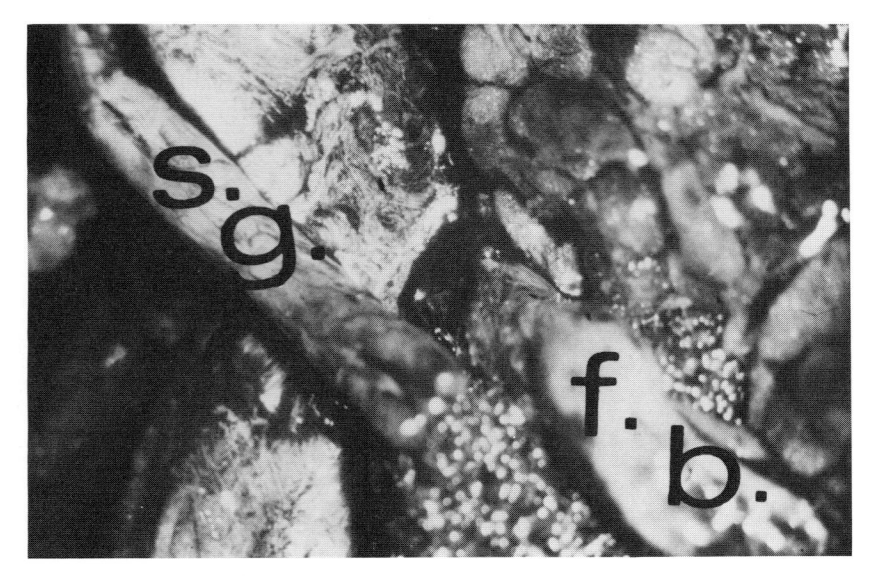

Fig. 24-12. Comparison of size of sural grafts, **s.g.**, and a branch of facial nerve, **f.b.**

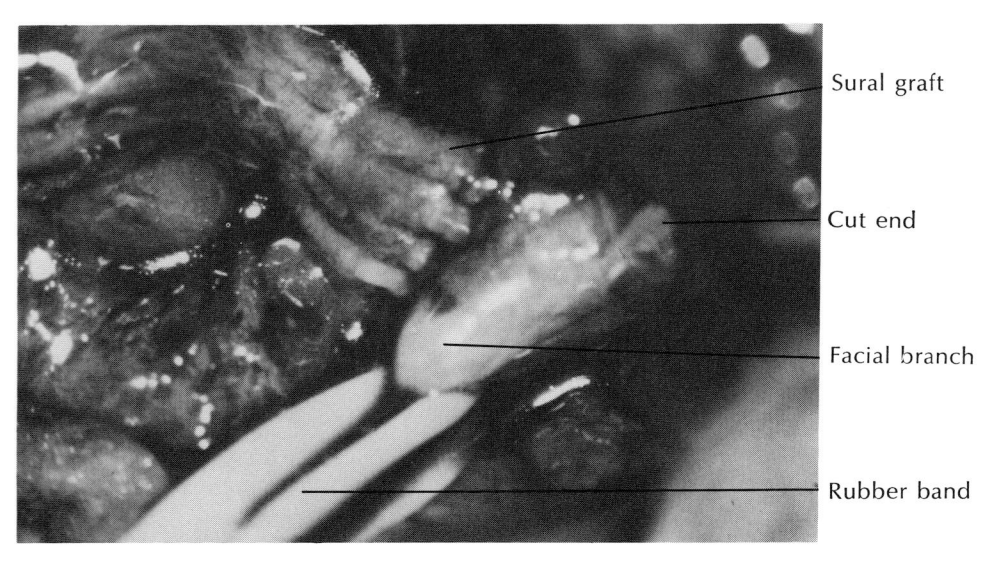

Fig. 24-13. Another comparison with a sural graft (demonstrating four little fascicles) and a thick branch (already severed) of facial nerve. They are nearly the same size.

case as many healthy nerve fibers as possible should be supplied for reinnervation and bud into the paralyzed muscles over the transplants. Comparing the main trunk of the facial nerve with a sural transplant, one can notice a relatively small difference in size in favor of the facial nerve. The question arises whether the cross section of facial nerve or of all its branches respectively are in fact large enough to supply, if occasion arises, three sural transplants without considerable weakening of the healthy supply area. The facial nerve is a predominantly motor nerve with a total of 8000 to 10,000 nerve fibers.[51] After branching off in the parotid, the nerve structure is fascicle-like with very little

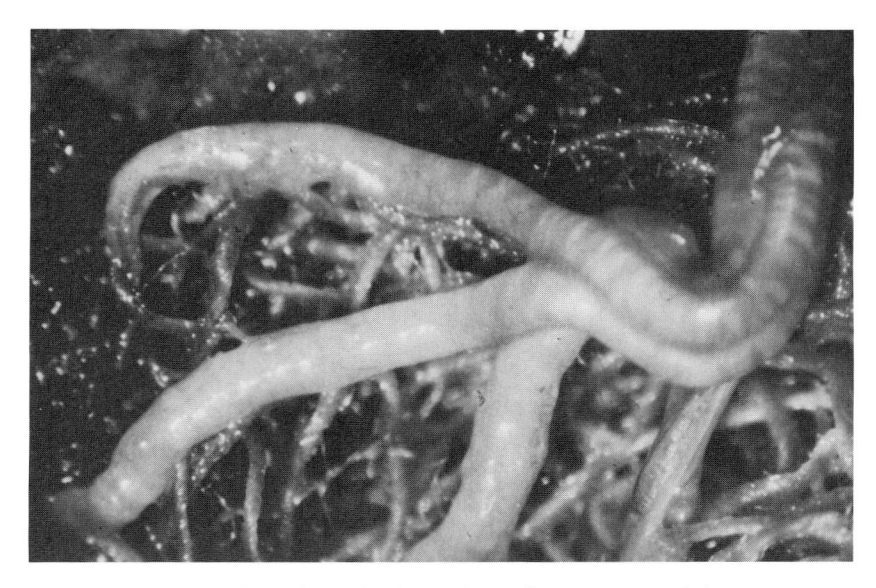

Cross-face nerve grafting—up to 12 months of seventh nerve disruption

Fig. 24-14. End of sural graft with three fascicles separated from each other.

epineural tissue. It is remarkable, however, what larger cross section all main branches of the nerve in a bundle amount to, in contrast to that of the trunk of the facial nerve. Once the abundant epineurium has been removed from a sural transplant, the 2 to 4 purely sensory fascicles are not much larger than one main branch of the facial nerve (Figs. 24-12 and 24-13). Therefore we have never had any difficulties in anastomosing the implanted sural transplants. The possibility of supplying a connection for this number of transplants also guarantees a selective reconstruction, since, if only one or two transplants were used for reanimation of the entire face in interfascicular fiber exchange considerable misinnervations would have to be taken into account. An additional factor favoring regeneration should also be mentioned: the sprouting of multiple processes from each axonal end bulb, a fact that guarantees the producing of a great number of new nerve fibers within a graft after an optimal anastomosis.

CONSTRUCTION OF ANASTOMOSIS

The first stage completes all the anastomoses between the selected intact facial fascicles and the fascicles of the sural grafts. The individual fascicles of the grafts (generally three or four) are separated from each other in a distance of 1 to 2 cm by resection of the epineurium (Fig. 24-14). They are then positioned in a loop in the direction to the little facial nerves so that no tension can occur. After the number and thickness of the sural fascicles is ascertained, an adequate number and size of facial fascicles already prepared must be severed. The selection was described previously (Fig. 24-15).

The nerve suturing is performed with Millesi's technique. For fascicular anastomoses, it is sufficient in most cases to use a single or at the most two perineural sutures with a 10-0 monofilament thread, so that the junction is sufficiently strong and yet allows the draining plasma to act as a glue to make the relaxed adjacent nerve endings adhere to each other (Fig. 24-16). *The most important point is to attain complete freedom from tension.* Sheaths of Millipore,[15] collagen tubes,[12,16] or silicone cylinders,[20,48,49] did not prove satisfactory, since these foreign bodies casused increased scarring with

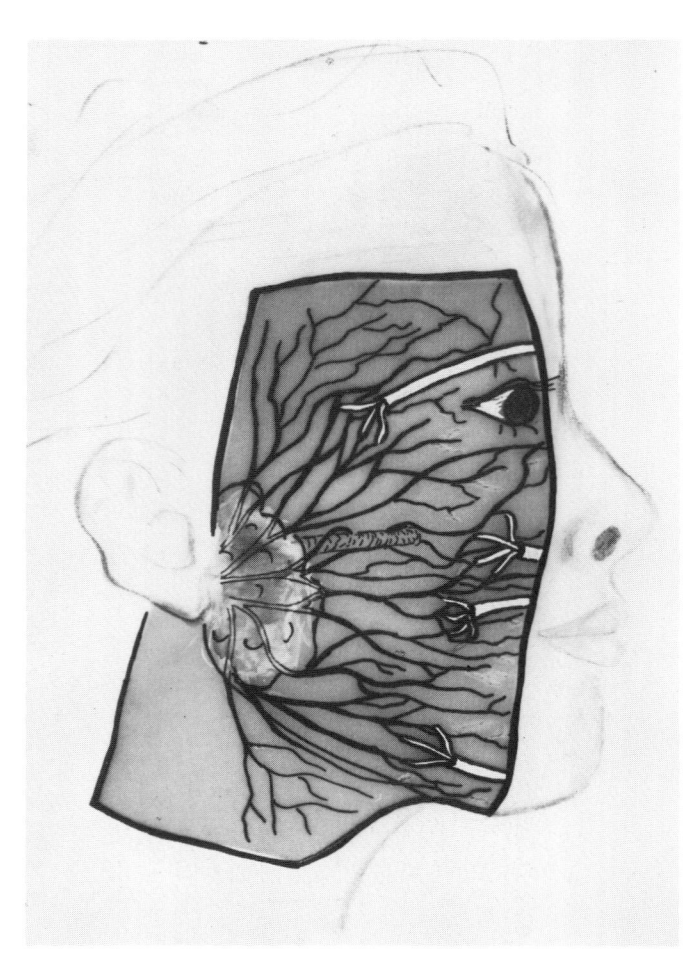

Fig. 24-15. Sketch of ramification of facial nerve (after Fujita, 1934) and anastomoses of sural transplants on healthy side of face.

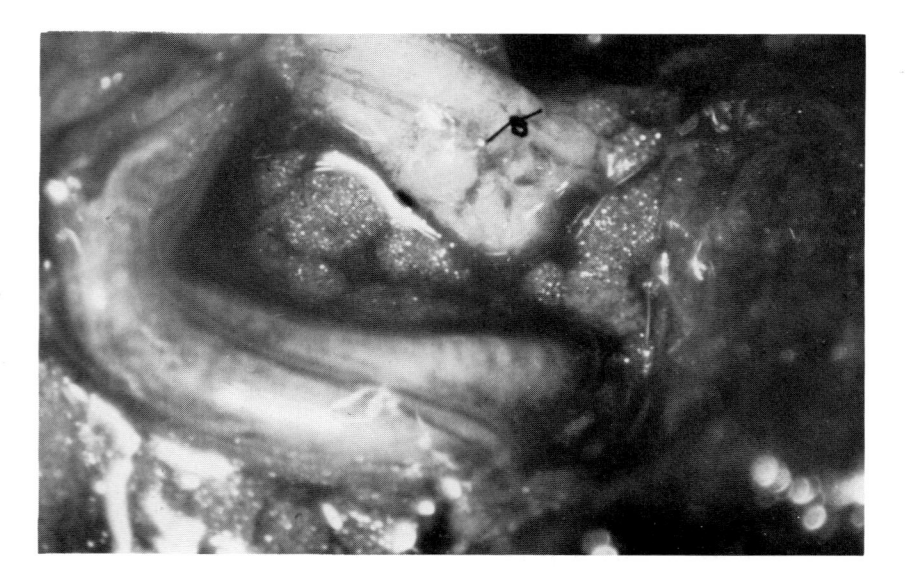

Fig. 24-16. Tension-free anastomoses of sural fascicles are situated in a loop with fascicles of facial nerve. One single suture is visible; the other sutures lie somewhat deeper.

strangulation interrupting axon budding. These methods were therefore discontinued.[9,16] (For further comments on nerve sutures see the Chapter by Millesi.)

After the suturing under the microscope has been performed with a magnification of 15 to 20, the sutures are covered with surrounding fat, which is fixed with thin catgut sutures. A small drain is inserted and the wound is closed.

Second operative stage

Four to 5 months later, the axons should have sprouted through the transplants across the face. This interval is chosen by experience of axon flow, which proceeds 1 to 3 mm a day.[64] The EMG might detect action potential along the sural graft signaling the progress of axon budding.

After careful general preoperative measures similar to the first stage, the operation is performed under general anesthesia and intubation. The incisions are made over the zygomatic arch in the direction to the lateral orbit, another 4 cm incision is made in a bow within the minimum tension lines of the skin in front of the parotid gland, and, if necessary, an incision over the mandible (Fig. 24-2). Another approach is by a face-lifting incision with extension submandibularly (Fig. 24-2). The skin is folded back and fixed with threads. The marking threads on the end of the grafts appear just under the skin surface (Fig. 24-7). The stumps of the sural nerve transplants can now be dissected out of the surrounding tissue. There should be thickening on their ends representing fibrous tissue and amputation neuromas, demonstrating the success of axon growth along the transplants (Fig. 24-17). Thus there is an additional criterion for proceeding to the second-stage procedure, since the presence of nerve fibers will guarantee regeneration of the facial nerve after suturing. The fascicles of the sural nerve transplants are separated again for a length of 1 to 2 cm, and one can see under the microscope which fascicle has formed a neuroma. In case of doubt a frozen section of each fascicle will demonstrate if enough nerve fibers are present. The sural fascicles are left long until the branches of the facial nerve are dissected.

The main fascial branches can be found best as they leave the parotid gland. Since we cannot use electrostimulation, one can only rely on anatomical features, and the branches should be found as it has been described previously in the anatomy. Following one buccal branch into the parotid gland, one meets other bigger buccal and zygomatic branches. If the division of the marginal branch is immediately proximal, exposure should be made in the area of the facial artery over the mandible. All facial branches that can be seen should be taken for connection and severed very deeply in the parotid gland. They are then dissected distally, including all divisions to the neighboring fascicles. The stumps are swung back and are brought near the corresponding endings of the sural grafts. If one facial fascicle nerve branch has a thicker size, it can be split into two fascicles to have a better match with the endings of the sural fascicles (Figs. 24-18 and 24-19). The anastomoses are performed in the same way as on the normal side of the face, using one or two sutures and no tension.

The suture lines are covered with surrounding fat tissue, the operating field is swabbed with an antibiotic solution, small drains are inserted, and the wound is closed with atraumatic stitches. A very light pressure bandage is applied. The extubation must be done very carefully without squeezing the cheek and pulling the lips. The surgeon should be present to supervise the maneuver.

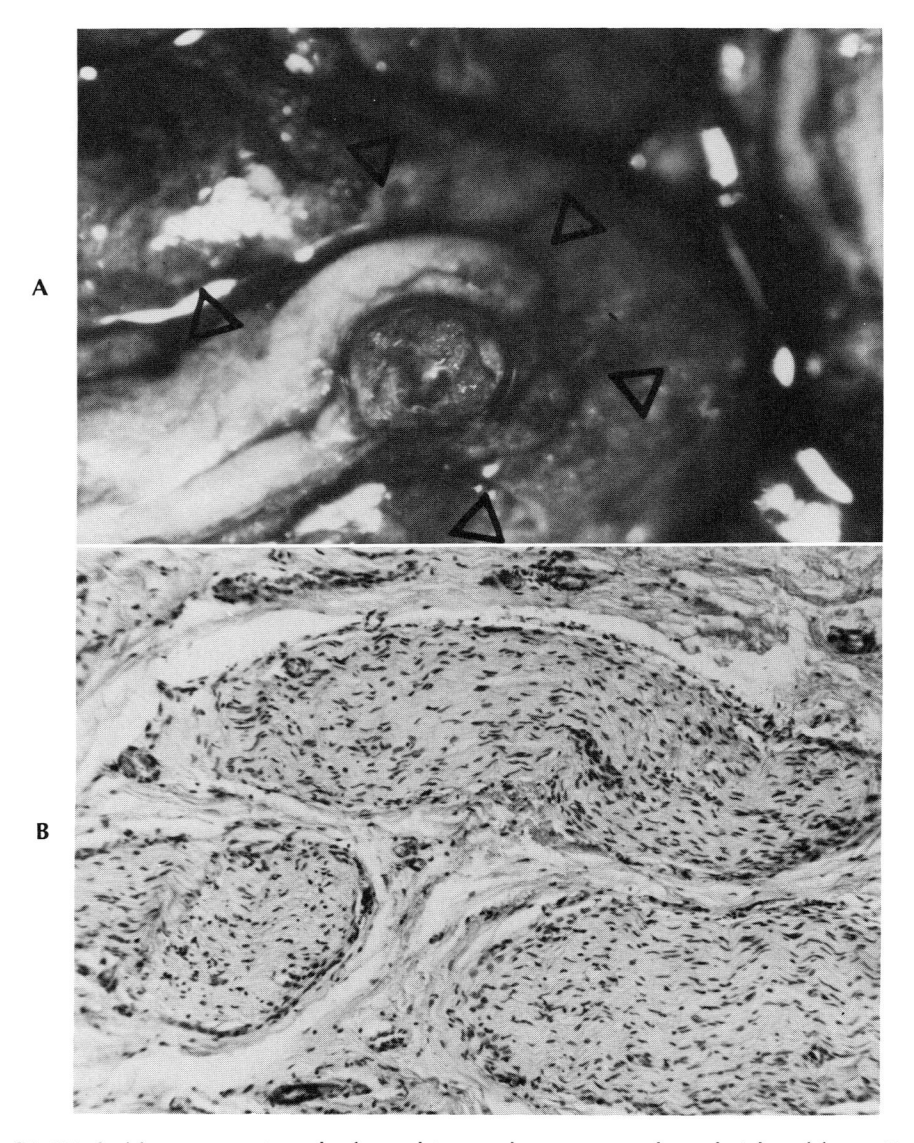

Fig. 24-17. A, Neuroma at end of sural transplant on paralyzed side of face. **B,** Histological picture of neuroma of **A.** Entwined nerve fibre bundles and connective tissue. (Hematoxylin and eosin, 100×; courtesy Dr. Albin Propst, Innsbruck, Austria.)

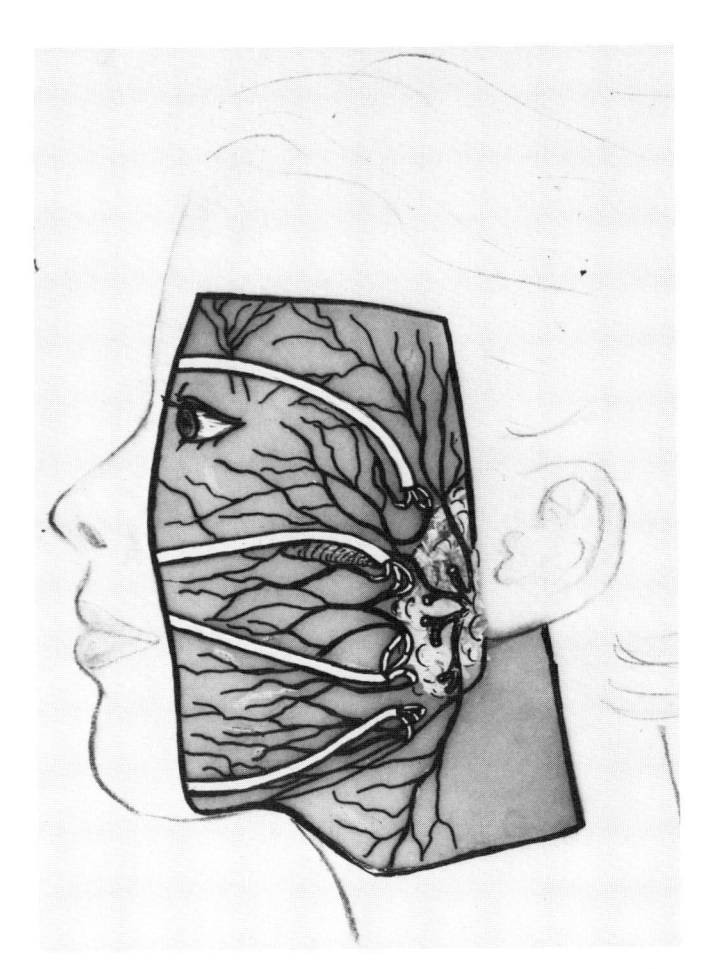

Fig. 24-18. Sketch of ramification of facial nerve and anastomoses of sural transplants on paralyzed face.

Reanimation of the paralyzed face

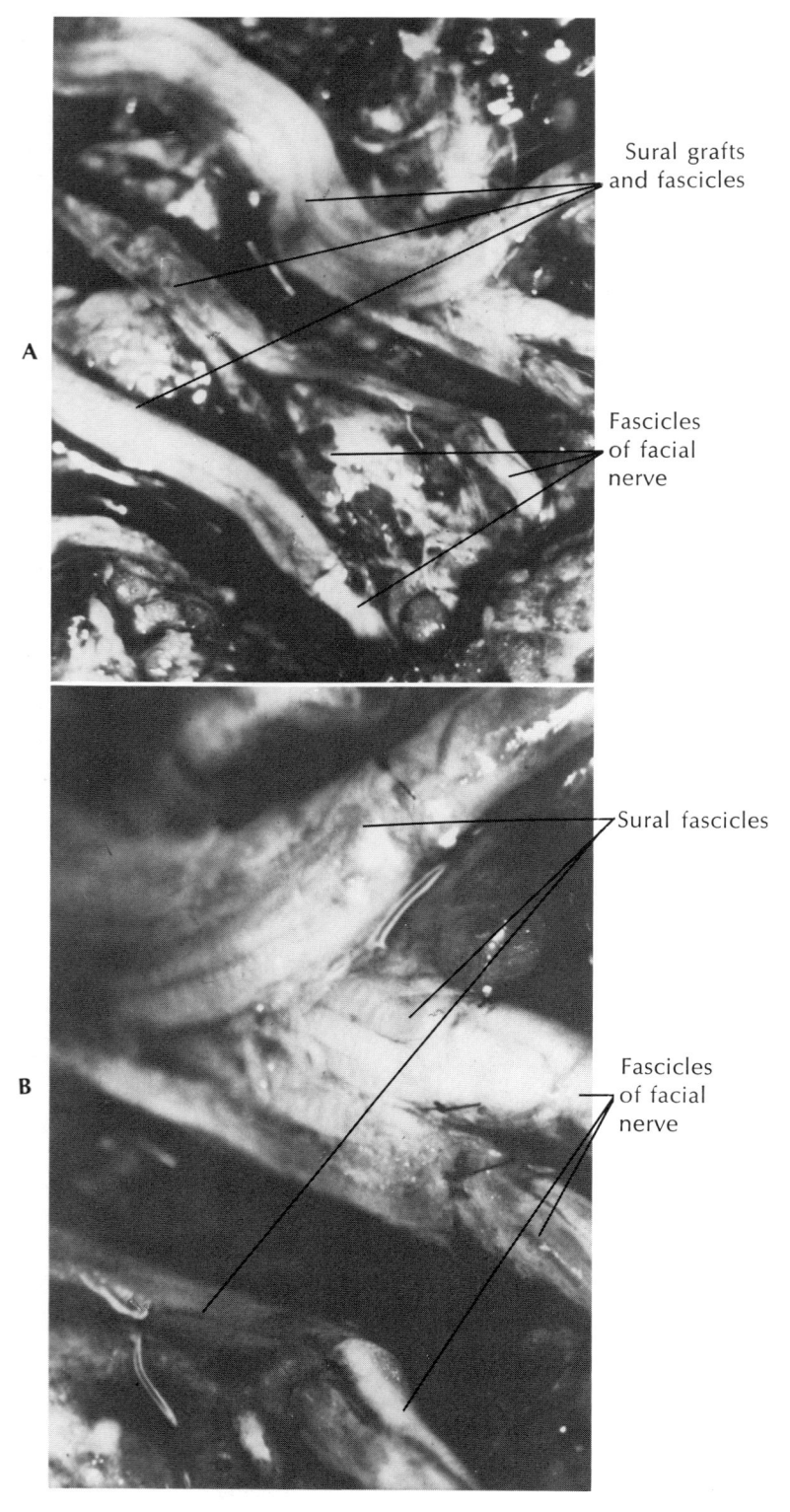

Fig. 24-19. A, Sural grafts and their fascicles and anastomoses with main branches of facial nerve. **B,** Section of **A** with anastomoses and higher magnification (about 20×).

Beside this optimal way of nerve anastomoses there might be cases, especially in the periorbital region, where the branches of the zygomatic ramus cannot be found. This may happen in small children or in the presence of scarring. In such a situation a direct neuromuscular innervation, as a result of the implantation of the distal nerve transplant into the muscle can be tried. For this purpose the ends of the sural graft is split and the epineurium is completely removed, so that the little fascicles are isolated. The fascicles are cut steplike and obliquely and implanted into the muscle that was pulled apart by blunt dissection before. The epineurium of the nerve is fixed then on the muscle with 8-0 nylon sutures. This ingrowth of axons with generating new end plates of reinnervating old ones is based on experimentation and clinical experience.[1,24,34,36,40,68] The same process also occurs in the axon budding out of the "cutaneous branches" of the graft as it has already been described.

Postoperative care and rehabilitating measures

The patient will receive antibiotics for 1 week and should have only liquid nutrition for the first days. He should not speak and is isolated alone in a room to eliminate temptation of doing so. There is no pain and narcotics are not needed. The drainage is removed after 2 days, the compression bandage after 5 days, and the stitches after 7 days. After 14 days electrophysiotherapy is started and is continued three times a week with exponential current at a strength of 20 to 60 milliamperes, with each group of muscles receiving a 2 to 3 minute dosage. The value of electrotherapy in retarding advancing muscle atrophy is still disputed.[35,38,42,43,73,80] However, the blood flow in the muscle is aided positively, and it helps to eliminate metabolic substances.[72] Therefore this measure, in addition to physiokinetic exercises before the mirror after the first signs of reinnervation, seems to me completely rational.

Application of cross-face nerve grafting

The main application is to reinnervate the paralyzed muscles within a certain period of time while the muscles are still capable of regeneration.

COMBINATIVE POSSIBILITIES

Free muscle transplantation for functional amelioration in permanent facial paralysis is discussed in Chapter 27. The following pages deal with combinative possibilities of the cross-face nerve grafting with myoplastic surgical methods. The following techniques, too recent to offer a substantial evaluation, must be mentioned as being a further potential in the future treatment of facial paresis:

1. Combination of cross-face nerve graft with a free muscle transplant
2. Combination of a cross-face nerve graft with transposed masseter or temporal muscles
3. Free muscle transplant and microvascular anastomosis as well as nerve connection to a cross-face nerve graft

Obviously no natural mimic function can be regained by the above methods. It is to be considered, however, an improvement in treatment insofar as the trigeminal nerve (fifth nerve) innervation to the masseter and temporalis muscles is now replaced by the facial nerve of the healthy normal opposite side of the face. Thus untoward facial movements caused by chewing movements (fifth nerve) are eliminated. For example,

Reanimation of the paralyzed face

mouth functions, necessitating opening or lifting or drawing sidewise when speaking or eating, need no longer be activated by an innervation stimulus of the trigeminal nerve but rather by a physiological function impulse of the facial nerve coming from the opposite side.

Combination of cross-face nerve graft with a free muscle transplant. In this combination of a free muscle graft connected to a supplying nerve from the end of a nerve graft fed by the healthy facial nerve of the opposite side, the transplanted muscle is no longer innervated by a nerve from the adjacent muscle fibers. The extensor digitorum brevis of the foot has proved to serve best in this procedure as described by Thompson. Here again, the first step to transplantation is a denervation of the muscle about 2 weeks prior to being moved. This denervation is performed in a place relatively proximal above the talocalcaneal joint in order to produce the long nerve stalk. The place of severance is marked with a colored thread for the second operation. (See Fig. 24-20.)

The extensor digitorum brevis consisting of several muscle sections can be used for lid closure and cheek function as described by Millesi and Samii.[55a] In this method, the extensor digitorum brevis of each foot is first denervated and then transplanted freely to the paralyzed half of the face. At the surgeon's disposal are a total of eight muscle sections, four of which are tightly attached to the zygomatic arch; two muscle sectors and their tendons, respectively, are led to the root of the nose along the free upper and lower lid margins where they are anchored in the periosteum; two muscle extensions and their tendons, respectively, are led to the right corner of the mouth and fixed there; four muscle extensions of the other extensor digitorum brevis (of the second foot) are implanted in the region of the upper and lower lips in the right cheek, with two tendons

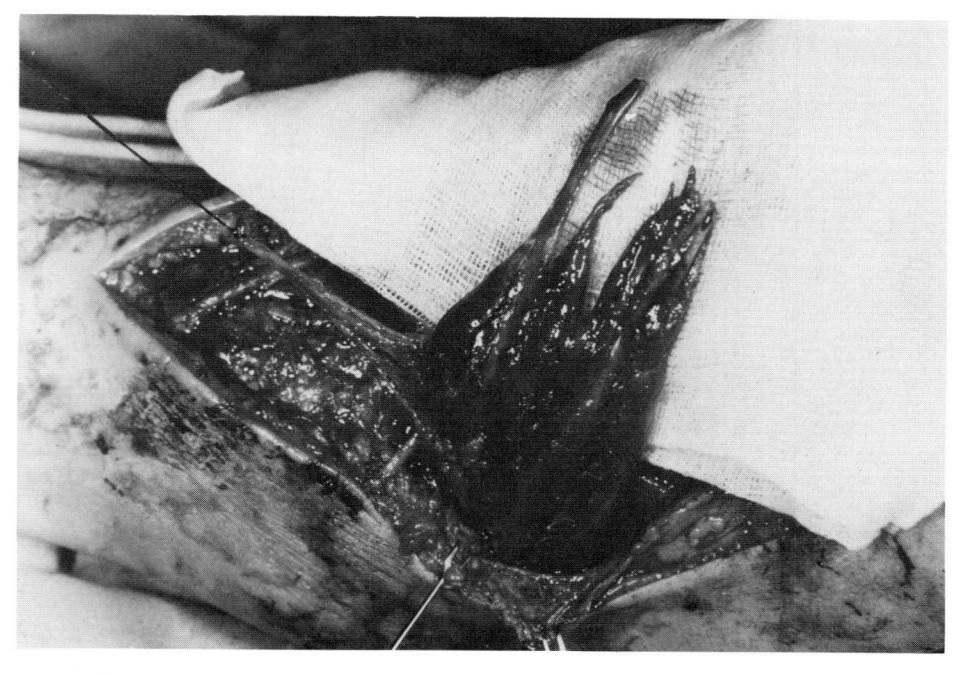

Fig. 24-20. Dissected extensor digitorum brevis muscle with tendons and the supplying nerve (left side with a thread).

Cross-face nerve grafting—up to 12 months of seventh nerve disruption

being anchored to the zygomatic arch and one in the center of both upper and lower lips, respectively.

The two muscles in the region of the lids close the lids when contracted. The remaining six muscles serve to activate the cheek as well as the upper and lower lips. The nerves leading to the muscles are connected with two sural grafts, which are first tunneled diagonally into the upper lip and connected with the fascicles of the healthy facial nerve of the other side of the face. The nerve transplant to the muscles in the zygomatic region must have a length of about 11 cm, the one leading to the cheek of about 8 cm. By this method, a functional amelioration in the lid and mouth regions of a 6-year-old boy was obtained after a one-sided congenital facial paralysis.

The combination of cross-face nerve grafting and free muscle transplantation in our experience applies only to the dynamic suspension of the cheek or lip.[6,36] Four months before the intended muscle transfer, a sural nerve graft is tunneled through the upper lip and connected with three or four fascicles from the rami buccales on the healthy side. The end of the nerve graft is marked with a thread in the vicinity of the nasolabial fold of the paralyzed side and deposited subcutaneously. The muscle of the entire extensor

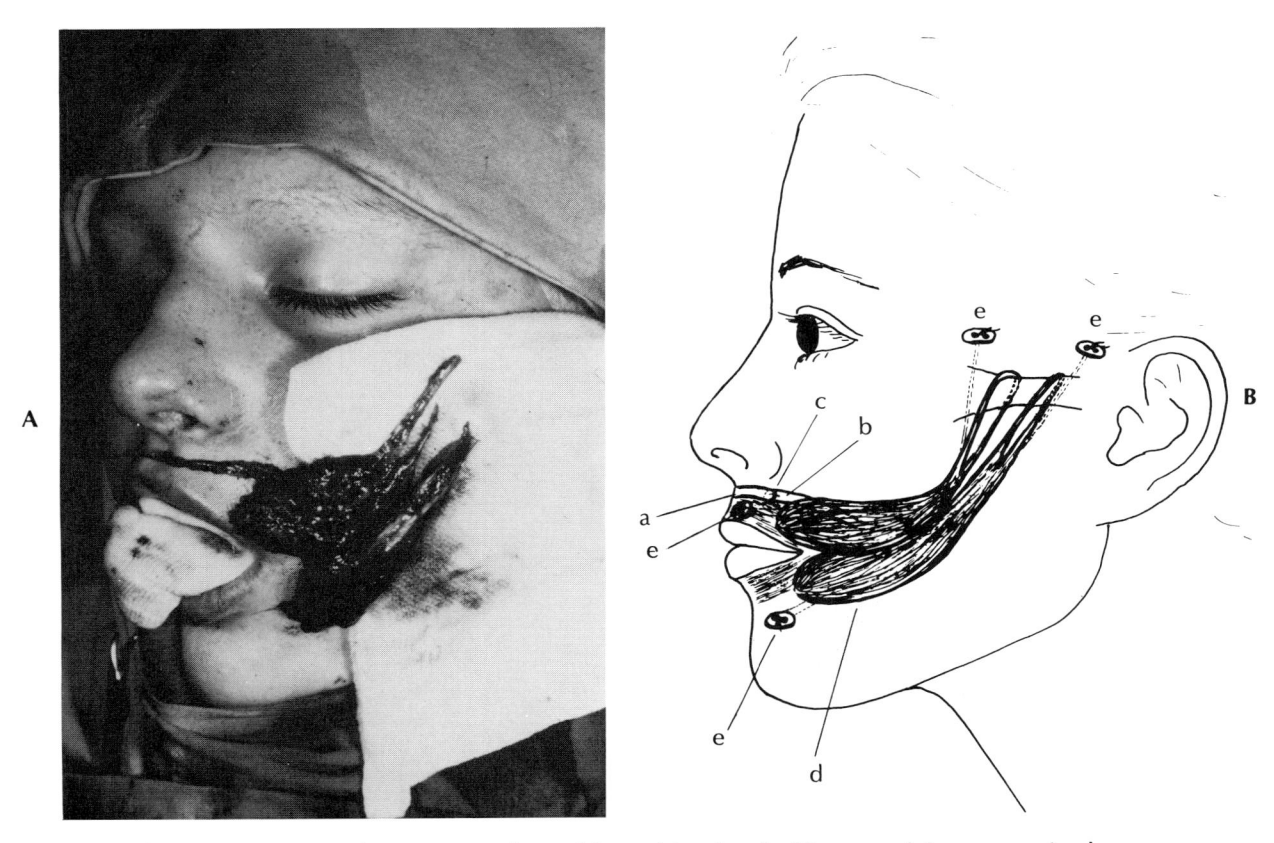

Fig. 24-21. A, Muscle-nerve graft positioned in cheek. The supplying nerve is shown in upper lip. **B,** Sketch showing extensor digitorum brevis, *d,* to zygomatic arch and corner of mouth. *a,* Sural nerves transplanted through upper lip being anastomosed, *c,* with nerve from extensor digitorum brevis, *b.* Through-and-through sutures attached through skin over buttons, *e.*

Reanimation of the paralyzed face

digitorum brevis denervated 2 weeks previously together with the supplying nerve is transposed into the cheek after the skin of the face is lifted by preauricular incision (a method used in face-lifting) and an auxiliary incision is made in the nasolabial fold. The muscle is then sewn into the commissure of the orbicularis oris. The free ends of the tendon are slung over the zygomatic arch and fixed in the tension required. The cross-face nerve graft is anastomosed with the nerve leading to the mouth (Fig. 24-21). Should a further lifting of the corner of the mouth be necessary after reinnervation of the muscle, one can perform the tightening process by shortening the tendons of the zygomatic arch. The cross-face operation must be done several months before the nerve graft to avoid muscle atrophy.

The methods described above have two disadvantages. First a rather voluminous muscle graft has to be transplanted, which causes a thickening of the cheek, and sec-

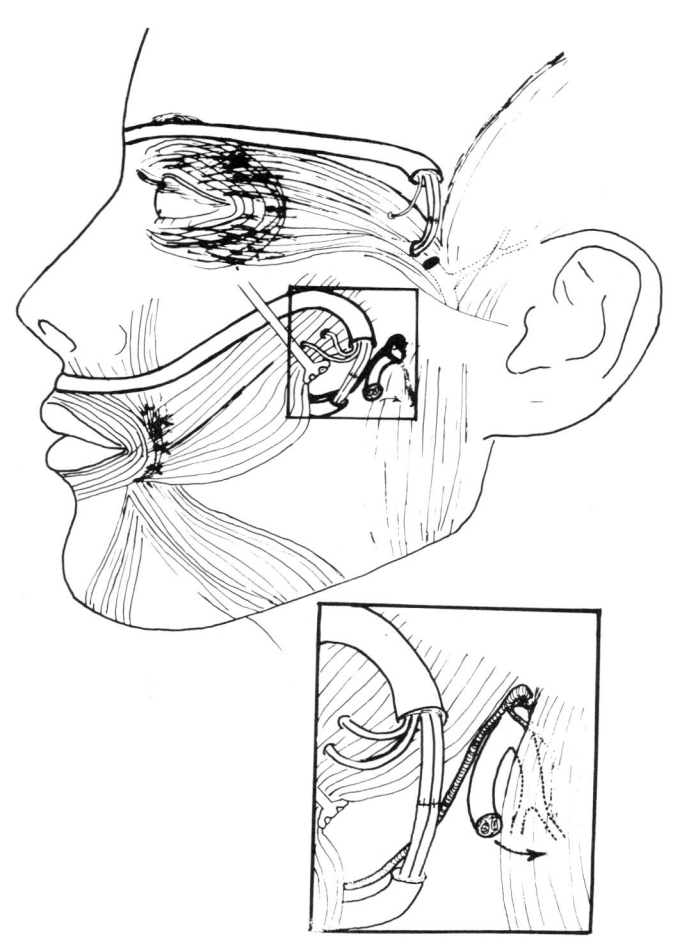

Fig. 24-22. Transposition of part of temporal muscle for eyelid function and masseter muscle for lifting paralyzed mouth. *Smaller drawing,* Anastomoses with sural nerve from healthy facial nerve of opposite face and part of masseteric nerve are shown. If masseter nerve is too small, two fascicles of sural nerve should be inserted into muscle itself. Cut end of masseteric nerve is put into remaining part of masseteric muscle. Nutrifying vessel is not damaged.

Cross-face nerve grafting—up to 12 months of seventh nerve disruption

ond, the muscle function is rather weak because of the fibrosis of the central muscle tissue caused by inadequate nourishment.

Combination of a cross-face nerve graft with transposed masseter or temporal muscles. By including muscles existent in the face for myoplastic operations, one can eliminate loss or the destruction of muscle fibers to a high degree. Motor power is supplied by the temporalis or masseter muscle, both being fed by the trigeminal nerve.

Freilinger[36] gives an account of the transposition of the central portion of the temporalis muscle into the corner of the paralyzed mouth with denervation of the said muscle. At the same time a sural nerve transplant is tunneled through the upper lip and anastomosed electively to the buccal ramus of the healthy facial nerve. The other end of this nerve graft is implanted directly into the transposed temporalis muscle. By direct neuromuscular innovation, a good lifting of the corner of the mouth in symmetry was noticed 6 months later in a patient.

In our method[5] the cross-nerve graft principle is combined with the muscle transposition of the temporalis and masseter muscles. Thus lid closure as well as the active lifting of the corner of the mouth independent of the innervation by the trigeminal nerve is effected.

According to the method described before in this chapter a sural nerve graft is transposed for the orbicular region and connected to the rami zygomatici of the healthy side by some fascicles. At the same time a graft is transplanted into the upper lip to provide muscle function. It is connected to three or four fascicles of healthy rami buccales. The nerve endings are deposited in the parotid region of the paralyzed side and marked. Four to 5 months later, the anterior portion of the temporalis muscle is split into two slips, threaded through the upper and lower lids, and fixed at the medial canthus. The deep temporal leading to the transposed muscle nerve is severed and connected to the

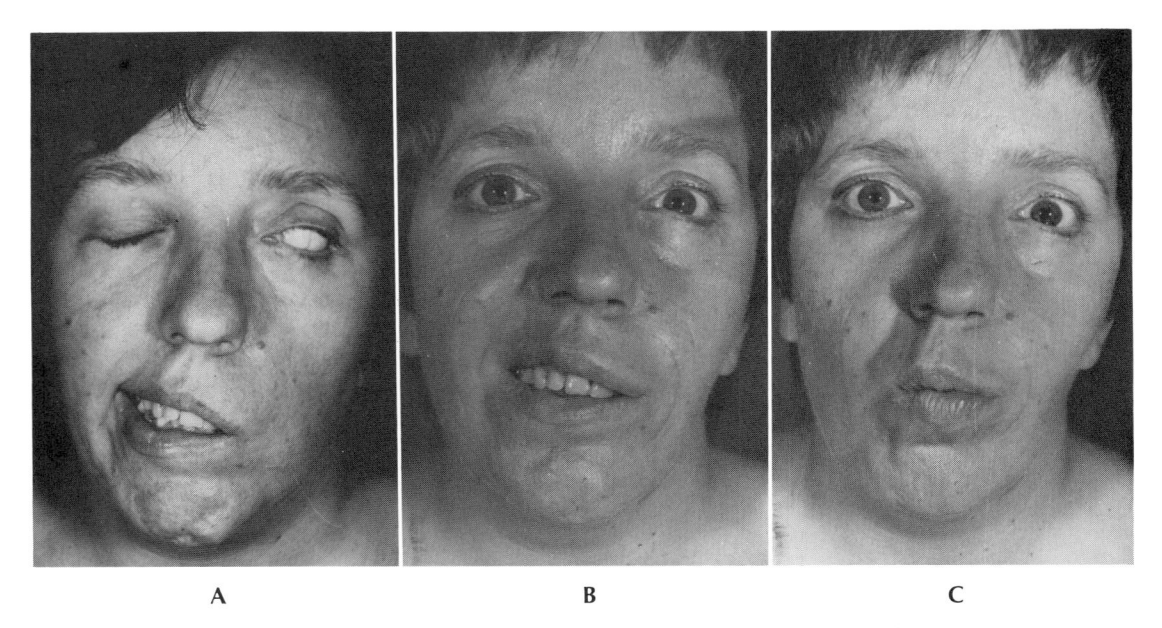

Fig. 24-23. A, Patient with long-standing facial paralysis. **B** and **C,** Same patient after masseter transposition, with good functional result, about half a year after operation.

end of the sural transplant fed by branches of the ramus zygomaticus from the healthy side.

In a similar fashion, the anterior portion of the masseter muscle is moved to the corner of the mouth where it is fixed to the commissure. The masseteric nerve serving the muscle is severed and connected to the end of the cross-face nerve graft coming from the healthy buccal branches. In one patient, we have noticed symmetry and good lifting of the corner of the mouth independent of chewing muscles (Figs. 24-22 and 24-23).

Free muscle transplant and microvascular anastomosis as well as nerve connection to a cross-face nerve graft. This method should be mentioned since both procedures can be performed separately. Harii et al. in 1976[39a] transplanted the gracilis muscle into the cheek and then passed it between the corner of the mouth and the temporal fascia. The muscle transplant was anastomosed to the temporal vessels and its nerve to the deep temporal nerve. Good function was obtained in two patients. Instead of anastomosing the graft to the trigeminal nerve, they could have connected it to a sural graft previously placed and joined with the branches of the buccal nerve on the healthy side. This would have given the patient more physiological movement in those cases where the facial nerve and muscles were absent on one side.

INDICATION

The reinnervation of the paralyzed facial muscles from healthy opposite facial nerves by means of the cross-face nerve transplantation effectuates a new method that allows a direct regeneration of the paralyzed face nerves. It must be stressed, however, that all other possibilities to restore the interrupted course of the facial nerve must be tried before nerve restitution in this way is to be considered. As previously stated, some patients have to put up with permanent paralysis despite the good results of modern facial surgery. Among these patients are cases of permanent palsy caused by idiopathic paralysis (about 10% of the patients show signs of "no recovery" after complete paresis[51]), paralysis caused by herpes zoster, or paresis after extensive tumor resection with extensive x-ray therapy. Beside medical problems concerned with the nerve itself, psychosocial problems, age of the patient, and his general condition must be taken into account. A 50-year-old patient in good physical condition can have the cross-face operation even if the regeneration of the nerve cannot be expected to grow to such extent as in younger patients.[64] In the coming years and in experience gained by recent methods, indications for many special surgical interventions will stand out even more clearly.

As of this time, the treatment of partial facial paralysis with this method is questionable. If a main branch of the facial nerve is paralyzed with impaired muscle function, one might be encouraged to try a selective graft for regeneration from the healthy side. However, the danger of an additional injury to facial branches must be considered. Relative indications might be mass movements after regeneration, serious facial spasm, or tic. In those cases, the branches of the facial nerve in the affected area of the face are severed completely and connected to the selected nerve fibers transplanted from the healthy side.

EMG is of great importance for verifying the results after cross-face nerve transplantation. Applying a direct stimulation to the facial nerve stem of the former para-

Cross-face nerve grafting—up to 12 months of seventh nerve disruption

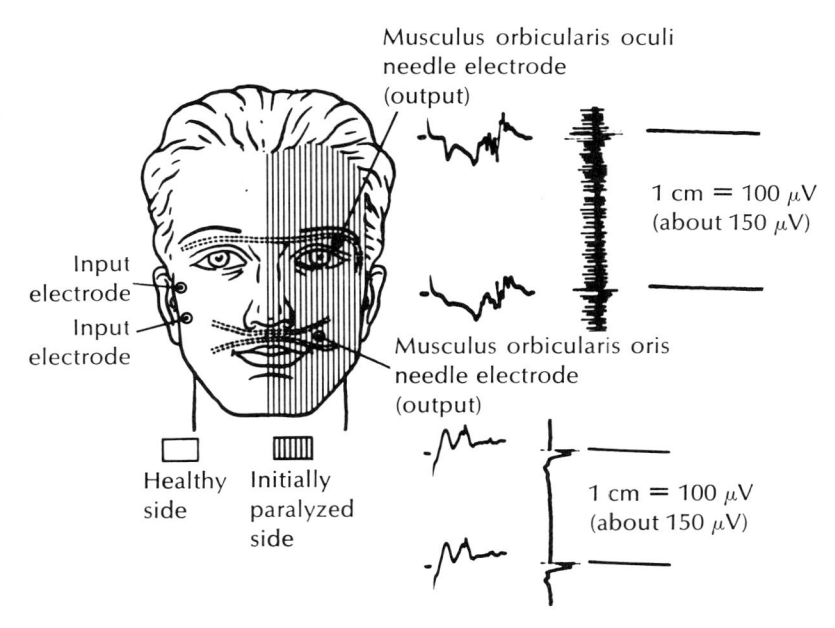

Fig. 24-24. Deflection of excitability response potential from the orbicularis oculi and oris muscles during electrical stimulation of facialis stem on healthy side. In both muscles, response potential is still low and clearly desynchronized.

lyzed face shows no response in the muscles. On the contrary, if the facial nerve stem on the healthy side of the face is stimulated, a good response by action potential from the originally paralyzed muscle shows conduction through the transplants and muscle reinnervation (Fig. 24-24). The registration of this conduction from the healthy face may not be possible by clinical observation because the excitability of the normal facial nerve is much higher and one cannot apply strong impulses to induce contraction on the opposite face, because of too much pain for the patient. By help of EMG one may find other sources of regeneration, such as fibers from the trigeminus or nerves from the contralateral side by means of a nerve graft.

The first signs of nerve regeneration can be detected by muscle activity along the transplant several weeks after the first operation using the EMG. The presence of a neuroma on the transplant ending about 4 to 5 months later is a further criterion of axon budding and allows a positive estimation for prognosis.

RESULTS

Our results are based on 15 patients who were treated with cross-face nerve transplantation since 1971. Table 2 shows the distribution of cause of paralysis, age and sex, and intervals between trauma and operation, as well as time of checkup after operation, respectively. The exact standards of results after facial restoration are far more difficult than in the other skeletal muscles. In the face we cannot use systems of grading expressing the motor function with numbers from 0 to 5. The emotional expression guaranteed by the coordinated innervation of the various facial muscle groups is more a subjective one, and we can record only tonus, symmetry, lid closure, and special

Reanimation of the paralyzed face

Table 2. Types of facial paralysis

Diagnosis	Age/sex	Interval (months) Trauma: CFNT (I + II)	Good	Satisfactory	Bad	In recovery	Follow-up (years)
Cerebellar tumor	34 ♀	13 (8 + 5)		X!			½
	6 ♀	18 (12 + 6)		X			3½
	50 ♀	16 (6 + 10)		X!			4½
	47 ♀	16 (10 + 6)		X!			2
	35 ♂	11 (3 + 8)				X	
	35 ♀	48	X (Masseter transplantation + CFNT)				1
Basocranial fracture + decompression	4 ♂	12 (7 + 5)	X				1
	21 ♂	15 (10 + 5)	X				3
	34 ♂	16 (8 + 8)	X				1½
	19 ♀	8				X	
Bell's palsy	32 ♂	14 (10 + 4)	X				4½
	50 ♂	11 years	(Masseter transplantation + CFNT)			X	
Extensive parotid malignancies + irradiation	48 ♂	16 (10 + 6)		X			1½
Radical operation of ear	53 ♂	24			X		5
	18 ♀	15 years			X		4½

CFNT, Cross-face nerve transplantation.
Good, Symmetry, active lifting of the angle of the mouth and cheek, lid closure almost perfect.
Satisfactory, Fair symmetry, cheek tone and slight lifting, lid closure two thirds.
Bad, None or little symmetry, little muscle action, poor lid closure.

movements of mouth and cheek. Despite relatively good muscle contraction, the impression of a natural emotional expression may be absent. The EMG cannot deliver objective conditions in this respect. There could be good muscle potentials detected even though the clinical gain of muscle function is poor. The reason could be, to a great extent, the muscle volume reinnervated. Continuous checking with the EMG after operation may give some hint as to whether reinnervation is progressing (Fig. 24-25).

From the beginning of treatment through the second-stage operation (Figs. 24-26 to 24-30) and a further time of regeneration in the main branches of the paralyzed facial nerve and to the onset of active muscle contraction, tonus can be expected within 7 to 8 months. Our experience shows that the continuity of regeneration takes a very long time and may not even be finished after 3 years.

There is still another observation after nerve transplantation to the facial nerve. Un-

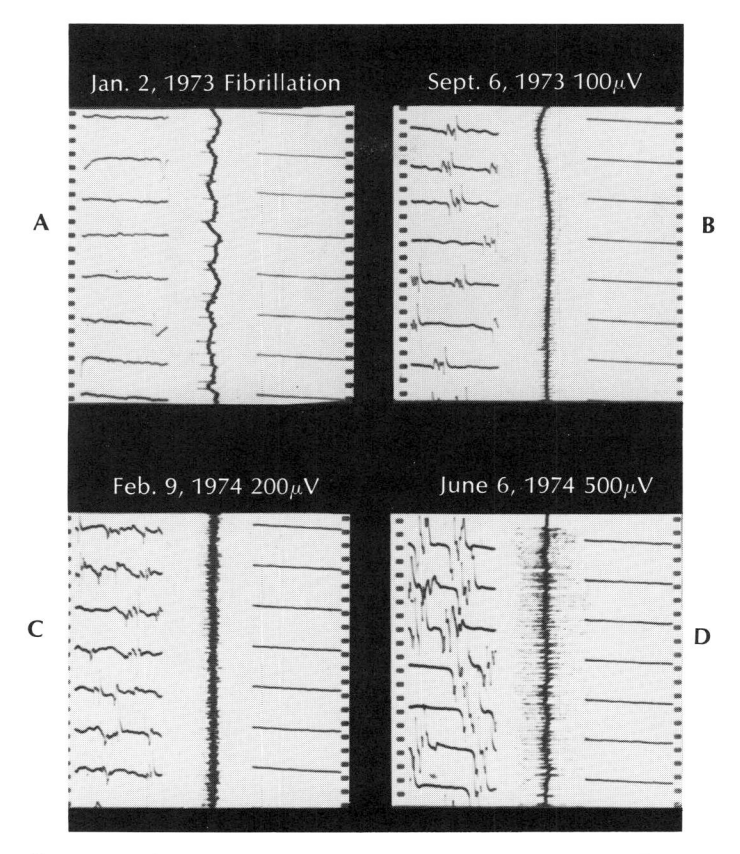

Fig. 24-25. Follow-up after cross-face nerve transplantation with EMG. **A,** Preoperatively good fibrillation potentials can be detected. **B** to **D,** Reinnervation pattern becomes more and more dense.

controlled movements and mass movements of different facial portions occasionally accompany rehabilitation. This manifestation applies especially to more centrally located lesions, and if numerous pathways are available for the budding nerve fibers to follow, the nerve fibers may extend to different facial regions besides the original desired area.

This phenomenon arises less frequently in cross-face nerve transplantation because individual nerve groups with specific innervation areas are connected with each other. What can be noticed, however, is synkinesis of muscle movements of the right and left half of the face. Mostly they refer to the same muscle groups, such that raising of the right healthy corner of the mouth could be accompanied by a movement in the lower eyelid of the paralyzed side. Synchronic movements of the corresponding muscle groups of the face does not appear to trouble the patient. Synkinesis usually disappears more or less to a degree where they are rarely recognizable. This is especially attributable to intensive physiotherapy before the mirror and is based on the experience in extremity muscle regeneration by an increasing subordination of previously defective muscle function to a directed formation of volition.[35]

Generally we must stress the fact that complete restitution of the face to the state before palsy can never be achieved, not even with ipsilateral facial nerve restoration.

Reanimation of the paralyzed face

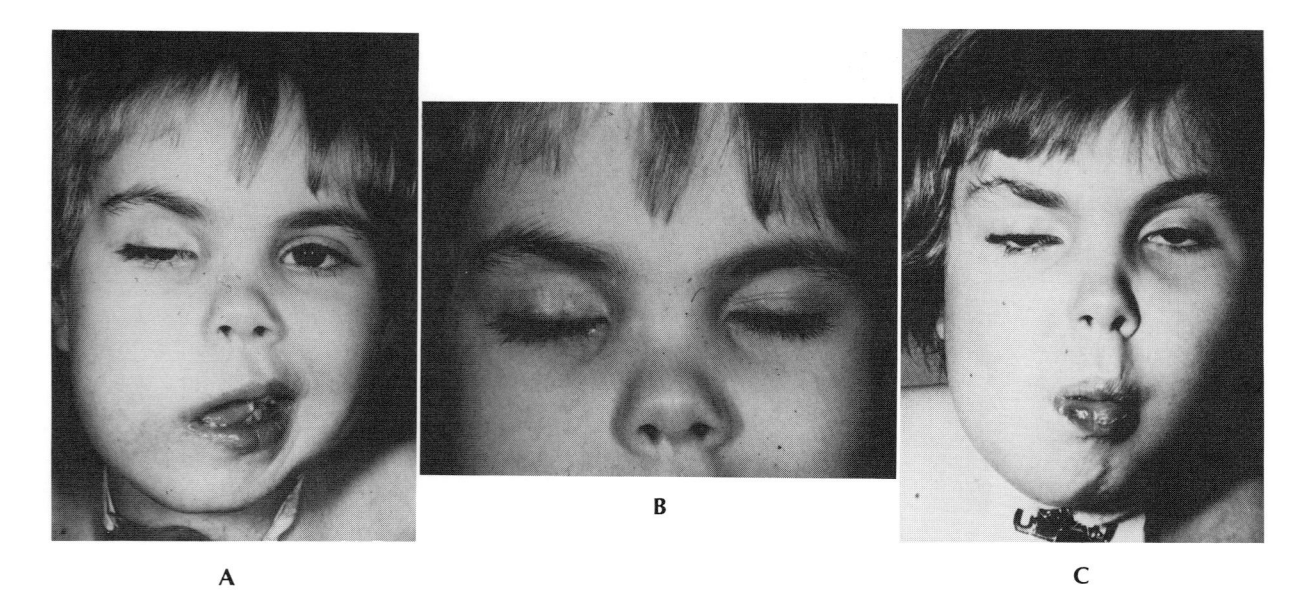

Fig. 24-26. **A,** Six-year-old child after operation of cerebellar tumor. Hypoglossus, glossopharyngeus, and facial palsy of right side of face. Primary lid spring into upper lid. **B,** Three years after operation: one graft in eye region with direct implantation of end of sural nerve into orbicularis oculi; one graft was implanted for restoration of function of mouth and cheek. Good lid closure. **C,** Same patient with relatively good muscle function of mouth. Continuous salivation has disappeared and there are no difficulties in eating.

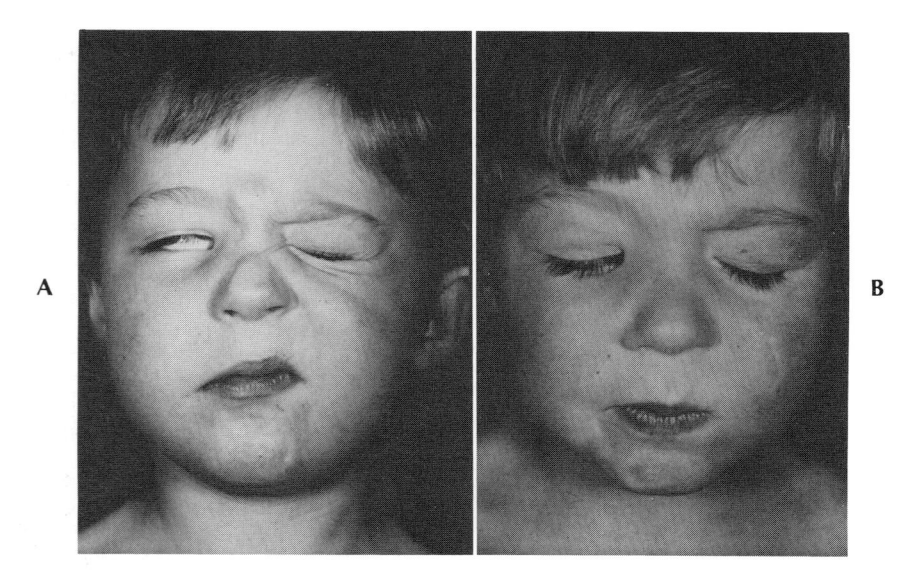

Fig. 24-27. **A,** Four-year-old boy after basocranial fracture and complete facial palsy on right side. **B,** Same patient 1 year after operation. There were implanted two grafts: one in the eye region and one for lip and cheek. Emotional expression just before crying is demonstrated clearly.

Cross-face nerve grafting—up to 12 months of seventh nerve disruption

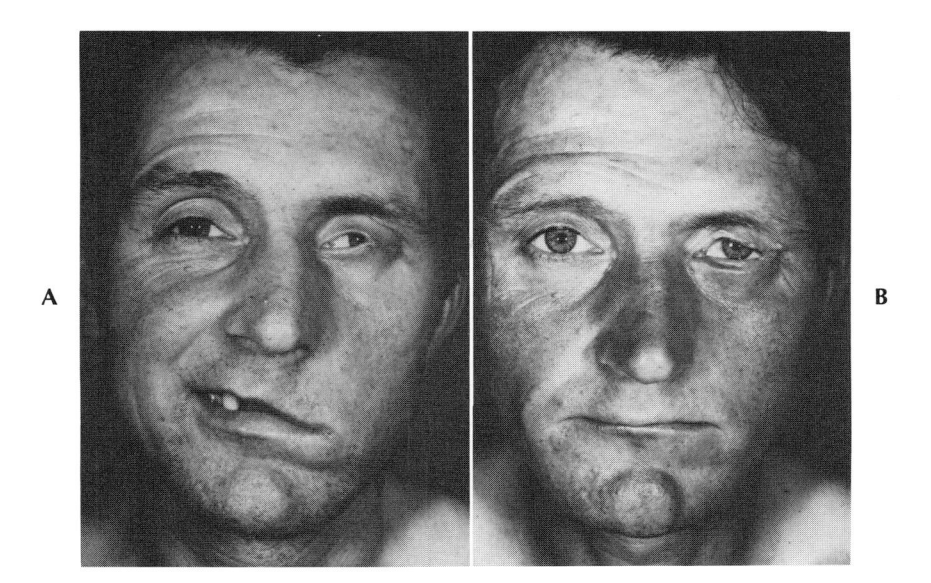

Fig. 24-28. A, Thirty-four-year-old patient after basocranial fracture and decompression in temporal bone. Complete facial palsy of left side of face and no spontaneous recovery. Lateral tarsorrhaphy removed and insert of Silastic membrane into lower lid as well as a lid spring into upper lid. **B,** Same patient with good return of function in all parts of the face, except frontal muscles.

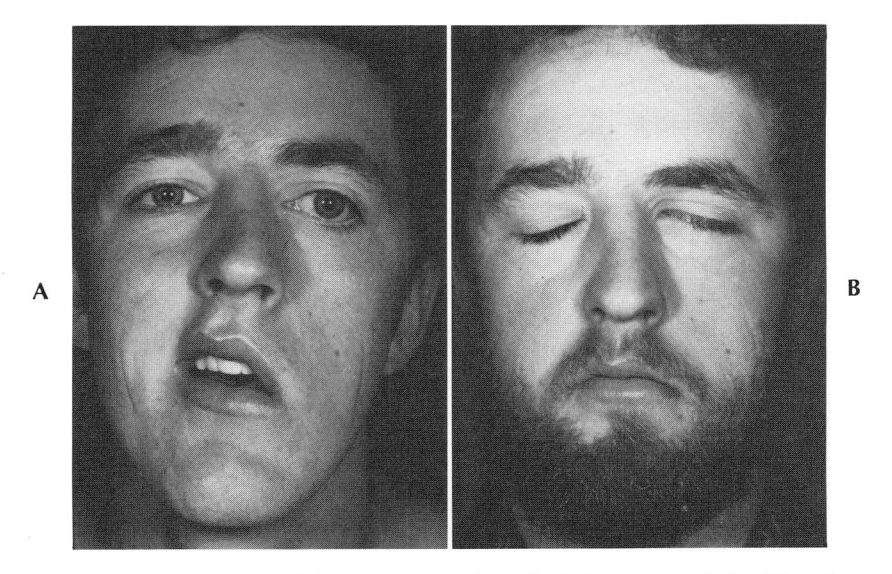

Fig. 24-29. A, Man, 21 years old, with complete facial palsy of left side after craniobasal fracture and decompression in the temporal bone (no recovery). Silastic membrane into the lower lid. **B,** Same patient 3 years after operation (three sural grafts in all segments of face). Good recovery.

Reanimation of the paralyzed face

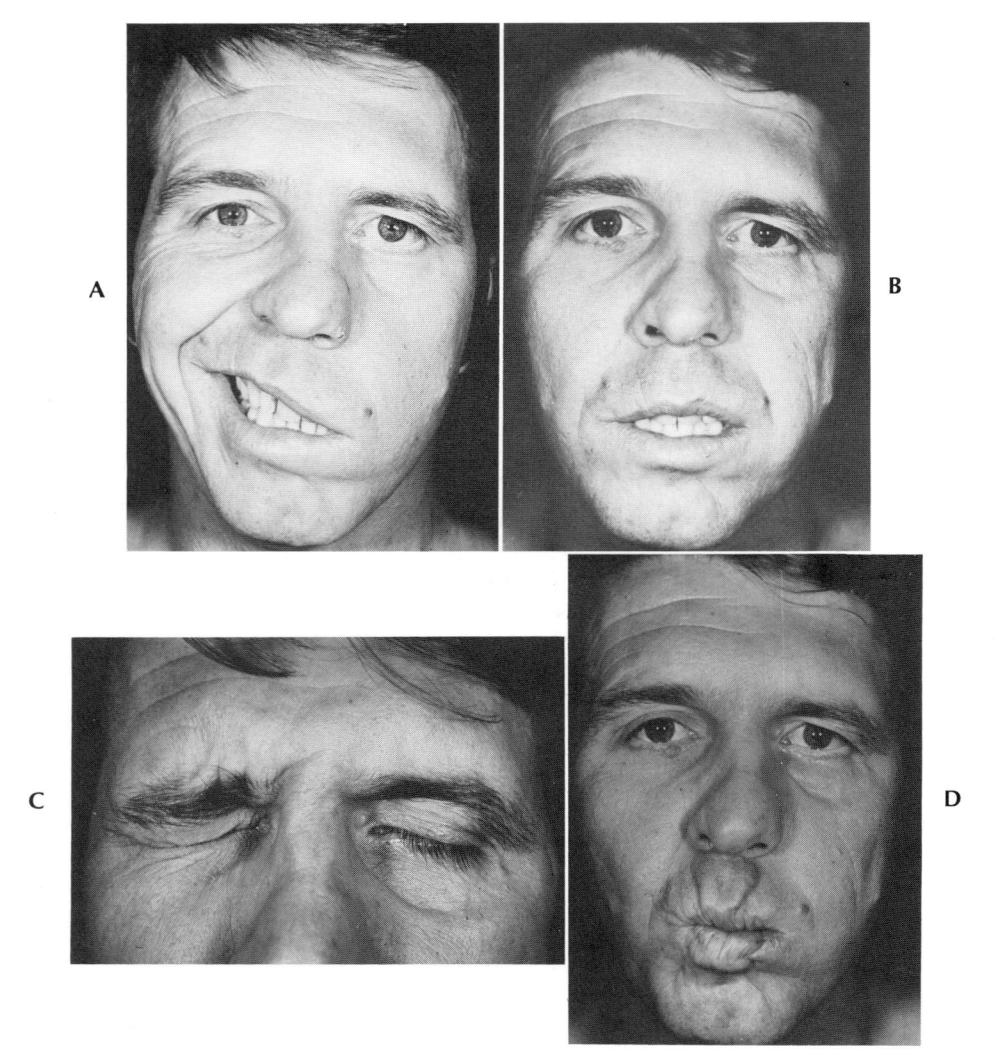

Fig. 24-30. A, Patient, 32 years old, with complete Bell's palsy. No recovery after decompression. Implantation of lid spring into the upper lid. **B,** Good recovery 5 years after operation (three grafts: one in the eye region, two in the upper lip). Even the natural folds of skin and symmetry of nose have reappeared. **C,** Lid closure in same patient. **D,** Same patient pointing the mouth.

There are some important facts that have to be considered before cross-face transplantation is performed, since they influence the result to a great extent:
1. State of degeneration of the facial muscle before operation
2. Time between nerve interruption and surgical nerve grafting
3. Presence of foreign bodies and scars from previous operations in the region of the contemplated anastomoses
4. Ability to find sufficient numbers of healthy fascicles on the normal side
5. Surgical and microsurgical technical faults
6. Preoperative and postoperative electrical and active physiotherapy

REFERENCES

1. Aitken, J. T.: Growth of nerve implants in voluntary muscle, J. Anat. **84:**38, 1950.
2. Anderl, H.: A simple method for correcting the ectropium, J. Plast. Reconstr. Surg. **49:** 156-159, 1972.
3. Anderl, H.: Nerventransplantation bei Facialisparese, Zurich, 1972, Jahrestagung der Schweizerischen Gesellschaft für Plastische und Wiederherstellungschirurgie.
3a. Anderl, H.: Reconstruction of the face through cross-face nerve transplantation in facial paralysis, Chir. Plastica (Berlin) **2:**17-46, 1973.
4. Anderl, H.: Rekonstruktive Eingriffe am peripheren Nerven mittels mikrochirurgischer Operationstechniken, Aktuelle Chir. **8:**285-292, 1973.
5. Anderl, H.: Cross face nerve transplantation in facial palsy. In Converse, J. M.: Reconstructive plastic surgery, Philadelphia, 1975, W. B. Saunders Co.
6. Anderl, H.: Cross face nerve transplantation in facial palsy (principle and further experience), Transactions of the Sixth International Congress for Plastic and Reconstructive Surgery, Paris, 1975, Manson.
7. Anderl, H.: Instrument for taking nerve grafts, Chir. Plastica (Berlin). (In press.)
8. Ballance, C., and Duel, A. B.: The operative treatment of facial palsy by the introduction of nerve grafts into fallopian canal and by other intratemporal methods, Arch. Otolaryngol. **15:**1-70, 1932.
9. Berger, A., Meissl, G., and Samii, M.: Experimentelle Erfahrungen mit Kollagenfolien über nahtlose Nervenanastomosen, Acta Neurochir. (Wien) **23:**141-149, 1970.
10. Bielschowsky, M., and Unger, E.: Die Überbrückung grosser Nervenlücken. Beiträge zur Erkenntnis der Degeneration und Regeneration peripherer Nerven, J. Physiol. Neurol. **22:**267, 1916-1918.
11. Böhme, P. E.: Die Parotischirurgie und ihre morphologischen Grundlagen, Stuttgart, 1966, Georg Thieme Verlag, p. 52.
12. Braun, R. M.: Comparative studies of neurorrhaphy and sutureless peripheral nerve repair, Surg. Gynecol. Obstet. **122:**15, 1966.
13. Buchthal, F.: Electromyography in paralysis of the facial nerve, Arch. Otolaryngol. **81:** 463, 1965.
14. Bunnell, S.: Suture of facial nerve within temporal bone with report of first successful case, Surg. Gynecol. Obstet. **45:**7, 1927.
15. Campbell, J. B.: Microfilter sheaths in peripheral nerve surgery: a laboratory report and preliminary clinical study, J. Trauma **1:** 139, 1961.
16. Campbell, J. B.: Discussion at the Tenth Congress of the SciCOT, Paris, Sept. 6-9, 1966.
17. Clodius, L.: (Contribution) Chir. Plast. et Reconstr. **8:**10, 1970.
18. Clodius, L.: Selective neurectomies to achieve symmetry in partial and complete facial paralysis, Br. J. Plast. Surg. **29:**43-52, 1976.
19. Conley, J. J.: Facial rehabilitation following radical parotid gland surgery, Arch. Otolaryngol. **66:**58, 1957.
20. Conley, J. J.: Treatment of facial paralysis, Surg. Clin. North Am. **51:** 1971.
21. Conley, J. J.: Salivary glands and the facial nerve, Stuttgart, 1975, Georg Thieme Verlag.
22. Dingman, R. O., and Grabb, W. C.: Surgical anatomy of the mandibular ramus of the facial nerve based on the dissection of 100 facial halves, Plast. Reconstr. Surg. **29:**268, 1962.
23. Dott, N. M.: Facial paralysis; restitution by extra–petrous nerve graft, Proc. Soc. Med. **51:**900, 1958.
24. Erlacher, P.: Direct and muscular neurotization of paralyzed muscles, experimental research, Amer. J. Orthop. Surg. **13:**22, 1915.
25. Esslen, E., and Magun, R.: Elektromyographie: Grundlage und klinische Anwendung, Fortschr. Neurol. Psychiatr. **26:**4, 1958.
26. Esslen, E.: Electrodiagnosis of facial palsy. In Miehlke, A.: Surgery of the facial nerve, Munich, 1973, Urban & Schwarzenberg.
27. Faure, J. L.: Traitement chirurgical de la paralysie facial par l'anastomose spinofacial, Rec. Chir. (Fr.) **18:**1098, 1898, and Sem. Med. (Fr.) 426, 1898.
28. Fisch, U. P.: Operations on the facial nerve in oto-neuro-surgical operations. In Yaşargil M. G.: Microsurgery, Stuttgart, 1969, Georg Thieme Verlag, p. 208.
29. Fisch, U.: Transtemporal surgery of the internal auditory canal, Adv. Otorhinolaryngol. **17:**203-240, 1970.
30. Fisch, U.: The surgical treatment of facial hyperkinesia. In Plastic and reconstructive surgery of the neck, Stuttgart, 1970, Georg Thieme Verlag.
31. Fisch, U.: Die Hypoglossus-Facialisanastomose, Med. Hyg. **31:**450-452, 1973.
32. Fisch, U.: Facial nerve grafting, Otolaryngol. Clin. North Am. **7:**517, 1974.
33. Förster, O.: Die Schussverletzungen der pe-

ripheren Nerven und ihre Behandlung, Z. Orthop. Chir. **36:**310, 1916.
34. Förster, O.: Handbuch der Neurologie von Bumke and Förster, Band VIII: Allgemeine neurologie, Berlin, 1936, Julius Springer Verlag.
35. Förster, O.: Handbuch der Neurologie von Bumke and Förster, Band III: Die Facialislähmung, Berlin, 1937, Julius Springer Verlag, p. 594.
36. Freilinger, G.: A new technique to correct facial paralysis, Plast. Reconstr. Surg. **56:** 44-48, 1975.
37. Fujita, T.: Über die periphere Ausbreitung des N. facialis beim Menschen, Morphol. Jahrb. **73:**578, 1934.
38. Gutmann, E., and Young, Z.: The reinnervation of muscles after various periods of atrophy, J. Anat. **78:**15-43, 1944.
39. Hakstian, N. R.: Funicular orientation by direct stimulation, J. Bone Joint Surg. (Am.) **50:**1178, 1968.
39a. Harii, K., Ohmori, K., and Torii, S.: Free gracilis muscle transplantation with neurovascular anastomoses for the treatment of facial paralysis, Plast. Reconstr. Surg. **57:** 133-143, 1976.
40. Hoffmann, H.: A study of the factors influencing innervation of muscles by implanted nerves, Aust. J. Exp. Biol. Med. Sci. **29:**289, 1951.
41. House, W. F., and Crabtree, J. A.: Surgical exposure of petrous portion of seventh nerve, Arch. Otolaryngol. **81:**506, 1966.
42. Kaeser, H. E.: Zur Frage der Elektrotherapie bei peripheren Lähmungen, Praxis **14:**438, 1969.
43. Kettel, K.: Surgery of the facial nerve, Arch. Otolaryngol. **81:**523-538, 1965.
44. Lexer, E.: Die gesamte Wiederherstellungschirurgie, Leipzig, 1931, Johannes Barth Verlag, vol. 2, p. 761.
45. Marino, H.: Paralysis des N. facialis, Fortschr. Kiefer. Gesichtschir. **2:**148, 1956.
46. McCormack, L. J., Cauldwell, E. W., and Anson, B. J.: The surgical anatomy of the facial nerve (with special reference to the parotid gland), Surg. Gynecol. Obstet. **80:** 620-630, 1945.
47. Michon, J.: Die Nervennaht unter dem Mikroskop, Handchirurgie **1,** 1969.
48. Miehlke, A.: Die Chirurgie des Nervus facialis, Munich, 1960, Urban & Schwarzenberg.
49. Miehlke, A.: Über den chirurgischen Wiederaufbau des Gesichtsnerven nach extratemporaler Läsion, Dtsch. Med. Wochenschr. **85:**506-510, 1960.
50. Miehlke, A., and Buske, A.: Die operative Freilegung der mittleren Schädelgrube und das Porus acusticus internus zur Behandlung interlabyrinthärer Läsionen des N. facialis, Chir. Plast. et Reconstr. **3:**37, 1967.
51. Miehlke, A.: Surgery of the facial nerve. Philadelphia, 1973, W. B. Saunders Co.
52. Millesi, H., Ganglberger, J., and Berger, A.: Erfahrungen mit der Mikrochirurgie peripherer Nerven, Chir. Plast. et Reconstr. **3:** 47, 1967.
53. Millesi, H.: Zum Problem der Überbrückung von Defekten peripherer Nerven, Wein. Med. Wochenschr. **9-10:**182, 1968.
54. Millesi, H., Berger, A., and Meissl, G.: Fascicular nerve grafting, using a microsurgical technique, Transactions of the Fifth International Congress of Plastic and Reconstructive Surgery, Chatswood, NSW, Aust., 1971, Butterworths Pty, Ltd., pp. 586-592.
55. Millesi, H., Berger, A., and Meissl, G.: Experimentelle Untersuchungen zur Heilung durchtrennter Nerven, Chir. Plastica (Berlin) **1:**174-206, 1972.
55a. Millesi, H., and Samii, M.: Erfahrungen mit verschiedenen Wiederherstellungsoperationen am N. facialis. In Höhler, H.: Plastische und Wiederherstellungschirurgie aus Klinik und Forschung, Stuttgart, 1975, F. K. Schattauer-Verlag, pp. 110-125.
56. Morel-Fatio, D., and Lalardrie, J. P.: Pallative surgical treatment of facial paralysis, The palpebral spring, Plast. Reconstr. Surg. **33:**446-456, 1964.
57. Mühlbauer, W. D., Segeth, H., and Viessmann, A.: Restoration of lid function in facial palsy with permanent magnets: Chir. Plastica (Berlin) **1:**295-304, 1973.
58. Mumentaler, M., and Schliack, H.L Läsionen peripherer Nerven, Stuttgart, 1965, Georg Thieme Verlag.
59. Rosenfalck, P., and Buchthal, F.: Studies on fibrillation potentials of denervated human muscle, Electroencephalogr. Clin. Neurophysiol. **22**(suppl.):130-132, 1962.
60. Rosenthal, W.: Die muskuläre Neurotisation bei Facialislähmung, Zentralbl. Chir. **24:** 489, 1916.
61. Rosenthal, W.: Die bleibende Facialislähmung und ihre Behandlung, Dtsch. Z. Chir. **223:**261, 1930.
61a. Samii, M.: Modern aspects of peripheral and cranial nerve surgery. In Krayenbühl, H., editor: Advances and technical standards in neurosurgery, Vienna, 1975, Springer Verlag, vol. 2, pp. 33-85.
62. Scaramella, L.: L'anastomosi tra i due nervi facciali, Arch. Otologia **82:**209-215, 1971.

63. Schröder, J. M., and Seiffert, K. E.: Untersuchungen zur homologen Nerventransplantation. 2. Morphologische Ergebnisse, Zentralbl. Neurochir. **33**:103, 1972.
64. Seddon, H.: Surgical disorders of the peripheral nerves, Edinburgh, 1972, E. & S. Livingstone, Ltd.
65. Smith, J. W.: Microsurgery of peripheral nerves, Plast. Reconstr. Surg. **33**:317, 1964.
66. Smith, J. W.: Microsurgery: review of the literature and discussion of microtechniques, Plast. Reconstr. Surg. **37**:227, 1966.
67. Smith, J. W.: A new technique of facial animation, Transactions of the Fifth International Congress of Plastic and Reconstructive Surgery, Chatswood, NSW, Aust., 1971, Butterworths Pty, Ltd., p. 83.
68. Steindler, A.: Direct neurotization of paralysed muscles: further study of the question of direct nerve implantation. Am. J. Orthop. Surg. **14**:707, 1916.
69. Struppler, A.: Myographie in der Facialis- und Handchirurgie, Chir. Plast. et Reconstr. **8**:3-8, 1970.
70. Sunderland, S.: Funicular suture and funicular exclusion in the repair of severed nerves, Br. J. Surg. **40**:580-587, 1953.
71. Sunderland, S.: Nerves and nerve injury, Edinburgh, 1968, E. & S. Livingstone, Ltd.
72. Sunderland, S.: Personal communication, 1976.
73. Taverner, D.: Electrodiagnosis in facial palsy, Arch. Otolaryngol. **81**:470, 1965.
74. Taverner, D.: Treatment of facial palsy, Arch. Otolaryngol. **81**:489, 1965.
75. Thompson, N.: Treatment of facial paralysis by free skeletal muscle grafts, Transactions of the Fifth International Congress of Plastic and Reconstructive Surgery, Chatswood, NSW, Aust., 1971, Butterworths Pty, Ltd., pp. 68-82.
76. Thompson, N.: Autogenous free grafts of skeletal muscle, Plast. Reconstr. Surg. **48**:11-27, 1971.
77. Thompson, N., and Gustavson, E.: The use of neuromuscular free autograft with microneural anastomosis to restore elevation to the paralysed angle of mouth in cases of unilateral facial paralysis, Chir. Plastica (Berlin) **3**:165-174, 1976.
78. Wilflingseder, P., and Anderl, H.: Indications for intermittent, palliative surgical measures and long-term results with alloplasties in facial paralysis, Arch. Ital. Otol. **82**:268-275, 1971.
79. Yaşargil, M. G., and Fisch, U.: Unsere Erfahrungen in der mikrochirurgischen Exstirpation der Akustikusneurinome, Arch. Ohrenheilkd. **194**:243, 1969.
80. Zülch, K. J.: Der Wert der konservativen Behandlung für die Restitution der gestörten Fascialisfunktion, Fortschr. Kiefer. Gesichtschir. **2**:132, 1956.

SECTION THREE

Late surgical treatment for facial paresis—after 12 months

25 Free muscle and nerve grafting in the face*

LARS HAKELIUS

The clinical application of free nerve and muscle grafting is described in detail. The placing of small muscles from the feet or arms against normal facial muscles encourages sprouting of nerves and blood vessels to the graft. The "taken" grafts regain motor function and activate movement to the paralyzed face.

---

*This chapter is based on the following papers:
Hakelius, L.: Transplantation of free autogenous muscle in the treatment of facial paralysis, Scand. J. Plast. Reconstr. Surg. **8:**220, 1974.
Hakelius, L., and Stålberg, E.: Electromyographical studies of free autogenous muscle transplants in man, Scand. J. Plast. Reconstr. Surg. **8:**211, 1974.

Free muscle and nerve grafting in the face

For long-standing facial paralysis two general principles of surgical treatment are currently in use. The first involves static suspension of the affected side of the face, which improves the balance of the face at rest. The second aims at dynamic reanimation of the paralyzed side. Several techniques for transposition of the masseter or temporal muscles have been used and some restoration of movement has been reported. With few exceptions, however, it is difficult to obtain acceptable results with these operations because these muscles are innervated by the trigeminal nerve, which gives at best uncoordinated movements. Besides, the transposed muscle has an unfavorable direction of the line of pull.

In 1971 Thompson[19] described a technique of free autogenous transplantation of skeletal muscle to the face to reanimate the paralyzed side of the face in patients with facial palsy.

A muscle deprived of motor nerve supply undergoes progressive atrophy. After suturing of the severed motor nerve, the muscle may have part of its function restored by reinnervation by growth of the proximal cut nerve ends. In partially denervated muscle, fibers can be reinnervated through collateral sprouting of nerve twigs from neighboring normal nerve fibers.[4,6] In man this type of reinnervation has been demonstrated in patients with neuromuscular diseases.[12,22] A pedicled flap of denervated skeletal muscle with an intact blood supply becomes reinnervated when placed in contact with normal muscle. This is well demonstrated clinically in the Abbe flap. Normal motor end plates have been demonstrated[18] and electromyographical studies have shown reinnervation of such flaps.[7,14]

Reinnervation of free muscle grafts is believed to occur by the ingrowth of nerve twigs from a normal recipient muscle. Kugelberg, Edström, and Abbruzzese[9] demonstrated that such collateral sprouting is hindered by connective tissue. It is thus important to remove the fascia of the graft before it is transplanted and to put the graft under the fascia of the recipient, but with facial muscles this is not an important consideration because they are not surrounded by fascia.[2]

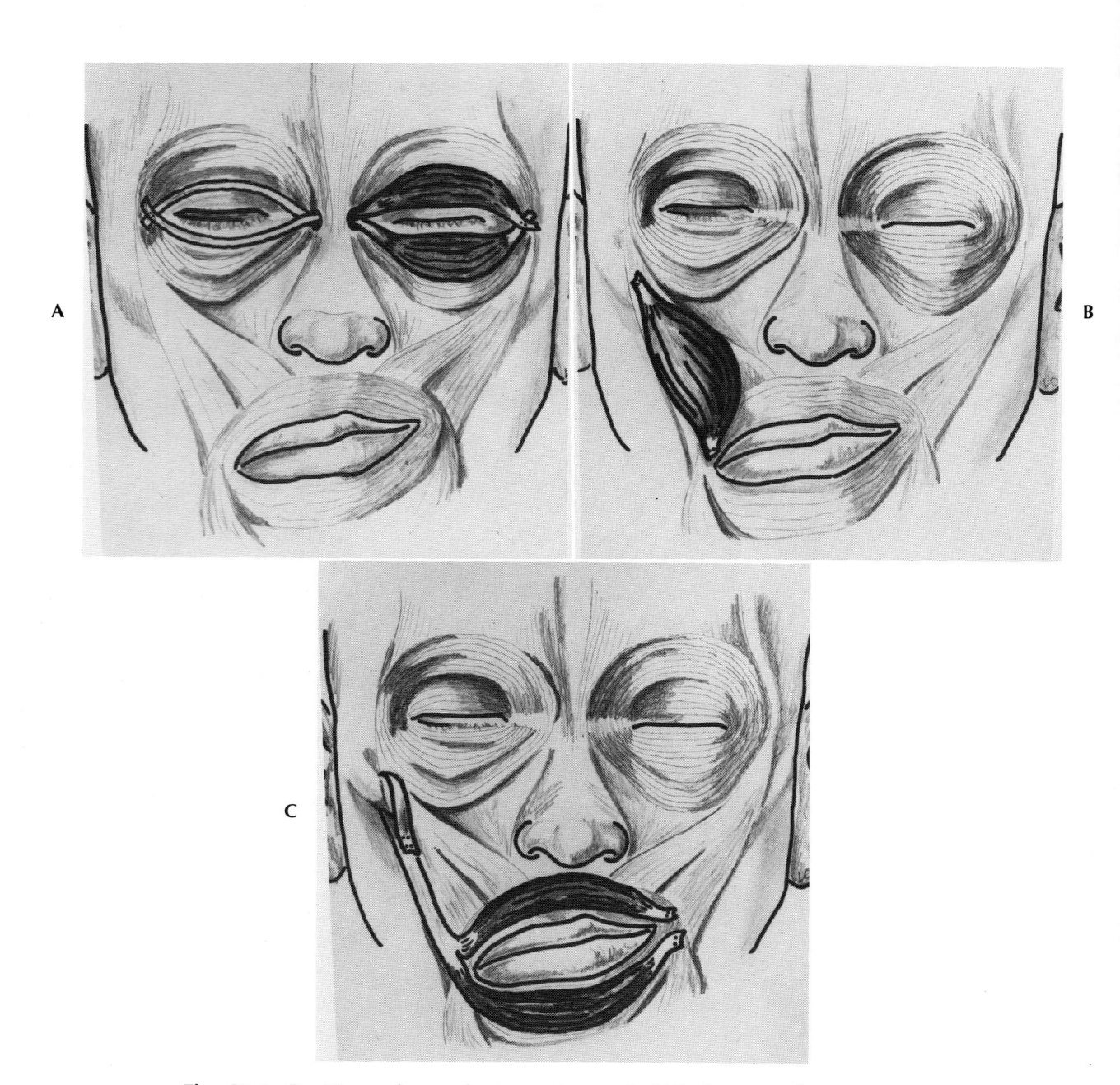

Fig. 25-1. Position of muscle transplants. **A,** Whole transplant in contact with a normal muscle. **B,** Whole transplant in contact with partially denervated muscle. **C,** Approximately half the transplant in contact with normal muscle.

In facial palsy several different muscle functions are disturbed. In free muscle grafting restoration is directed selectively to a single function with each transplantation.

The transplants are placed in one of three different positions, each in close relationship to the muscles from which reinnervation is expected. In one group, the muscle belly of the graft is placed with its whole length in contact with normal muscle. This technique is used for total paralysis of the eyelids (Fig. 25-1, *A*). In a second group, the transplant is positioned with its whole length on a partially paralyzed muscle in an attempt to strengthen that muscle (Fig. 25-1, *B*). In a third group, approximately half the transplant is placed in contact with healthy muscle. This is used for the treatment of unilaterally denervated orbicularis oris muscle (Fig. 25-1, *C*).

Operative techniques

The operative techniques are principally those developed by Thompson.[20] They are described here with some modifications. I have experience with this technique in about 100 transplantations.

SELECTION AND DENERVATION OF MUSCLE TRANSPLANTS

Four different muscles have been used as grafts: the extensor digitorum brevis of the foot, the palmaris longus, the plantaris, and the superficial flexor of the fourth finger. The latter two muscles were used because of aplasia of the palmaris longus. These four muscles were chosen for transplantation because they are of sufficient size for facial grafting and their removal causes little or no functional impairment.

For eyelid transplantation, the extensor digitorum brevis muscle was used exclusively, since at least two of its four muscle bellies correspond in size to the recipient. The extensor digitorum brevis often shows a reduction of motor units in normals, but rarely to a significant degree before the age of 60.[10] The extensor digitorum brevis muscles were studied with preoperative EMGs, and only normal or minimally denervated muscles were used.

The palmaris longus is most suitable for encircling the mouth. In addition, the plantaris and the superficial flexor digitorum muscles were also used; the extensor digitorum brevis is usually too short for this purpose.

The denervation of the donor muscle was performed 2 to 3 weeks before grafting, with use of a bloodless field and an electrical nerve stimulator to locate the correct motor nerve. One to 2 cm of the nerve was then resected.

The motor nerve of the palmaris longus branches from the median nerve usually just above the level of the elbow. Occasionally it courses together with the motor nerve to the pronator teres or the flexor carpi radialis. To be certain that only the palmaris branch is divided, the tendon is initially sectioned at the wrist near its junction with the palmaris aponeurosis. With the severed end of the tendon held in a hemostat, it is possible to observe isolated contractions of the muscle belly on electrical stimulation of the correct motor nerve.

The extensor digitorum brevis muscle is supplied by the deep peroneal nerve emerging on the dorsum of the foot from beneath the lower border of the inferior extensor retinaculum, usually just lateral to the dorsalis pedis artery. It divides into two branches at varying levels: the lateral branch supplies the extensor digitorum brevis only, whereas the medial branch is the cutaneous nerve of the lateral side of the first

Reanimation of the paralyzed face

toe and the medial part of the second. The nerve is exposed through a 2 cm longitudinal incision over the dorsalis pedis artery. The motor nerve is found just distal to the inferior extensor retinaculum, whence it disappears under the extensor digitorum brevis muscle belly of the first toe. It lies deep and close to the bone. Electrical stimulation causes extension of the four medial toes. The motor branch is resected.

The plantaris muscle is innervated from the tibial nerve. The nerve is found in the popliteal fossa just above the level where the tibial nerve passes deep to the tendinous arch of the soleus muscle. Before the nerve is sectioned, the tendon is cut close to its insertion on the os calcaneus, medial to the Achilles tendon. Electrostimulation is then used to determine its motor innervation.

The superficial flexor digitorum muscles are innervated by branches from the median nerve, usually as it courses between the two heads of this muscle. The nerve branch to the muscle of the fourth finger is localized in a similar manner as described above.

MUSCLE GRAFTING IN EYELID PARALYSIS

The principle of this operation is threefold: (1) to get the transplant innervated from the normal orbicularis oculi muscle, (2) to pass the tendons of the grafts through a tunnel in the bony portion of the nose, and (3) to place the tendons subcutaneously along the margins of the paralyzed eyelids and suture them to the lateral palpebral ligament (Fig. 25-1, A). Contraction of the normal orbicularis oculi muscle should then produce a simultaneous contraction of the grafts, resulting in lid closure on the opposite, paralyzed side.

The facial surgery is divided into two stages. In the first stage a tunnel through the nose is created. A sagittal incision, about 2.5 cm long, is made from the glabella over the ridge of the nose. The nasal bones are exposed at the level of the medial canthi of the eyes, and a transverse resection is made in the bony framework, with careful preservation of the nasal mucosa. The bone is chiseled out en bloc and preserved for later replacement. On each side, a more limited resection of the nasal bone is carried down to the plane of the eyelids. Parts of the septal bone are also removed to the same level so that a straight channel across the nose may be created, ending subcutaneously on both sides. A silicone rod 4 mm in diameter enclosed by a free vein graft with the intima against the rod is placed in the groove. The section of bone removed initially is then replaced to complete a tunnel, and the wound is sutured. Denervation of the donor muscle is also made at this stage.

Two to 3 weeks later, the denervated extensor digitorum brevis muscle is transplanted. Through short transverse incisions just proximal to the interdigital spaces, the tendons are severed near their distal attachments. The four muscle bellies with their tendons attached are then dissected free through a supplementary curved incision, starting over the middle of the third metatarsal bone and ending over the lateral side of the cuboid bone. Two of the muscle bellies are selected as transplants, and their surrounding fascia is carefully removed.

Dissection of the eyelids is facilitated by infiltration with lidocaine (Xylocaine) 0.5% with epinephrine. On the normal side, short incisions are made at the lateral canthus and medially over the end of the palpable rod previously inserted. These incisions are connected by subcutaneous undermining in the plane of the orbicularis oculi. The larger of the two grafts is then pulled subcutaneously along the lower lid and the smaller one in a similar way along the upper lid. The ends of the muscle bellies are sutured to the periosteum at the lateral border of the orbit. The silicone rod is now removed, with the vein graft still in place, and the tendons of the grafts are pulled through the nasal tunnel. Short incisions at the medial and lateral canthi are made on the paralyzed side, and the tendons of the transplants are passed subcutaneously along the margin of the upper and lower eyelids. In this maneuver the tendons are crossed medially so that the tendon from the muscle graft in the upper eyelid is passed along the margin of the lower eyelid on the paralyzed side. The ends of the tendons are sutured to the lateral palpebral ligament under slight tension. In most cases the tendons have to be lengthened. A tendon from one of the rejected muscle bellies is used for this purpose. The skin incisions are closed with 5-0 nonabsorbable sutures, and a compression bandage is applied for 48 hours.

In cases later in the series, I have used only the muscle graft placed in the lower eyelid on the normal side with its tendon running in the upper eyelid of the paralyzed side. To prevent ectropion of the paralytic lower eyelid, a tendon is transplanted along its upper margin.

MUSCLE GRAFTING IN PARALYSIS OF ORBICULARIS ORIS MUSCLE

The intention of the operation is to encircle the mouth with a muscular graft, thereby reinnervation from the normal half of the orbicularis oris muscle is obtained (Fig. 25-1, *C*). Such an operation can restore the sphincter function only and no effect is expected for the elevation of the angle of the mouth. The denervated donor muscle (usually palmaris longus) is removed, together with its tendon, and the surrounding fascia is excised. The muscle transplant is split longitudinally, parallel with the lay of its fibers, as far as the tendinous attachment.

Through an incision at the angle of the mouth on the paralyzed side, each half of the muscle is passed subcutaneously in bluntly dissected tunnels through the upper and lower lips to the healthy angle of the mouth. On the paralyzed side the muscle-tendon portion of the graft is firmly sutured to the deep tissues with nonabsorbable sutures; on the opposite side the muscle is sutured to the subcutaneous tissue. The tendon of the transplant is passed subcutaneously to the zygomatic arch and fixed around this bone to give static support, keeping the mouth in a balanced position when the face is at rest. The entire operation is carried out through two small perioral incisions and a third over the zygomatic arch.

MUSCLE GRAFTING IN PARTIALLY PARALYZED MUSCLE

The muscle-grafting procedure has also been used to strengthen weak, partially denervated facial muscles. The transplant is then placed on the affected muscle and receives its new innervation from this bed. The most common aim of this application of the graft is to strengthen the elevators of the angle of the mouth. (Fig. 25-1, *B*). It can even be used for strengthening of the lower lip muscle, the eyelid muscle, and the frontalis muscle. Muscle grafts are introduced through small incisions over the ends of the affected muscles and placed subcutaneously over the recipient muscles under slight tension.

Clinical material and results

The first 30 muscle transplantations (MT) to the face were performed in 23 patients, and they have been thoroughly followed up. Age, sex, duration of the paralysis, and degree of denervation prior to operation are shown in Table 3. At operation these patients were 15 to 67 years old (average 45.6 years), and the observation time after surgery ranged from 2 to 18 months (average 9.5 months). A distorted facial appearance and functional disturbances were the major problems for these patients.

Fourteen patients treated for eyelid paralysis preoperatively suffered from lagophthalmos of 4 to 12 mm. All of them complained of watering of the unprotected

Table 3. Data of 30 muscle transplants in 23 patients

Muscle transplantation number (MT)	Initials of patient	Age at operation	Sex	Duration of paralysis (months or years)	Degree of denervation preoperatively (EMG)	Type of operation*	Muscle used as graft†	Follow-up time (months)
1	ET	22	m	22 y	Pronounced	2	p.l.	18
2	LF	60	m	2 y	Total	3	p.l.	18
3	HA	61	f	3 m	Total	1	e.d.b.	16
4	HA	61	f	4 m	Total	3	p.l.	15
5	DL	41	f	2 y	Moderate	2	e.d.b.	16
6	LS	25	f	21 y	Moderate	2	p.l.	15
7	HS	62	m	15 m	Total	1	e.d.b.	14
8	HH	64	m	8 y	Total	1	e.d.b.	14
9	KE	40	f	2 y	Moderate	1	e.d.b.	16
10	KE	41	f	3 y	Moderate	2	p.g.	4
11	OE	48	m	5 y	—	1	e.d.b.	14
12	OE	48	m	5 y	—	3	p.l.	11
13	WA	24	f	24 y	Pronounced	3	p.	12
14	ÅM	50	f	3 m	Total	1	e.d.b.	11
15	JI	22	f	10 y	Total	1	e.d.b.	8
16	SS	52	m	3 y	Total	1	e.d.b.	9
17	SS	53	m	3 y	Total	3	p.l.	3
18	CI	35	f	8 y	Total	1	e.d.b.	8
19	CI	35	f	8 y	Total	3	f.d.s.	3
20	LK	60	m	5 m	Total	1	e.d.b.	6
21	LK	60	m	8 m	Total	3	p.l.	3
22	JH	22	m	5 y	Moderate	2	e.d.b.	7
23	BG	15	f	4 y	Total	3	e.d.b.	4
24	BK	60	f	2 m	—	1	e.d.b.	8
25	BK	61	f	6 m	—	3	p.l.	4
26	JA	67	f	13 y	Total	1	e.d.b.	14
27	ÖE	32	f	11 y	Total	1	e.d.b.	2
28	CH	66	f	2 y	Pronounced	2	e.d.b.	5
29	WK	16	m	2 y	Slight	2	e.d.b.	4
30	SE	66	f	2 y	—	1	e.d.b.	2

*1 = the whole transplant in contact with a normal muscle; 2 = the whole transplant in contact with a partially denervated muscle, and 3 = approximately half of the transplant in contact with a normal muscle.

†e.d.b. = Extensor digitorum brevis; f.d.s. = flexor digitorum superficialis of the fourth finger; p. = plantaris; p.l., palmaris longus.

eye and constant irritation, caused by exposure conjunctivitis. They were also distressed about their wide-eyed appearance. Nine cases treated for paralysis of the orbicularis oris muscle, in addition to cosmetic embarrassment, complained of dribbling and accidental biting of the cheek and lips as well as difficulties in articulation. All of them were unable to whistle and had difficulty in keeping water in the mouth when brushing their teeth. Seven patients with partial paralysis complained mainly of the cosmetic distress.

A preoperative EMG investigation was carried out in all but three patients so that the degree of denervation in the muscles intended for improvement by transplantation could be estimated (Table 3). The patients not investigated with EMG preoperatively had undergone surgery for intracranial tumors (two cases) and tumor of the parotid gland (one case) when the facial nerve had to be sectioned. The muscles were thus totally denervated prior to reconstructive surgery.

Movements of the grafts were first observed about 6 to 8 weeks after grafting. The earliest contractions were noted in the small grafts placed on the normal orbicularis oculi muscle. As a rule, movements in the grafts around the mouth occurred about 12 weeks after grafting. There was continued improvement in the function of the grafts over the following 6 months.

EYELID PARALYSIS

Twelve patients were observed for more than 3 months after eyelid repair. In 10 of these cases, improvements were striking (Fig. 25-2). The synchronization of movements of the normal and paralyzed eyelids was good, and the eyelids were closed during sleep. On forced contraction, six patients demonstrated a persistent lagophthalmos of 0 to 1 mm, and four patients had 2 to 3 mm, when the head was in a prone position. Complete relief of epiphora was obtained in two cases, and the remaining eight were considerably improved. Exposure conjunctivitis healed completely in six cases and rapid improvement was obtained in the remaining four. The patients ex-

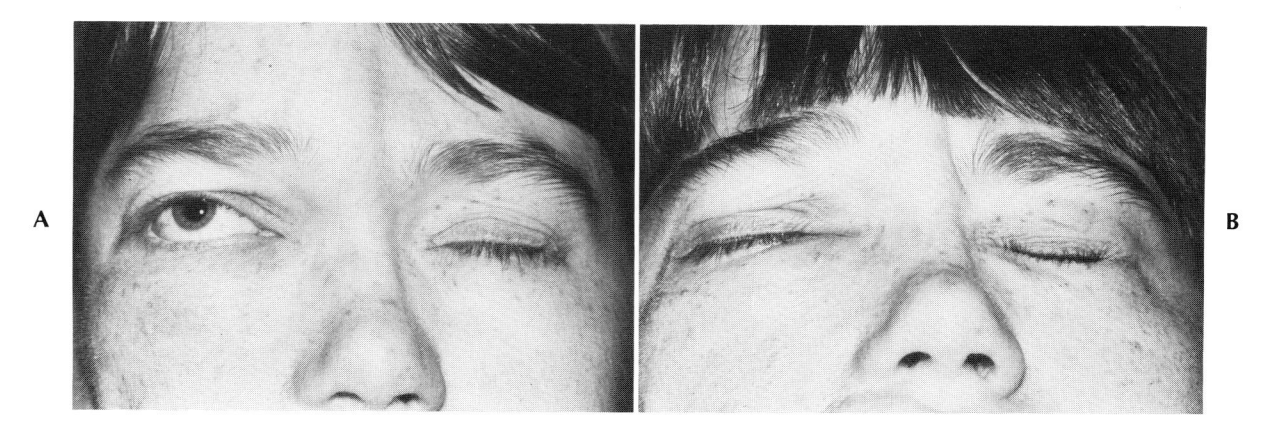

Fig. 25-2. A 22-year-old woman (MT 15), born with lymphangioma on right side of face. Repeated surgical excisions caused a total facial paralysis approximately 10 years ago. **A,** Before surgery, attempting to close the eyelids. **B,** 5 months after grafting of the extensor digitorum brevis muscle to left (normal) orbicularis oculi. Note contracting grafts laterally in eyelids on left side.

Reanimation of the paralyzed face

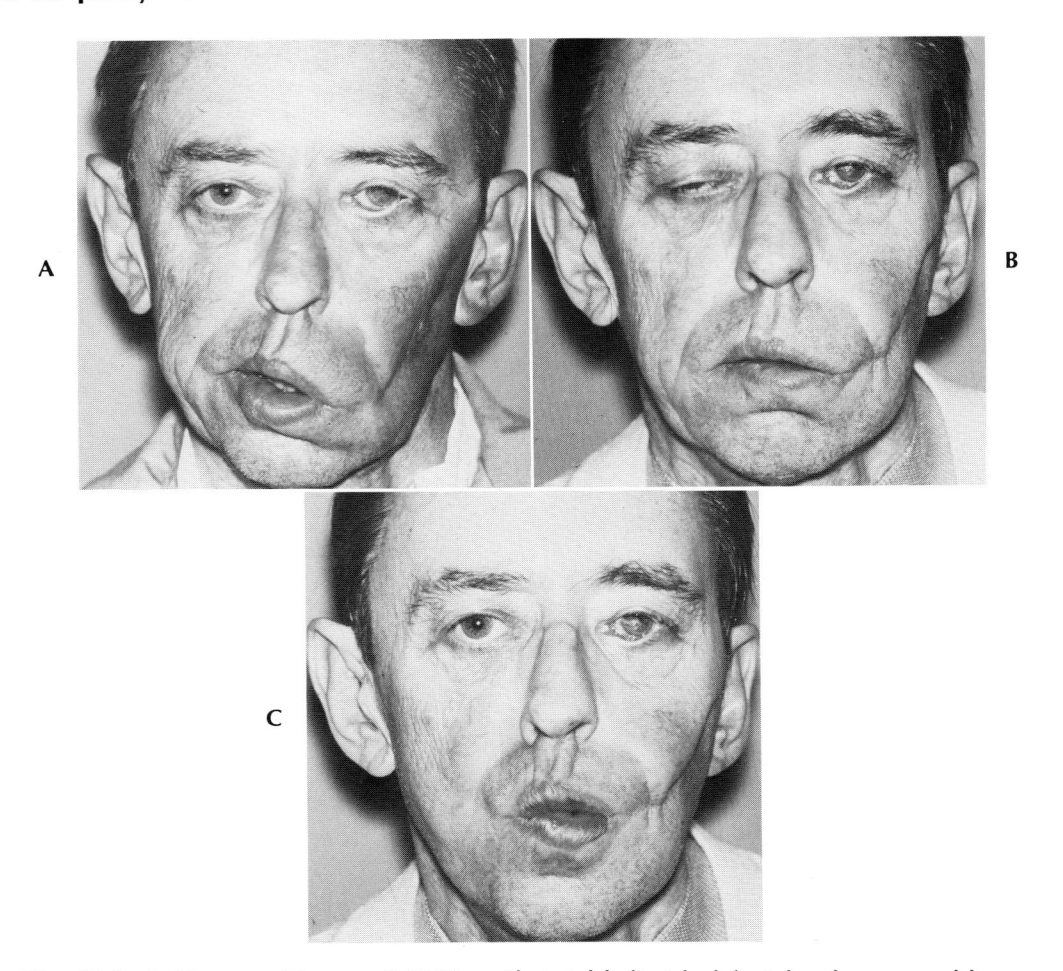

Fig. 25-3. A 60-year-old man (MT 2), with total left-sided facial palsy caused by operation for neurinoma of acoustic nerve 2 years earlier. **A,** Before surgery. **B,** 8 months after transplantation of palmaris longus muscle to orbicularis oris and static support of angle of mouth using tendon of transplant. **C,** Pursing the lips.

pressed great satisfaction that their pronounced gazing appearance had been corrected or improved.

When the normal orbicularis oculi muscle was contracted, the grafts could be felt subcutaneously except in the upper eyelid of muscle transplantation number (MT) 3. In none of the cases did the transplant distort the contour of the normal eye region. In MT 9 and MT 27 the palpebral fissure on the paralyzed side became smaller than that on the normal side because the tendons were too tight. Correction of the tension in these cases is made. MT 3 and MT 7 were failures because of infection in the nose tunnel and subsequent tendon necrosis. The tendon ruptures were confirmed at a later exploration.

PARALYSIS OF ORBICULARIS ORIS MUSCLE

Nine patients, treated for paralysis of the orbicularis oris, were observed for 3 months or more. All of them showed improvement of sphincteric action on pursing

Free muscle and nerve grafting in the face

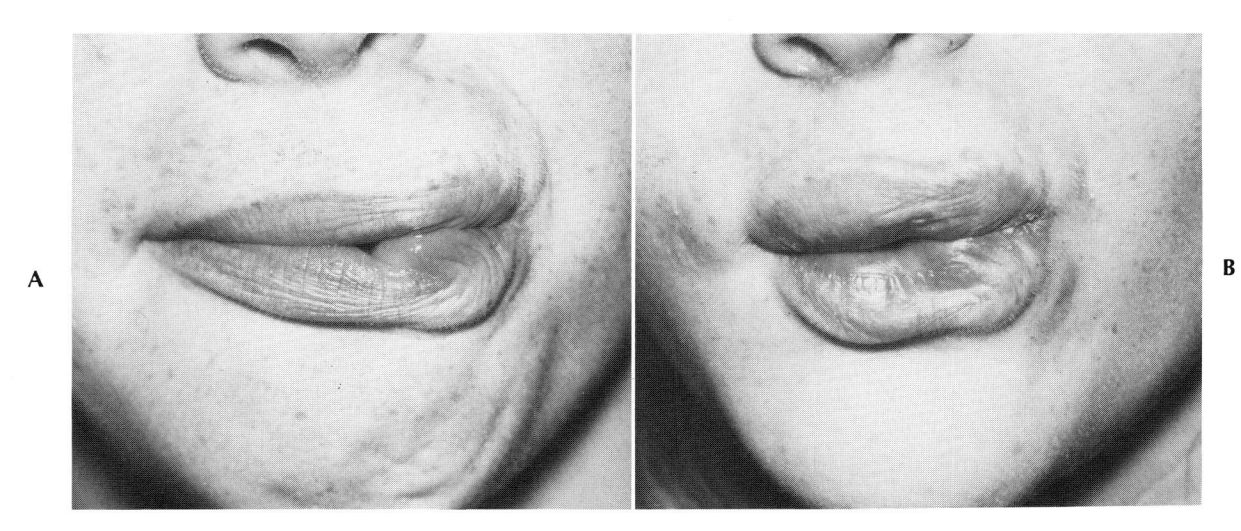

Fig. 25-4. Girl, 15 years of age (MT 23), with Bell's palsy, 4 years earlier involving only right side of orbicularis oris muscle and to a minor degree elevators of angle of mouth. **A,** Before surgery, attempting to purse the lips. **B,** Pursing the lips 4 months after transplantation of extensor digitorum brevis, with graft encircling mouth.

the lips, and six can whistle, an ability that was previously impossible (Figs. 25-3 and 25-4). The strength of the orbicularis oris on closure has improved and was demonstrated by the patient's ability to blow out the cheeks and hold water in the mouth, such as when brushing the teeth. All patients considered their speech improved. The accidental biting of cheeks and lips has disappeared in seven patients and is less frequent in the other two (MT 4 and 25). Dribbling was eliminated in seven cases and decreased in two (MT 4 and MT 19). At the follow-up, all patients but one (MT 4) spontaneously expressed a feeling of natural movement and liveliness in the tissues around the mouth. The poorest result, clinically and electromyographically, was obtained in MT 4, where most of the graft seemed to have undergone resorption. The static support for the paralyzed angle of the mouth, created in eight cases, added balance of the mouth to the resting face.

PARTIALLY PARALYZED MUSCLES

Seven cases, treated for partial paralysis, were observed for more than 3 months. In three of them, the elevators of the mouth were strengthened. The result was excellent in one patient; in the second, lifting of the angle of the mouth was evidently improved; and in the third no change was noted (MT 2). In the last case, even though movements were not restored, the cheek obtained a more rounded contour because of the bulk of the transplant and the symmetry of the face was thereby improved.

In one case, where the paretic orbicularis oculi of the lower lid was strengthened (MT 29), the patient complained preoperatively of persistent watering of the eyes and chronic irritation. He had developed a minor paralytic ectropion of the eyelid and was unable to protect the eye with normal blinking. Postoperatively all the symptoms have abated, and the patient is very content.

Reanimation of the paralyzed face

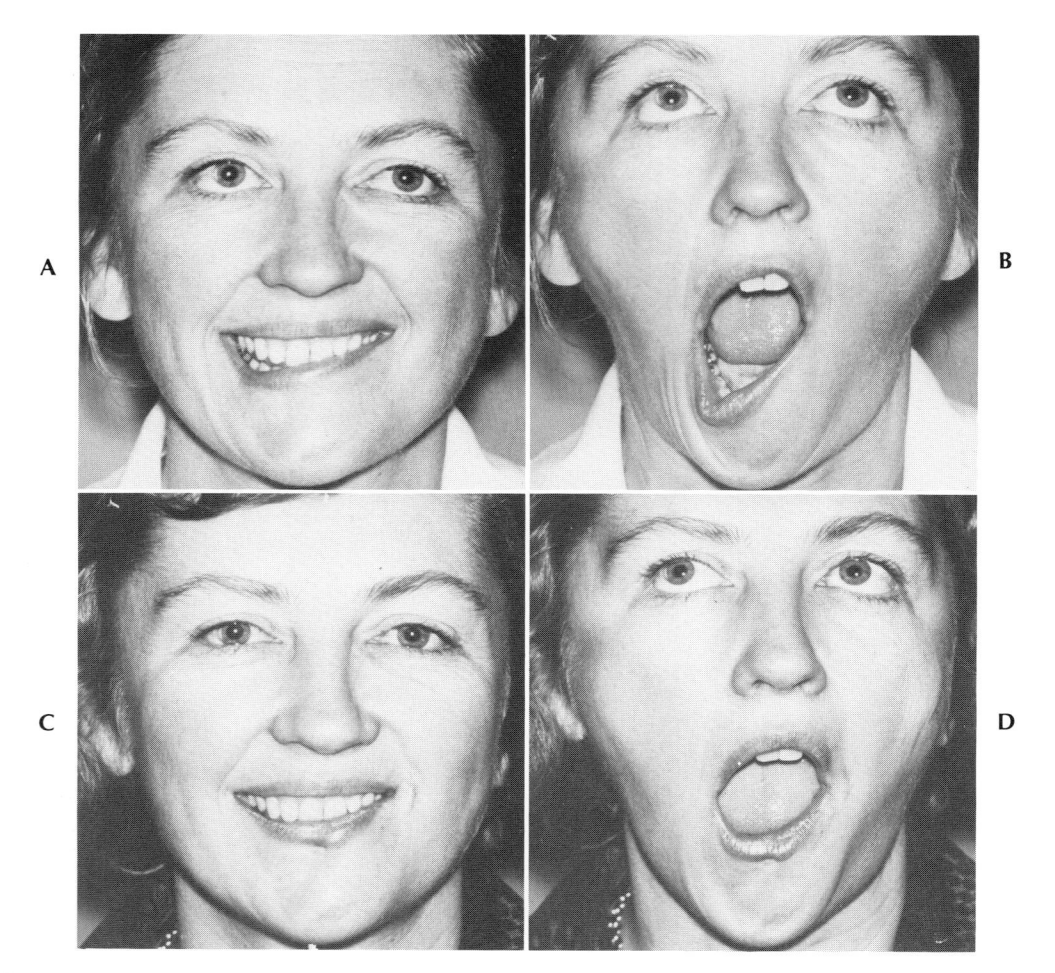

Fig. 25-5. Woman, 41 years of age (MT 5), with damage of nerve branches to orbicularis oris muscle of lower lip and quadratus muscle on right side after operation for parotid tumor 2 years earlier. EMG showed moderate degree of denervation in affected part of orbicularis oris before (**A** and **B**), and 6 weeks after (**C** and **D**), grafting of one belly of extensor digitorum brevis muscle to partially denervated left, lower part of orbicularis oris.

A strong improvement in appearance was achieved in the patient (MT 5) where orbicularis oris in the lower lip was strengthened (Fig. 25-5).

The transplantation of the extensor digitorum brevis to the frontalis muscle in MT 22 was a failure as far as restoring normal wrinkling of the forehead. When this patient closes his eyes, concomitant elevation of the eyebrow occurs, along with wrinkling of the forehead (Fig. 25-6). The explanation for this peculiar synchronized action apparently is that reinnervation originated from the undamaged orbicularis oculi that reinnervated the paralyzed frontalis. From this muscle the graft in turn was reinnervated.

In MT 28 prolonged infection damaged the transplants. Nevertheless, lip contraction was well restored. Parts of the transplant in the cheek also survived and allowed increased movement of the angle of the mouth.

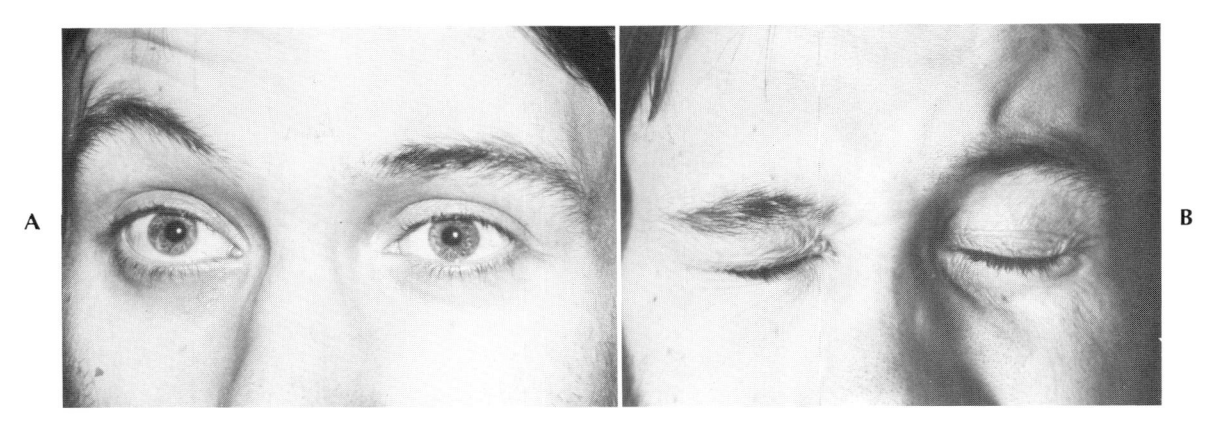

Fig. 25-6. Man, 22 years old (MT 22), with partial denervation of left frontalis muscle caused by operation for progenia 5 years earlier and with transplant of extensor digitorum brevis to forehead of left side made 7 months previous to present photograph. **A,** Attempting to wrinkle the forehead. **B,** Closing the eyelids. Note contraction of graft of forehead, which causes elevation of eyebrow.

Electromyographical methods and results

Twenty-six of the 30 muscle transplants to the face, performed in 21 patients, were followed with conventional electromyography (EMG) and with single-fiber EMG[17] from 2 months to 1 year after transplantation. The patients' age range was 16 to 67 years (average 43.5 years).

The position of the recording electrode in relation to the transplant was of crucial importance. Normally, the graft was easily seen and felt and the needle inserted with the guidance of a palpating finger. When the needle was moved, movements of the graft were often observed. Recordings obtained from surrounding muscle showed a different type of EMG activity.

Recordings were made from at least three different electrode positions; spontaneous activity had to be seen in two electrode positions to be accepted.

CONVENTIONAL ELECTROMYOGRAPHY

Signs of denervation (fibrillation action potentials and positive sharp waves) were seen in 20 out of 24 investigations up to 1 month after grafting. The occurrence of the spontaneous activity decreased with time and was only exceptionally seen after 4 months (Fig. 25-7). In three cases, the spontaneous activity was still present after 6 to 12 months. This occurred in one case with a postoperative infection of the graft. This graft was placed in toto on the healthy orbicularis oculi muscle. Reinnervation had taken place in a part of the muscle. The two other transplants were placed partly on a healthy orbicularis oris muscle. After 8 and 9 months, respectively, denervation activity was present in the most lateral parts of the grafts. At 12 months, denervation activity had disappeared.

Voluntary activity could be recorded in 15 of 24 transplants up to 1 month after grafting. At the 2- to 3-month follow-up, all 25 examined grafts showed signs of reinnervation.

Reanimation of the paralyzed face

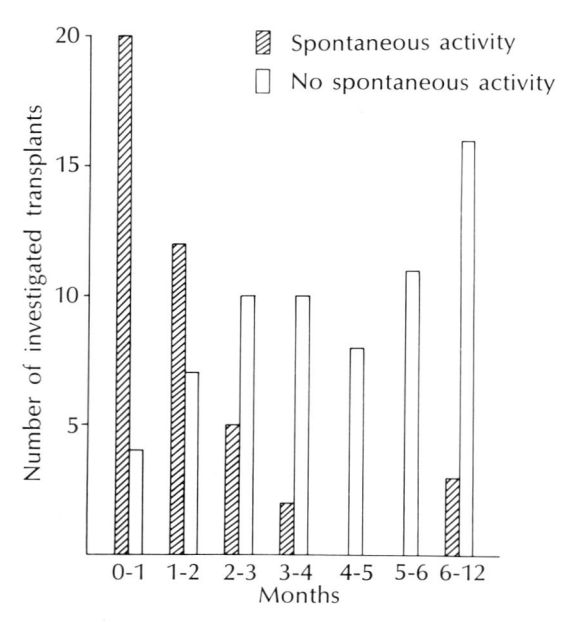

Fig. 25-7. Number of transplants showing spontaneous EMG activity.

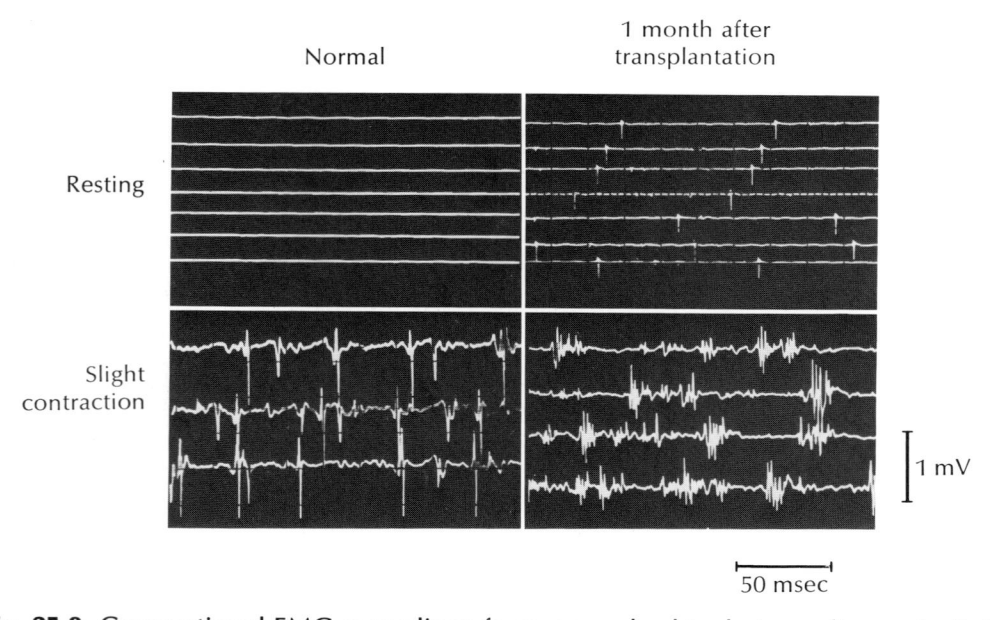

Fig. 25-8. Conventional EMG recordings from normal orbicularis oculi muscle *(left)* and graft *(right)* 1 month after transplantation. Fibrillation potentials (at rest) and low polyphasic action potentials on slight contraction are seen in transplant.

Action potential shape. The motor action potentials, recorded at voluntary activity after 1 month, were either relatively simple or polyphasic (Fig. 25-8). The number of components in the recorded motor action potentials increased during the first months and in later controls polyphasic potentials were always the dominant type. In normal facial muscles the incidence of polyphasic potentials is about 5%[3] and the potential duration is 2.28 ± 0.3 msec (range 0.8 to 6 msec).[15] Despite the small size of the transplant, it was not possible to obtain a sufficient number of action potentials to make an accurate measurement of their mean duration. The impression was, however, that the duration increased during the first months parallel with the complexity. In 11 out of 17 transplants, durations longer than 6 msec were common at investigations 3 to 5 months after the grafting. The maximal duration measured was 80 msec. No further increase was observed after the sixth month; instead the duration tended to become shorter.

The amplitude of action potentials was usually 50 to 500 μV for the individual motor unit during the first 2 months and about 200 to 1000 μV at 12 months, which were similar to values obtained from the underlying muscle.

Interference pattern. Initially, activity from only a few motor units was recorded at maximal efforts, but after 3 months a relatively large number of motor units could be activated. The interference pattern at maximal contraction increased during the first 6 months and was hereafter relatively unchanged. At follow-up 11 to 12 months after grafting, the interference pattern at maximal contraction was discrete in three, dense but still reduced in eight, and full in two of the 13 cases.

The amplitude of the highest action potentials at maximal contraction was much lower than that obtained from the surrounding or underlying normal muscle. This was particularly evident in the early stages (amplitude 200 to 2000 μV), but the amplitude progressively increased and at the 1-year control it was 500 to 5000 μV, which is within the range of normal.

Generally speaking, the interference pattern was more reduced in the upper eyelid than in the lower and similarly less in the upper than in the lower lip. This was not merely ascribed to the time delay in reinnervation in the upper eyelid and upper lid. This difference remained even after follow-up many months later.

In the first group, where the whole transplant was placed in contact with the normal muscle, the same degree of reinnervation was found throughout the whole graft. Signs of reinnervation were seen in eight out of 10 cases at the 1-month control. After 1 year the interference pattern was slightly reduced in the six cases that were studied.

In the second group the graft was superimposed on a partially denervated muscle. There was difficulty in ascertaining the position of the recording electrode in the graft, as the underlying muscle too had shown reinnervation preoperatively. Signs of graft reinnervation were seen after 1 month in three of the six cases. In the other three, reinnervation was recorded at 6, 8, and 10 weeks, respectively. Three cases were followed for 1 year. In two of them a full interference pattern was obtained, but in one it was discrete. This case had the first signs of reinnervation at 10 weeks. There was a pronounced denervation in the recipient muscle. In two patients the graft was placed on the normal orbicularis oris and the partially denervated zygomaticus. Reinnervation took place from both of these muscles. From the same electrode position a different EMG pattern could be obtained, depending on whether the patient activated the graft by contracting the orbicularis oris muscle or the zygomatic muscle.

In the third group only half of the transplant was in contact with the healthy muscle. The part of the muscle placed on the paretic side was investigated. Reinnervation first appeared in the vicinity of the part of the graft that was in contact with the recipient. Six cases out of nine showed reinnervation at 1 month. After 1 year, two had

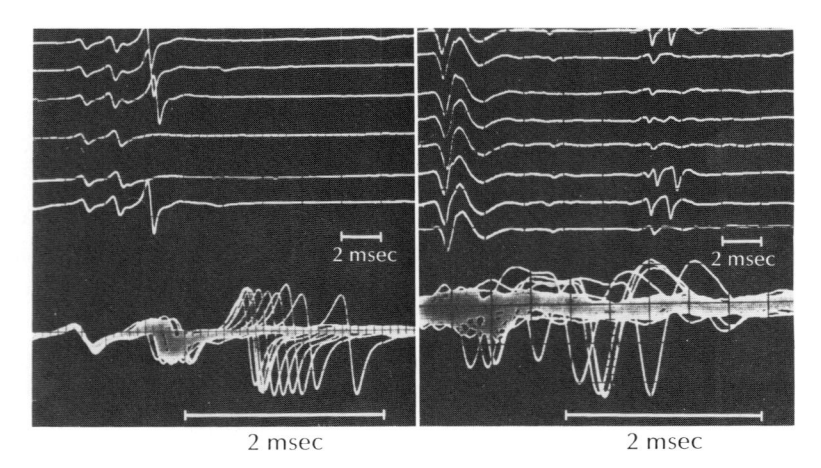

Fig. 25-9. Relatively unstable action-potential complexes 1 month *(left)* and 6 months *(right)* after grafting. Left part shows blocking of last component and increased jitter. Right part shows paired (neurogenic) blocking. In lower parts of illustration, 10 successive action potentials are superimposed.

a reduced and two a discrete interference pattern of the four transplants investigated. Even the most lateral parts of the grafts were reinnervated.

SINGLE-FIBER ELECTROMYOGRAPHY

In the recordings made after 1 month (five cases), there was an increased jitter and blockings of single action potentials or sometimes paired blockings, indicating impulse failure in the terminal nerve twigs. During the first 6 months the action potential complexes became more stable. This increased stability was seen after 2 months, but blockings were still present after 6 months and, exceptionally, after 1 year (Fig. 25-9).

The fiber density of the motor unit was increased in four of five cases at 1 month and in all cases investigated after 4 months. Usually 3 to 7 fibers per electrode surface were seen. In many recordings more than 10 fibers (up to 20 within the electrode uptake radius of 200 μm) were incorporated in the same motor unit.

In a number of recordings, independent of time after the transplantation, it was observed that the patient had difficulty in keeping a constant innervation frequency. The motor neuron could not be activated for more than a short period and this recurred in a phasic manner.

Conclusion

Good results for eyelid-closure restoration are reported after temporalis transfer,[1] use of a spring inserted in the upper eyelid,[11] or insertion of permanent magnets[13] or weights[16,8] in the eyelids. Compared to these methods for restoration of the paralyzed eyelids, the results after grafting are superior. In addition free muscle grafting offers a synchronized and reflex lid closure on both sides, and no foreign material has to be deposited subcutaneously. A method for restoration of the sphincteric function of the orbicularis oris muscle has not been described before. In these conditions muscle transplantation thus offers unique possibilities for restoration.

In patients with unilateral facial paralysis and total absence of voluntary activity in the muscles concerned with elevation of the angle of the mouth, it is not possible to restore function with free muscle grafting only because reinnervation of the graft cannot occur.

Freilinger[5] has solved this problem by first inserting a cross-face nerve graft sutured to normal facial nerve filaments on the normal side, and several months later the free end of the nerve graft was implanted into a newly transplanted skeletal muscle graft on the paralyzed side. Thompson and Gustavsson[21] have refined this muscle-nerve grafting by transplanting the muscle as a free graft together with its motor nerve, the latter being anastomosed to filaments of the facial nerve on the uninvolved side.

REFERENCES

1. Andersen, J. G.: Surgical treatment of lagophthalmus in leprosy by the Gillies temporalis transfer, Br. J. Plast. Surg. **14:**339, 1961.
2. Benninghoff, A.: Lehrbuch der Anatomie des Menschen, Munich, 1954, Urban & Schwarzenberg, vol. 1, p. 539.
3. Buchthal, F., and Rosenfalck, P.: Action potential parameters in different human muscles, Acta Psychiat. Scand. **30:**126, 1955.
4. Edds, M.: Collateral regeneration of residual motor axons in partially denervated muscles, J. Exp. Zool. **113:**517, 1950.
5. Freilinger, G.: A new technique to correct facial paralysis, Plast. Reconstr. Surg. **56:** 44, 1975.
6. Hoffman, H.: Local reinnervation in partially denervated muscle: a histo-physiological study, Aust. J. Exp. Biol. Med. Sci. **28:**383, 1950.
7. Isaksson, I., Johanson, B., Petersén, I., and Selldén, U.: Electromyographic study of the Abbe and fan flaps, Acta Chir. Scand. **123:** 343, 1962.
8. Jobe, R. P.: A technique for lid loading in the management of the lagophthalmus of facial palsy, Plast. Reconstr. Surg. **53:**29, 1974.
9. Kugelberg, E., Edström, L., and Abbruzzese, M.: Mapping of motor units in experimentally reinnervated rat muscle, J. Neurol. Neurosurg. Psychiatry **33:**319, 1970.
10. McComas, A. J., Fawcell, P. R. W., Campbell, M. J., and Sicca, R. E. P.: Electrophysiological estimation of the number of motor units within a human muscle, J. Neurol. Neurosurg. Psychiatry **34:**121, 1971.
11. Morel-Fatio, D., and Lalardrie, J. P.: Contribution a l'étude de la chirurgie plastique de la paralysie facial. Le ressort palpebral, Ann. Chir. Plast. **7:**275, 1962.
12. Morris, C. J.: Human skeletal muscle fibre type grouping and collateral reinnervation, J. Neurol. Neurosurg. Psychiatry **32:**440, 1969.
13. Mühlbauer, D., Segeth, H., and Viessmann, A.: Restoration of lid function in facial palsy with permanent magnets, Chir. Plastica (Berlin) **1:**295, 1973.
14. de Palma, A. T., Leaville, L. A., and Baron Hardy, S.: Electromyography in full thickness flaps rotated between upper and lower lips, Plast. Reconstr. Surg. **21:**448, 1958.
15. Petersén, I., and Kugelberg, E.: Duration and form of action potential in the normal human muscle, J. Neurol. Neurosurg. Psychiatry **12:**124, 1949.
16. Smellie, G. D.: Restoration of the blinking reflex in facial palsy by a simple lid-load operation, Br. J. Plast. Surg. **19:**279, 1966.
17. Stålberg, E., and Ekstedt, J.: Single fibre EMG and microphysiology of the motor unit in normal and diseased human muscle. New Dev. Electromyogr. Clin. Neurophysiol. **1:** 113, 1973.
18. Thompson, N., and Pollard, A. C.: Motor function in Abbe flaps, Br. J. Plast. Surg. **14:**66, 1961.
19. Thompson, N.: Autogenous free grafts of skeletal muscle, Plast. Reconstr. Surg. **48:** 11, 1971.
20. Thompson, N.: Treatment of facial paralysis by free skeletal muscle grafts. In Transactions of Fifth World Congress of Plastic and Reconstructive Surgery, London, 1972, Butterworth & Co. (Publishers) Ltd., p. 66.
21. Thompson, N., and Gustavsson, E. H.: The use of neuromuscular free autografts with microneural anastomosis to restore elevation to the paralyzed angle of the mouth in cases of unilateral facial paralysis, Chir. Plastica (Berlin) **3:**165, 1976.
22. Wohlfart, G.: Collateral regeneration in partially denervated muscles, Neurology **8:**175, 1958.

26 Entire temporalis muscle transposition

LEONARD R. RUBIN

The entire temporalis muscle substitutes for the paretic muscles on the affected side to activate the eyelids, cheeks, and lips in a one-stage procedure. The detailed operation is described and illustrated with sketches.

There can be no comparable substitute for a paralyzed facial motor apparatus. The subtly controlled facial movements of each side are the result of 20 contracting muscles, blended and muted by the superficial fascia. Surgical procedures to improve facial function have concentrated on the use of the muscles of mastication to supply an alternate motor power train. The temporalis muscle supplied by the fifth cranial nerve is rarely paretic and makes an excellent facial contracting force.

In 1933, Gillies transplanted the anterior portion of a temporalis muscle to activate the corners of the mouth and nasolabial folds.[1] Fascia lata was used as tendon for the needed length beyond the ends of the muscle (Fig. 26-1, *G*). In 1938, Sheehan[2] included the eyelid in a similar fashion. Anderson,[3] in 1951, modified Gillies technique by employing temporalis fascia instead of the fascia lata to activate eyelids. In 1952, McLaughlin[4] detached the coronoid process of the mandible leaving the bone attached to the temporalis tendon (Fig. 26-1, *M*). A sling of fascia lata was placed around the lips to simulate an orbicularis oris and was then inserted into a hold in the coronoid process, which in turn was elevated by the entire temporalis muscle (Fig. 26-1, *M*).

The most commonly used procedure by plastic surgeons has been a static sling of fascia lata[5] threaded around the mouth and fastened to the zygomatic arch to give support to the lips and the nasolabial fold (Fig. 26-1, *F*). The anterior portion of the masseter muscle has also been used to give tone to the upper lips (Fig. 26-1, *N*). Unfortunately, the line of contraction is poor when compared to the temporalis pull (*T*, temporalis muscle; *M*, masseter muscle) (Fig. 26-2).

Entire temporalis muscle transposition

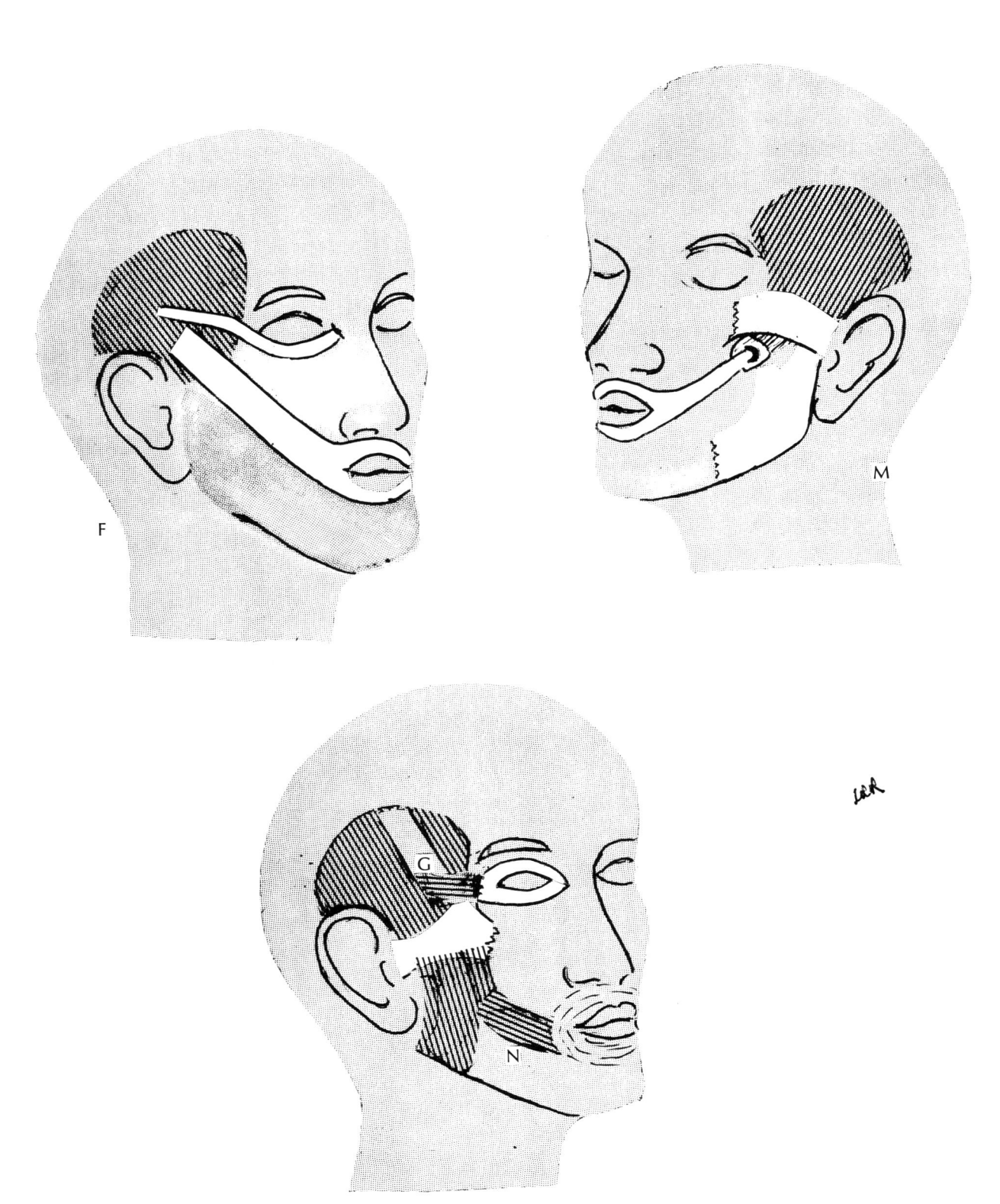

Fig. 26-1

Reanimation of the paralyzed face

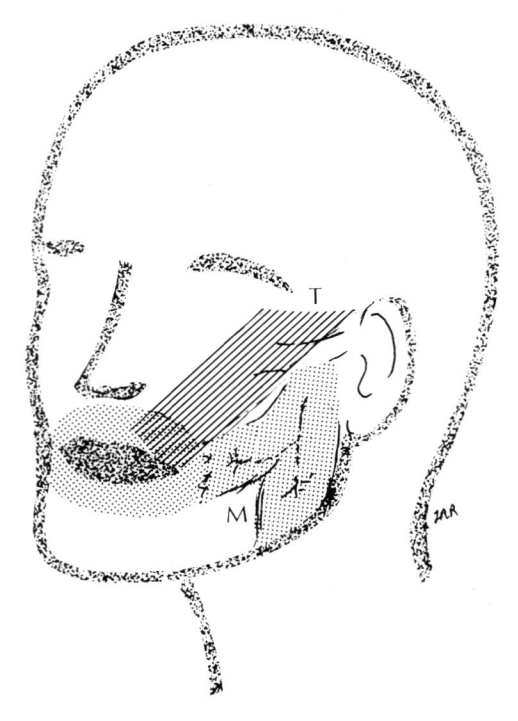

Fig. 26-2

In 1966, I presented a paper[5] describing bilateral temporalis muscle transplantation with temporal fascia added as tendons to activate the eyelids, cheeks, upper lips, and nasolabial folds. Almost all the muscle is used in this one-stage procedure. The operation is still being used as described in 1966 with very little change. Animation of the face can be accomplished in a one-stage procedure, in about 3 hours of operating time.

Before describing my technique, a few paragraphs describing the anatomy of the temporalis muscle is needed to familiarize the reader with its anatomical structure.

Anatomy of temporalis muscle

The temporalis muscle is a fan-shaped, thick, broad muscle occupying the temporal fossa on the external surface of the skull's temporal bone. It is covered with a dense, firm fascia. The muscle fibers are attached to the periosteum of the temporal fascia and converge to pass under the zygomatic arch, inserting finally into the anterior border of the coronoid process. The muscle is covered by a dense fascia continuous with the deep fascia rising from the neck. The fascia envelops the mandible, the facial muscles, and the zygomatic arch. At the superior border of that arch, it fuses to form the thick sheet covering the muscle up to the superior temporal line, where it merges into the galea of the scalp.

The function of the temporalis muscle is to assist in elevating the mandible by contracting its fibers. It also aids in its protrusion and retraction. The temporalis-muscle nerve supply is derived from the temporal branch of the motor division of the fifth cranial nerve. The anatomical division of the temporal nerve is fortuitous in that it splits into three separate branches innervating the anterior, middle, and posterior belly of the muscle. The nerve is found in the midlevel of the zygomatic arch where it divides into its three branches, each penetrating the muscle at about the junction of its lower one third and upper two thirds. Thus the muscle can be freed from the temporal bone down to the upper level of the zygomatic arch without injuring the nerve supply.

The technique of the temporal muscle transfer in facial paralysis is possible because of the attachment of the upper one half of the muscle to the temporal bone above the level of the zygomatic arch. When the superior part of the muscle is freed from the bone and draped over the zygomatic arch, the lower one half has sufficient attachment to the temporal bone to contract and serve as a motor apparatus to raise the lips and corner of the mouth and activate the eyelids. In most cases, the length of the draped muscle is insufficient to reach the nasolabial fold and the lips. The temporal fascia can then act as tendons to reach and insert into the upper lip, corner of the mouth, lower lip, and the eyelids.

Before starting the operation, the surgeon must examine the patient's smile on the normal side. In Chapter 1, I described three types of smiles produced by the dominant muscles of the lips and the corners of the mouth. The surgeon can locate, on the normal side, the exact position of major muscle pull and plan to place the temporalis muscle and its fascial tendons into the exact mirror image on the affected side. *These points of attachment must be predetermined prior to the operation.*

Reanimation of the paralyzed face

Technique of temporalis transposition procedure

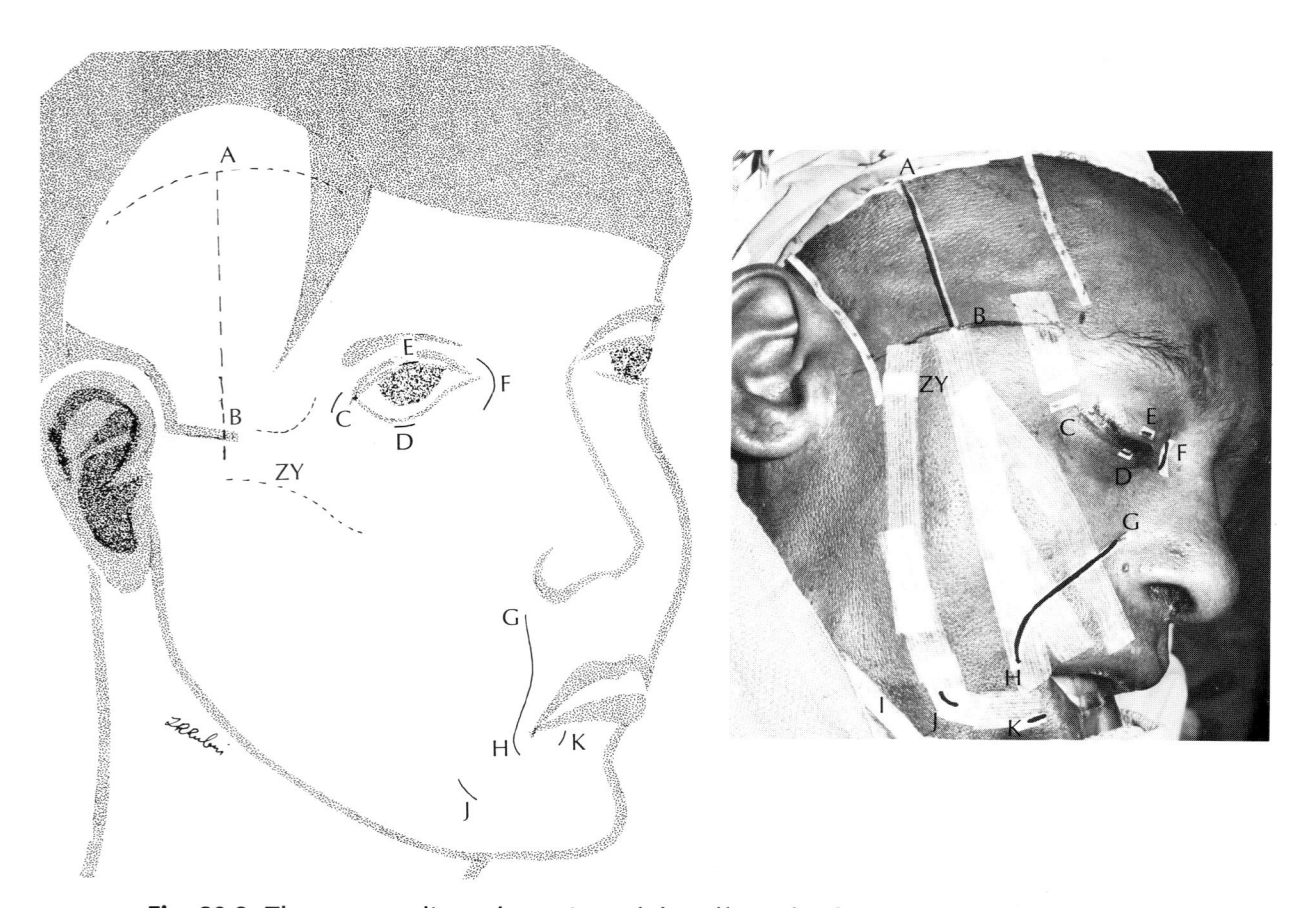

Fig. 26-3. The temporalis scalp region of the affected side is prepared by cutting of the hair close to the scalp, with shaving being unnecessary. All planned incisions are drawn on the scalp and face with gentian violet. A line is marked out corresponding to **AB**. This will denote the first incision to expose the temporal fascia. The line **AB** starts at the superior temporal line (which indicates the limits of the superior border of the temporal muscle) to the upper border of the zygomatic arch. In an elderly person, the marking will be made in the preauricular area similar to that of a face lift. This can allow the removal of redundant skin. The drawn line **GH** is at the new nasolabial fold and corresponds to the normal-side nasolabial fold. **F** will show the contemplated incision to expose the inner canthus. **D** and **E** are placed in the middle of the upper and lower lids, respectively, just below the lid margins. **C** is curved just lateral to the outer canthus. **K** is in the wrinkle lines of the lower lip about 2 cm medial to the corner of the mouth. **J** is in the wrinkle lines of the cheek approximately 3 cm below and lateral to the corner of the mouth.

Entire temporalis muscle transposition

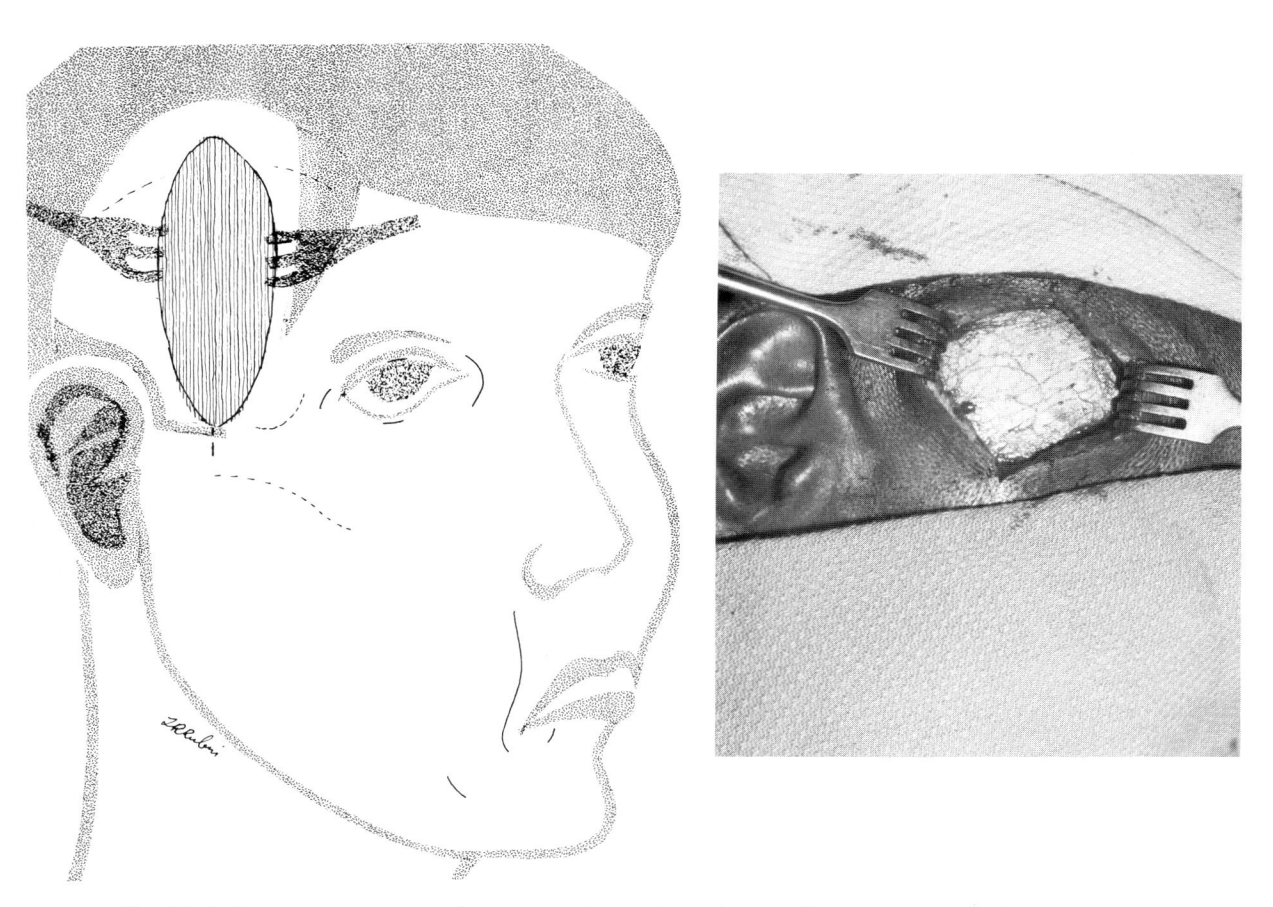

Fig. 26-4. Drapes are sutured to the scalp with 3-0 black silks to ensure hair coverage. An incision is made through the scalp skin to the depth of the deep fascia. The fascia exposed looks like a thick white-gray film.

Reanimation of the paralyzed face

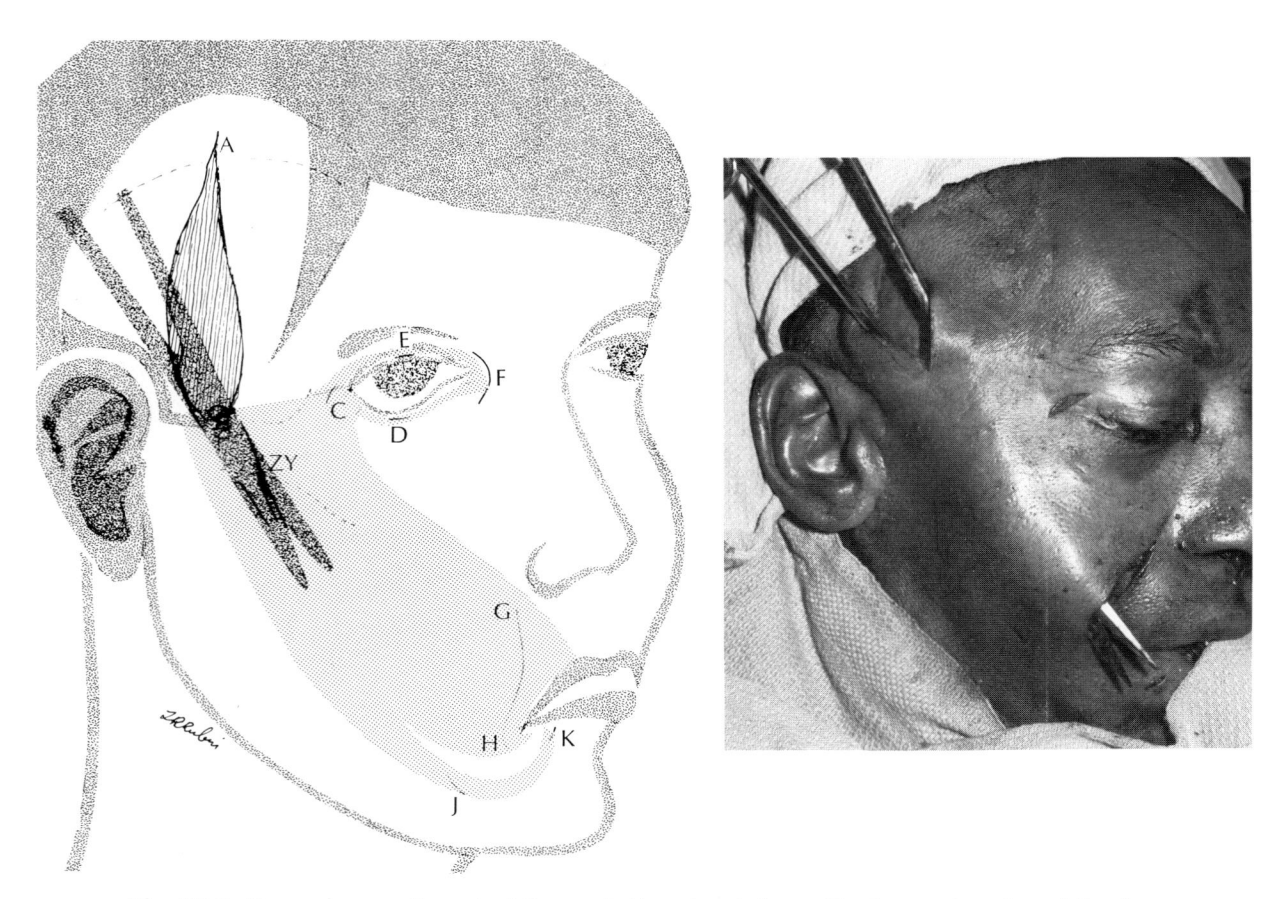

Fig. 26-5. Tunnels are dissected through the cheek from the lower border of the incision and superficial to the zygomatic arch down to the nasolabial fold, the upper lip, corner of the mouth, and portions of the lower lip as shown in the *shaded areas*. An incision is made in the skin just lateral to the outer canthus in the lines of the face, **C.** Horizontal incisions, no more than 3 mm, are made through the skin of the upper and lower eyelids in the midarea just above and below the eyelashes, **D** and **E.** Another incision is made medial to the inner canthus to expose the medial inner canthal ligaments, **F.** An incision is made in the nasolabial fold, **G** and **I,** to match the shape and location of the normal nasolabial fold. This incision runs from 1 cm below the alar nasolabial fold junction to the level of the corner of the mouth. The incision in this area goes into the deep tissue and will allow the exit of the scissors making the tunnel from the zygomatic arch. Incision **J** is made in the cheek along the facial lines as shown. It measures about 1 cm in length. **K** is a vertical incision in the lower lip about 2 cm medial to the corner of the mouth and just below the vermilion tissue. It is no more than 1 cm long.

Entire temporalis muscle transposition

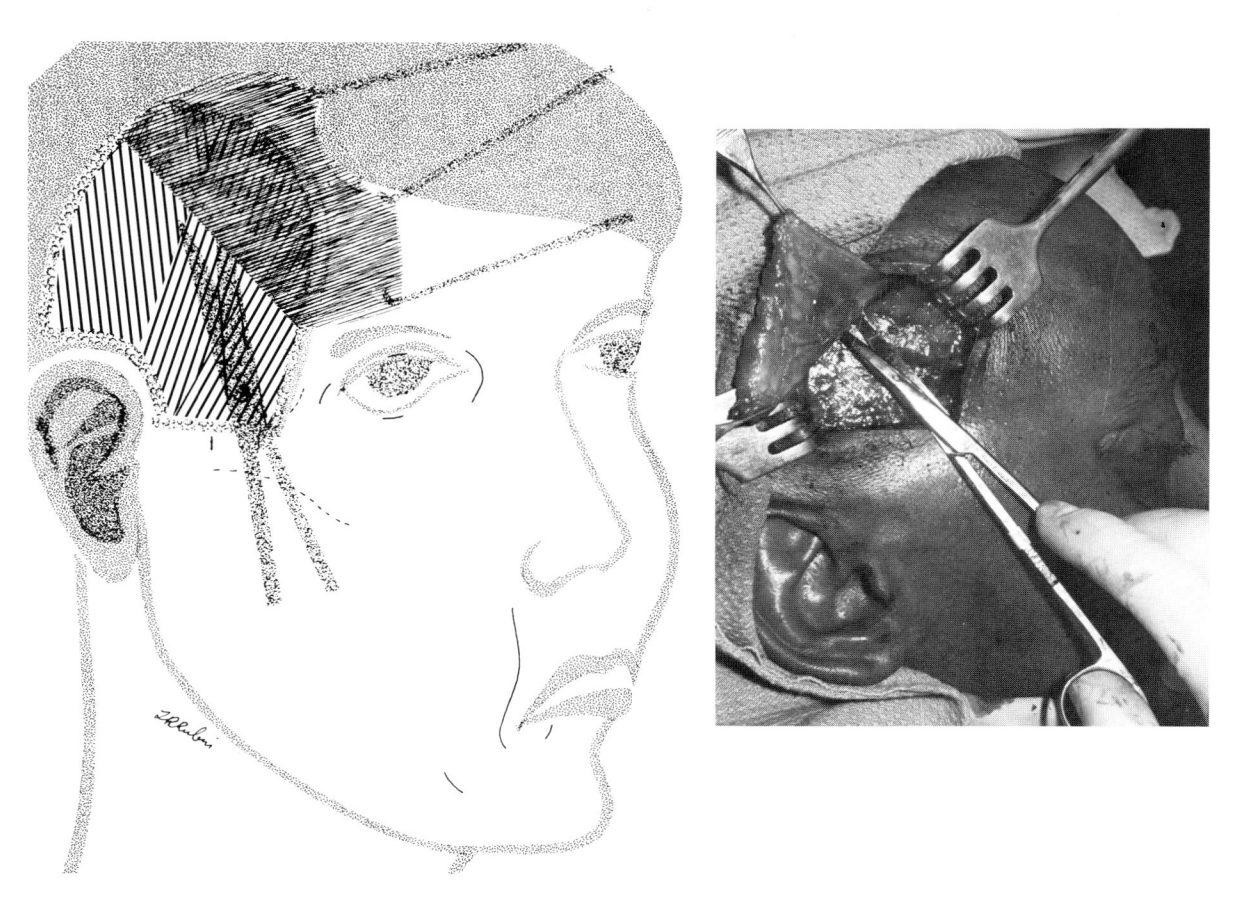

Fig. 26-6. This sketch shows the scalp removed from the area of the temporalis muscle to help illustrate the surgical technique. In the operation performed, good exposure of the fascia and the muscle can be obtained by use of broad, blunt retractors to hold back the scalp. The sketch shows a flap of deep temporal fascia being lifted off the muscle as a sheet. A first incision is made horizontally at the level of the zygomatic arch. Two vertical incisions are then made through the fascia anteriorally and posteriorly, creating a flap based superiorly. The anterior vertical incision is level with the outer canthus of the eye, and the posterior incision is made behind the helix of the ear. The fascia is lifted off the muscle by blunt dissection almost to the height of the superior temporal line where it is left attached to the underlying muscle. A horizontal incision is cut above the temporal line through the fascia to the bone joining each vertical incision to create a rectangular flap of muscle and fascia.

Reanimation of the paralyzed face

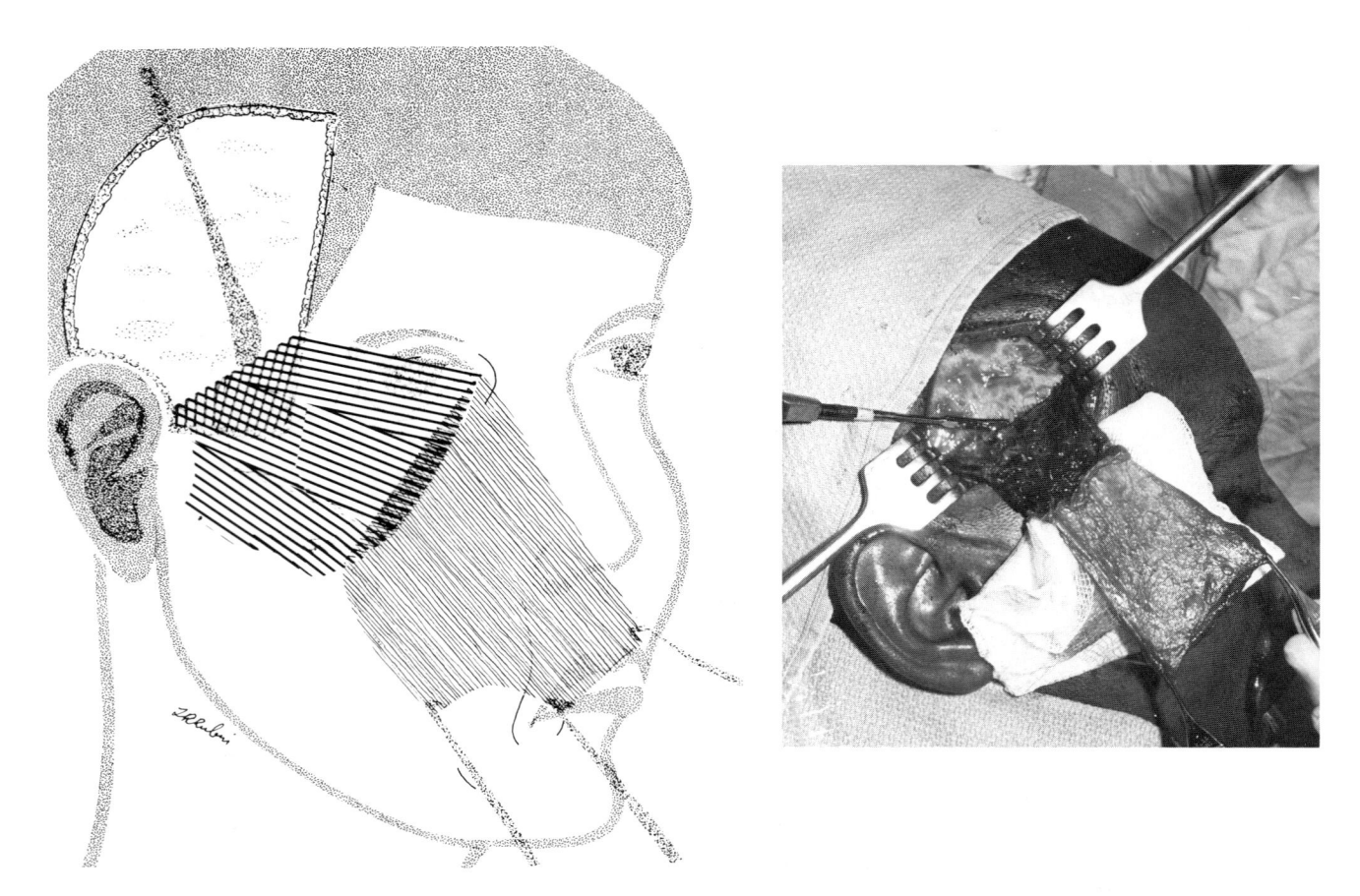

Fig. 26-7. With a blunt instrument, the muscle is stripped downward off the temporal bone. The muscle flap is the same size as the overlying fascial flap. The stripping is carried downward to the level of the upper border of the zygomatic arch with the attached fascia held gently by the assistant using fine hooks. It is most important not to strip the muscle below the level of the zygomatic arch, since the nerve entering the muscle is located halfway down the width of the zygomatic arch and is subject to injury.

Entire temporalis muscle transposition

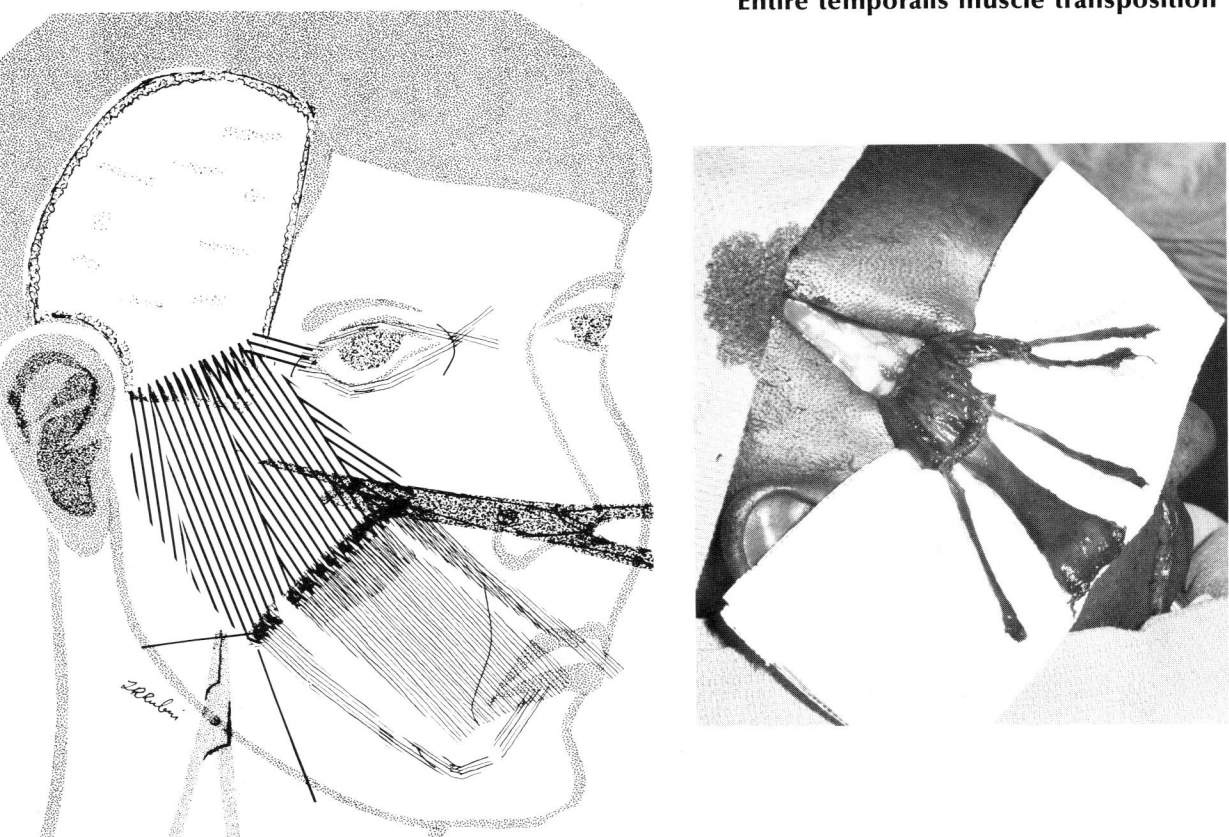

Fig. 26-8. After the muscle is draped over the arch, it becomes obvious that it could not reach the lips or the inner canthi of the eyelids. The fascia now takes the role of tendons. On the medial side, two narrow strips of fascia are cut, each 4 mm wide. They will serve as tendons for the eyelids. The motor muscle for these fascial strips to the eyelids is now cut from the medial aspect of the temporalis muscle flap and is no more than about 8 mm wide. The fascia attachment is reinforced with white 4-0 Mersilene mattress sutures. The remaining fascia is now divided into three parts:

1. A strip medially of about 5 mm wide is used to activate the upper lip and substitutes for the levator superioris portion of the quadratus labii superioris muscle. (This strip is used if the patient has demonstrated a dominant canine smile.)
2. A 5 mm wide strip is placed most laterally to serve as a long tendon to thread through the cheek and fasten to the lower lip.
3. The remaining intervening fascia, which is about 4 cm wide, is used to activate the nasolabial fold, lateral portions of the upper lip, and the angle of the mouth.
4. *The junctions of each fascial strip to the muscle must be reinforced with many white 4-0 Mersilene mattress sutures.* Many sutures are used to ensure a firm union. One should test the strips by pulling them taut, making sure that there is no separation of the fascia from the muscle. These junctions must withstand firm stretching when they are inserted into their new position.

Reanimation of the paralyzed face

Fig. 26-9. Strips of the fascia acting as tendons are tested for proper length to the desired areas. Note the two tendons for the eyelids. They must be long enough to fasten to the inner canthus. The strip to the lower lip is too short to reach its destination, requiring additional length by suturing of an extra piece to the end. Care must be made to ensure that the suturing is beyond the cheek incision **J,** where the tendon turns upward toward the lip. Point **J** acts as a pulley, and if the lengthening strips are sutured proximal to the pulley, it could be snagged when the muscle is contracted.

The tendons have been threaded through the tunnels. The tendons to the eyelids must be very close to the lid margins. A suture of 5-0 Mersilene is usually placed in the soft tissue around the tendons to keep the tendons close to the margins, and it avoids slipping down of the lids. This could produce an ectropian when the tendons are tightened. The strips are threaded under and around the medial canthus and intertwined after being pulled *taut*. They are sutured into the inner canthus with 4-0 white Mersilene. The sketch shows the strips coming through the medial incision after being threaded under the medial inner canthal ligaments.

The medial strip to the upper lip will be fastened to the mirror position of the levator superioris on the normal side. The wide strip is attached to the lip laterally, to the corner of the mouth, and to the lateral portion of the lower lip. It is sutured to the deep fascia, remaining muscle, or dermis, if need be, with 4-0 white Mersilene mattress sutures. If one *sutures under tension,* two dull rakes are used to pull the cheek upward while the pull on the tendons is downward, stretching the muscle as much as possible.

The tendon to the lower lip is pulled upward around the pulley in the cheek and then sutured to the lower lip, which is held in a neutral position. This tendon will act as a restraining force to exert counterpull to the upward force at the mouth angle. The temporalis muscle can be seen in the sketch as a bulge above the level zygomatic arch. This bulge is unavoidable and makes the face somewhat asymmetrical in the region of the zygomatic arch. The sketch also shows a silicone shaped block being inserted above the muscle to fill the temporal fossa, which had been occupied by the temporalis muscle.

Entire temporalis muscle transposition

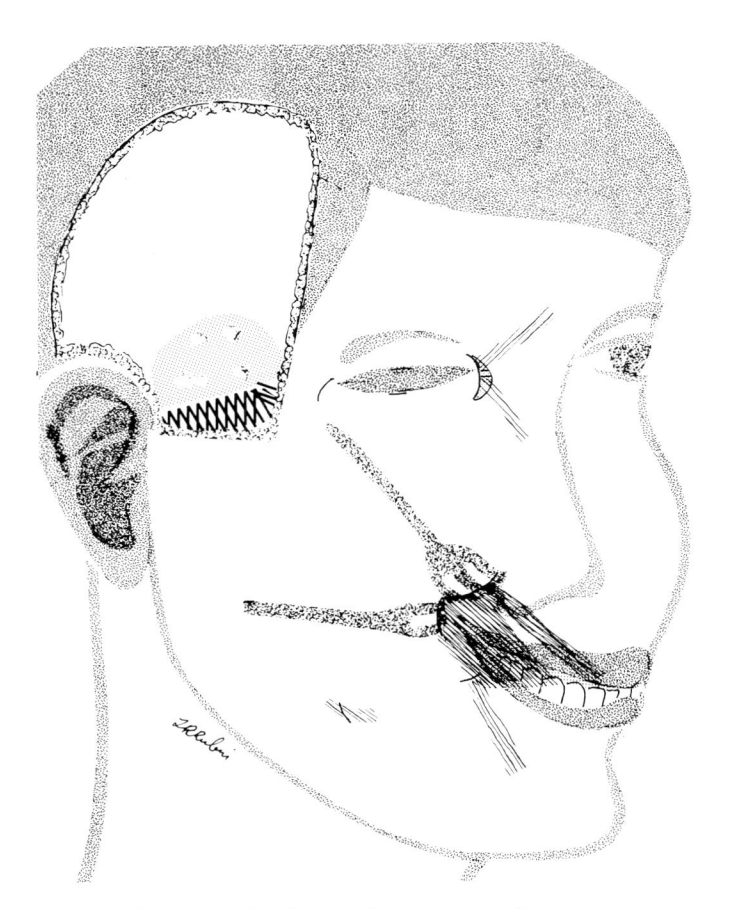

Fig. 26-9, For legend see opposite page.

Reanimation of the paralyzed face

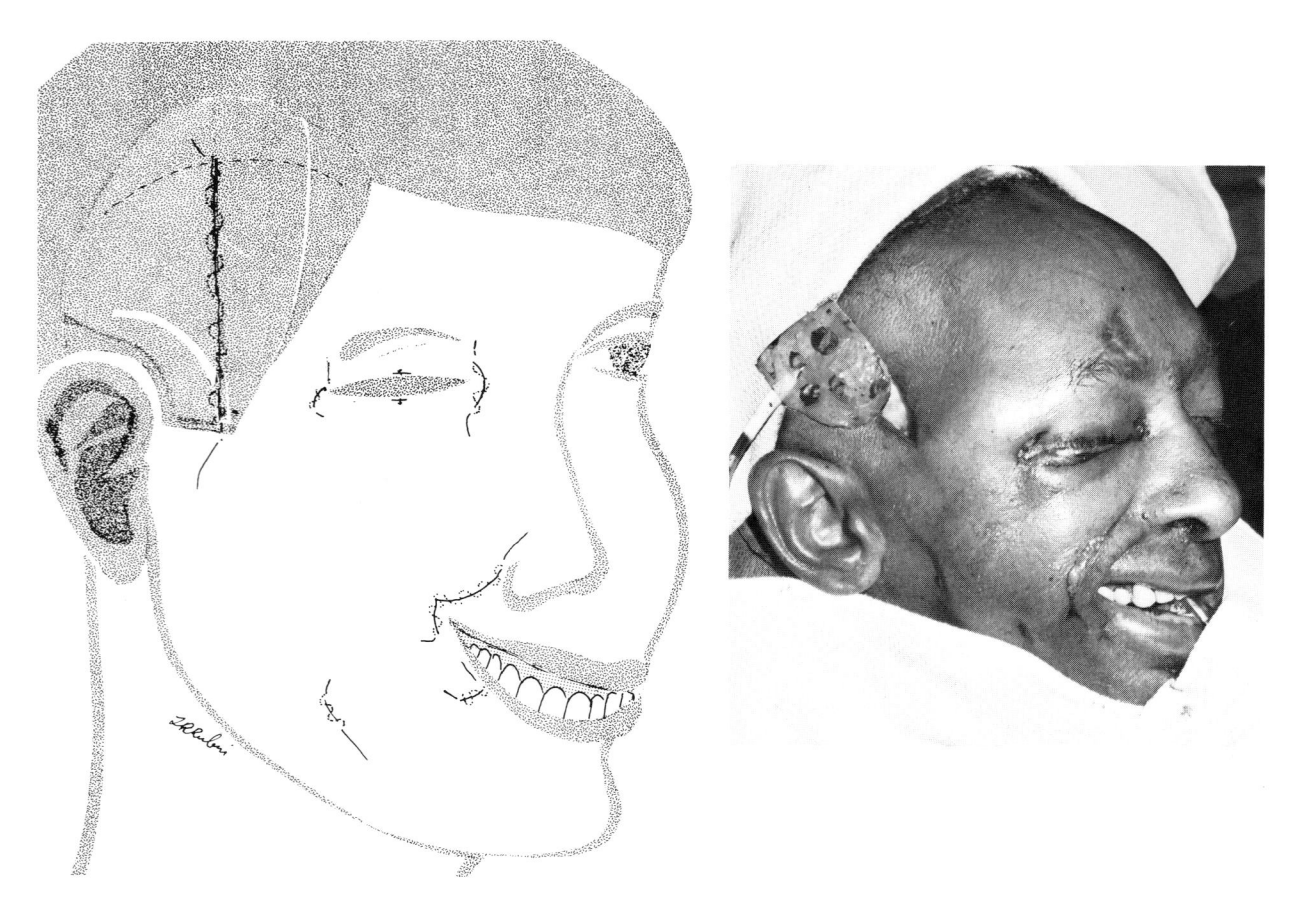

Fig. 26-10. The tendons have been pulled taut and sutured under tension to the inner canthi, the upper lip, angle of the mouth, and lower lip. All face skin wounds have now been closed with 4-0 Dexon for the deep tissue and 5-0 nylon pull-out subcuticular stitches for the superficial skin. The defect in the temporal fossa created when the muscle is turned downward is filled with a soft silicone block carved at the table. Holes are made in the block to allow scar tissue invasion for fixation.

The final closure of the scalp is made with 3-0 interlocking continuous black silk sutures. The sketch shows a suction tube being placed deep in the face and the scalp pocket to evacuate any residual hematoma. The tube is removed in 24 to 48 hours. A tight pressure dressing is placed over the entire cheek to help close the space created by the extensive undermining.

Entire temporalis muscle transposition

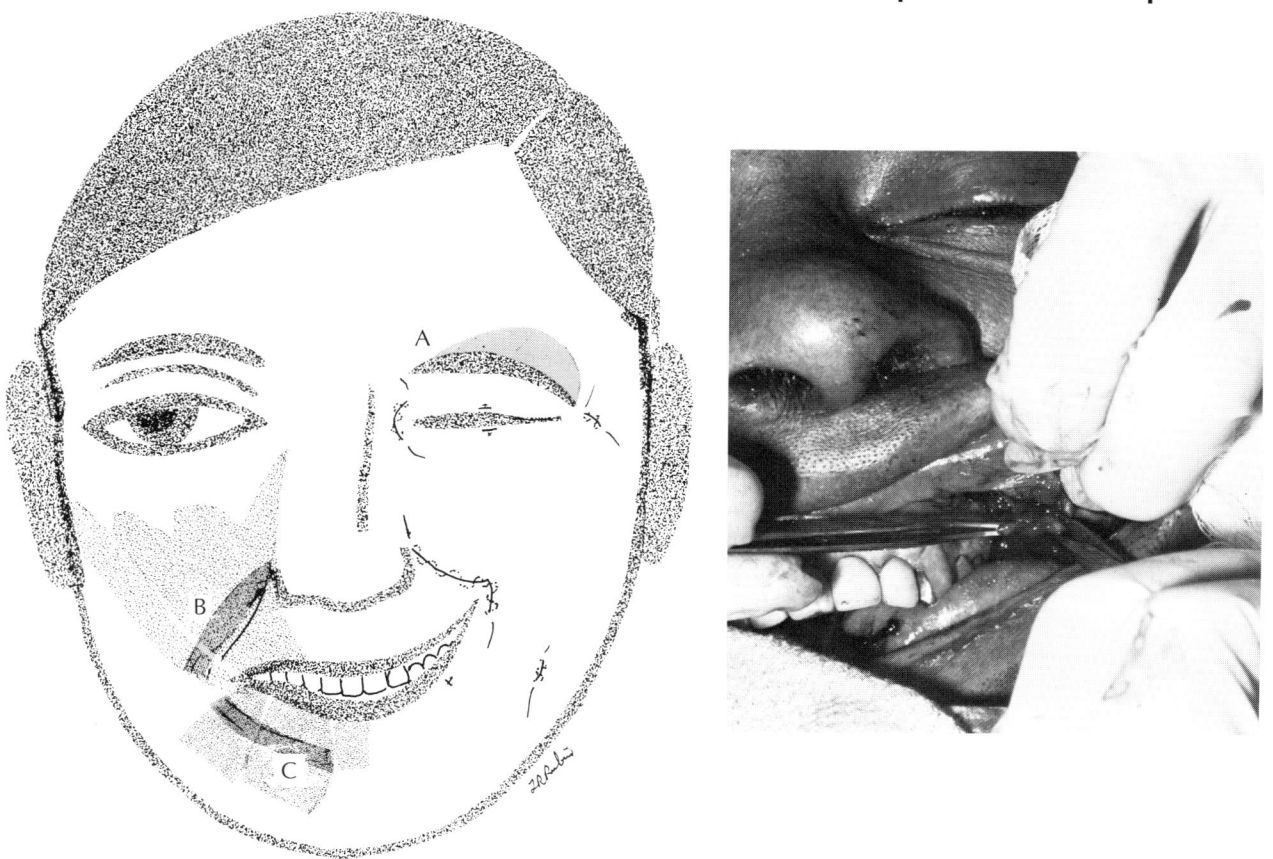

Fig. 26-11. When skin closure is completed on the paralyzed side, attention is shifted to the normal side. Weakening of the dominant muscle is needed to equalize the disproportionate contracting force of the normal side as compared to the weak temporalis contractions. After one has predetermined which muscles are dominant, a curving incision is made in the mouth mucosa above the orbicularis on the normal side, exposing the quadratus labii superioris and the zygomaticus major muscles, **B.** About 0.5 cm is excised from each muscle just as it reaches the orbicularis oris. The muscle will contract and separate immediately. A similar incision is made in the mucosa of the lower lip, exposing the quadratus labii inferioris and the triangularis **C,** the major depressors of the lower lip and corner of the mouth. A 0.5 cm strip is removed from each of these muscles. The *dark lines* in the sketch show the lines of excision. There is little fear of paralysis. Considerable weakening only creates a more pleasant balance. As time goes on, muscle reattachment occurs and the contracting forces on the normal side start approaching their original contractions. However, if moderate excisions are made, the lessened contracting force is beneficial. The mucosal wounds are sutured with 4-0 Dexon sutures, which need no removal.

The sagging of the eyebrow is corrected by removal of a crescent of skin above the brow, **A.** One can determine the amount of skin to be taken by pulling the brow upward to the best level to correspond to the normal eyebrow shape. It is advisable to overcorrect the brow height. The shape of the skin patch removed seems best suited when cut as shown in the sketch. The incision is made just at the brow line, and the final closure with a pull-out of 4-0 nylon subcuticular sutures leaves but a minimal scar.

Reanimation of the paralyzed face

Postoperative course

The immediate postoperative course creates an extremely edematous face. The eyelids are shut tightly. All the teeth are exposed in an extreme grimace. The nasolabial fold and the corner of the mouth are pulled upward and backward. The soft pressure dressings are removed by the fourth day. Several more days will elapse before the eyelids start functioning. Levator function will slowly open the upper lids. The corner of the mouth and the nasolabial fold will return to a normal position covering the teeth within approximately 10 days.

Muscle movements become apparent within 24 to 48 hours after surgery and continue to function with greater efficiency as the patient, clenching his teeth, stimulates the temporalis contractions. The full muscle function may take about 1 year to be completed. Edema of the face persists for months. During this time, the patient must observe himself in front of a mirror and practice exposing his teeth in an expression of happiness or pleasure that can now be called a smile. This can always be accomplished by clenching the teeth tightly on the affected side. After the edema subsides, the muscle contracts the upper lip and the nasolabial fold to a greater degree since the edema of the facial tissue is no longer a restricting force. The greater the overcorrection of the smile at the time of surgery by stretching the temporalis muscle, the greater will be the excursion when the patient clenches his teeth.

A number of our patients have, in time, been able to control movements of eyes and mouth independently. It is our feeling that some of this independent action may take place because of changes in the brain, or, that the three branches of the nerve to the temporalis muscle may be sufficient to cause the different portions of the muscle to move independently.

Pitfalls to be avoided

1. The possibility of a weak or underdeveloped temporalis muscle exists. Testing must be done beforehand to ensure the temporalis function. If the fifth nerve is injured, the operation obviously cannot be performed. If the muscle is weak, the patient can strengthen it by active exercise such as clenching his teeth continuously or chewing gum. Several months of exercise prior to the surgery may be needed to obtain the increased strength.
2. The temporalis fascia, acting as tendons, must be carefully sutured to the muscle to reinforce the junctions since the fascia and the muscle must be pulled taut in extreme tension.
3. The tendons threading through the eyelids must be at the lid margins. Failure can cause ectropion as the tendons slip beyond the margins to evert the eyelids. The author has found that a 4-0 Dexon suture may often act as a tunnel check in the mideyelid incision area to help hold the marginal position.
4. Facial configuration must be carefully planned before surgery. Proper placement of the nasolabial fold incision can create a pleasant, normal result. By predetermining the optimal direction of the pull, one can place the muscle and its fascia in the mirror position of the normal side to develop a pleasant smile when all muscles contract simultaneously.

The temporalis transplantation procedure as described has one definite limitation. It does not provide for a coordinated, synchronized, balanced face during speech.

However, a solution is in sight. Our recent work with dogs have confirmed the principle of neural neurotization (see Chapter 15). The implantation of a free nerve graft into a denervated muscle will stimulate nerve-end axon sprouting and reanastomosis with the neuromuscular junction. A sural nerve anastomosed with buccal fascicles of the opposite normal side can be threaded across the face and inserted into the belly of the temporalis muscle that has been transplanted to activate the face. This may be done only after the functioning temporalis muscle has had its fifth-nerve motor function cut at least 2 weeks prior to the implantation. Whereas the possibility exists of doing a direct nerve anastomosis to the end of the fifth nerve as it enters the temporalis, the logistics of suturing under microscope makes it a most difficult approach.

Summary

I have described a comparatively simple procedure by using the temporalis muscle and its overlying thick fascia, acting as tendons, to provide a dynamic motor force to activate the paralyzed upper portions of the face including the eyelids. The temporalis muscle is innervated by the fifth cranial nerve, which is rarely paretic. The temporal muscle transplantation has been a satisfactory motor apparatus for the facial paralysis as demonstrated by the photographed cases. Many static procedures using fascia lata have been described in textbooks. I believe these should not be used under any circumstances since the results leave a face fixed and immobile instead of giving it a dynamic, moving expression.

The temporalis muscle transposition has one great limitation. It does not make for a synchronized face during speech. New techniques of nerve grafting have brightened the picture for a solution to this problem.

Reanimation of the paralyzed face

CASE 1

Patient is a 51-year-old white male who had an acoustic nerve neuroma removed 25 years previously with resultant complete left-side facial paralysis. Nerve studies showed no activity.

A, Preoperative view with patient in repose. The clouded eyeball was unrelated to his paralysis.

B, Preoperative view of patient trying to smile and close his left eyelid.

C, Postoperative view, 1 year after temporalis muscle transposition. The eyelids contract and the patient smiles when he tenses his left jaw. By practice in front of the mirror, he has been able to correlate and balance his smile.

D, The patient in repose.

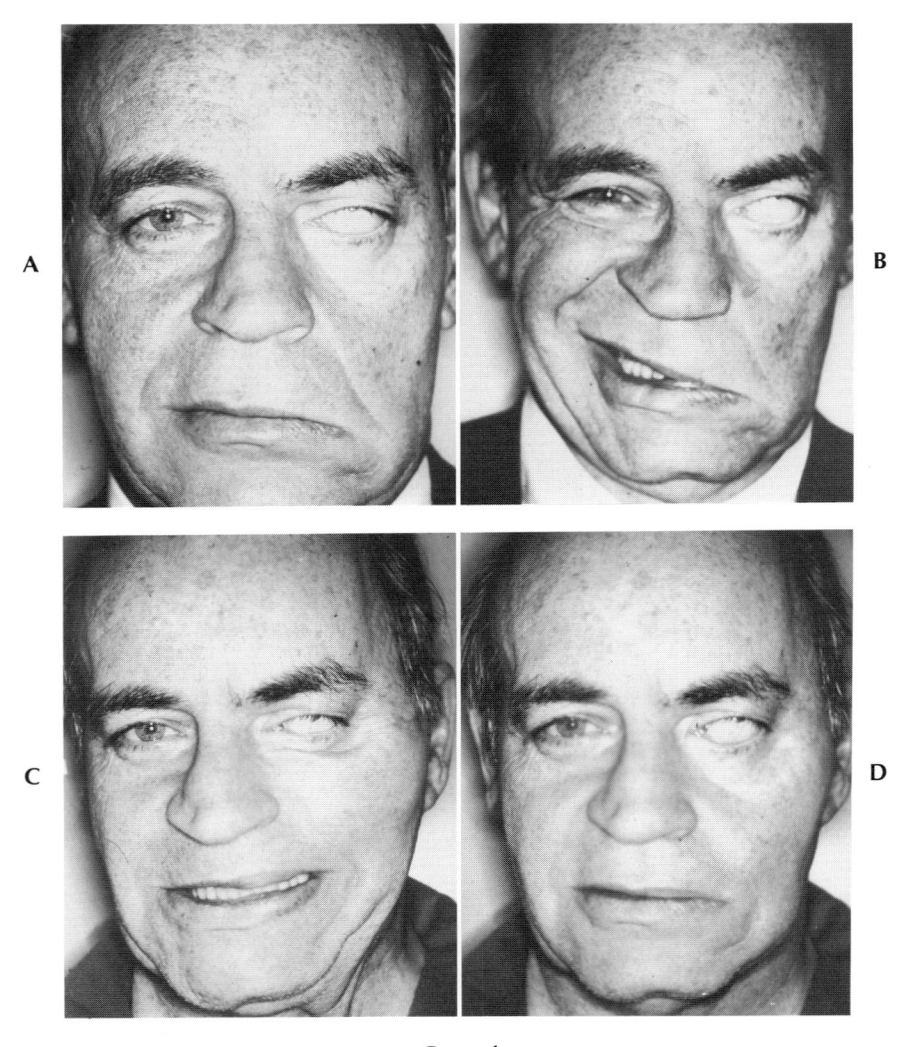

Case 1

Entire temporalis muscle transposition

CASE 2

An 18-year-old white female who suffered severe cerebral damage after a fractured skull. She had been unconscious for several weeks. She was left with a permanent facial paralysis as well as a partial hemiplegia. The accident had occurred 18 months prior to taking of the photographs. Eight months previously, the patient had a partial masseter muscle implant to the corner of the mouth and a fascia lata sling from the mouth to the temporalis muscle by another surgeon. Electronic testing just prior to present operation showed complete absence of seventh nerve function on the paralyzed face.

A, Preoperative view of the patient trying to smile and close her right eyelid.

B, The patient with face in repose. Note the thick pad in the right cheek lateral to mouth corner. This is the masseter muscle attachment to the mouth corner done 8 months previously.

C and **D,** Postoperative views in repose and smiling after temporalis muscle transplant to cheeks, lips, and eyelids. The patient also had weakening of the levator superioris muscle on the normal side. Patient is now able to close her eyelids.

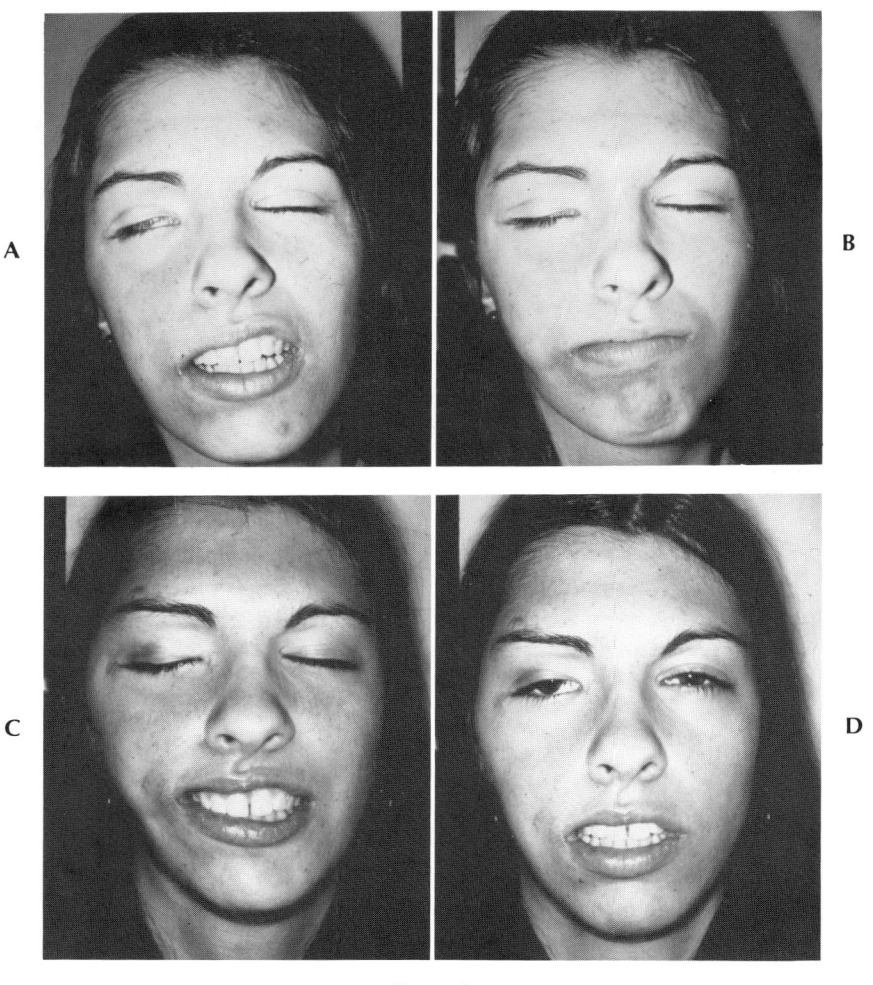

Case 2

Reanimation of the paralyzed face

CASE 3

Patient is a 23-year-old white housewife who had a radical parotidectomy 2 years before being seen. Her facial nerve was completely removed in the radical dissection. A neck dissection was performed at the same time followed by extensive x-ray therapy. Electrical studies showed no evidence of any nerve regrowth. The paralysis was complete for the left affected side.

A, Preoperative view in repose.
B, The patient trying to close her left eye.
C, The patient trying to smile.
D, Postoperative view of the patient in repose 1 year after surgery.
E, Postoperative view showing a balanced controlled smile.
F, Postoperative view showing patient smiling and closing her eyelids. Repeat electronic studies showed no facial nerve recovery on the affected side.

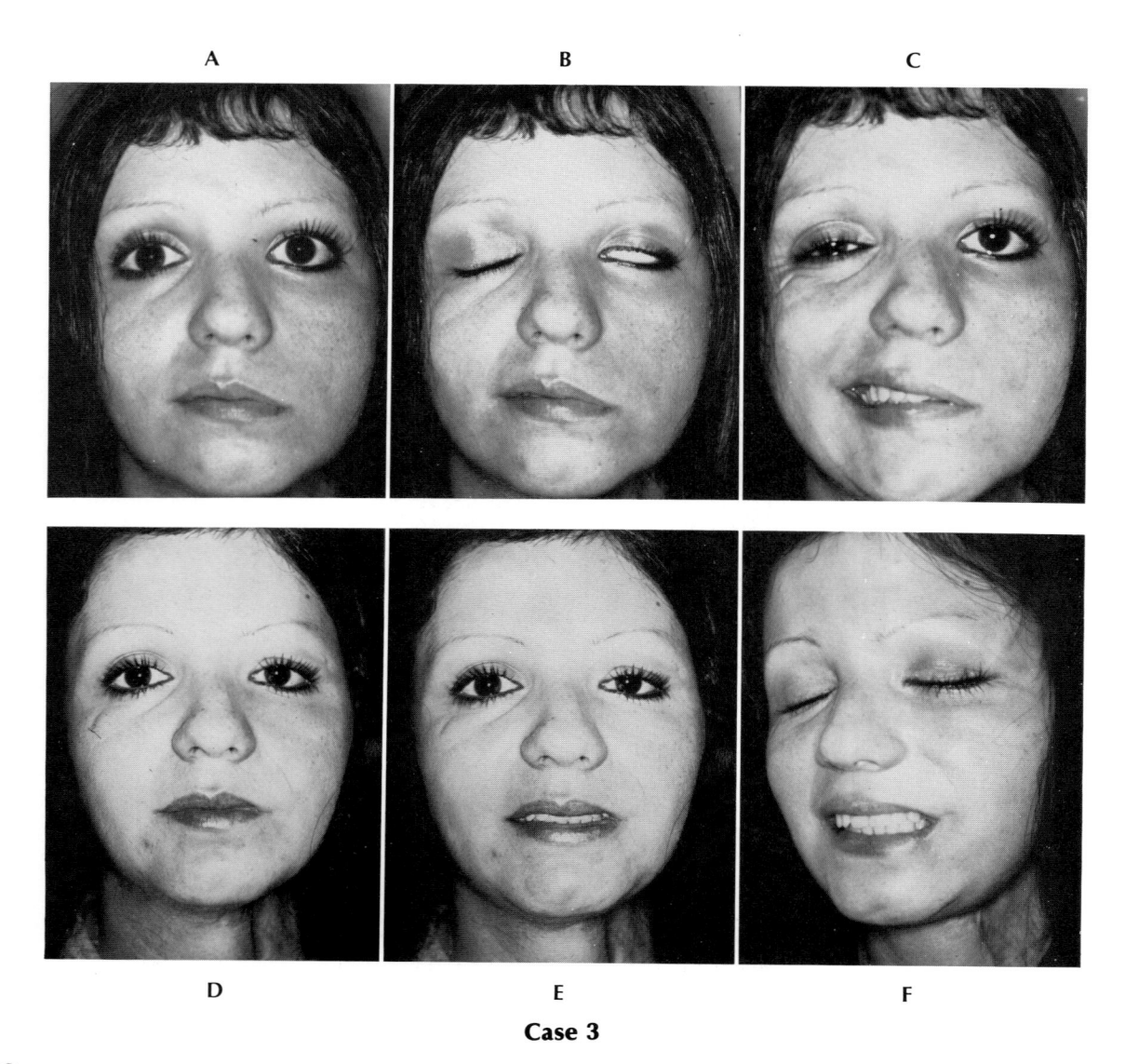

Case 3

Entire temporalis muscle transposition

CASE 4

Patient is a 22-year-old white male who was born with a unilateral complete facial paralysis (Möbius syndrome). Electronic stimulation showed no activity in the buccal and marginal branches and limited activity of the zygomatic branches.

A, Preoperative view of the patient trying to smile. He could not close his eyelids tightly.
B, The patient in repose.
C, Postoperative view 1 year after a temporalis muscle transplant. The patient in repose.
D, The patient smiling and closing his left eye at the same time.

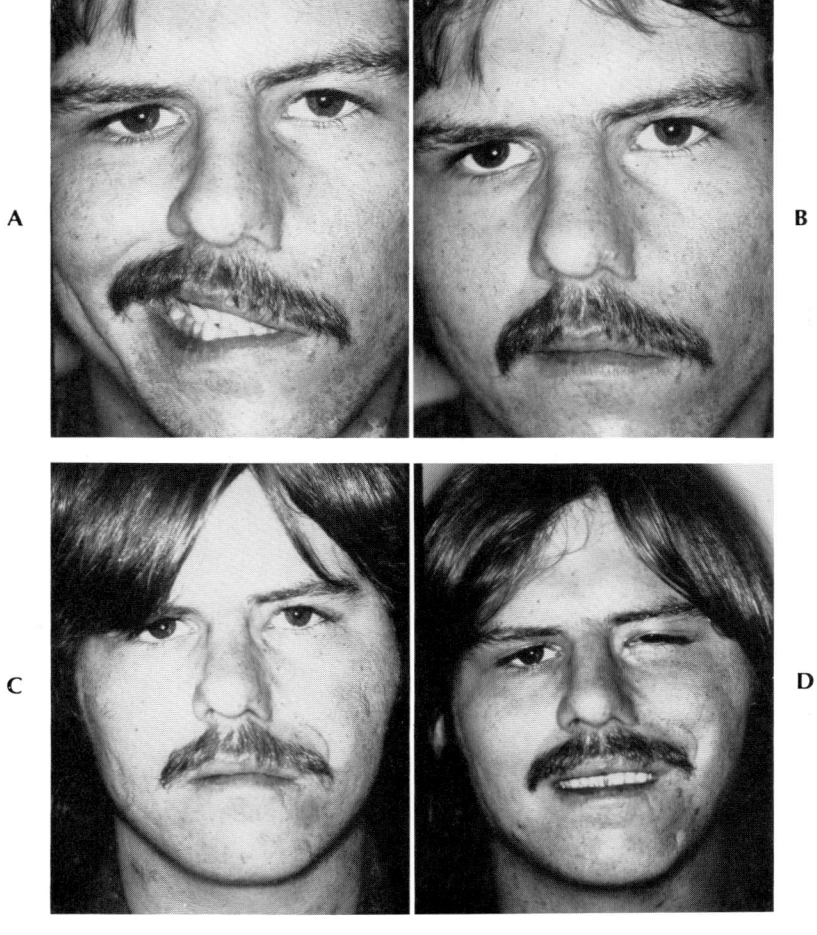

Case 4

Reanimation of the paralyzed face

CASE 5

A 56-year-old housewife who had an acoustic nerve tumor removed approximately 3 years prior to a temporal muscle transposition. Electronic studies showed muscle degeneration and no nerve regeneration prior to temporalis muscle operation.

A and **B,** Patient attempting to smile and close her eyes.

C, Patient in repose.

D and **E,** Patient has had the temporalis muscle transplantation and the removal of about 1 cm of the levator superioris and zygomaticus major muscles on the normal side.

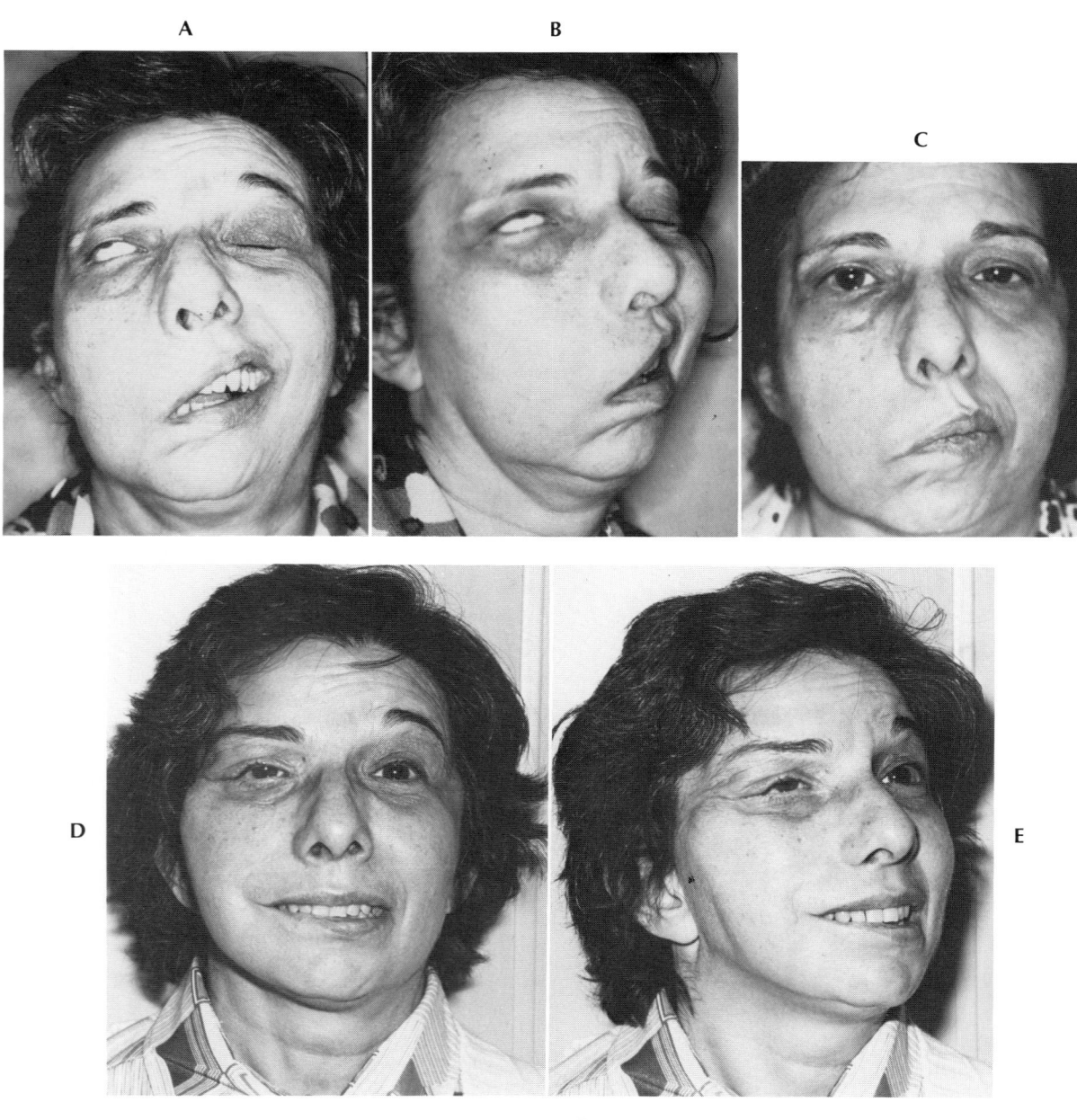

Case 5

REFERENCES

1. Anderson, J. G.: Surgical treatment of lagophthalmos in leprosy by the Gillies temporalis transfer, Br. J. Plast. Surg. **14**(4):339, 1961.
2. Converse, J. M.: Reconstructive plastic surgery, Philadelphia, 1964, W. B. Saunders Co., pp. 1154-1162.
3. Gillies, H. D.: Facial paralysis, Proc. Roy. Soc. Med. **27**:1372, 1934.
4. McLaughlin, C. R.: Surgical support in permanent facial paralysis, Plast. Reconstr. J. **11**:203, 1953.
5. Rubin, L. R., Bromberg, B. E., and Walden, R. H.: Congenital bilateral facial paralysis, Möbius syndrome, surgical animation of the face, Transactions of the Fourth International Congress on Plastic and Reconstructive Surgery, Amsterdam, 1969, Excerpta Medica Foundation, pp. 740-746.
6. Sheean, J. E.: Manual of reparative plastic surgery, New York, 1938, The Macmillan Co.

27 Free muscle grafts by microneurovascular techniques

KITARO OHMORI
KIYONORI HARII

Muscle grafts to the face survive by microneurovascular anastomosis with use of the microscope. The muscles replace the facial muscles that have atrophied. The suturing of blood vessels and nerves ensures a functioning and surviving graft.

Free muscle grafts by microneurovascular techniques

Transfer of free muscles by microneurovascular surgery for facial paralysis is one of the ideal methods of treatment. We previously reported on two cases of unresolved Bell's palsy treated by transfer of free gracilis muscles to the face and their grafting by use of microneurovascular anastomoses.[4] That was the world's first published report describing clinical neurovascular anastomoses used successfully to connect a transferred muscle while enabling the muscle to retain its function. The success has added a new dimension to the treatment of facial paralysis and muscle paralyses in other parts of the body. This chapter describes the technique as a method of treating facial paralysis caused by a muscular defect.

Removal, transfer, and emplacement of free muscle by neurovascular anastomoses, like the various free flap transfers we have described in the past,[1-3,5,6] consists of two important elements—microsurgical techniques and the neurovascular base of the donor site.

Selection of donor muscle

The ideal donor muscle would be nourished by a pair consisting of an artery and a vein that can be anastomosed and would be free from multiple innervation. Another condition is that sacrifice of the donor muscle should not result in a functional disorder in the donor site. A number of muscles meet these conditions. We use the gracilis muscle for large donor requirements and the extensor brevis muscle of the foot for smaller requirements.

Microsurgical techniques

The microsurgical techniques required in a free muscle transfer are divided into microvascular surgery and microneurosurgery, of which the technical aspects are discussed elsewhere in this book. The technical difficulty in the transfer lies primarily in adjustment of the differences in vessel diameter between donor site and recipient site and in the number and size of funiculi between the two sites. In nerve anastomoses, the motor nerve must be properly selected.

Anatomical base of donor muscles

GRACILIS MUSCLE

The gracilis muscle is located most superficially in the adductor muscle group of the thigh. It originates from the medial margin of the lower half of the body of the pubis and from the upper half of the pubic arch and inserts into the medial surface of the upper end of the tibia.

The main nourishing vessels of this gracilis muscle mostly emerge directly from the deep femoral vessels (sometimes these nourishing vessels originate from the medial circumflex femoral vessels and their junction with the deep femoral vessels), but all of them run between the adductor longus and adductor brevis muscles to enter the muscle belly at the proximal third of the gracilis muscle and can nourish the whole muscle.

There are one or two more small nourishing vessels that enter this muscle at the middle and distal third, but they are not necessary for inclusion with this muscle for microvascular anastomoses.

The motor supply of the gracilis muscle is derived from the motor branch of the obturator nerve, which descends between the adductor longus and brevis muscles. The motor nerve, as the only such nerve for this muscle, innervates the gracilis muscle accompanied by the nourishing vessels (Fig. 27-1).

EXTENSOR BREVIS MUSCLE

The extensor brevis muscle usually has four muscle bellies. Located in the dorsal aspect of the foot, this muscle originates on the dorsal side of the tarsal bone and inserts in the base of the proximal phalanx or the expansion hood of the toes, or in both areas.

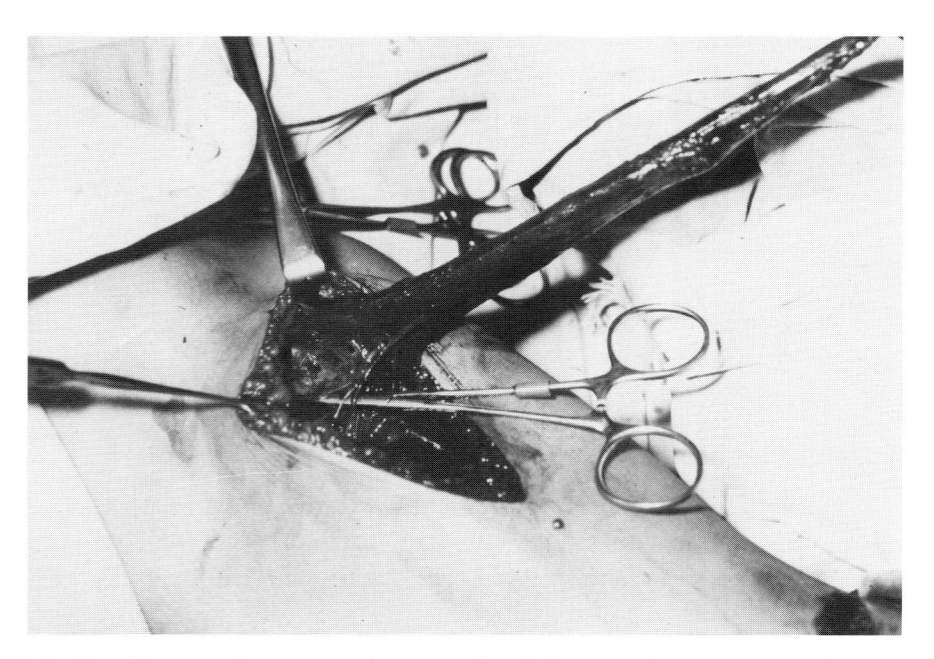

Fig. 27-1. Gracilis muscle is raised in an island form with main nourishing vessels of this muscle and motor branch of obturator nerve. (From case 2.)

Free muscle grafts by microneurovascular techniques

The nourishing vessels for the extensor brevis muscle originate from the lateral tarsal artery, which is one of the terminal branches of the anterior tibial vessels. Innervation of the extensor brevis muscle is provided by the lateral portion of the anterior tibial nerve, which serves as the motor nerve (Fig. 27-2).

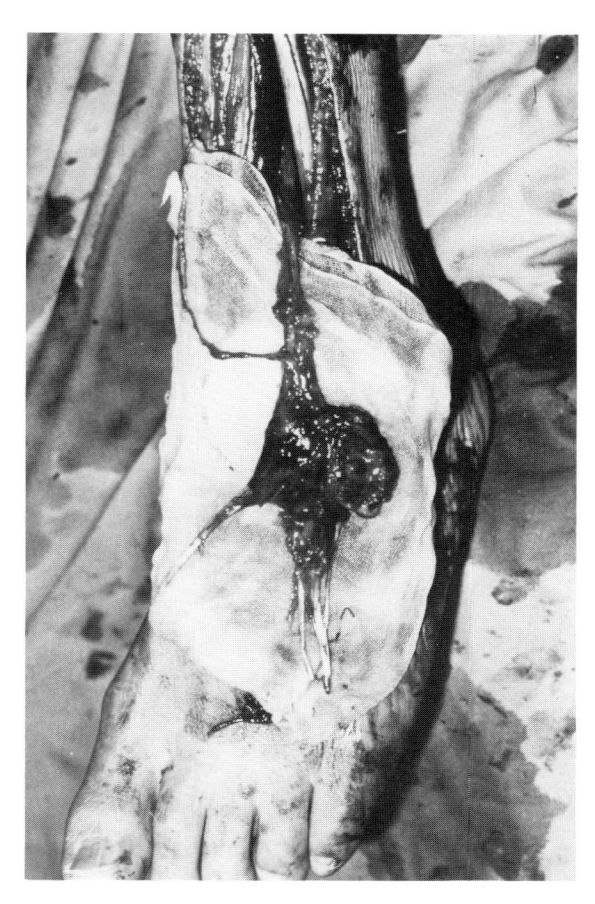

Fig. 27-2. Extensor brevis muscle is raised in an island form with anterior tibial vessels and anterior tibial nerve as pedicle.

Reanimation of the paralyzed face

CASE 1

A 23-year-old female with partial facial paralysis caused by traumatic damage of the facial muscle in the left cheek region (Fig. 27-3) had a traffic accident 7 years before undergoing surgery. In primary care soon after the accident, the damaged left eyeball and inferior orbital rim were removed, together with soft tissues including the muscle of the left cheek. The chief complaint of this patient was the inability to create the left nasolabial fold. To treat this patient, neurovascularized free muscle transfer was performed, with the left extensor brevis muscle as the donor muscle.

Operation. Through a preauricular incision, the superficial temporal vessel was exposed and hinged down to prepare the recipient vessels. The zygomatic branch of the facial nerve was prepared as the motor nerve of the recipient site, and then the recipient bed was prepared for the muscle to be transferred (Fig. 27-4).

Through a Z incision of the dorsal aspect of the foot, the left extensor brevis muscle was exposed and this muscle, with the tendon toward all toes, was raised as an island, with the anterior tibial vessel as the vascular pedicle and the anterior tibial nerve as the motor nerve of the donor muscle. During this maneuver, the extensor brevis muscle was reflected to check its nourishing vessels, which are the lateral tarsal vessels, and the dorsal artery of the foot was ligated distal to the origin of the lateral tarsal artery (Fig. 27-5).

The anterior tibial nerve is anatomically divided into the medial and lateral portions. The lateral portion is described as the motor nerve of the extensor brevis muscle. Clinically, however, the whole anterior tibial nerve was removed with the donor muscle, and the motor nerve of the donor site was selected by means of an electric stimulator.

Muscle transfer and microneurovascular anastomosing. After Heifetz's neurosurgical clips were applied to the pedicle vessels of the donor muscle, the pedicle vessels were severed and the freed extensor brevis muscle was transposed. The proximal end of this muscle was sutured to the periosteum of the remaining zygomatic bone and surrounding soft tissue, and the four tendons of this muscle were sutured to the upper lip and the nasolabial fold (Fig. 27-6).

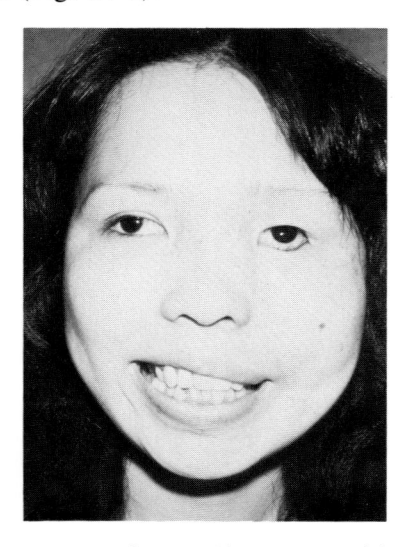

Fig. 27-3. Case 1. Preoperative condition. She was unable to create the L-nasolabial fold.

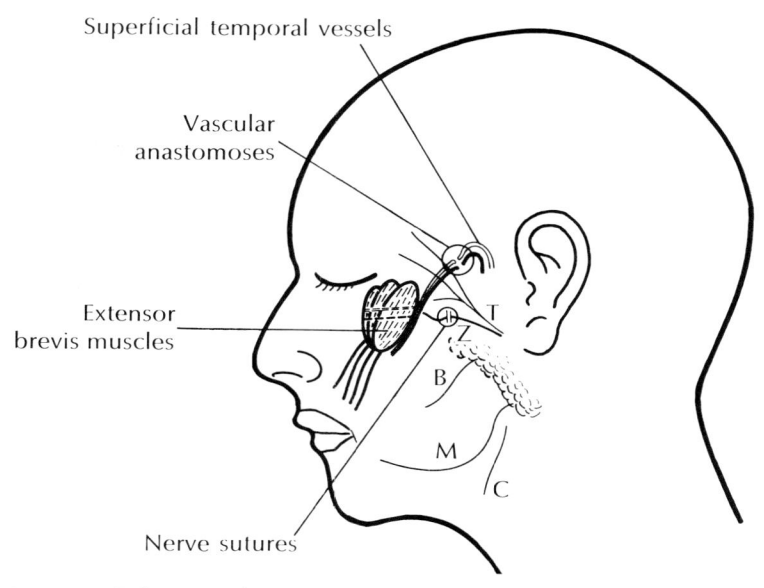

Fig. 27-4. Case 1. Schema of operative procedure. Nerves: *T*, temporal; *Z*, zygomatic; *B*, buccal; *M*, mandibular; *C*, cervical.

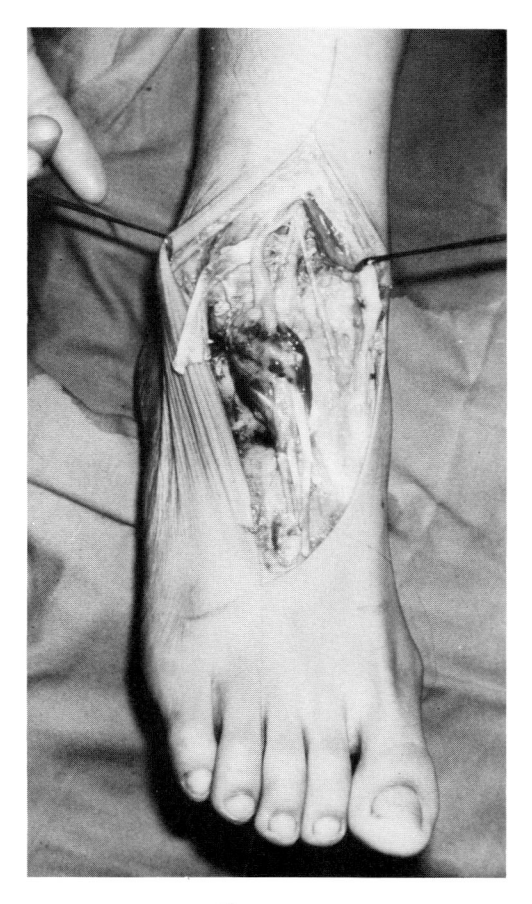

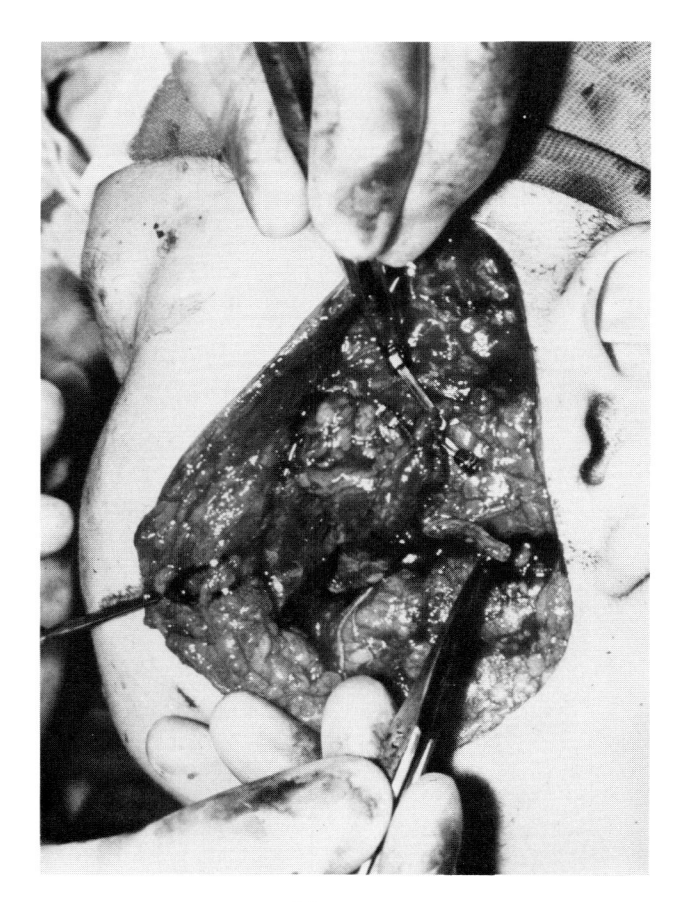

Fig. 27-5

Fig. 27-6

Fig. 27-5. Case 1. Extensor brevis muscle was raised in an island form with anterior tibial nerve and vessels as pedicle.

Fig. 27-6. Case 1. Shown are anterior tibial vessels with Heifetz's clips, anterior tibial nerve picked up by forceps, and proximal portion of transferred muscle.

After fixation of the muscle in the recipient bed, with the application of microvascular surgery, the muscle was revascularized. After proper blood circulation in the muscle was assured, the motor nerve was anastomosed.

Result. Up to 3 months after the surgery, the muscle bulk was palpated, but no voluntary contraction occurred. At 4 months, a twitch of the transferred muscle was observed. At 6 months, voluntary contraction of the muscle was observed clearly. The electromyogram at 8 months showed positive volitional waves (Fig. 27-7). At 8 months and thereafter, no increase in muscular contraction was observed (Fig. 27-8).

Reduction of the muscle volume occurred up to 2 months after the surgery. At 8 months, no abnormal prominence was observed even in the stage of muscle contraction. However, the muscle was palpated throughout the period of follow-up.

Muscle power on this side was weaker than that on the right (the normal) side, but it was enough to create a nasolabial fold. In this case, the strongest muscle contraction was observed when the eye was closed tightly (Fig. 27-9).

By this operation, the drooping sensation of the left cheek disappeared and the patient was satisfied with the result.

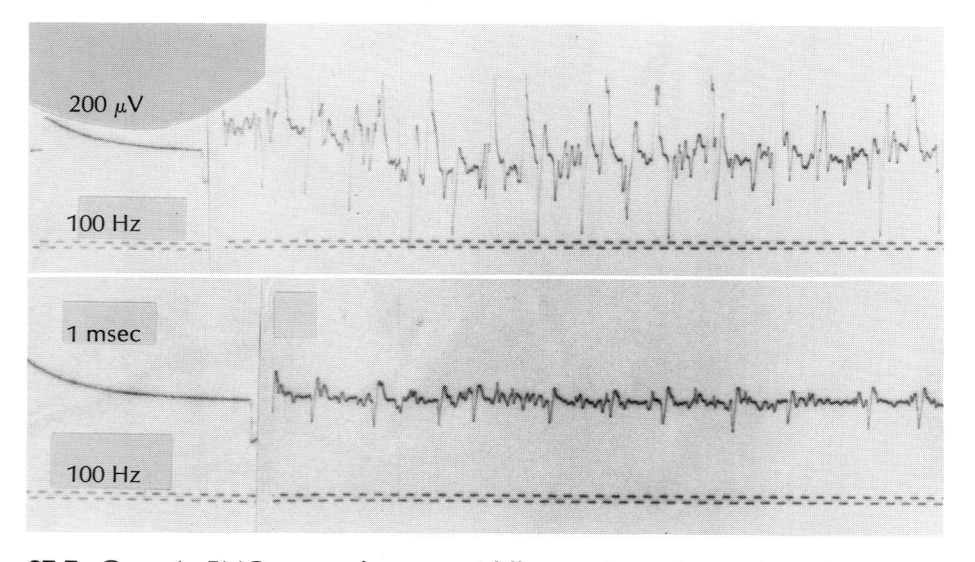

Fig. 27-7. Case 1. EMG was taken at middle portion of transferred muscle with positive pattern of volitional activity.

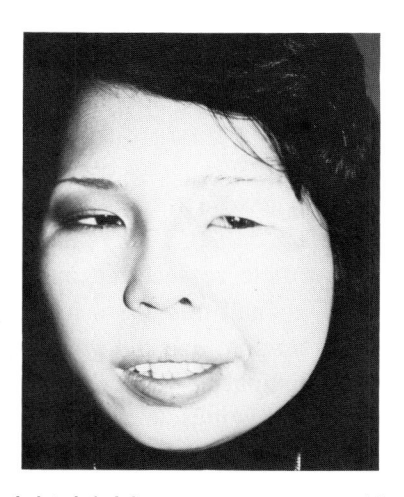

Fig. 27-8. Case 1. Left nasolabial fold was reconstructed by voluntary contraction of transferred muscle.

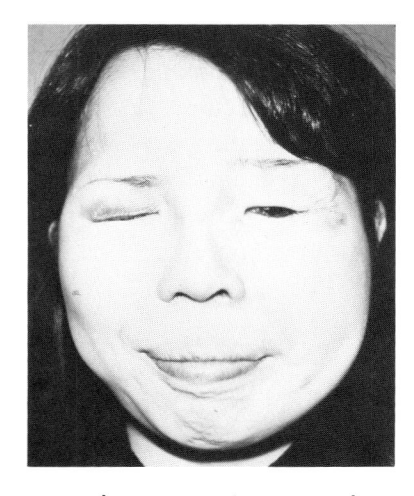

Fig. 27-9. Case 1. Strongest muscle contraction was observed when eye was closed tightly.

Reanimation of the paralyzed face

CASE 2

A 6-year-old girl had complete facial paralysis caused by surgical excision of a large cavernous lymphangioma in the right hemifacial region. This facial paralysis was caused by excision of the tumor with the facial muscles. This case of facial paralysis was ascribed to muscle defect. For treatment, the gracilis muscle was selected as the donor muscle, transferred, and grafted by microneurovascular technique (Fig. 27-10.)

Operation. Through a preauricular incision, superficial temporal vessels and the right buccal branch of the facial nerve were prepared as the nourishing vessels and motor nerve of the recipient site. Then, through a longitudinal incision of approximately 10 cm length on the medial side of the thigh, the proximal half of the gracilis muscle and the pedicle vessels and motor nerve of this muscle were exposed. This was followed by a small transverse incision made on the medial side of the knee to sever the gracilis tendon, and the gracilis muscle was pulled out in the proximal direction. The gracilis muscle was raised in an island form, with the nourishing vessels and motor nerve of this muscle as the pedicle (Fig. 27-1).

Muscle transfer and microneurovascular anastomosing. After Heifetz's neurosurgical clips were applied to the pedicle vessels of the donor muscle, the pedicle vessels were severed and the freed gracilis muscle was transposed (Fig. 27-11).

As in case 1, this donor muscle was not irrigated. After the proximal end of the gracilis muscle was fixed in the recipient bed, the distal end of this muscle was divided into two parts; one was inserted into the upper lip and the other into the lower lip, and both were fixed with a proper tension. Microneurovascular technique was applied to repair the artery and vein of both sites, and after the muscle was revascularized, the nerves were sutured.

Result. Up to 3 months after the surgery, the muscle bulk was palpated, but no voluntary contraction occurred. At 4 months, a twitch of the transferred muscle with slight voluntary contraction was observed. The power of this muscle had increased after 7 months. Maximum contraction of the transferred muscle was observed at 10 months (Fig. 27-12). The volume of the transferred muscle gradually decreased, but it was palpated throughout the period of follow-up.[4a]

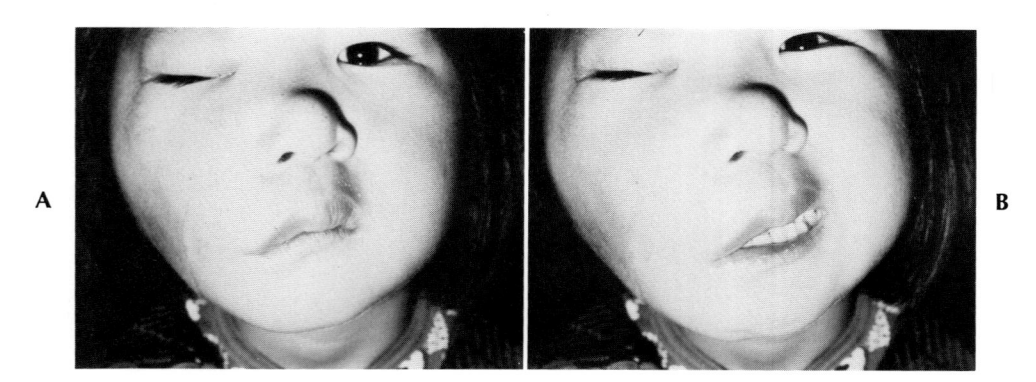

Fig. 27-10. Case 2. Preoperative condition. After excision of lymphangioma, no recurrence was observed but tumor still remains at right lower eye lid. Typical facial paralysis was observed on her right hemifacial region. **A,** Static. **B,** Smiling.

Free muscle grafts by microneurovascular techniques

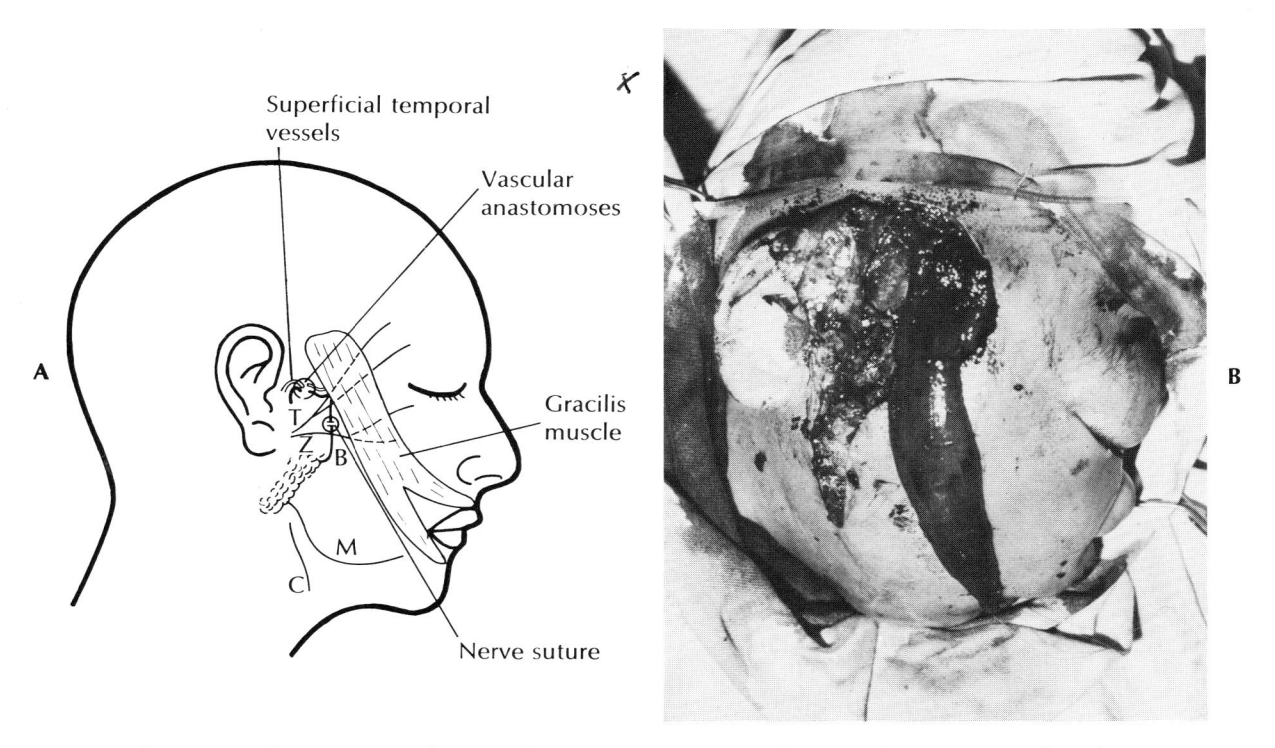

Fig. 27-11. Case 2. **A,** Schema of operation. **B,** Gracilis muscle transposed to face.

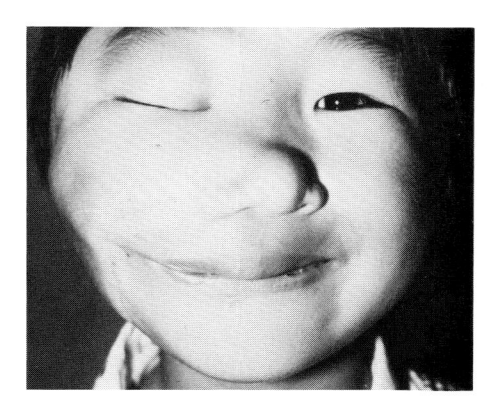

Fig. 27-12. Case 2. Final result of this patient smiling.

Reanimation of the paralyzed face

Discussion

Repair of the blood flow and reinnervation of the motor nerve are indispensable factors after the transfer of a muscle that has a proper motor function for reanimating a paralyzed muscle.

To repair blood flow in a muscle, which is a tissue vulnerable to ischemia, we use microvascular surgery. By this technique, the transferred muscle is revascularized in a minimum ischemic time (60 to 90 minutes) on the table.

To repair the motor nerves of the recipient site and donor site, we apply funicular suture to both nerves.

It is observed clinically that the muscle thus transferred by our method, discussed previously in this chapter, recovers its function at about 4 months after surgery and the recovery of function reaches a maximum at about 8 months. These clinical signs are correlated to the recovery based on electron microscopic and optical microscopic findings as well as on electromyograms.

However, muscles transferred by this technique decrease in volume in the process of reinnervation. Even when muscular function is recovered to a maximum at 8 months or thereafter, the transferred muscle has never been observed to recover the original muscle belly volume prior to surgery. Control of the muscle belly volume of the transferred muscle is related to the control of muscle functions to be recovered, such as muscle power and excursion.

Whereas in case 1, a small muscle, the extensor brevis muscle, was transferred, in case 2, a large muscle, the gracilis muscle, was used. In our clinical experience, the final muscle power was larger in the case where the larger muscle was transferred, even though the same type of healthy facial nerve was selected as the motor nerve in the recipient site. Therefore, we carefully select the motor nerve of the recipient site and use a larger donor muscle to make sure that the transferred muscle recovers sufficient power.

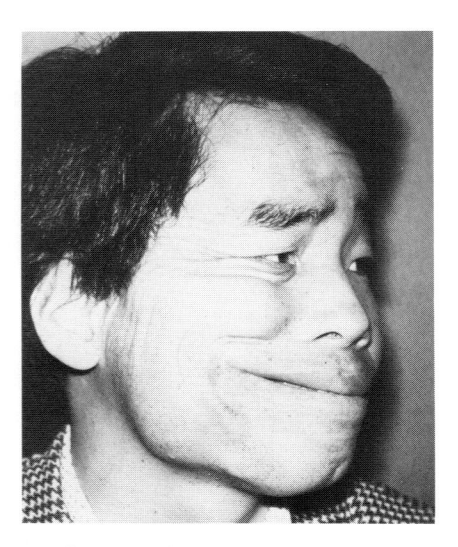

Fig. 27-13. In this case, gracilis muscle was transferred with superficial vessels and deep temporal nerve in recipient site, respectively. (Case reported in Plast. Reconstr. Surg. **57**[2]:133, 1976.)

Fig. 27-13 shows the maximum muscle power and excursion that was obtained in the cases of muscle transfer we have experienced so far. Such excessive power recovery is controlled by partial excision of the transferred muscle.

Although Thompson[7] suggests the need for denervation before transfer in his method of muscle transfer, we have succeeded in muscle transfer without preoperative denervation of the donor muscle. Nevertheless, control of the volume, power, and excursion of the transferred muscle involves a number of problems yet to be resolved. In the near future, if research in muscle transfer enables postoperative muscle power to be predicted before surgery, it would contribute much to the treatment of muscle paralysis by this procedure.

Summary

This chapter has described the technique of free skeletal muscle removal, transfer, and grafting by microneurovascular anastomoses, with two cases treated successfully for facial paralysis caused by muscular defects.

A number of methods have been proposed for treating muscle paralysis depending on the cause and the onset course. The effects have also been discussed.

The muscle transfer described here has been made possible by recent advances in microsurgical techniques and, as such, leaves much to be desired. We believe that, depending on further research, the surgery can be applied to muscle paralysis in different parts of the body as well.

REFERENCES

1. Harii, K., Ohmori, K., and Ohmori, S.: Free deltopectoral skin flaps, Br. J. Plast. Surg. **27:** 231, 1974.
2. Harii, K., Ohmori, K., and Ohmori, S.: Successful clinical transfer of ten free flaps by microvascular anastomoses, Plast. Reconstr. Surg. **53:**259, 1974.
3. Harii, K., Ohmori, K., Torii, S., Murakami, F., Kasai, Y., Sekiguchi, J., and Ohmori, S.: Free groin flaps, Br. J. Plast. Surg. **28:**225, 1975.
4. Harii, K., Ohmori, K., and Torii, S.: Free gracilis muscle transplantation, with microneurovascular anastomoses for the treatment of facial paralysis, Plast. Reconstr. Surg. **57:** 133, 1976.
4a. Harii, K.: Free muscle transplantation with microneurovascular anastomoses. In Daniller, A. I., and Strauch, B.: Symposium on microsurgery, St. Louis, 1976, The C. V. Mosby Co.
5. Harii, K., and Ohmori, K.: Free skin flap transfer, Clin. Plast. Surg. **3:**111, 1976.
6. Ohmori, K., and Harii, K.: Transplantation of a toe to an amputated finger, The Hand **7:**134, 1975.
7. Thompson, N.: Autogenous free grafts of skeletal muscle, Plast. Reconstr. Surg. **48:**11, 1971.

28 Surgical treatment of bilateral facial paresis (Möbius syndrome)

LEONARD R. RUBIN

The temporalis muscles on both sides of the face serve as substitute motor mechanisms to activate the paralyzed face. The operation is performed in one stage.

The surgical correction of congenital bilateral facial paresis has never been vigorously pursued until 1966 when I[4] described the use of most of the temporal muscles on each side of the face to supply a dynamic motor apparatus for facial animation. Prior to this time, the surgical treatment was less than enthusiastic, since the multiple congenital deformities associated with the facial diplegia added to the customary poor results found in activating any paralytic face. Standard methods of treatment were the use of slings made of fascia lata, dermis, wire, and nylon to give static support for the expressionless face.[2] Since both sides of the face were involved, a blank more or less symmetrical appearance resulted. I describe this facies in Chapter 4.

The fifth nerves and the temporalis muscles are rarely affected in the Möbius syndrome, although in a large series studied, Henderson[3] found a weakness of the fifth nerve in several of his cases.

In Chapter 26, I describe in detail the surgical technique of activating one side of a paralytic face by use of most of the temporalis muscle. The same technique applied to both sides of the face can be used to animate the congenital bilateral patient in a one-stage operation. Prior to the operation, a complete electronic testing of both temporalis muscles must be done to ensure muscle function of each side. Technically, the operative procedure should be performed with two teams of surgeons to expedite surgical time. Experienced surgeons need to allow 4 hours to complete the procedure. The reader should review the sketches in Chapter 26 to understand the technique of treatment of unilateral facial paralysis.

Surgical treatment of bilateral facial paresis (Möbius syndrome)

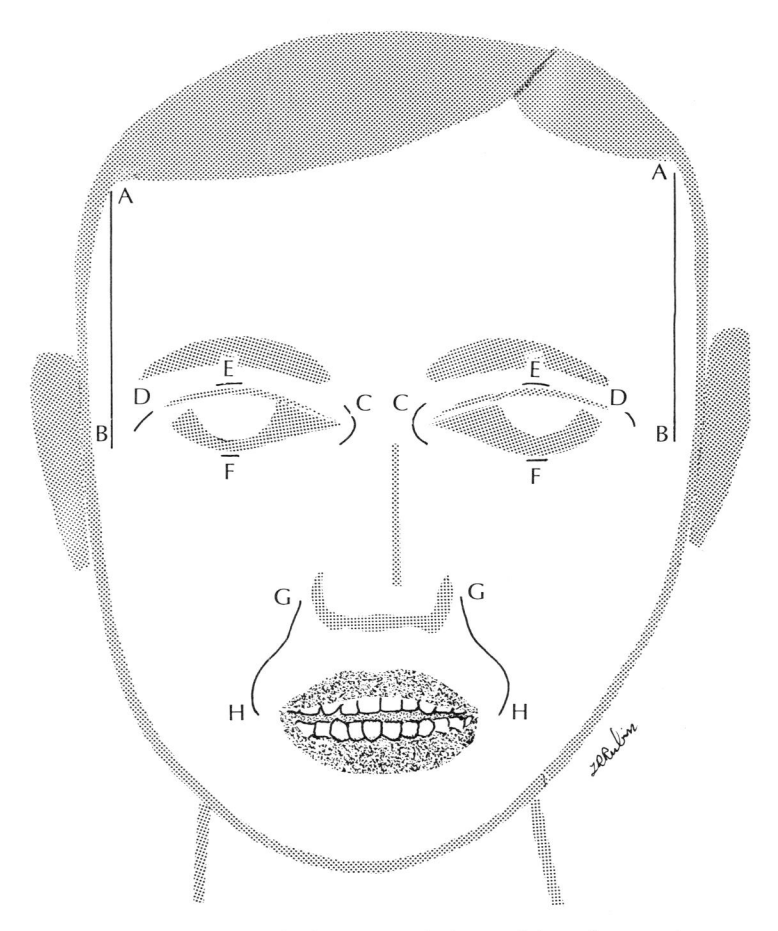

Fig. 28-1. Lines of incisions needed to treat bilateral facial paresis.

Incisions **AB.** Vertical incisions to expose the temporal fascia and the underlying temporal muscle.

Incisions **C.** Overlying the upper canthus ligament.

Incisions **D.** Lateral to the outer canthus in the wrinkle lines of the face.

Incisions **EF.** One cm lines running horizontally just below and above the lid margins.

Incisions **GH.** Curving lines simulating normal nasolabial folds.

Reanimation of the paralyzed face

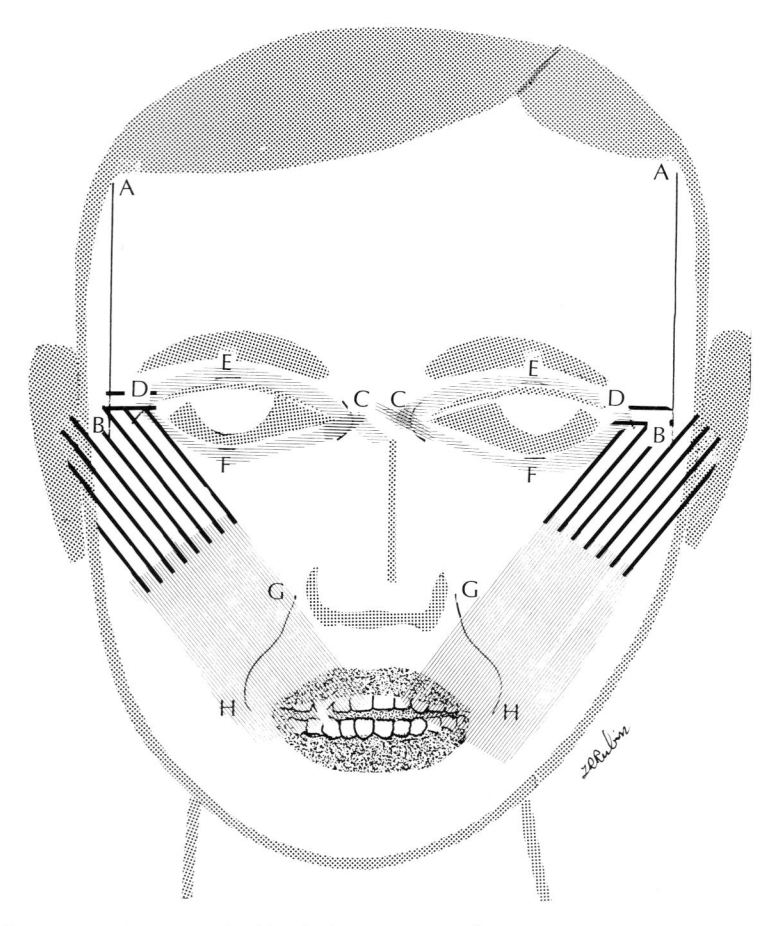

Fig. 28-2. The superior one half of the temporalis muscle on each side has been stripped off the temporal bone and draped over the zygomatic arch. Since the muscles are not long enough to reach their needed destination, the overlying deep fascia, cut into strips, will act as tendons. The sketch shows two strips attached to a muscle flap to activate the eyelids. Each strip will be threaded through the margins of the eyelids to weave under and around the inner canthus. The remainder of the temporalis muscles and the fascial tendons will go downward and inward toward the nasolabial folds and the upper lip to simulate the actions of the quadratus labii superioris and the zygomaticus major. NOTE: Reinforcing mattress sutures 4-0 Mersilene must be placed at the junction of the fascia and the muscles. This is a *must* in the technique since the muscles and tendons will be sutured under great tension. Review the detailed technique in threading these tendons in Chapter 26.

Surgical treatment of bilateral facial paresis (Möbius syndrome)

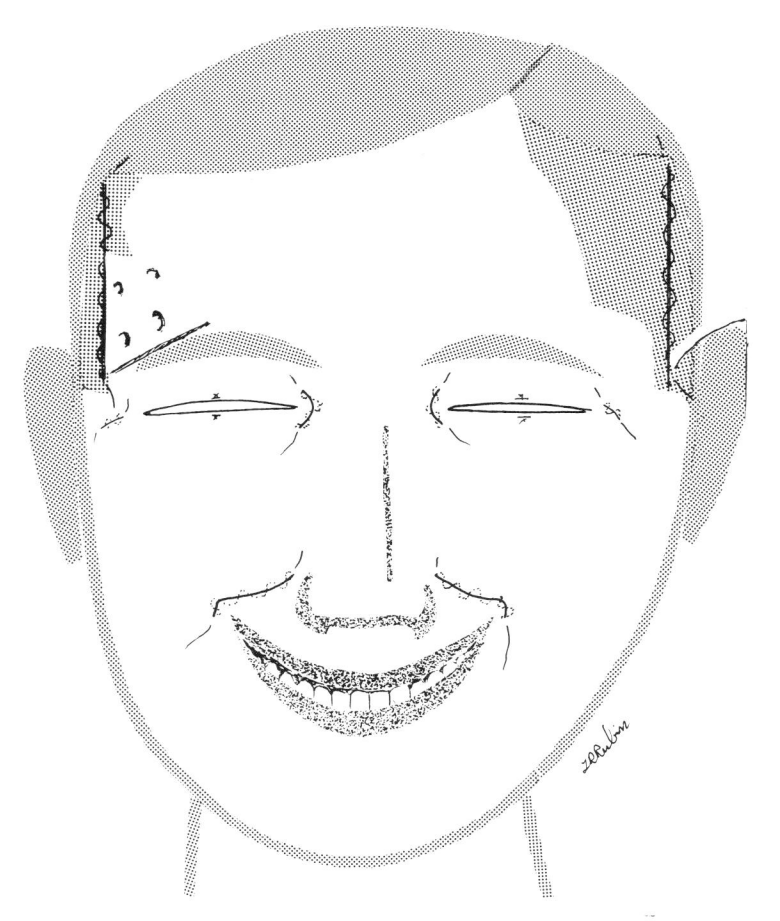

Fig. 28-3. The final result after the temporalis muscles and their fascial tendons have been inserted is shown. The eyelid strips are tightly interdigitated under and around the inner canthi. At the end of the operation, they are shut tightly. New nasolabial folds are formed by insertion of the fascial tendons into the dermis of the upper lip at the mucocutaneous lines and the corners of the mouth simulating the action of the quadratus labii superioris and the zygomaticus major muscles. Since one encounters replacement fatty tissue for muscle in the congenital paralytic face,[3] there is great difficulty in suturing the tendons under tension. The dermis is the only firm tissue for attachment. *The key to successful results is suturing under great tension.* At the end of the operation, all the gingivae of the maxilla should be exposed as the upper lip and the corner of the mouth are pulled upward and outward. The final skin suturing is done with a subcuticular pull-out suture to minimize the scarring.

Reanimation of the paralyzed face

Discussion

The use of the temporalis muscle and their overlying fascia can offer a dynamic muscle force to animate the blank expressionless face. It is now accepted that the victim of the Möbius syndrome is devoid of facial muscles in the upper three fourths of the face and that the seventh nerve is usually intact.[3] Most of the cases we have encountered have had muscles and nerve function in the lower lip.[4] The temporalis muscles activating the mouth and the eyelids have but limited functions since they act in mass contraction. Unfortunately, a new regime of learning has to be instituted to teach these people the act of smiling and expressing their emotions by direct facial expressions. This can only be accomplished by practice in front of a mirror. The operation is best suited to adults and children over 12 years of age. We have performed the operation on three children and have found that their short attention span and lack of purpose left little for concentration to learn the act of smiling. The patients have to be taught to bite down hard to move their temporalis muscles to obtain a smile. After an indeterminable period of time, the movements become easier and the "bite-down" need is lessened to a clenching or tightening of the jaws.

It is conceivable that as more is learned about nerve transposition and grafting, one might be able to neurotize the temporalis muscle by grafting segments of sural nerve from the seventh nerve as it exits from the facial canal. This would indeed bring coordination movements to the paralytic victims of the Möbius syndrome.

CASE 1

The patient is a 15-year-old white male with paralysis of the forehead, eyelids, and midface. The lower lip is normal. Sixth and ninth nerve paresis is apparent. The patient has an abnormal left hand with the loss of fingers and hypoplasia of the palm.

A, The patient tries to smile and close his eyelids. Note action of the lower lip.
B, The patient in repose. Note the failure to obtain lateral gaze.
C, Postoperative picture of the patient 1 year later. The patient in normal repose.
D, The patient smiling.
E and **F,** Four years later, the patient in repose and smiling.

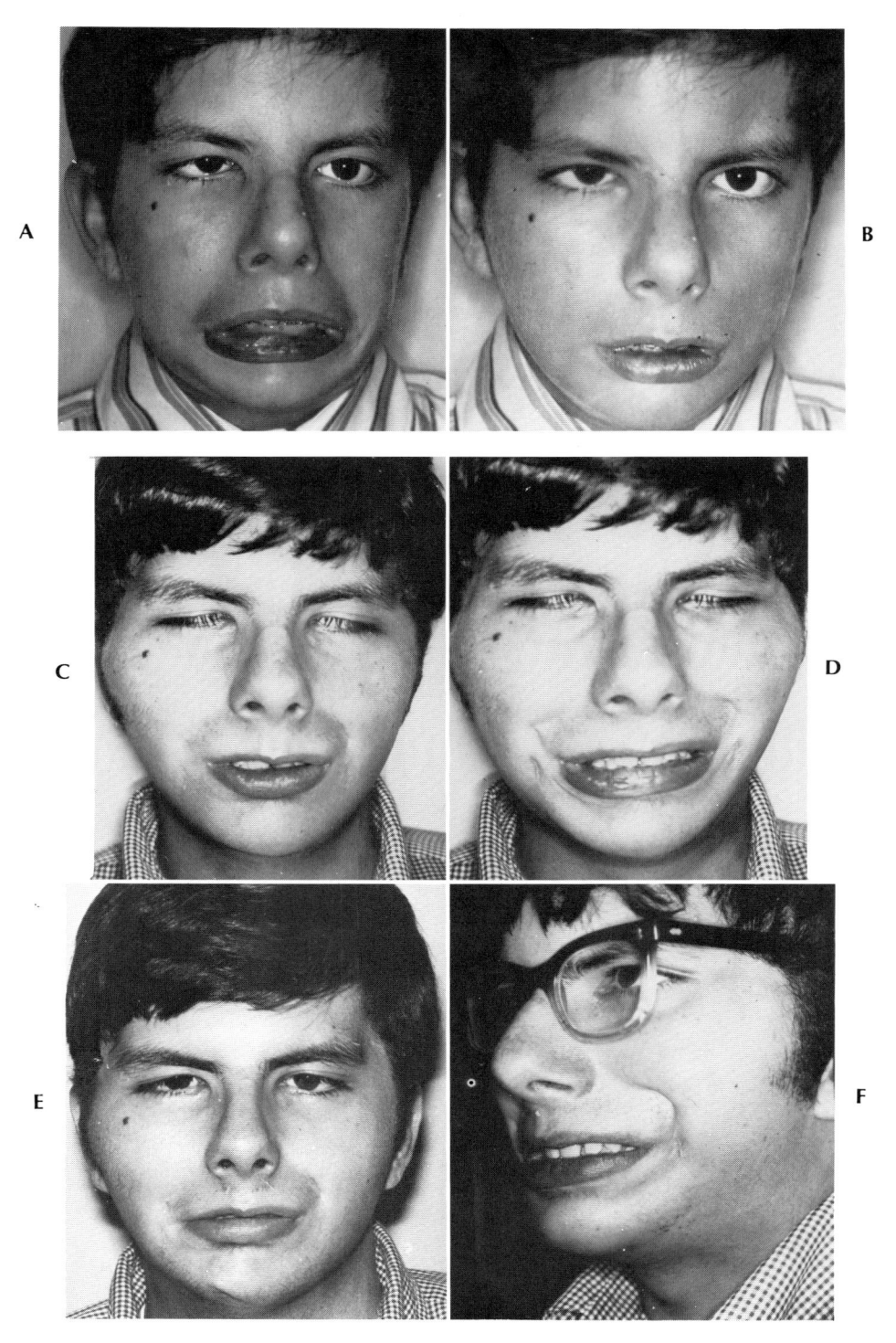

Surgical treatment of bilateral facial paresis (Möbius syndrome)

Case 1

Reanimation of the paralyzed face

CASE 2

An 8-year-old white female has paresis of her forehead, eyelids, and midface. The lower lip has good function. She has sixth nerve involvement with lateral rectus difficulties. The ninth nerve, which affects speech, is partially involved. The extremities are normal.

A, The child tries to smile and close her eyelids.

B, The child in repose.

C and **D,** Postoperative views 1 year after the temporalis transplants. She can smile readily. However, eyelid closure is not total. The patient rolls her eyeballs upward to effect sleep. She shows the spread of her facial scars. Being dark skinned, they are hyperpigmented and very apparent. As mentioned in the text, the results in children under 12 years never come up to expectations.

E, Four years later in repose. The scars are lighter in color but still spread. They will be improved when she reaches the age of 16 years.

F, The patient in repose and smiling. The temporalis muscle contractions are good. However, she states she does little exercising or practicing. Corrective surgery in children cannot produce the good results found in the adult. It is difficult to motivate a child to practice continuously.

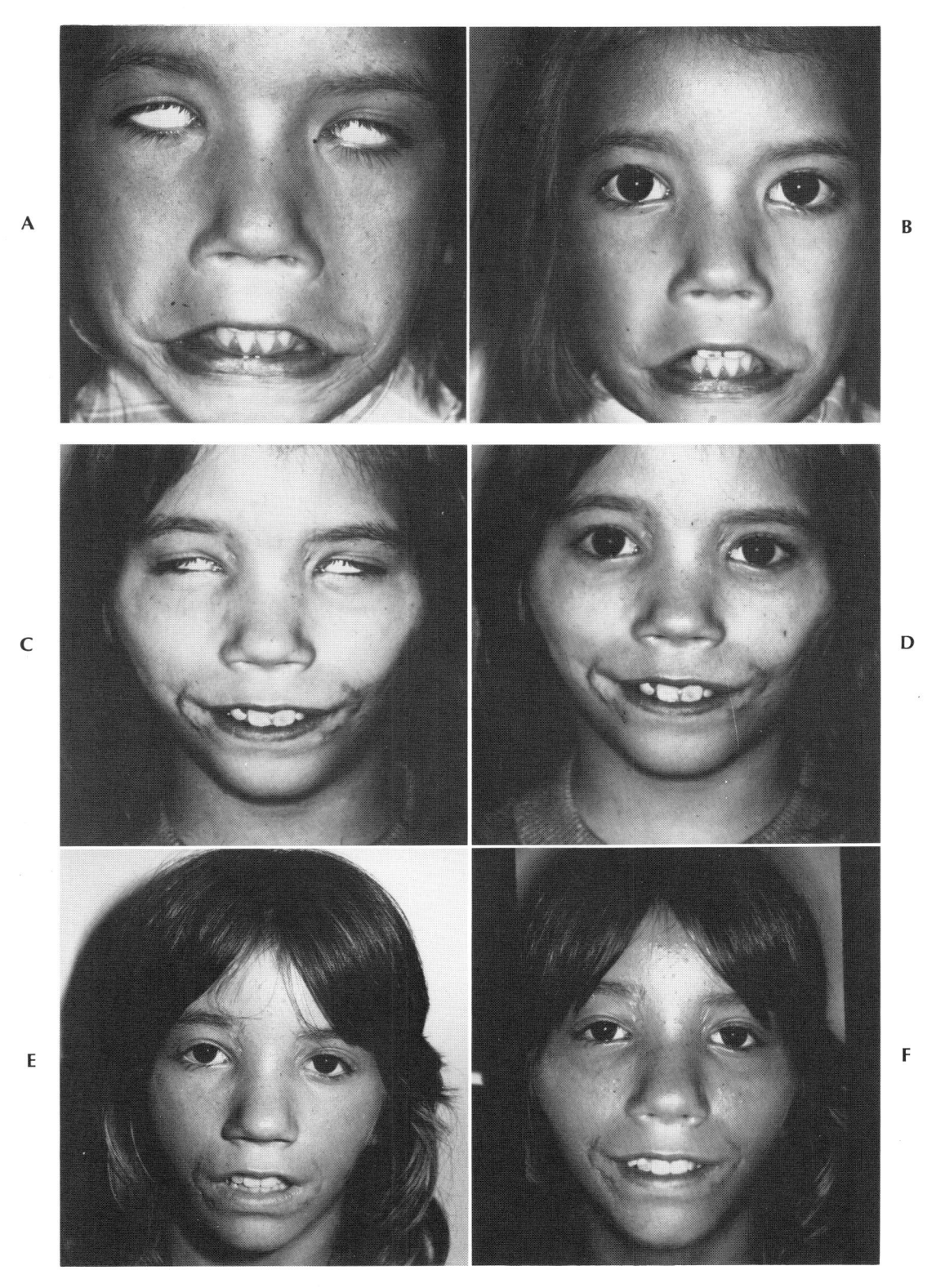

Surgical treatment of bilateral facial paresis (Möbius syndrome)

Case 2

335

Reanimation of the paralyzed face

CASE 3

An 18-year-old white female has paresis of the forehead, eyelids, midface, and right lower lip. She has associated sixth nerve paralysis and involvement affecting her speech.

A, Preoperative view when patient was asked to smile. Note the action of the lower lips showing the facial nerve to be intact and the muscles to the lower lip being normal.

B, The patient is trying to close her eyes. The lids are immobile and the eyeballs roll upward.

C, One year after surgery. The patient is smiling with eyes open. The right lower eyelid tendon is slipped away from the lid margin causing an ectropion.

D, The patient is smiling and closing her eyelids.

E, Ten years later. The patient has retained her ability to smile. The right lower eyelid still shows the mild ectropion. The patient wanted no further surgery.

F and **G,** The patient smiling. She is capable of closing her eyes without smiling. She does not clench her teeth to smile, but rather tenses her lower jaws. This act is done unconsciously.

Surgical treatment of bilateral facial paresis (Möbius syndrome)

Case 3

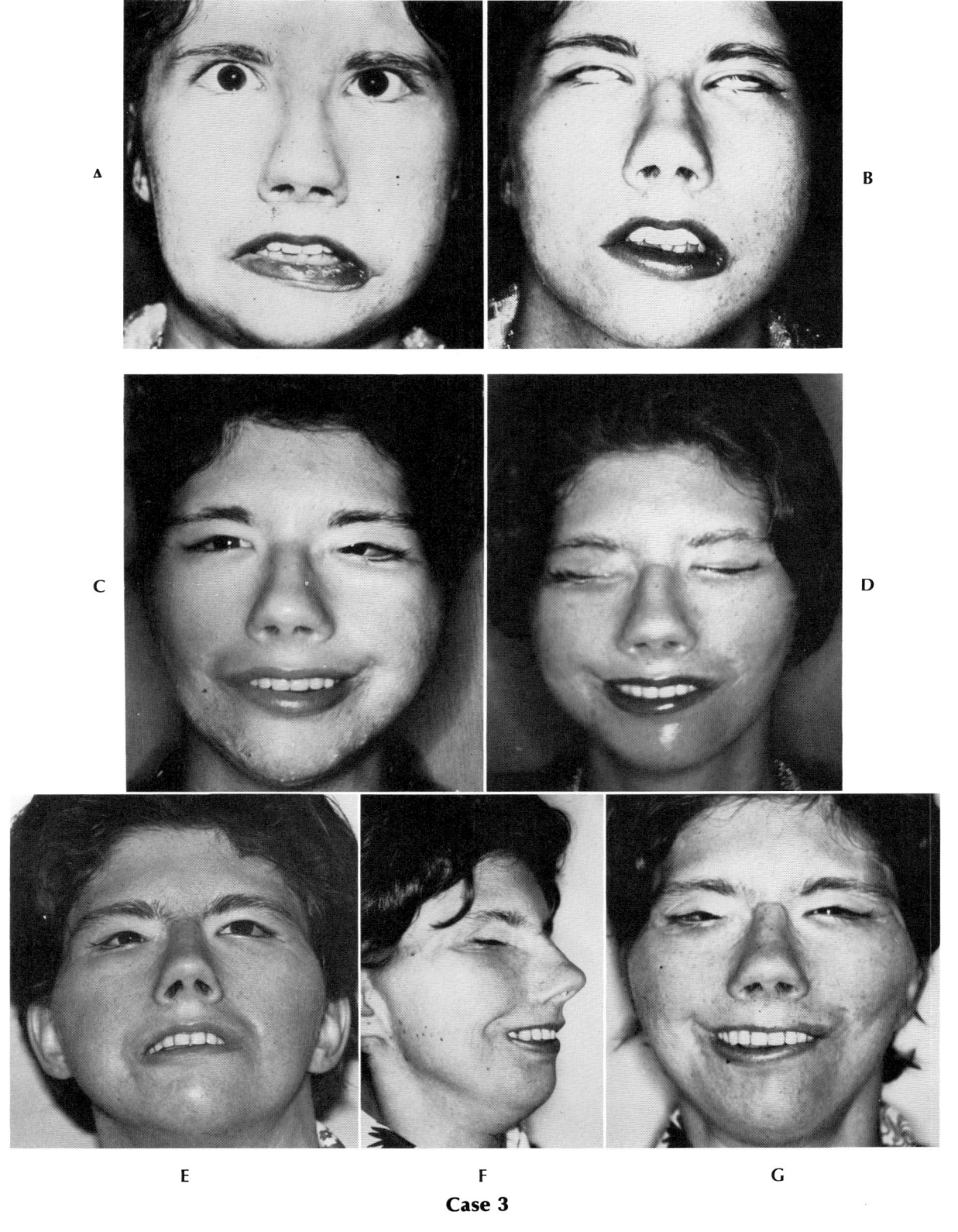

Reanimation of the paralyzed face

CASE 4

A 4-year-old white male has complete facial paresis including the lower lip. The sixth and ninth nerves were involved. He had no legs and feet starting below the knees.

A, The patient is trying to smile and close his eyelids.
B, One year after surgery. He can close his eyelids and smile.
C, Prosthetic legs. The patient had no difficulty learning to walk.
D, The patient 10 years later in repose. The patient has a moderate smile. He can close each eye or smile on each side at will. However, the patient admits he never practices smiling and that any movement he makes is done unconsciously.

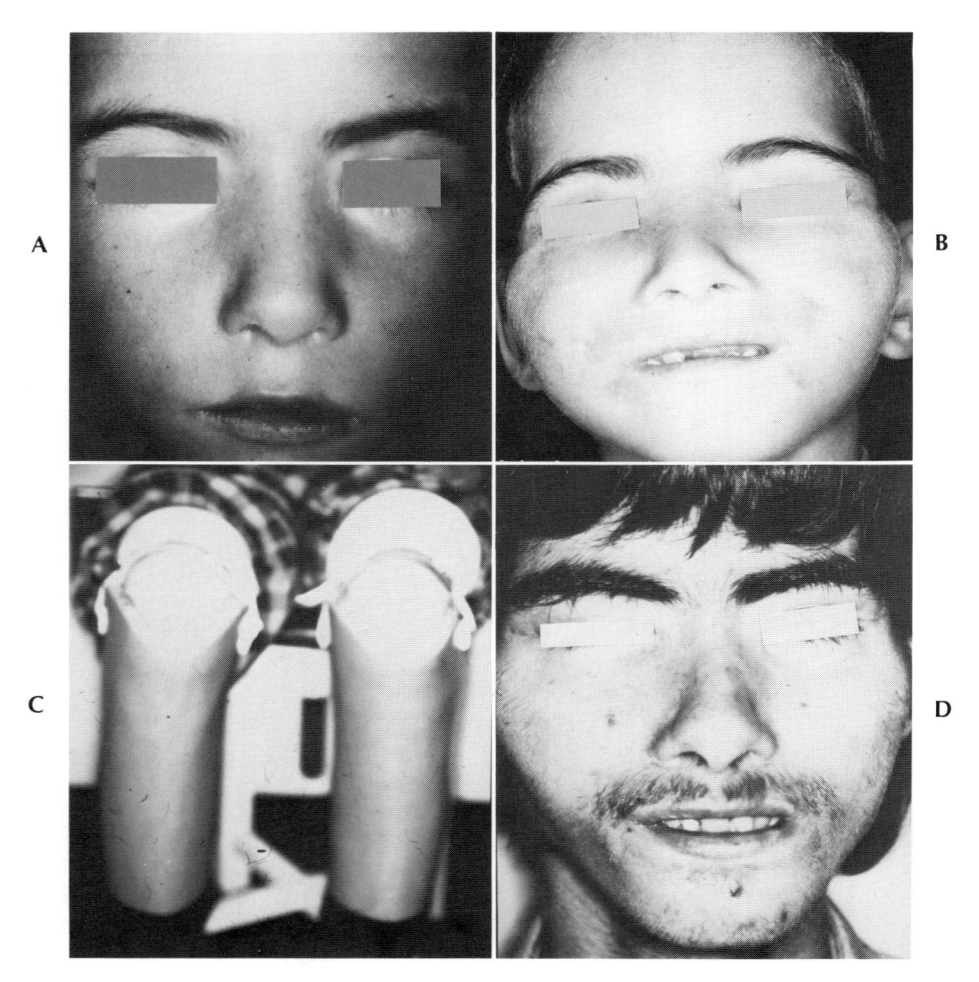

Case 4

REFERENCES

1. Converse, J. M.: Reconstructive plastic surgery, Philadelphia, 1964, W. B. Saunders Co., pp. 1154-1162.
2. Henderson, J. L.: Congenital facial diplegia, clinical features, pathology and etiology, Brain **62:**381-403, 1939.
3. Pitner, S. E., Edwards, J. E., and McCormick, W. F.: Observations on pathology of the Moebius syndrome, J. Neurol. Neurosurg. Psychiatry **28:**362, 1965.
4. Rubin, L. R., Bromberg, B. E., and Walden, R. H.: Congenital bilateral facial paralysis, Möbius syndrome, surgical animation of face, Transactions of the Fourth International Congress on Plastic and Reconstructive Surgery, Amsterdam, 1969, Excerpta Medica Foundation, pp. 740-746.

29 Partial facial paresis

LEONARD R. RUBIN

The treatment of partial facial weakness is not only difficult but may often convert the partial paresis to a complete paralysis. There are many choice techniques to improve a partial facial weakness, and several of the most commonly used techniques are described. However, the reconstructive surgeon must always ask himself, "What are the dangers of making the patient worse?"

Improving the partially paralyzed face taxes the inventiveness of the reparative surgeon. What should be done and what can be done without damaging the surrounding normal functioning structures?

Partial and complete weakness of sections of the face may be found after Bell's palsy, parotid tumor removal, trauma to the distal branches of the seventh nerve, removal of tumors of the face, such as cavernous hematoma, and other iatrogenic causes in the temporal canal and the cranium. Once satisfied with time allowance for maximum nerve and muscle recovery, a thorough quantitative electronic study must be made to confirm the maximum recovery. Only then should the areas be reevaluated for possible surgical intervention.

FOREHEAD

Complete isolated injury to the frontal branches of the facial nerves are rather uncommon. As a rule, recovery is usually complete over a period of time. However, we have seen cases where paresis has persisted over years with no return of function. The most common causes have been direct trauma and iatrogenic causes such as surgery to the parotid gland and face-lifting. The physical appearance of the affected eyebrow sags to a lower level than the opposite normal side, giving the patient a heavy bloodhound type of appearance. The horizontal creases disappear from the forehead and make those of the opposite side more apparent.

TREATMENT

Very little has been done to surgically animate the paralyzed frontal muscle. The efforts have been made primarily to equalize both sides by one or two methods:

Partial facial paresis

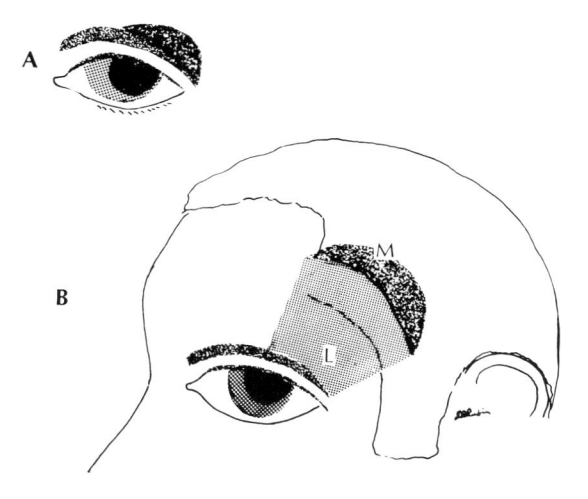

Fig. 29-1. **A,** Elevation of paretic eyebrow by removal of crescent of skin above lateral half of affected eyebrow. **B,** Elevation of paretic eyebrow by removal of crescent of scalp, *M,* and undermining of forehead skin, *L,* to level of affected eyebrow. By suturing of scalp at *M,* brow is pulled upward. Advantage of this procedure over that of **A** is the hidden scar in scalp.

1. Elevate the affected eyebrow by removing crescents of forehead over the affected eyebrow or by removing a crescent in the scalp after extensive undermining to the supraorbital ridge (Fig. 29-1, *B*).
2. Paralyze the opposite normal side by removing large segments of frontalis muscle through a scalp coronal incision or by actually finding the nerve to the frontal muscle and excising a portion. As a rule, the patients, once informed of all the consequences of frontal nerve paresis, prefer having the crescents removed from the eyebrow (Fig. 29-1, *A*) or from the scalp on the affected side rather than going to the normal side. Whereas the elevation of the brow might sag again in the future and require a repeat procedure, paralysis of the opposite side produces drooping of the eyebrow on both sides with a bilateral hound-dog appearance.

EYELIDS

Localized paresis of the eyelids can be caused by local tumors, parotid tumors, trauma, or senile weakness. The nerve innervation to the orbicularis oculi muscle is rich, and cross-linking of fine nerve filaments usually ends with good muscle function. However, for persistent paresis of the lower lids, many surgical procedures have been devised. I wish to make known my dissatisfaction with the use of foreign bodies such as weights, magnets, and slings of nylon, Dacron, or Teflon. Anything less than a dynamic, living replacement of function can be considered a temporary measure giving inadequate results and, more likely than not, causing further damage as the foreign materials are rejected through the thin overlying skin. The procedures of choice at the present time are as follows:

1. A partial temporalis muscle may be transplanted to the lids after the technique of Gillies and the modifications by Anderson (Fig. 29-2).

Reanimation of the paralyzed face

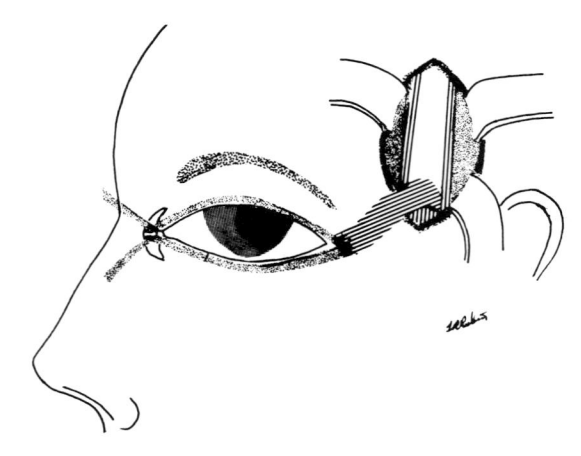

Fig. 29-2. Dynamic activation of paretic eyelids by swinging of a strip of temporalis muscle and attached temporalis fascia to create a pursestring action (after Anderson). Technique of exposure of muscle and temporal fascia and threading through eyelids to inner canthus can be reviewed in Chapter 26.

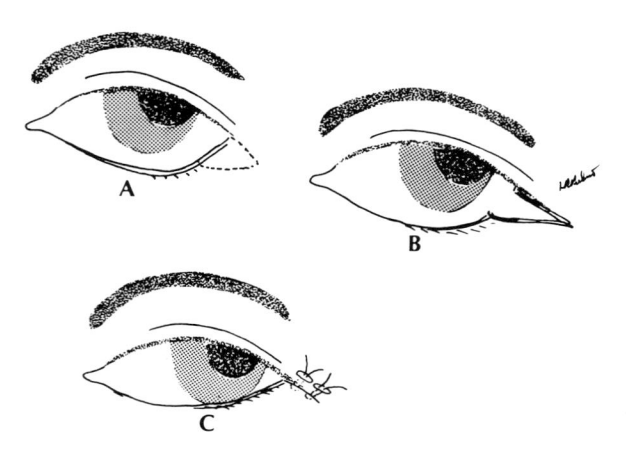

Fig. 29-3. Relief of paretic lower eyelid ectropion by shortening of lid margin. A, Triangle of skin muscle and tarsus. B, Triangle removed. C, Lid margin is restored at level of outer canthus. Two 5-0 nylon pullout sutures pass through a piece of rubber dam and hold repaired wound. After dam was removed 10 days later, scar had become invisible and appearance of eyelids is normal.

2. A lateral canthoplasty may be made either by the McLaughlin procedure or by a through-and-through wedge resection of the lower eyelid at the outer canthus (Fig. 29-3). Both of these procedures are done merely to take up the slack for ectropion or eyelid sagging.
3. Of great interest is the work being done by Anderl with nerve grafting. This technique may be utilized with greater success after the experience with direct nerve implantation into the muscle as performed by McCoy and Rubin (see Chapter 15).

Partial facial paresis

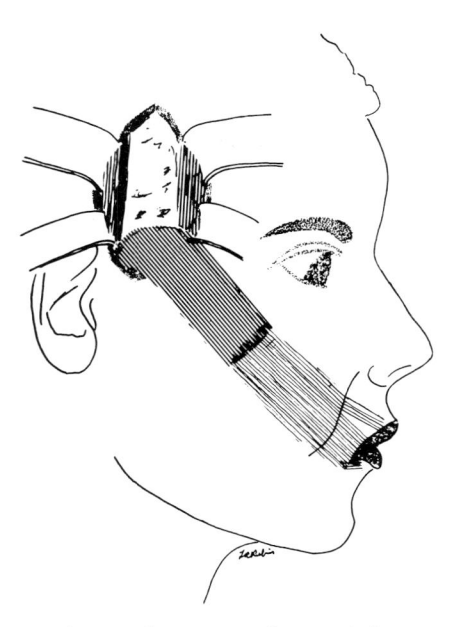

Fig. 29-4. Elevation of upper lip and corner of mouth by transposition of portion of temporalis muscle. Details on exposure and transposition of temporalis muscle can be studied in Chapter 26.

CHEEK AND UPPER LIP PARESIS

Partial weakness of the cheek and the upper lip is most commonly seen after recovery from Bell's palsy. The decision to improve the facial movement requires great surety of purpose. Surgical intervention may increase the weakness to a total paresis. The options open to the surgeon are as follows:

1. One may do a face-lifting in the older patient, plicating the deep fascia toward the zygomatic arch and elevating the corner of the mouth.
2. A selective elevation of the corners of the mouth and the upper lip by a temporalis muscle and fascia transposition can be done (Fig. 29-4).
3. Plications of the elevators of the corners of the mouth and the upper lip can be made (Fig. 29-5).
4. Muscles on the normal side can be weakened by partial excision (Fig. 29-6).

FACE LIFT

Little improvement can be had with a face-lift procedure plicating the deep fascia to the zygomatic arch. The procedure is useful for older persons but certainly not applicable to the young child or the teenager. In time, the skin and fascia will stretch and the condition will probably reoccur.

TEMPORALIS MUSCLE TRANSPOSITION

A selected area of temporalis muscle and fascia can be attached to the corner of the mouth and the upper lip to dynamically activate the angle of the mouth and the upper lip. This procedure must be reserved for a serious paresis. The danger of tearing

Reanimation of the paralyzed face

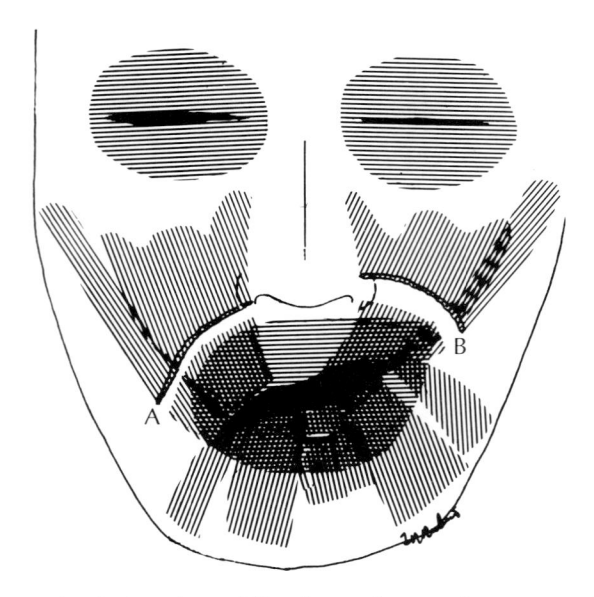

Fig. 29-5. Facial muscle balancing. Plication of muscle on weak side is usually associated with selective myectomy on normal side. **A,** Technique of muscle plication. Incision along nasolabial fold will expose levators of upper lip and zygomaticus major as they join orbicularis oris. Muscles are cut about 1 cm above orbicularis and then resutured at a much higher level greatly overcorrecting and exaggerating smile mechanism. This can be seen in Fig. 29-6, C. Muscles are sutured with braided 4-0 nylon or 4-0 Mersilene.

B, Selective myectomy is accomplished on normal side and through mucosal incision in cheek corresponding to external nasolabial fold.

Quadratus labii superioris and the zygomaticus major are exposed as they insert into the orbicularis. Removal of approximately 1 to 2 cc of muscle allows superior portions to retract upward and backward.

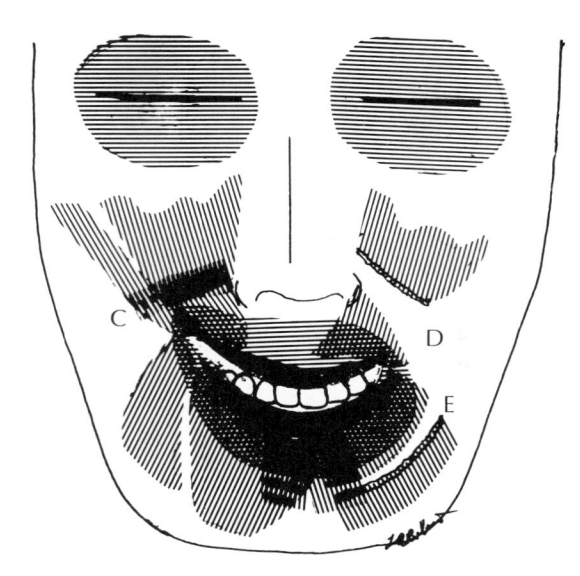

Fig. 29-6. In a similar fashion, lower lip muscles can be cut to equalize paretic lower lip. Muscles to be cut must be predetermined after careful observance of patient's normal smile as described in Chapter 1.

Partial facial paresis

the delicate nerve fascicles going to the forehead and the eyelids is great. The dissection through the face must be kept at a most superficial level (Fig. 29-4). (For details on technique, consult Chapter 26.)

PLICATION OF THE ELEVATORS OF MOUTH AND UPPER LIP

This procedure is relatively easy. An incision along the nasolabial fold will expose the zygomatic major and the levators of the upper lip as they join the orbicularis oris. The muscles can be cut for approximately 1 cm above their insertion and resutured at a much higher level, with great overcorrection and exaggeration of the smile mechanism. The muscles are sutured with 4-0 Mersilene, and the wound is closed in layers. Within several days, the muscles stretch and the mouth returns to a normal level (see Fig. 29-5).

WEAKENING OF OPPOSITE, NORMAL SIDE BY SELECTIVE MYECTOMY

The presence of a weakened lip and cheek produces an increased tone and overaction of the so-called normal side, resulting in an even greater imbalance and abnormal appearance. Weakening of the normal side can be accomplished by *selected neurectomy*. However this is most difficult to accomplish because of the extensive anastomosing branching between the distal branches of the facial nerve. Of greater benefit is the *selected myectomy,* easily accomplished through a mucosal incision. A very careful analysis of the muscles involved making the patient's smile will demonstrate which muscles on the normal side should be excised. The nasolabial fold is marked out and a similar line is placed in the mucosa of the mouth. With use of local 1% lidocaine (Xylocaine), incisions are made through the mucosa to allow viewing of the insertions of the quadratus labii superioris and the zygomaticus major. By dissection upwards for approximately 1 cm or so, each muscle can be seen easily and a section of approximately 1 cm can be removed. This will allow the superior portion of each muscle to retract upward. The immediate result appears to be pronounced weakness on the normal side, with improvement of the movements on the abnormal side. However, as weeks go by, the weakness of the normal side is lessened, and within several months, mouth motion is diminished but appears normal. The greatest fault in the procedure is the fear of causing a paresis on the normal side and not removing enough muscle (Fig. 29-6).

LOWER LIP

Partial paresis of the lower lip by injury to the marginal branch of the facial nerve can be iatrogenically produced in removal of a parotid tumor, face lift, reduction of a fractured mandible, neck dissections, and so forth. Direct trauma, of course, is also another possibility. The procedures for correction are varied and must be weighed very carefully. One can decide to do no surgical procedure at all, particularly for a very mild, partial weakness. However, for the persistent weakness, the patient must be offered the following:
1. Selected weakening of the depressors of the corner of the mouth and of the lower lip on the normal side.
2. A neurectomy of the marginal branch of the facial nerve.
3. Selected nerve grafting as described by Anderl.

Reanimation of the paralyzed face

Most weaknesses of the lower lip are permanent since the anastomosing of the fine filaments of the buccal branches is not present in the marginal branch. A surgical injury to the lower branch is most often permanent, resulting in a drooping of the lower lip. When confronted with the alternative, the patient will usually choose the surgical procedure that is usually least drastic for the so-called cure. Weakening of the muscles on the normal side is an office procedure and can easily be done through mucosal incisions. As in the upper lip, approximately 1 cm of muscle is removed (Fig. 29-6).

A neurectomy of the marginal branch on the opposite side to equalize the lower lip is not well received by most informed patients. However, should the patient insist, exposure of the nerve is very simple since it is usually found just above the inferior margin of the mandible 1 cm anterior to the facial artery and vein as they cross the inferior border of the mandible. An excision of approximately 1 cm of nerve will ensure a paresis on the normal side giving an equality to the lower lip. The lower lip will certainly droop and most patients are usually unhappy.

Selected nerve grafting has not been performed by me, but according to the principles of Anderl, it is most feasible if the time from surgical injury to the time of nerve grafting has not been too great and muscle degeneration has not occurred.

Summary

The partially paralyzed face presents a great challenge to the surgeon. The question to be answered is, Can I improve the patient or will I make him worse? Carefully selected procedures in certain cases can improve the condition and equalize facial movements. Several cases are being presented to show what can be done.

CASE 1

Partial facial paresis

This case illustrates the use of eyebrow-lifting for frontal nerve paresis and the improvement of the ectropion of the lower lid after paresis. The patient is a 55-year-old male who underwent a removal of an acoustic nerve tumor 3 years previously resulting in a complete left facial nerve paresis with considerable soft-tissue atrophy. A temporalis muscle transposition was successful in elevating the upper lip and the angle of the mouth, but was not sufficient for the eyebrow droop or the paretic lower-lid ectropion.

A and **B** show the patient after temporalis transposition. The patient is now shown with a crescent of forehead above the lateral aspect of the eyebrow having been removed. The brow lift was successful but the temporalis transposition to the eyelids was inadequate because of fascial strip tendon slippage. The lower lid still shows a paretic ectropion.

C and **D** demonstrate the excellent lid result after removal of a through-and-through triangle of the lower lid at the most lateral margin (see Fig. 29-3).

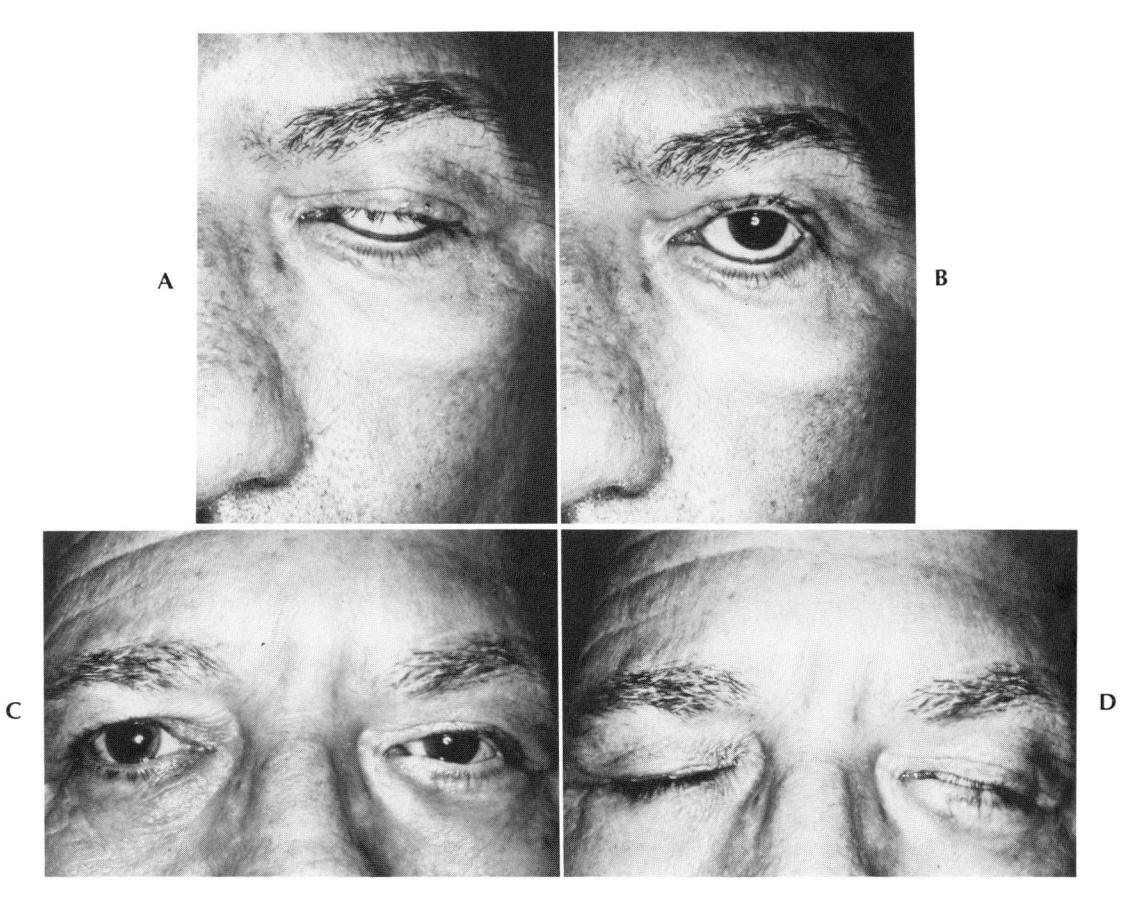

Case 1

Reanimation of the paralyzed face

CASE 2

This patient is a 22-year-old female who had an extensive expanding hemangioma removed surgically at the age of 4 months. This left her with a paresis of the upper lip and the corner of the mouth.

A and **B** show the patient in repose and smiling with a noticeable defect seen in the cheek and a partial paralysis of the upper lip and the corner of the mouth.

C and **D** show the patient in repose and smiling after having had a partial temporalis transposition to the upper lip and the corner of the mouth (Fig. 29-4). Selective myectomy of the lateral portions of the elevators of the upper lip and the zygomatic major were performed at the same time (see Figs. 29-5 and 29-6). The selection of muscles to be cut on the normal side was carefully predetermined by observation of the patient's smile and assessment of the value of severing the muscles that caused abnormal movement. The added bonus of the temporalis transposition was to furnish bulk and fill the defect of the cheek.

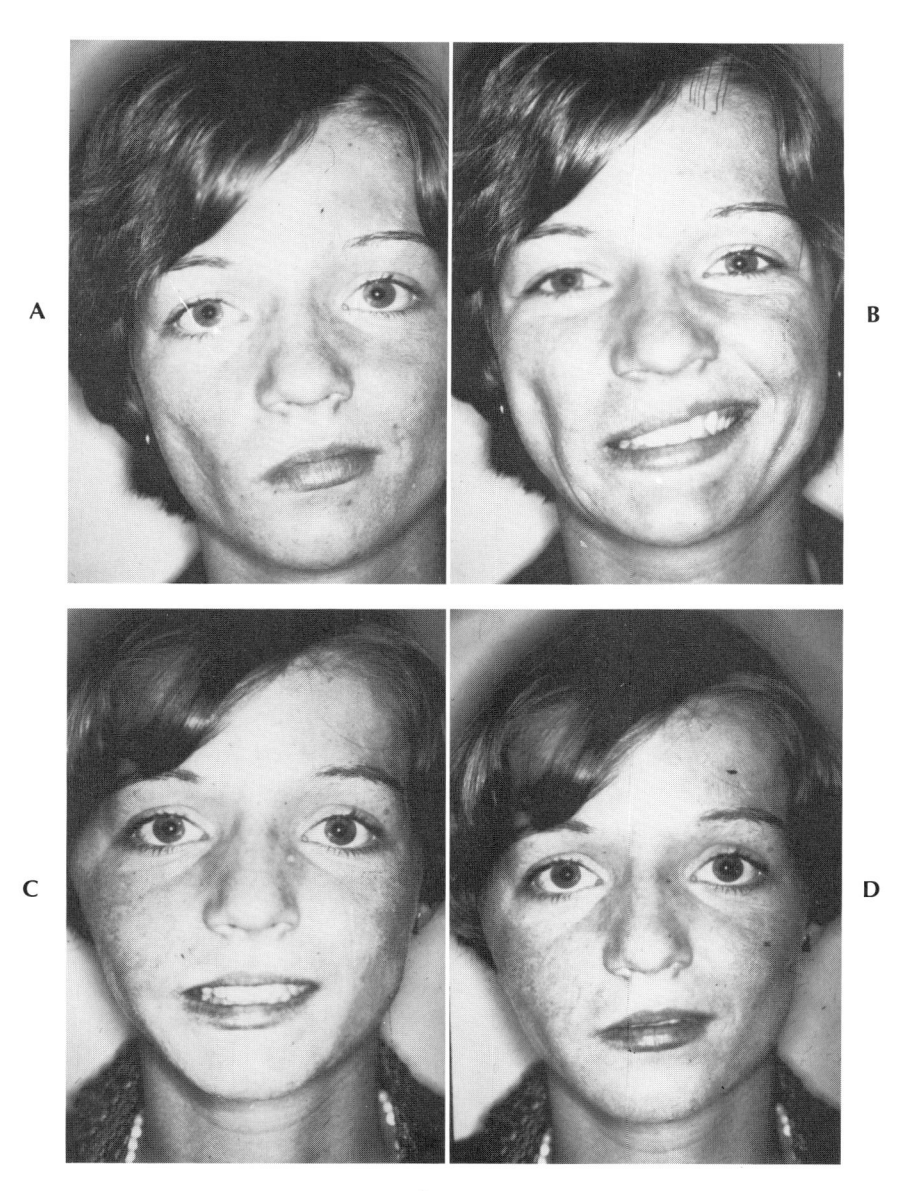

Case 2

Reanimation of the paralyzed face

CASE 3

The patient is a 36-year-old male who suffered an attack of polio when he was a child. He recovered almost all of his facial motion but was left with a partial weakness of the right cheek. His lips were strongly everted and distorted. (this may have been partially based on a genetic background).

- **A** and **B** show the patient in repose and smiling. Electronic testing showed good nerve conduction to the levators to the upper lip and the corners of the mouth.
- **C** and **E** show the patient postoperatively after having had plication of the elevators of the upper lip and mouth corner on the affected side, selected myectomy on the normal side, and revision of the thick abnormal lip vermilion border of the upper and lower lips.

Case 3

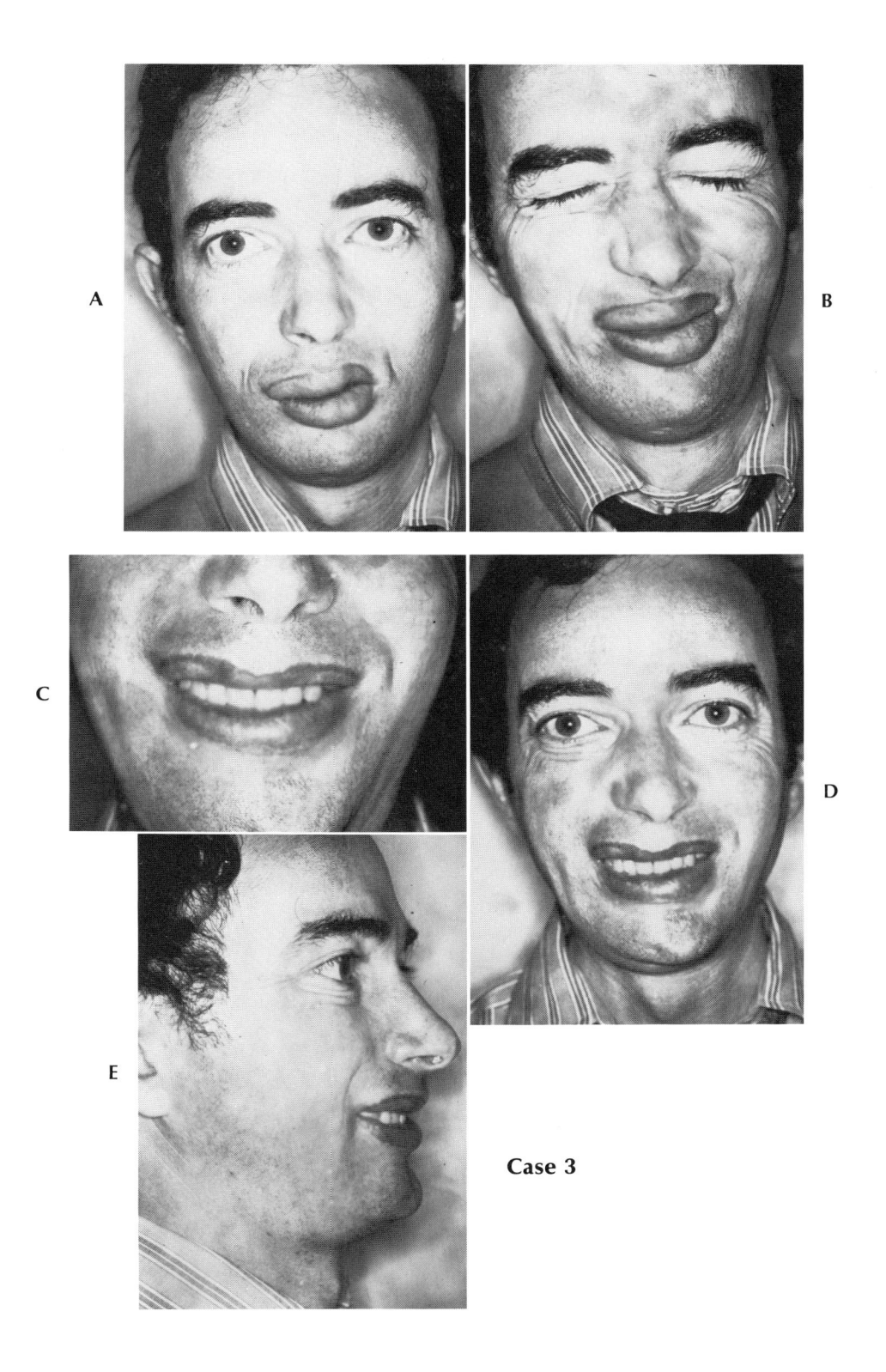

REFERENCES

1. Anderson, J. G.: Surgical treatment of lagophthalmos in leprosy by the Gillies temporalis transfer, Br. J. Plast. Surg. **14:**339-1961.
2. Edwards, B. F.: Bilateral temporal neurotomy for frontalis hypermobility, Plast. Reconstr. Surg. **19:**341, 1957.
3. Rubin, L. R., Bromberg, B. E., and Walden, R. H.: Congenital bilateral facial paralysis, Möbius syndrome, surgical animation of the face, transactions of the Fourth International Congress on Plastic and Reconstructive Surgery, Amsterdam, 1969, Excerpta Medica Foundation, pp. 740-746.

Index

A

A band of myofibrils, 30, 31
Abbe flap, 279
Ablation, radical, of parotid gland, 225-226
Accessory nerve in spinofacial anastomosis, 241
Acetylthiocholine, 140
Acland's clips, use of, in microvascular suturing, 177, 187
Acoustic nerve, paresis after tumor of, 286; *see also* Acoustic neuroma
   partial, 347
   temporalis muscle transposition for, 314
Acoustic neuroma, 75, 105
   facial nerve in, 60
      destruction of, 211
   growth of, 57, 60
   retrolabyrinthine suboccipital craniectomy for, 58-59, 61-63
      left, 212-213
      preservation of hearing in, 61
   sural nerve grafts after removal of, 215
   temporalis muscle transplantation for paralysis after surgery for, 310
Action potential shape of muscle after grafting, 290-292
Adenocarcinoma as cause of facial paresis, 76
Adenoid cystic carcinoma as cause of facial paresis, 76
Adenosine triphosphatase, 33-34
   myofibrillar, 138, 140, 141-144, 148, 149
   myosin, effects of cross-innervation on, 116
   reduction of, effect of electrical stimulation on, 199
   staining, muscle types determined by, 113-116
Adventitectomy in microvascular anastomosis, 183, 184
Aging process, effect of, on wrinkles of face, 4
Allografts, nerve, disadvantages of, 127
Amplification, equipment for, in electromyography, 93
Amplitude of action potentials after free muscle graft, 291
Amyotrophic lateral sclerosis
   spontaneous potentials in, 94
   Z line dissolution in, 37-38
Anastomosis(es)
   construction of, in cross-face nerve graft, 257-259
   intrafascicular, 213, 214
   microvascular
      arterial, 182-187
      end-to-side, 189, 190
      in extensor brevis muscle graft, 320-322
      in gracilis muscle graft after lymphangioma excision, 324
      radical patency test of, 186, 187
      techniques of, 178-190
      venous, 187-188
      of vessels of different diameters, 189
   of rami buccales with ramus marginalis, 244
   of rami buccales with ramus zygomaticus, 244
   scarring between, as factor in two-stage cross-face nerve grafting, 247

Anatomical direction of grafts in cross-face nerve grafting, 255
Anatomical location, diagnosing site of nerve disruption by
   anatomical description, 99-100
   appraisal of facial nerve function, 100-101
   central or supranuclear lesions, 102-107
Anatomical variations in smiles, 18
Anatomy
   considerations of, in cross-face nerve grafting
      healthy side, 243-244
      paralyzed side, 244-245
   of donor muscles for graft by microneurovascular technique, 318-319
   of facial expression, 2-20
   of facial nerve, 99-100
      surgical, 21-27
         composition, 21-23
         course and relationships, 23-27
         variability of, 26-27
   of temporalis muscle, 297
Anodal stimulation of tongue, threshold to, 91
Antibiotics after cross-face nerve grafting, 263
Aorta, rat, dissection of, 181, 182
Application of nerve grafts in facial nerve surgery, 134-135
Approach, surgical, to facial nerve within parotid gland, 80
Arms, defects of, in Möbius syndrome, 49
Arterial anastomosis, microvascular, 182-187
Artery, rat femoral, anastomosis of, 188
ATPase; *see* Adenosine triphosphatase
Atrophy
   degree of, as factor in electrotherapy, 199
   denervation, loss of myofilaments in, 37
   effect of galvanic stimulation on, 198
   postdenervation, 35
   tongue, after hypoglossal crossover, 230
Auditory meatus, internal
   and geniculate ganglion, diagnosing lesions between, 102, 104, 105
   and pons, lesions between; *see* Cerebellopontine angle, neoplasms of
Auditory-palpebral reflex, assessment of, 101
Auricular nerve, 245
   cable graft of, in facial trauma, 237
   in cross-face nerve grafting, 251
Auriculotemporal syndrome, 107
Autogenous nerve grafting in radical parotidectomy, 226-228
Autografts, nerve, 251
Autologous nerve grafting
   basic considerations in, 127-128
   superiority of, 251
Axon(s)
   growth of
      in direct neuromuscular innervation, 263
      from healthy to paralyzed side of face, 254

Index

Axon(s)—cont'd
  growth of—cont'd
    in hypoglossal crossover, 229
    neuroma as evidence of, 259, 260
    in sural graft, 247
  regeneration of, electrical stimulation and, 198
  sprouting of
    irregularity of, 131
    in reinnervation, 111-116
    scar tissue as obstacle to, 127
Axonolysis in nerve repairs under tension, 127
Axonotmesis
  in Bell's palsy, 206
  in local injury, 236
Axoplasm, manufacture of, after nerve interruption, 218
Axoplasmic membrane, loss of sodium-pump capability of, 218
Axoplasmic transport of factors in muscle reinnervation, 111-112

B

Balancing of facial muscles in partial paresis, 344
Bard-Parker surgical blade, 222
Basal cell epithelioma as cause of facial paresis, 76
Basocranial fracture, cross-face nerve graft after, 270, 271, 272
Bell's palsy
  changes in taste threshold in, 91
  conduction-latency measure in, 87, 88, 89
  degree of paralysis as factor in recovery, 201
  edema in, 195-196
  effect of partial restitution of nerve fibers in, 243
  electrical stimulation in treatment of, 202, 205
  as emergency, 197
  etiological factors in, 54, 106
  gross nerve excitability in, 90-91
  medical treatment of, 201-203
  misdiagnosis of, 71
  partial paresis after, 340
    of cheek and upper lip, 343
  strength-duration curves in, 84, 86, 87
  surgical treatment of, 204-210
    arguments for, 195-196
    cross-face nerve graft in, 270, 272
    facial nerve decompression in, 207-209
    free muscle graft in, 287
    rationale of, 205-207
    transfacial crossover in, 228
Bell's phenomenon, 106
Benign tumors causing facial paresis, 74-75
Biangulation, types of, in microvascular anastomosis, 184
Bilateral facial paresis, surgical treatment of, 328-329
Bleeding, control of, in facial trauma, 235
"Blink burst" in regeneration, 96-97
Blink reflex, assessment of, 101
Blood flow, repair of, after free muscle graft, 326
Blood supply
  in autologous nerve grafting, 127-128
  of facial nerve, 22-23
Bone
  nasal, resection of, in muscle graft for eyelid paralysis, 282
  removal of, in surgery for Bell's palsy, 208, 209
Branches
  of cervical plexus as donors in nerve grafting, 134
  of facial nerve; *see* specific branches
Buccal branch of facial nerve, 222, 267
  anastomosis of, with marginal and zygomatic branches, 244
  anatomy of, near parotid gland, 245
  in cross-face nerve grafting, 243
    of healthy side, 244
    in second operative stage, 259
Buccal region, cross-face nerve grafting in
  incision in, 250-251
  positioning of graft in, 254, 255

Buccinator muscle
  in facial anatomy, 13
    upper part of, 14, 15
  innervation of, 250
Bulk, muscle, after experimental minced-muscle grafting, 159-160
Büngner's bands, 251

C

Cable graft of auricular nerve in facial trauma, 237
Café-au-lait spots, 74
Caninus in facial anatomy, 13-15
Canthoplasty, lateral, for partial paresis of eyelids, 342
Capillaries in whole muscle grafting, 148, 149
Caput angulare in facial anatomy, 14, 15
Carcinoma
  mucoepidermoid, of parotid gland, 226
  squamous cell, as cause of facial paresis, 76
Carcinomatosis, meningeal, 105
Cell, muscle, structure and function of, 29-31
Cellular changes, early postdenervation, 35-39
Cellular events in muscle regeneration, 117
Central or supranuclear facial paralysis, 102-107
Cephalic herpes as cause of lower motor neuron facial palsy, 54-55
Cerebellar tumor, cross-face nerve graft for, 270, 272
Cerebellopontine angle, neoplasms of
  acoustic neuroma, 58-63
  diagnosis of, 105
  ependymomas, 64
  epidermoid, 64, 67-69
  meningiomas, 64
  metastatic, 69
  neurofibromas, 64-66
Cerebrospinal-fluid otorrhea as complication of surgery for Bell's palsy, 209
Cervical plexus in nerve grafting
  branches of, as donors, 134
  in radical parotidectomy, 226
Cervical spine injury, possibility of, in facial trauma, 236
Checkerboard pattern of type I and II muscle fibers, 113, 114
Cheek(s)
  graft of extensor digitorum brevis for function of, 264
  and mouth, muscles of region of, 12-13
  partial paresis of
    face lift for, 343
    myectomy of normal side for, 344, 345, 348, 348, 350, 351
    plication of elevators of mouth and upper lip for, 344, 345, 350, 351
    temporalis muscle transposition for, 343, 345
  position of muscle-nerve graft in, 265
Chin, incision in, for positioning cross-face nerve graft, 251, 252, 253
Chin region, positioning of cross-face nerve graft in, 254, 255
Cholesteatoma, 55, 72
  as cause of facial palsy, 106
Cholinesterase in end plates, 145
  after reinnervation, 112
Cholinesterase-positive plaques in whole muscle grafting, 146, 147
Chorda tympani syndrome, 107
Chordoma as cause of facial paresis, 76
Chromatolytic hypertrophy of nerve cell body, 222
Chronaxy, measurement of, 82-84
Ciliary bundle, 7
Circulating cell as possible source of myoblasts, 157
Clamps for microvascular suturing, 176-177
Clinical examination of muscle before cross-nerve grafting, 246
Clips for microvascular suturing, 177
Clotting, fibrin, coaptation by, in nerve grafting, 129
Coaptation, fascicular, in nerve grafting, 129-130

Index

Cobbett's asymmetric biangulation, 184
Collateral sprouting
 in free muscle graft, hindered by connective tissue, 279
 of healthy axons, type grouping as a result of, 116
 nerve, 139
 in reinnervation, 111-116
Combinative possibilities of cross-face nerve grafting, 263-268
Combined middle fossa–transmastoid approach in surgery for Bell's palsy, 208-209
Complications of surgery for Bell's palsy, 209
Composition of facial nerve, 21-23
Compressor naris in facial anatomy, 11
Computer technology, diagnostic techniques from, 82
Condition, general physical, of patient, as factor in cross-face nerve grafting, 246
Conduction-latency measurements in diagnosing site of nerve disruption by electronic methods, 87-90
Congenital facial palsy, 55; see also Möbius syndrome
Congenital keratoma as cause of facial paresis, 75-76
Conjunctivitis, exposure, 285
Connective tissue
 after experimental minced-muscle grafting, 160-162
 collateral sprouting hindered by, 279
 proliferation of, after nerve interruption, 218, 219, 220
 in whole muscle grafting, 149, 150
Contemporary concepts in free nerve and muscle grafting
 free minced-muscle grafting, 156-165
 free whole muscle grafting, 136-155
 fundamentals of microvascular suturing, 174-192
 nerve-end implantation into a denervated muscle, 166-173
 reinnervation and regeneration of striated muscle, 110-123
 technique of free nerve grafting in the face, 124-135
Continuous regeneration, 116-117
Contractile properties of reinnervated muscles, reversal of, in cat, 113
Conventional biangulation, 184
Corda tympani, diagnosing lesions distal to, 102, 104, 105-106
Corrugator supercilii
 effects of, on expression, 8
 in facial anatomy, 6-9
Cortical representation of forehead and eyelid musculature, 103
Corticosteroids in treatment of Bell's palsy, 202, 203, 205
Corticotrophin in treatment of Bell's palsy, 203
Course and relationships of facial nerve, 23-27
 variability of, 26-27
Coverings of facial nerve, 22
Craniectomy, retrolabyrinthine suboccipital, 58-64
Cranium, surgical causes of facial paresis in, 57-70
Crocodile tears
 as complication of Bell's palsy, 205
 syndrome of, 107
Crossed innervation, 96
Cross-face nerve grafting
 application of, 263-274
  combinative possibilities, 263-268
  indication, 268-269
  results, 269-274
 combined with transposed masseter or temporal muscles, 267-268
 first operative stage
  buccal region, 250-251
  construction of anastomosis, 257-259
  marginal region, 251
  orbital region, 247-250
  positioning of grafts, 251-257
  preparation of nerve grafts, 251
 history of, 243
 operation, 246-247
 postoperative care and rehabilitative measures, 263
 preoperative investigation and measures, 245-246

Cross-face nerve grafting—cont'd
 second operative stage, 259-263
 special anatomical considerations, 243-245
Cross-innervation
 effects of
  on muscle fiber types, 113
  on myosin, 116
 experiments in, 139
Crossover
 hypoglossal, in parotidectomy, 229-231
 motor nerve, 242
 spinal accessory, 229
 transfacial, in paresis in malignant tumors of parotid gland, 228
Cutaneous femoral nerve, 134, 251
Cutaneous antebrachii medialis as donor in nerve grafting, 134
2-Cyanobutylacrylate, glue technique with, in nerve grafting, 129

D

Decompression, facial nerve, in Bell's palsy
 approaches and technique in, 207-209
 results of, 196
Dedifferentiation
 metabolic, in denervated muscle fiber, 40
 of muscle, 157
Degeneration
 postdenervation, 35, 217-218
 wallerian
  in complete transection of nerve, 236
  in nerve autografts, 251
Dehydrogenase activity of muscle fiber, 33-34
Delayed repair of neural defect, advantages of, 220-221
Demyelization, localized, in neurapraxia, 236
Denervating diseases
 reinnervation of muscle fibers in, 112
 type grouping of muscle fibers in, 113-114
Denervation
 in Bell's palsy, testing, 206, 207
 chronaxy value in, 82
 of donor muscle in free muscle graft, 281
 pathophysiology of
  normal skeletal muscle structure and function, 29-35
  postdenervation changes in muscle fiber and motor end plate, 35-40
 preoperative, free muscle graft without, 327
 results of experimental muscle transplantation after, 151-153
 and selection of muscle grafts, 281-282
 signs of, after free muscle grafting, 289
Depressor labii inferioris, 16, 17
Depressor septi in facial anatomy, 11
Depressors of angle of mouth, 16, 17
Diabetes, 246
Diagnosing site of nerve disruption
 by anatomical location
  anatomical description, 99-100
   appraisal of facial nerve function, 100-101
   central or supranuclear lesions, 102-107
 by electronic methods, 81-97
  electromyographic recording, 91-97
  testing by stimulation, 82-91
Diagnostic techniques, computer technology and, 82
Dilator naris in facial anatomy, 11
Disadvantages of combined free muscle and cross-face nerve graft, 266-267
Discontinuous regeneration, 116-117
Dissection
 microsurgical, of small vessels, 181-182
 to obtain sural nerve graft, 251

Index

Distal tubule(s)
 after nerve interruption, 218
 connective tissue invasion of, 220
 shrinking of, 222
Donor muscles for free muscle graft by microneurovascular techniques
 anatomical base of, 318-319
 denervation of, 281-282
 extensor digitorum brevis of foot as, 281-282
 flexor digitorum superficialis for, 282
 palmaris longus as, 281
 plantaris as, 282
 selection of, 317
Donor nerves in nerve grafting, 134
Dorsalis pedis artery, 281
Double hump–camel swelling in partial nerve transection, 236
Drug therapy for Bell's palsy, 202-203, 205
Dual innervation of muscle, establishment of, 112

E

Ear
 infections of, as cause of lower motor neuron facial palsy, 55
 radical operation of, cross-face nerve graft after, 270
Ectropion, 304
 after temporalis muscle transposition, 308
 for Möbius syndrome, 336
 of paralytic lower eyelid, prevention of, 283
 shortening of lid margin for, 342, 347
Edema
 in Bell's palsy
  drugs for reduction of, 202
  as factor in surgery for, 195-196
  surgical treatment of, 205, 208, 209
 after temporalis muscle transposition, 308
Effects of local tension on nerve regeneration, 126-127
Elasticity of nerve tissue, force needed to overcome, in neurorrhapy, 126
Electromyography
 after cross-face nerve grafting, 270-271
 after free muscle graft(s)
  conventional, 289-292
  to create nasolabial field, 322
  single-fiber, 292
  in verifying results, 268-269
 before cross-face nerve grafting, 246
 in Bell's palsy, 206
 in diagnosing site of nerve disruption, 91-97
 in nerve-end implantation into denervated muscle, 171
 preoperative, in free muscle and nerve graft, 285
 showing fibrillations in palsy complete after 2 weeks, 196-197
 single-fiber, recording of, 93
 in survey of whole muscle grafting, 140, 151
Electron microscopy of reinnervated motor end plates, 113
Electroneuromyography laboratory, 92
Electronic methods, diagnosing site of nerve disruption by, 81-97
Electrophysiotherapy after cross-face nerve grafting, 263
Electrostimulation
 selection of facial fascicles by, in cross-face nerve grafting, 244, 249
 in treatment of Bell's palsy, 202, 205
Electrotherapy
 beneficial effects of, 198
 controversies concerning, 197-198
 factors in effectiveness of, 199
Elevators
 of corner of mouth, 14, 15
 of mouth and upper lip, plication of, for partial paresis, 344, 345, 350, 351
Embryonal rhabdomyosarcoma as cause of facial paresis, 76
Emotional central facial paresis, 103
Emotional expression after cross-face nerve graft, 272
Encephalomeningomyelitis, Ramsay Hunt syndrome as, 71

End plate(s), 222
 after nerve interruption, 218
 cholinesterase in, after reinnervation, 112
 formation of
  and nerve implantation, 112
  in whole muscle grafting, 144-147
 postdenervation changes in
  atrophy and degeneration, 35
  early cellular, 35-39
  histochemical, 39-40
  hypertrophy, 39
  target fibers, 40
 potentials in electromyography, 94
 reinnervated, electron microscopy of, 113
 structure and function of, 32-33
Endomysial connective tissue in whole muscle grafting, 149, 150
Endomysial tubes in muscle regeneration, 120
Endoneurium of facial nerve, 22
End-to-side microvascular anastomosis, 189, 190
Enzyme, mitochondrial oxidative, in denervated muscle, 39, 40
Enzyme-constitution, studies of change in, in whole muscle grafts, 139-140
Ependymomas arising from fourth ventricle, 64
Epicranius
 effect of, on expression, 8
 in facial anatomy, 6, 7
Epidermoid carcinoma as cause of facial paresis, 76
Epidermoid tumor of cerebellopontine angle, 64, 67-69
Epinephrine, 282
Epineural sutures, 214
 coaptation by, in nerve grafting, 129
Epineurium of facial nerve, 22
 and sural graft, 257
Epiphoria, 103, 106
 relief of, 285
Epithelioma, basal cell, as cause of facial paresis, 76
Epitympanum in surgery for Bell's palsy, 208
Ergotamines in treatment of Bell's palsy, 203
Etiological factors
 in Bell's palsy, 54, 106
 in Möbius syndrome, 50-51
Etiology of disruption of the facial neuromuscular motor unit
 congenital facial paresis, 44-52; *see also* Möbius syndrome
 diagnosing site of nerve disruption
  by anatomical location, 98-108
  by electronic methods, 81-97
 medical causes including Bell's palsy, 53-56
 surgical causes
  in cranium, 57-70
  in parotid gland, 79-80
  in temporal canal, 71-78
Evaluation
 of facial injury, 235-236
 of nerve regeneration, 237
Excitability, gross nerve, electronic testing of, 90-91
 and pain, 269
Excitability test, facial nerve, in Bell's palsy, 206, 207
Exercises in treatment of Bell's palsy, 202
Explosion, mine, facial trauma caused by, 238, 239
Expression, facial
 anatomy of, 2-20
 effects on
  of depressors of lower lip, 16, 17
  of elevators of corner of mouth, 14, 15
  of muscles of forehead and eyelids, 8
  of muscles of region of mouth and cheeks, 12-13
  of muscles of region of nose, 10
 in examination of motor function, 100
Extensor brevis muscle
 anatomy of, 318-319
 graft of, to create nasolabial fold, 320-323

Index

Extensor brevis muscle—cont'd
   nourishing vessels for, 319
Extensor digitorum brevis of foot for muscle graft
   combined with cross-face nerve graft, 264-267
   denervation of, 281-282
   in eyelid paralysis, 282-283
   to frontalis muscle, 288
Extratemporal facial nerve, intraneural topography of, 130, 131, 132
Extremities, malformation of, in Möbius syndrome, 49
Extubation after second stage of cross-face nerve graft, 259
Eye
   care of, in Bell's palsy, 202
   and mouth, localized paresis about, muscle-tendon onlay grafts for, 233-234
Eyebrow, sagging of, 340-341
   correction of, 307
   removal of skin crescent to elevate, 341, 347
   unilateral, paralyzing normal side in, 341
Eyelid(s)
   after cross-face nerve graft for Bell's palsy, 274
   closure of
      draft of extensor digitorum brevis for, 264
      innervation of, by ramus zygomaticus, 244
      missing, before cross-face nerve grafting, 246
      by orbicularis muscle, 249
   difference in interference patterns of, after free muscle graft, 291
   and forehead, muscles of region of, 6-9
      cortical representation of, 103
   function of, graft of temporal muscle for, 266
   lower, orbicularis oculi of, clinical condition after strengthening of, 287
   paralysis of
      free muscle grafting for, 282-283
         clinical condition after, 285-286
         selection of muscle for, 281
      partial, 341-342
      preoperative clinical condition in, 284-285

F

Face lift for partial paresis of cheek and upper lip, 343
Facial nerve
   anatomical description of, 99-100
      surgical, 21-27
         composition, 21-23
         course and relationships, 23-27
         variability of, 26-27
   appearance of, in retrolabyrinthine suboccipital craniectomy, 62-64
   appraisal of function of, 100-101
   approach to, in acoustic neuroma, 61-62
   assessment of, in temporal bone fractures, 77
   branches of, within parotid gland, 244-245; *see also* specific branches
   communications of trigeminal nerve branches with, 244
   destruction of, in acoustic neuromas, 211
   diagnosis of impaired function of, 101-102
   electromyography of; *see* Electromyography
   establishing continuity of, in temporal canal
      appropriate action according to location of injury, 222
      methods of repair, 222
      processes that continue after nerve interruption, 217-220
      timing of operation, 220-222
   excitability test of, in Bell's palsy, 206, 207
   extratemporal, intraneural topography of, 130, 131, 132
   injury to branches of, 222
   in Möbius syndrome, 46, 47-48
   in parotidectomy for malignant tumor, 225-226
   preservation of, in surgery for acoustic neuroma, 61
   relationship to parotid gland, 79, 80, 99-100
   signs and symptoms denoting site of interruption of, 102

Facial nerve—cont'd
   and sural grafts, comparison of size of, 256
   surgical approaches and technique in decompression of, in Bell's palsy, 207-209
   stretching of, in acoustic neuroma, 60
   terminal branches of, within parotid gland, 80
   testing of, by stimulation, 82-91
   tumors of, as cause of facial paresis, 73-74
   zygomatic plexus of, in cross-face nerve grafting, 249
Faciofacial anastomosis; *see* Cross-face nerve grafting
Fallopian canal, courses of facial nerve in, 23, 24
Fascia
   acting as tendons in temporalis muscle transposition of, 304-305
      for Möbius syndrome, 330, 331
   exposure of, in temporalis muscle transposition, 299
   facial, anatomy of, 3-4
   lata, sling of, to support lips and nasolabial fold, 296-297
   removal of, from muscle, in temporalis muscle transposition, 301
   superficial, in facial muscle contractions, 3-5
   as tendons in temporalis muscle transposition, 303
Fascial stripping in muscle transfer, 233
Fascicles
   dissection between, in nerve grafting, 128
   marking of, in cross-face nerve grafting, 250
Fascicular coaptation
   of facial nerve near stylomastoid foramen, 130, 131, 132
   in nerve grafting, 129-130
Fasciculations in electromyography, 94, 95
Fatty tissue, replacement, for muscle in congenital paresis, 331
Fiber(s)
   muscle
      effect of reinnervation and cross-innervation on types of, 113
      postdenervation changes in
         atrophy and degeneration, 35
         early cellular, 35-39
         histochemical, 39-40
         hypertrophy, 39
         target fibers, 40
      striated, types of, 33-34
   nerve, intraneural orientation of, 131-134
   types and disposition of, facial, 21-22
Fiber density, increased, of motor unit after free muscle graft, 292
Fibrillation potentials in electromyography, 94-95
Fibrillations shown by electromyography in palsy complete after 2 weeks, 196-197
Fibrin clotting, coaptation by, in nerve grafting, 129
Fibroblasts in regenerative processes after nerve interruption, 218
Fibrosis
   of central muscle tissue in muscle graft, 267
   end-stage muscle, muscle transfer for, 233
   of muscle fibers, preoperative, in cross-face nerve grafting, 245
   and revascularization in whole muscle grafting, 147-151
Flexor carpi radialis, 281
Flexor digitorum superficialis of fourth finger for free muscle graft in face, 281, 283
   denervation of, 282
Focus of regeneration in rhabdomyolysis, 119
Forehead
   and eyelids, muscles of region of, 6-9
      cortical representation of, 103
   movement of, after nerve grafting in parotidectomy, 228
   partial paresis of, 340-341
   wrinkling of, 288
Foreign bodies, use of, in paresis of lower eyelids, 341
Fourier analysis, 82, 92

Index

Fracture
    basocranial, cross-face nerve graft after, 270, 271, 272
    skull, temporalis muscle transposition after, 311
    temporal bone, as cause of facial paresis, 76-77
Fragments, minced, regeneration of whole muscles from, 118
Free muscle graft; *see* Muscle graft(s)
Free nerve graft; *see* Nerve graft(s)
Frontalis muscle
    anatomical direction of, in cross-face nerve graft, 255
    effect of, on expression, 8
    in facial anatomy, 6, 7
    graft of extensor digitorum brevis to, 288
Function
    nerve, recovery of, after primary suturing in facial trauma, 237
    and structure of muscle fiber, correlation of, 33
Functional zones of face, most important, 243
Fundamentals of microvascular suturing, 174-191

G

Galea aponeurotica, 7
Galvanic stimulation
    in examination before cross-face nerve grafting, 246
    history of use of, 197-198
    immediately after paresis, 194-200
Gaze, lateral, in intrapontine lesions, 104
Gazing appearance, correction of, 286
Gelatin foam, use of, in nerve anastomosis, 214
    in fallopian canal, 222
Geniculate ganglion
    diagnosing lesions at, 102, 104, 105
    diagnosing lesions distal to, 102, 104, 105
    and internal auditory meatus, diagnosing lesions between, 105
Geniculate neuralgia; *see* Ramsay Hunt syndrome
Giant cells, multinucleated, after minced-muscle grafting, 160
Glabella, incision in, to position cross-face nerve grafts, 251
Glioma(s)
    distal, 218
    pontine, 69
Glomus tumor as cause of facial paresis, 74-75
Glue technique in nerve grafting, 129
Glycolytic activity of muscle fiber, 33-34
Glycolytic metabolism, muscle fibers with, 138
Golgi tendon organ, 33
Golgi-Mazzoni corpuscle, 33
Gracilis muscle
    anatomy of, 318
    graft of
        after lymphangioma excision, 324-325
        in cheek, 268
Graft; *see* Muscle graft(s); Nerve graft(s)
Granulomatous infections as cause of lower motor neuron facial palsy, 55
Guillain-Barré syndrome and lower motor neuron facial palsy, 55; *see also* Landry-Guillain-Barré syndrome
Gustatory hyperhidrosis syndrome, 107

H

H zone of myofibrils, 30, 31
Halothane anesthesia, 247
Handling of tools in microvascular anastomosis, 178-179
Hanke-Büngner bands in autologous nerve grafting, 127
Healthy side in cross-face nerve grafting, anatomical considerations in, 243-244
Hearing
    deficit in
        in acoustic neuroma, 57, 60
        as complication of surgery for Bell's palsy, 209
    preservation of, in surgery for acoustic neuroma, 61
Heifetz's neurosurgical clips, 177, 320, 321
Hemangioma, partial paresis after, 348, 349
Hematoma, cavernous, partial facial paresis after, 340

Hemorrhage
    control of, in facial trauma, 235
    into facial nerve or facial canal, 106
Herpes zoster
    geniculate, as cause of lower motor neuron facial palsy, 54-55
    of geniculate ganglion, 105
    oticus, as cause of facial paresis, 71, 72
    palsy caused by
        electronic diagnosis of site of disruption in, 87-88
        permanence of, 268
Histamine in treatment of Bell's palsy, 203
Histochemical change(s)
    indicating reinnervation of grafted muscle, 153
    postdenervation, in muscle fiber, 39-40
Histochemical methods in survey of whole muscle grafting, 140
Histochemical transformation of muscle fibers in reinnervation, 116
Histochemistry, in survey of whole muscle grafting, 141-144
    experimental studies of, 139-140
    and reinnervation, 138-139
Histological methods in survey of whole muscle grafting, 140
History
    of cross-face nerve grafting, 243
    of nerve-end implantation into denervated muscle, 167-169
    of striated muscle grafting, 157-158
    of use of galvanic stimulation, 197-198
Hunt's syndrome, 71
Hydergine in treatment of Bell's palsy, 203
Hyperacusis in assessment of facial nerve function, 101, 102, 105
Hypertension
    associated with Bell's palsy, 54
    causing hemorrhage into facial nerve or facial canal, 106
Hypertrophic scar as result of heating under tension, 126
Hypertrophy
    chromatolytic, of nerve cell body, 222
    postdenervation, 39
Hypoglossal nerve, grafting of, 135
    in parotidectomy, 229-231
    in spinofacial anastomosis, 241
Hypoglossofacial anastomosis, 214

I

I band of myofibrils, 30, 31
Idiopathic paralysis, permanent, 268
Idiopathic peripheral facial paralysis; *see* Bell's palsy
Implements for microvascular suturing, 175-178
Incisions
    in cross-face nerve grafting
        in buccal region, 250-251
        in marginal region, 251
        in orbital region, 247-250
        in second operative stage, 259
    for gracilis muscle graft after lymphangioma excision, 324
    for graft of extensor brevis muscle to create nasolabial fold, 320
    for muscle graft in eyelid paralysis, 282, 283
    for temporalis muscle transposition, 298, 299, 300, 301
    for Möbius syndrome, 329
Indication for cross-face nerve grafting, 268-269
Infections
    causing facial paralysis in temporal bone, 71-73
    as cause of lower motor neuron facial palsy, 54-55
    postoperative, damaging muscle grafts, 288
Injury, facial; *see* Trauma
Innervation
    crossed, 96
    dual, of muscle, establishment of, 112
Interdigitation, muscle, in parotidectomy, 227, 231-232
Interfascicular dissection
    of facial nerve near stylomastoid foramen, impossibility of, 130

Index

Interfascicular dissection—cont'd
  in nerve grafting, 128
Interfascicular technique of nerve grafting, 129-130
Interference pattern after free muscle graft, 291-292
Internal acoustic meatus, course of facial nerve in, 23, 24
Interruption, nerve, processes that continue after, 217-220
Intracanalicular lesions, diagnosing site of, 105-106
Intracranial tumor, paralysis caused by surgery for, 285
Intrafacial lesions, peripheral, diagnosing, 106-107
Intrafascicular anastomosis, 213, 214
Intraneural nerve fiber orientation, 131-134
Intraneural topography of extratemporal facial nerve, 130, 131, 132
Ischemia in Bell's palsy, 205
  vasodilators for, 203, 205
Isolation of patient after cross-face nerve grafting, 263

K

Keratoma
  associated with chronic suppurative otitis media, 72
  congenital, 75-76

L

Lacrimal portion of orbicularis oculi, 7
Lagophthalmos, 103, 104, 106
  postoperative, 285
  preoperative, 284
Landry-Guillain-Barré syndrome, 55, 106
Langer's lines, 3-5
Legs, defects of, in Möbius syndrome, 49
Levator labii superioris
  dominance of, in smile, 19
  in facial anatomy, 14, 15
Levator palpebrae superioris
  effect of, on expression, 8
  in facial anatomy, 9
Lid; see Eyelid(s)
Lid magnets, 246
Lid spring, 272, 273, 274
  as temporary measure, 246
Lidocaine, 345
  in dissection of eyelids, 282
  for spasm in microvascular anastomosis, 183
Lifesaving procedures in facial trauma, 235, 236
Lingua plicata in Melkersson-Rosenthal syndrome, 55
Lip(s)
  fascia lata sling to support, 296-297
  lifting, 244
  lower
    depressors of, 16, 17
    function of, in Möbius syndrome, 46, 47-48
    partial paresis of, 345-346
  muscles affecting bulk and shape of, 12, 13
  pursing, 244, 286-287
    after cross-face nerve graft, 274
  upper
    elevators of, 14, 15
    incision in, for positioning cross-face nerve graft, 251, 252, 253
    partial paresis of
      face lift for, 343
      myectomy of normal side for, 344, 345, 348, 349, 350, 351
      plication of elevators of mouth and upper lip for, 344, 345, 350, 351
      temporalis muscle transposition for, 343, 345
Lip region, positioning of cross-face nerve graft in, 254, 255
Lipids, visualization of, in studies of whole muscle grafting, 140
Local preoperations as factor in cross-face nerve grafting, 246
Localization of disorder in Bell's palsy, 207
Lock type of needle driver for microvascular anastomosis, 180

Logarithmic form for recording values from strength-duration curve, 85, 86
Longitudinal fractures of temporal bone, 76-77
Low molecular weight dextran for edema in Bell's palsy, 202
Lower motor neuron facial palsy, etiology of, 54-55
Lymphangioma, paralysis caused by excision of, 285
  gracilis muscle graft for, 324-325

M

Magnets, lid, 246
Malignant external otitis as cause of facial paresis, 72-73
Malignant tumors as cause of facial paresis, 76
Mandible, deformities of, in Möbius syndrome, 49
Mandibular branch of facial nerve, 222
Marginal branch of facial nerve
  anastomosis with buccal branches, 244
  in cross-face nerve grafts, 243
    of healthy side, 244
    of paralyzed side, 245
    in second operative stage, 259
  neurectomy of, in partial paresis of lower lip, 345, 346
Mass movements
  accompanying rehabilitation after cross-face nerve grafting, 271
  after regeneration as indication for cross-face nerve graft, 268
Massage in treatment of Bell's palsy, 202
Masseter muscle, transposition of
  combined with cross-face nerve graft, 267-268
  to corner of mouth, 311
  disadvantages of, 279
  to give tone to lips, 296
  for lifting mouth, 266
  in muscle interdigitation, 227, 231-232
Masticatory muscles, tightening of, in muscle interdigitation, 232
Mastoid segment of facial nerve, variability of, 26
Mastoidectomy, 222
  in surgery for Bell's palsy, 208
Mastoiditis
  chronic, as cause of facial palsy, 106
  discovery of, in surgery for Bell's palsy, 196
Mastoid–middle fossa exposure of facial nerve, 25
Mattress sutures, Mersilene, in temporalis muscle transposition, 303, 304
  for Möbius syndrome, 331
McLaughlin procedure for lateral canthoplasty, 342
Mechanism of facial expression and pathophysiology of degeneration
  anatomy of facial expression, 3-20
  pathophysiology of denervation in facial neuromuscular motor unit, 28-42
  surgical anatomy of facial nerve, 21-27
Medical treatment of Bell's palsy, 201-203
Melkersson-Rosenthal syndrome, 55
Meningeal carcinomatosis, 105
Meningioma(s)
  as cause of facial paresis, 75
  cerebellopontine angle, 64
Meningitis, tuberculous, 105
Mental defects in Möbius syndrome, 49
Mentalis in facial anatomy, 16, 17
Mersilene mattress sutures in temporalis muscle transposition, 303, 304
  for Möbius syndrome, 331
Metastic tumors as cause of facial paresis, 76
Microforceps for microvascular suturing, 176
  handling of, 179-180
Microinstruments for microvascular suturing, 175-177
Microneurovascular techniques, free muscle grafts by, 316-327
Microscissors, 214
  in adventitectomy, 183, 184
  for microvascular suturing, 176
Microscope, operating, for microvascular suturing, 175, 176

Index

Microsurgical dissection of small vessels, 181-182
Microsurgical techniques in free muscle graft, 317
Microvascular anastomosis, techniques of, 178-190
Microvascular suturing, fundamentals of, 174-191
Midepitympanum in surgery for Bell's palsy, 208
Millesi's technique for nerve suturing, 257
Mimetic muscles in muscle interdigitation, 231-232
Minced-muscle graft(s); *see* Graft(s), minced-muscle
Mitochondria, postdenervation changes in, 38
Mitochondrial oxidative enzyme in denervated muscle, 39, 40
Möbius syndrome, 44-52, 55, 105
    clinical characteristics of, 47-49
    definition of, present-day, 45
    discussions on etiological factors in, 50-51
    historical background of, 45-47
    temporalis muscle transposition for, 312, 328-339
Modified asymmetric biangulation, 184
Molding process in minced-muscle grafting, 158
Monocytes; *see* Myoblasts
Mononuclear myoblasts; *see* Myoblasts
Monofilament nylon for microvascular suturing, 177, 222
Mononeuritis involving cranial nerve, 54
Mosaic pattern of type I and II muscle fibers, 113, 114
Motor end plates; *see* End plate(s)
Motor nerve, reinnervation of, after free muscle graft, 326
Motor neuron disease
    atrophic muscle fibers in, 115
    size grouping of muscle fibers in, 114
Motor unit(s)
    definition of, 139
    increased fiber density of, after free muscle graft, 292
    reduction of, in normal extensor digitorum brevis, 281
    size of, in partially denervated muscle, 111
    structure and function of, 34-35
Mouth; *see also* Lip(s)
    cheeks, muscles of region of, 12-13
    corner of, transposition of temporalis muscle into, 267
    depressors of angle of, 16, 17
    elevators of corner of, 14, 15
    graft of masseter muscle of lifting, 266
    palmaris longus as graft encircling, 281
    pursing of, 244, 286-287
        after cross-face nerve graft, 274
    and upper lip, plication of elevators of, for partial paresis, 344, 345, 350, 351
Movement
    excessive, after hypoglossal crossover, 229-231
    mass
        after cross-face nerve grafting, 271
        as indication for cross-face nerve grafting, 268
    return of, after nerve grafting in parotidectomy, 228
Mucoepidermoid carcinoma of parotid gland, 226
Multiple sclerosis, facial paralysis in, 104
Muscle(s)
    dedifferentiation of, 157
    denervated, nerve-end implantation into, 166-173
        historical review of, 167-169
        materials and methods in, 170-171
        results of, 172
    facial, survival time of, without innervation, 245-246
    of forehead and eyelids, cortical representation of, 103
    graft of; *see* Muscle graft(s)
    histochemistry of, in survey of whole muscle grafting, 141-144
    interdigitation of, in parotidectomy, 227, 231-232
    involvement of, in Möbius syndrome, 47-48
    minced; *see* Muscle graft(s), minced
    movements of, after temporalis muscle transposition, 308
        for Möbius syndrome, 332-338
    partially paralyzed, clinical condition after strengthening of, 287-288
    preoperative state of, in cross-face nerve grafting, 245-246
    regeneration of; *see* Regeneration

Muscle(s)—cont'd
    reinnervation of; *see* Reinnervation
    size of, after experimental minced-muscle grafting, 159-160
    strength of, after experimental minced-muscle grafting, 160-162
    striated
        historical background of grafting of, 157-158
        mammalian, histochemistry and reinnervation, 138-139
    structure and function of
        correlation of, 33
        fiber types, 33-34
        motor end plate, 32-33
        motor unit, 34-35
        muscle cell, 29-31
        muscle spindle, 33
        sarcolemma, 31-32
Muscle cell, structure and function of, 29-31
Muscle contractions, skin lines and, 5
Muscle disease, human, regeneration in, 119
Muscle fiber
    effect of reinnervation and cross-innervation on types of, 113
    postdenervation changes in
        atrophy and degeneration, 35
        early cellular, 35-39
        histochemical, 39-40
        hypertrophy, 39
        target fibers, 40
Muscle graft(s)
    after 12 months, 278-293
        clinical material and results, 284-288
        electromyographical methods and results, 289-292
        operative techniques, 281-283
    combined with cross-face nerve graft, 264-267
    in eyelid paralysis, 282-283
    selection of muscle for, 281
    gracilis, after lymphangioma excision, 324-325
    by microvascular techniques, 316-327
        anatomical base of donor muscles, 318-319
        case histories, 320-325
        discussion, 326-327
        microsurgical techniques, 317
        selection of donor muscles, 317
    minced-muscle, 156-165
        experimental, 159-162
        favorable ambiance for, 158-159
        historic background of striated muscle grafting, 157-158
        principle of, 157
        regeneration of whole muscle from, 118
    and nerve-end implantation into denervated muscle, 168
    in paralysis of orbicularis muscle, 283
    in parotidectomy, 232-234
    in partial paralyzed muscle, 283
    regeneration in, 118-119
    selection and denervation of, 281-282
    of temporalis muscle; *see* Temporalis muscle, transposition of
    whole muscle, 136-155
        experimental studies of, 139-140
        histochemistry and reinnervation in, 138-139
        history of, 137
        results of, 140-151
Muscle spindles
    after experimental minced-muscle grafting, 160
    new, in whole nerve grafting, 144
    in normal muscle, 141
    reinnervation of, 116
    structure and function of, 33
Muscle-tendon onlay grafts, 233-234
Muscular dystrophy
    action potentials in, 96
    discontinuous regeneration in, 119
Myectomy, selective, weakening of normal side by, in partial paresis, 344, 345, 348, 349, 350, 351

Index

Myelin coat, breakup of, after nerve interruption, 218
Myoblast(s)
  in muscle regeneration
    in human muscle disease, 119
    of whole muscles from minced fragments, 118
  origin of, 117-118, 157
  peak of, after trauma, 117
Myofibrils, structure of, 29-30
Myofilamentogenesis, debate about, 117
Myofilaments
  loss of, in denervation atrophy, 37
  in muscle regeneration, 117
Myonuclei as possible origin of myoblasts, 118, 157
Myoplastic surgical methods, combination of, with cross-face nerve grafting, 263-268
Myosin, effects of cross-innervation on, 116
Myotonia, action potentials in, 95
Myotubes, fusion of myoblasts into, 117

N

NADH-tetrazolium reductase, 138, 140, 141, 144
NADH-TR; see NADH-tetrazolium reductase
Nasalis in facial anatomy, 11
Nasolabial fold(s)
  in facial expression, 4
  free muscle graft to create, 320-323
Nasolacrimal reflexes, 101
Needle driver
  handling of, 179-180
  lock or ratchet type, 180
  spring-handled, 176
Needles, atraumatic, for microvascular suturing, 177
Neoplasms of cerebellopontine angle, 57-70
Nerve(s)
  accessory, in spinofacial anastomosis, 241
  acoustic, paresis after tumor of, 286; see also Acoustic neuroma
    partial, 347
    temporalis muscle transposition for, 314
  auditory, appearance of, in retrolabyrinthine suboccipital craniectomy, 62-64
  auricular, 245
    cable graft of, in facial trauma, 237
    in cross-face nerve grafting, 251
  cutaneous antebrachii medialis, 134
  cutaneous femoral, 134, 251
  diagnosing site of disruption of
    by anatomical location
      anatomical description, 99-100
      appraisal of facial nerve function, 100-101
      central or supranuclear lesions, 102-107
    by electronic methods, 81-97
  facial; see Facial nerve
  grafting; see Nerve graft(s)
  gross excitability of, electronic testing of, 90-91
  hypoglossal, grafting of, 135
    in parotidectomy, 229-231
    in spinofacial anastomosis, 241
  implantation of
    and formation of new end plates, 112
    and reinnervation, 111-116
  inferior alveolar, grafting after resection of, 135
  innervating gracilis muscle, 318
  lesions, peripheral, 106
  pathophysiology of injury of, 236
  processes that continue after interruption of, 217-220
  resections of, in malignant tumors of parotid gland, 225
  suitable as donors in nerve grafting, 134
  sural, as donor in nerve grafting, 134, 215
  trigeminal
    communications of facial nerve with branches of, 244
    grafting in lesions of, 135

Nerve(s)—cont'd
  ulnar, effect of galvanic stimulation on paralysis of, 197
  vestibular, acoustic neuroma arising from, 58-59
Nerve cell, proteosynthetic ability of, 218
Nerve cell body, chromatolytic hypertrophy of, 222
Nerve fibers, intraneural orientation of, 131-134
Nerve graft(s)
  after twelve months, 278-293
    clinical material and results, 284-288
    electromyographical methods and results, 289-292
    operative techniques, 281-283
  application of nerve grafts in facial nerve surgery, 134-135
  of auricular nerve in facial trauma, 237
  autologous
    basic considerations in, 127-128
    superiority of, 251
  cross-face; see Cross-face nerve grafting
  delay in reinnervation after, 214
  disadvantage of, 125
  effects of local tension on nerve regeneration, 126-127
  hypoglossal, 135
    crossover in parotidectomy, 229-231
  as inferior to neurorrhaphy, 125
  interfascicular technique of, 129-130
  intraneural nerve fiber orientation, 131-134
  intraneural topography of extratemporal facial nerve, 130, 131, 132
  length of, 128
  by microscope in cranium, 211-216
  for partial paresis
    of eyelids, 342
    of lower lip, 345, 346
  positioning of, in cross-face nerve grafting, 251-257
  preparation of, in cross-face nerve grafting, 251
  provision of nerve grafts, 134
  in radical parotidectomy, 226-228
  steps in
    coaptation, 129-130
    preparation of stumps, 128
  transfacial, in paresis in malignant tumors of parotid gland, 228
Nerve stimulator, surgical use of, 237
Nerve supply
  of depressors of lower lip, 16, 17
  of elevators of corner of mouth, 14, 15
  of forehead and eyelids, 8
  of region of mouth and cheeks, 12-13
  in region of nose, 10
Nerve tissue, elasticity of, 126
Nerve-end implantation into denervated muscle, 166-173
Nervus; see Nerve(s)
Neural neurotization with temporalis muscle transposition, 309
Neuralgia, geniculate; see Ramsay Hunt syndrome
Neurapraxia
  in Bell's palsy, 206
  in local injury, 236
Neurectomy for partial paresis
  of lower lip, 345, 346
  weakening of normal side, 344, 345
Neurinoma of acoustic nerve, paralysis caused by surgery for, 286
Neurofibroma(s)
  of cerebellopontine angle, 64-66
  involving facial nerve as cause of facial paresis, 73-74
  of von Recklinghausen, 74
Neuroma
  acoustic
    facial nerve in, 60
    destruction of, 211
    growth of, 57, 60

Index

Neuroma—cont'd
  acoustic—cont'd
    retrolabyrinthine suboccipital craniectomy for, 58-59, 61-63
      left, 212-213
        preservation of hearing in, 61
        sural nerve grafts after removal of, 215
        temporalis muscle transposition for paralysis after surgery for, 310
  after immediate neurorrhaphy, 221
  at end of sural graft, 259, 260
  as evidence of axon growth in sural graft, 247
  in prognosis after cross-face nerve graft, 269
  proximal, production of, after nerve interruption, 218, 219
  stump, resection of, 126, 127
Neuromuscular diseases, reinnervation in, 279
Neurorrhaphy
  in facial trauma, 237
  immediate, neuroma formation after, 221
  methods of, within temporal canal, 222
  nerve graft as inferior to, 125
Neurotization, neural, 168-169
  in cross-face nerve grafting, 255
  with temporalis muscle transposition, 309
Neurotmesis in facial trauma, 236
Nicotinic acid in treatment of Bell's palsy, 203
Nissl bodies after nerve interruption, 218
Nondegenerative lesions, electromyographic determination of, 197
Nose, muscles of regions of, 10-11
Nuclear or intrapontine lesions, 104-105
Nuclei, sarcolemmal, postdenervation changes in, 35-36
Number of transplants necessary in cross-face nerve grafting, 255-256

O

Obturator nerve, 318
Occipital, effect of, on expression, 8
Ocular involvement in Möbius syndrome, 48
Onlay grafts, muscle-tendon, 233-234
Overactivity, muscle, after hypoglossal crossover, 229-231
Operative techniques in free muscle and nerve grafting for long-standing paralysis, 281-283
Ophthalmic needle drivers for microvascular suturing, 176
Orbicularis oculi
  in central or supranuclear lesions, 102, 103
  closure of eyelid by, 249
  in facial anatomy, 7
  function of, positioning of cross-face nerve graft for, 253-254
  innervation of, 341
  normal, innervation of graft from, 282
Orbicularis oris
  effects of, on expression, 12, 13
  innervation of, 250
    in Bell's palsy, 287
      preoperative clinical condition in, 285
    grafting for, 283
      clinical condition after, 286-287
      position of graft in, 280, 281
Orbicularis oris reflex, assessment of, 101
Orbital region, cross-face nerve grafting in
  incisions for, 247-250
  positioning of graft in, 253-254
Orbital tomograms in evaluations of facial trauma, 236
Origin of myoblastic cell, 117-118
Oscilloscope, storage recording latency measurements, 89
Otitis
  malignant external, as cause of facial paresis, 72-73
  media
    chronic, necessity for surgery in palsy caused by, 195
    suppurative, as cause of facial paresis, 72
Otorrhea, cerebrospinal fluid, as complication of surgery for Bell's palsy, 209

Oxidative activity of muscle fiber, 33-34
Oxidative enzymes, fibers rich in, 138, 140, 141

P

PAS reaction; see Periodic acid–Schiff reaction
Palate, soft, paresis of, in Möbius syndrome, 48
Palmaris longus in free muscle graft encircling mouth, 281, 283
Paralysis
  complete after 2 weeks, fibrillations shown by electromyography in, 196-197
  completeness of, in Bell's palsy, 201
  long-standing
    psychological attitudes of patients with, 230-231
    principles of surgical treatment of, 279
  partial, caused by trauma, extensor brevis muscle graft for, 320-323
  ulnar nerve, effect of galvanic stimulation on, 197
Paralyzed side in cross-face nerve grafting, anatomical considerations in, 244-245
Paramedian muscles, reinnervation of, 242
Paresis, facial
  congenital; see Möbius syndrome
  galvanic muscle stimulation immediately after, 194-200
  localized, about eye and mouth, muscle-tendon onlay grafts for, 233-234
  in malignant tumors of parotid gland, management of, 224-234
  medical causes of, 53-56
  surgical causes of
    in cranium, 57-70
    in parotid gland, 79-80
    in temporal canal
      infectious processes, 71-73
      trauma, 76-78
      tumors, 73-76
Parotid area, injury to, repair of, by nerve grafting, 133-134
Parotid gland
  branches of facial nerve within, 244-245
  frontal margin of, as landmark in cross-face nerve grafting, 245
  management of paresis in malignant tumors of, 224-234
    free nerve grafting, 226-228
    hypoglossal crossover, 229-231
    muscle interdigitation, 227, 231-232
    muscle transfer, 232-234
    transfacial crossover, 228
  relationship to facial nerve, 99
  Stenson's duct of, 245
  surgical causes of facial paresis in, 79-80
  tumors of, 106, 285
    cross-face nerve graft after, 270
    paralysis caused by surgery for, 288
    partial, 340
Parotidectomy, temporalis muscle transposition after, 312
Partial facial paresis, 340-352
  case histories, 347-352
  causes of, 340
  of cheek and upper lip, 343
  of eyelids, 341-342
  of forehead, 340-341
  of lower lip, 345-346
  temporalis muscle transposition for, 343-345
Passavant's cushion, absence of, in Möbius syndrome, 48
Patency test, radical, of microvascular anastomosis, 186, 187
Pathological conditions influencing variations in smile, 18
Pathophysiology of nerve injury, 236
Patient, reassurance of, in treatment of Bell's palsy, 202
Perimysial connective tissue in whole muscle grafting, 149, 150
Perineurium of facial nerve, 22
Periodic acid–Schiff reaction, 140
Periorbital region, scarring in, 263
Peripheral intrafacial lesions, diagnosing, 106-107

Index

Phosphorylase
  activity
    of muscle fiber, 33-34
    in studies of whole muscle grafting, 140
  muscle fibers rich in, 138
Phrenic nerve in spinofacial anastomosis, 241
Physical condition, general, of patient as factor in cross-face nerve grafting, 246
Physiotherapy after cross-face nerve grafting, 271
Planning facial configuration before surgery in temporalis muscle transposition, 308
Plantaris muscle for free muscle graft, 281
  denervation of, 282
Plaques, cholinesterase-positive, in whole muscle grafting, 146, 147
Plastic stage in minced-muscle grafting, 157
Platysma muscle
  in facial anatomy, 16, 17
  involvement of, after nerve grafting in parotidectomy, 228
Plication of elevators of mouth and upper lip for partial paresis, 344, 345, 350, 351
Poliomyelitis, facial paralysis in, 104-105
  partial, 350, 351
Polymyositis, discontinuous regeneration in, 119
Polytomograms in diagnosis of facial nerve tumors, 74
Pons and internal auditory meatus, lesions between; see Cerebellopontine angle, neoplasms of
Pontine gliomas, 69
Position of surgeon in microvascular anastomosis, 178-179
Positioning of grafts
  in cross-face nerve grafting, 251-257
  muscle, for long-standing paralysis, 280-281
Positive waves in electromyography, 94, 95
Postdenervation changes in muscle fiber and motor end plate
  atrophy and degeneration, 35
  early cellular, 35-39
  histochemical, 39-40
  hypertrophy, 39
  target fibers, 40
Postdenervation hypertrophy, 39
Postoperative care after cross-face nerve grafting, 263
Postoperative course after temporalis muscle transposition, 308
Prednisone in treatment of Bell's palsy, 203
Preoperations, local, as factor in cross-face nerve grafting, 246
Preoperative investigation and measures in cross-face nerve grafting
  general condition, 246
  local preoperations, 246
  state of muscle, 245-246
Preparation
  of nerve grafts, cross-face, 251
  of scalp region in temporalis muscle transposition, 298
Principle(s)
  of minced-muscle grafting, 157
  of surgical treatment for long-standing facial paralysis, 279
Priority, order of, in treatment of patient with facial trauma, 236
Procaine in treatment of Bell's palsy, 203
Procerus
  effect of, on expression, 8
  in facial anatomy, 6-9
Processes that continue after nerve interruption, 217-220
Progenia, partial paralysis caused by surgery for, 289
Prognosis, methods of determining, in Bell's palsy, 206
Pronator teres, 281
Proteosynthetic ability of nerve cell, 218
Proximal neuroma, production of, after nerve interruption, 218, 219
Pseudomonas aeruginosa, 73
Psychological attitudes of patients with long-standing facial paralysis, 230-231
Pterygoid muscles in muscle interdigitation, 231-232

Pursing lips, 244, 286-287
  after cross-face nerve graft, 274

Q

Quadratus labii
  inferioris
    exposure of, in temporalis muscle transposition, 307
    in facial anatomy, 16, 17
  superioris
    exposure of
      in selective myectomy, 345, 348
      in temporalis muscle transposition, 307
    in facial anatomy, 14, 15
    innervation of, 250

R

Radical patency test of microvascular anastomosis, 186, 187
Ramification(s)
  in end plate formation, 144-146
  of facial nerve
    and anastomosis with cross-face sural graft
      on healthy side, 258
      on paralyzed side, 261
    effect on reinnervation of paramedian muscles, 242
    peripheral, of branches, 243-244
Ramsay Hunt syndrome, 71, 105
  as cause of lower motor neuron facial palsy, 54-55
Ratchet type of needle driver for microvascular anastomosis, 180
Razor blade, surgical use of, 237
  in neurorrhaphy, 222
Reaction of degeneration after nerve interruption, 217-218
Reanimation of paralyzed face
  immediate or early treatment
    establishing facial nerve continuity in temporal canal, 217-223
    management of facial nerve paresis in malignant tumors of parotid gland, 224-234
    medical treatment for Bell's palsy, 201-203
    nerve grafting by microscope in cranium, 211-216
    present-day concepts of surgical treatment for Bell's palsy, 204-210
    primary nerve suturing of severed motor nerves in facial trauma, 235-240
    value of galvanic muscle stimulation immediately after paresis, 194-200
  intermediate (4 months to 1 year), cross-face nerve grafting, 241-277
  late (after 12 months)
    entire temporalis muscle transposition, 294-315
    free muscle grafts by microneurovascular techniques, 316-327
    free muscle and nerve grafting in face, 278-293
    partial facial paresis, 340-352
    surgical treatment of bilateral facial paresis (Möbius syndrome), 328-339
Reassurance of patient in treatment of Bell's palsy, 202
Recovery of nerve function after primary suturing in facial trauma, 237
Red muscle fibers, 138-144
  in minced-muscle grafting, 158
Reflex function of facial nerve, examination of, 101
Reflex tearing, test of, in Bell's palsy, 207
Regeneration
  after cross-face nerve graft, detection of, 269
  continuous and discontinuous, 116-117
  effects of local tension on, 126-127
  in human muscle disease, 119
  nerve, evaluation of, 237
  spontaneous, as factor in two-stage cross-face nerve grafting, 247

Index

Regeneration—cont'd
  of striated muscle
    cellular events in, 117
    continuous and discontinuous, 116-117
    factors necessary for successful, 120
    free muscle grafts, 118-119
    in human muscle disease, 119
    origin of myoblastic cell, 117-118
    of whole muscles from minced fragments, 118
Regenerative processes after nerve interruption, 218
Rehabilitating measures after cross-face nerve grafting, 263
Reinnervation, muscle
  chronaxy values in, 83
  delayed, 112
    after nerve grafting, 214
  in denervating diseases, 112
  effect of galvanic stimulation on, 198
  effect of, on muscle fiber types, 113
  of muscle grafts, 279
    electromyographic signs of, 291-292
    histochemical change indicating, 153
    of motor nerve after free muscle graft, 326
  and nerve implantation, 111-116
    delayed reinnervation in, 112
    effects of cross-innervation on muscle fiber types in, 113
    effects of cross-innervation on myosin in, 116
    electron microscopy of motor end plates in, 113
    experimental, 111-112
    and formation of new end plates in, 112
    reinnervation of muscle spindles in, 116
    type grouping in, 113-116
  origin of myoblastic cell in, 117-118
  and regeneration of striated muscle, 110-123
    histochemistry of, 138-139
  of whole muscle grafts, experimental studies of, 139-140
Repair, methods of, in temporal canal, 222
Residual abnormalities after Bell's palsy, 201, 205
Retrolabyrinthine suboccipital craniectomy
  for acoustic neuroma, 58-59, 61-63
  appearance of facial and auditory nerves in, 62-64
Revascularization and fibrosis in whole muscle grafting, 147-151
Rheobase of muscle, determining, with chronaximeter, 83
Rhabdomyosarcoma, embryonal, as cause of facial paresis, 76
Rhabdomyositis, focus of regeneration in, 119
RNA
  in cytoplasm after nerve interruption, 218
  of denervated fibers, 38

S

Sagging of eyebrow, 340-341
  correction of, 307
  removal of skin crescent to elevate, 341, 347
  unilateral, paralyzing normal side in, 341
Salt in assessment of sensory function of facial nerve, 100-101
Saphena magna as guide in obtaining sural nerve graft, 251
Sarcoidosis, facial palsy occurring with, 55
Sarcolemma
  effect of injury on, 117
  importance of integrity of, in complete regeneration, 117
  postdenervation changes in, 38
  structure and function of, 31-32
Sarcolemmal nuclei, postdenervation changes in, 35-36
Sarcoplasm
  degeneration of, 117
  of motor end plate, 32-33
  of muscle fiber, 30-31
Sarcoplasmic reticulum
  hypertrophy of, after nerve section, 38
  in muscle regeneration, 117

Satellite cell(s)
  in normal muscle, 31, 32
  number of, in denervated muscle, 36
    increased, 118-119
  as possible origin of myoblasts, 118, 157
Scalp, closure of, in temporalis muscle transposition, 306
Scalp region, preparation of, for temporalis transposition procedure, 298
Scar, hypertrophic, as result of healing under tension, 126
Scarring
  between anastomoses as factor in two-stage cross-face nerve grafting, 247
  caused by foreign bodies in nerve suturing, 257, 259
  in periorbital region, 263
  as problem in minced-muscle grafting, 158-159
Schirmer test, 101
  in Bell's palsy, 207
Schwann cell(s)
  in autologous nerve grafting, 127
  proliferation of, 251
  after nerve interruption, 218
Schwann cell process(es), 33
  postdenervation changes in, 36-37
  in reinnervated motor end plates, 113
Schwann cell sheaths in collateral nerve sprouting, 112
Schwannoma as cause of facial paresis, 73-74
  vestibular, 75
SDH; see Succinic dehydrogenase
Secretory function of facial nerve, examination of, 101
Selection of donor muscle for free muscle grafting by microneurovascular techniques, 317
Selective myectomy, weakening of normal side by, in partial paresis, 344, 345, 348, 349, 350, 351
Sensory function of facial nerve, examination of, 100
Sheathing, nerve, at time of neurorrhaphy, 237
Signs and symptoms denoting site of facial nerve interruption, 102
Single fiber electromyography after free muscle grafting, 292
Size, muscle, after experimental minced-muscle grafting, 159-160
Size grouping of muscle fibers in progressive denervating diseases, 114
Skin, rigidity of, in preoperative clinical examination, 246
Sling sutures, 213, 214
Slurring of speech after hypoglossal crossover, 230
Smile(s)
  analysis of, in planning myectomy on normal side in partial paresis, 345
  dominant canine, in temporalis muscle transposition, 303
  factors influencing variations in, 18
  matching normal side of, in temporalis muscle transposition, 297
  types of, 19
Smiling, after temporalis muscle transposition for Möbius syndrome, 332-338
Sodium-pump capability of axoplasmic membrane, loss of, after nerve interruption, 218
Spasm
  facial
    as indication for cross-face nerve grafting, 268
    regeneration of nerve in, 242
  vessel, in microvascular anastomosis, 183
Speech
  slurring of, after hypoglossal crossover, 230
  after temporalis muscle transposition, 308, 309
Spinal accessory crossover, 229
Spinal muscular atrophy, Z line dissolution in, 37-38
Spindles, muscle
  after experimental minced-muscle grafting, 160
  new, in whole nerve grafting, 144
  in normal muscle, 141

Index

Spindles, muscle—cont'd
  reinnervation of, 116
  structure and function of, 33
Spinofacial anastomosis, 214, 241-242
Splinting in treatment of Bell's palsy, 202
Spontaneous activity, electromyographic recording of, 93-95
  after free muscle grafting, 289, 290
Spontaneous regeneration as factor in two-stage cross-face nerve grafting, 247
"Spontaneous return" of facial movements after muscle interdigitation, 231
Sprouting
  axon
    irregularity of, 131
    scar tissue as obstacle to, 127
  collateral
    in free muscle graft, hindered by connective tissue, 279
    nerve, 139
    in reinnervation, 111-116
Squamous cell carcinoma as cause of facial paresis, 76
Stapedius muscle, diagnosing lesions distal to, 102, 104, 105
Stay sutures in microvascular anastomosis, 183, 184
  venous, 187
Stellate block in treatment of Bell's palsy, 203
Stenson's duct in identification of ramus buccalis, 245
Sternocleidomastoid muscle, transfer of, 233
Stimulation, anodal, of tongue, threshold to, 91
Strength
  msucle, after experimental muscle grafting, 160-162
  tensile, of fibrin clotting, 129
Strength-duration curves in diagnosing site of nerve disruption by electronic methods, 84-87
Strengthening
  of orbicularis oculi, clinical condition after, 287
  of partially denervated muscle, graft for, 283
  position of graft in, 280, 281
Stripping of muscle from bone in temporalis muscle transposition, 302, 330
Stroke, transfacial crossover in, 228
Structure and function of muscle fiber, correlation of, 33
Stump(s)
  neuroma, resection of, 126, 127
  preparation of, in nerve grafting, 128
  proximal nerve, identification of, 237
Stylomastoid foramen
  facial nerve exposure after exit from, 25
  tumor of parotid gland approaching, 226-227
Subneural apparatus
  visualization of, 140, 145, 146
  in whole muscle grafting, 145-147
Succinic dehydrogenase, 138, 140, 141
Sudan black B stain, 140
Suppurative otitis media as cause of facial paresis, 72
Supramaximal stimulus in latency measurements, 87
Supranuclear or central lesions, 102-107
Supranuclear palsy, recognition of, 53
Sural nerve grafts, 243
  anastomoses of, with facial nerve branches, 258, 261, 262
  cross-face, 251
    anatomical direction of, 255
    combined with free muscle graft, 265-268
    positioning of, 251-257
    preparation of, 251
  and facial nerve, comparison of size of, 256
  neuroma as evidence of axon growth in, 247
  in transfacial crossover in malignant tumors of parotid gland, 228
Surgeon's position in microvascular anastomosis, 178-179
Surgical techniques in primary suturing of nerves in facial trauma, 237

Surgical approach to facial nerve within parotid gland, 80
Surgical causes of facial paresis in cranium, 57-70
Surgical treatment of facial paresis
  bilateral, 328-339
  long-standing, principles of, 279
Surgical treatment
  of Bell's palsy, 204-210
    arguments for, 195-196
    cross-face nerve graft in, 270, 272
    facial nerve decompression in, 207-209
    free muscle graft in, 287
    rationale of, 205-207
    transfacial crossover in, 228
  decision about, in particular case, 195-197
  timing of, 220-222
Suture(s)
  epineural, coaptation by, in nerve grafting, 129
  materials for, microvascular, 177-178
    in nerve grafting in radical parotidectomy, 226
  Mersilene mattress, in temporalis muscle transposition, 303, 304
    for Möbius syndrome, 331
  number required in microvascular anastomosis, 186
  sling, 213, 214
  stay, 183, 184
    in venous anastomosis, 187
  subcuticular, in temporalis muscle transposition, 306
  technique of, 179-180
Suturing
  in cross-face nerve grafting, 257-259
  microvascular, fundamentals of
    anastomosis of vessels of different diameters, 189
    arterial anastomosis, 182-187
    end-to-side anastomosis, 189
    implements, 175-178
    microsurgical dissection of small vessels, 181-182
    surgeon's position and handling of tools, 178-179
    suture technique, 179-180
    technique of anastomosis, 180-181
    venous anastomosis, 187-188
  under tension in temporalis muscle transposition, 304
    for Möbius syndrome, 331
Swallowing, difficulty in, after hypoglossal crossover, 230
Swelling
  double hump–camel, in partial nerve transection, 236
  facial, in Melkersson-Rosenthal syndrome, 55
Synchronization of eyelid movement, 285
Syndrome of crocodile tears, 107
Synkinesis
  of muscle movements after cross-face nerve grafting, 271
  as residual abnormality after Bell's palsy, 201, 205

T

Target fibers in denervation atrophy, 40
Tarsorrhaphy, 228
  lateral, 246
Taste in assessment of sensory function of facial nerve, 100-101
Taste threshold, changes in, in Bell's palsy, 91
Tearing, reflex, test of, in Bell's palsy, 207
Tears, artificial, use of, in Bell's palsy, 202
Technique(s)
  of free nerve grafting in face; see Nerve graft(s)
  of microvascular anastomosis, 178-190
  and surgical approaches in facial nerve decompression in Bell's palsy, 207-209
  suture, in microvascular anastomosis, 179-180
  of temporalis transposition procedure, 298-307
    for Möbius syndrome, 329-331

Index

Temporal bone
　fracture of, as cause of facial paresis, 76-77
　radical resection of, in malignant tumors of parotid gland, 228
　stripping of muscle from, in temporalis muscle transposition, 302, 330
Temporal canal
　establishing facial nerve continuity in
　　appropriate action according to location of injury, 222
　　methods of repair, 222
　　processes that continue after nerve interruption, 217-220
　　timing of operation, 220-222
　surgical causes of facial paresis in
　　infectious processes, 71-73
　　trauma, 76-78
　　tumors, 73-76
Temporal nerve, anatomy of, 297
Temporalis muscle
　anatomy of, 297
　as contracting force, 296
　electromyographic study of, 96
　graft of, for eyelid function, 266
　in muscle interdigitation, 231-232
　transposition of, 294-315
　　after acoustic neuroma, 310
　　case histories, 310-314
　　combined with cross-face nerve graft, 267-268
　　disadvantages of, 279
　　after fractured skull, 311
　　for Möbius syndrome, 328-339
　　　smiling in, 332-338
　　for partial paresis
　　　after acoustic nerve tumor, 342
　　　of cheek and upper lip, 343, 345
　　　of eyelids, 341, 342
　　　after hemangioma, 348, 349
　　pitfalls to be avoided in, 308-309
　　postoperative course, 308
　　technique of procedure, 298-307
　　underdeveloped, 308
Temporofrontal branch of facial nerve, 245
Tendons
　fascia as, in temporalis muscle transposition, 303
　　testing of, 304-305
　in free muscle graft for eyelid paralysis, 283
　in minced-muscle grafting, 159
Tensile strength of fibrin clotting, 129
Tension
　importance of freedom from, in nerve suturing, 257
　local, effects of, on nerve regeneration, 126-127
　in muscle regeneration, 120
　suturing under, in temporalis muscle transposition, 304
　　for Möbius syndrome, 331
Terminal axon of motor end plate, 32
　postdenervation changes in, 36-37
Terminal innervation ratio, 116
Testing fascia acting as tendon in temporalis muscle transposition, 304-305
Thread for microvascular suturing, 177
Thrombus formation, factors in, in microvascular anastomosis, 183, 185, 186
Tibial nerve, anterior, 319, 320
Tic
　as indication for cross-face nerve graft, 268
　posttraumatic, 107
　regeneration of nerve in, 242
Time
　between injury and recovery, effect of galvanic stimulation on, 198
　operating, reduction of, by two-stage operation, 247
Timing of operation to repair neural defect, 220
Tinell-Hoffman sign, 244
Tissue, connective; see Connective tissue

Tissue adhesive, use of, in nerve anastomosis, 214
Tomograms, orbital, in evaluation of facial injury, 236
Tone
　after cross-face grafting, 270
　after nerve graft in radical parotidectomy, 228
Tongue
　atrophy of, after hypoglossal crossover, 230
　in Möbius syndrome, 48
　threshold to anodal stimulation, 91
Tools, handling of, in microvascular anastomosis, 178-179
Topographic location of fibers of facial nerve, 23
Topography, intraneural, of extratemporal facial nerve, 130, 131, 132
Transfacial crossover in paresis in malignant tumors of parotid gland, 228
Transfer, muscle, in parotidectomy, 232-234
Translabyrinthine approach for acoustic neuroma, 61
Transmastoid approach in facial nerve decompression for Bell's palsy, 207-208
Transverse fracture of temporal bone, 76
Trauma
　as cause of facial paresis, 55, 77-78
　　partial, 340
　　in temporal canal, 76-78
　as cause of peripheral nerve lesions, 106
　causing disruption of facial nerve within parotid gland, 79-80
　evaluation of, 235-236
　extensor brevis muscle graft for partial paralysis caused by, 320-323
　parotid, nerve grafting repair of, 133-134
　timing of cross-face nerve grafting after, 246
Trigeminal nerve, 263, 267, 268, 269
　communications of facial nerve branches with, 244
　in Möbius syndrome, 48
　transposition of muscles innervated by, 279
Trigeminal reflex, assessment of, 101
Tuberculous meningitis, 105
Tubulization of suture site in nerve grafting, 129
Tumor(s)
　acoustic nerve, paresis after
　　partial, 347
　　temporalis muscle transposition for, 314
　as cause of facial paresis
　　extrinsic, 74-76
　　in temporal bone, 73-76
　cerebellar, cross-face nerve graft for, 270, 272
　malignant, of parotid gland, management of paresis in, 224-234
　of middle ear, discovery of, in surgery for Bell's palsy, 196
　partial facial paresis after removal of, 340
　surgery for paralysis caused by, 285
　　parotid, 288
Tunnels, dissection of, in temporalis muscle transposition, 300
Twitching as complication of Bell's palsy, 205
Tympanic bone fractures, 77
Tympanic segment of facial nerve, variability of, 26
Type grouping, 139
　of muscle fibers, 113-116, 139
　in survey of whole muscle grafting, 143

U

Ulnar nerve paralysis, effect of galvanic stimulation on, 197
Ultrafine caliber monofilament nylon for microvascular suturing, 177
Urea for edema in Bell's palsy, 202

V

Value of galvanic muscle stimulation immediately after paresis, 194-200
van Gieson stain, 140, 150, 151
Varicella-zoster DNA virus as cause of Ramsay Hunt syndrome, 71

Index

Vasodilators in treatment of Bell's palsy, 203, 205
Vein, rat femoral, anastomosis of, 189
Venous anastomosis, microvascular, 187-188
Vessels
    of different diameters, anastomosis of, 189
    small, microsurgical dissection of, 181-182
Vestibular schwannoma, 75
Virus
    in etiology of lower motor neuron facial palsy, 55
    varicella-zoster DNA, as cause of Ramsay Hunt syndrome, 71
Volitional central facial paresis, 103
Volume, muscle
    deficiency of, preoperational, 246
    reduction of, after extensor brevis muscle graft, 322
Voluntary activity, muscle, in electromyograph, 95-97
von Recklinghausen, neurofibroma of, 74

W

Wallerian degeneration
    in autologous nerve grafting, 127, 251
    in complete transection of nerve, 236
Weakening
    of depressors of corner of mouth for partial paresis of lower lip, 345, 346
    of muscle on normal side
        by selective myectomy, 344, 345, 348, 349, 350, 351
    in temporalis muscle transposition, 307
Weck surgical blade, 222
Weight loss in denervated muscle, effect of electrical stimulation on, 199
Whistling, postoperative, 287
White muscle fibers, 138-144
    in minced-muscle grafting, 158
Whole muscle grafting, free, survey of, 136-155
    experimental studies of, 139-140
    histochemistry and reinnervation in, 138-139
    history of, 137
    results of, 140-151
Winking, 102
Wohlfart-Kugelberg-Welander syndrome, myofibril changes in, 37-38
Wrinkles, facial, variations in anatomy of, 4-5
Wrinkling of forehead, 288

X

X-ray therapy and tumor resection, paralysis caused by, 268
Xylocaine; *see* Lidocaine

Z

Z lines
    changes in, in denervation atrophy, 37
    dissolution of, in spinal muscular atrophy and amyotrophic lateral sclerosis, 37-38
    of myofibrils, 30, 31
Zeiss operating microscope (OPMi-6), 175, 176
Zones of regeneration in minced-muscle grafting, 158
Zygomatic arch
    fixing muscle graft around, 283
    stripping muscle above, in temporalis muscle transposition, 302, 330
Zygomatic branch of facial nerve, 222, 263, 267
    anastomosis of, with buccal branch, 244
    in cross-face nerve grafts, 243
        anatomical direction of, 255
        of healthy side, 244
        in second operative stage, 259
    in transfacial crossover, 228
Zygomatic plexus of facial nerve in cross-face nerve grafting, 249
Zygomaticus muscle(s)
    exposure of, in temporalis muscle transposition, 307
    major
        dominance of, in smile, 19
        exposure of, in selective myectomy, 345, 348
        in facial anatomy, 14, 15
    minor, in facial anatomy, 14, 15